At a Glance

T0252316

Color Atlas of Pathology

Pathologic Principles · Associated Diseases · Sequela

Ursus-Nikolaus Riede, M.D.
Professor of Pathology

Martin Werner, M.D.
Professor and Chairman

Department of Pathology
University of Freiburg, Germany

1017 illustrations – 835 in color, 113 electron micrographs

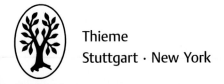

Thieme
Stuttgart · New York

Library of Congress Cataloging-in-Publication Data

Riede, Ursus-Nikolaus, 1941–
  [Taschenatlas der allgemeinen Pathologie. English]
Color atlas of pathology : pathologic principles and associated diseases-sequela / Ursus-Nikolaus Riede ; with cooperation by Gabriele Koehler, Marzenna Orlowska-Volk, Georg Schwarzkopf ; [translated by John Grossman].
  p. ; cm.
Includes index.
ISBN 3-13-127781-5 (alk. paper) –
ISBN 1-58890-117-3 (alk. paper)
1. Pathology–Atlases.
[DNLM: 1. Pathology–Atlases. QZ 17 R551t 2004a] I. Title. RB33.R5313 2004
616.07'022'2–dc22
                                    2004009449

This book is an authorized translation of the German edition: Taschenatals der allgemeinen Pathologie, edited by U.N. Riede. Published and copyrighted 1998 by Georg Thieme Verlag, Stuttgart, Germany.

Translated by: John Grossman, Berlin and Carole Cürten, Freiburg

© 2004 Georg Thieme Verlag
Rüdigerstraße 14, D-70469 Stuttgart, Germany
http://www.thieme.de
Thieme New York, 333 Seventh Avenue, New York, N. Y. 10001, U.S.A.
http://www.thieme.com
Cover design: Thieme Marketing

Typesetting by Mitterweger & Partner Kommunikationsgesellschaft mbH, Plankstadt

Printed and bound in India by Replika Press Pvt. Ltd.

ISBN 3-13-127781-5
ISBN 1-58890-117-3
                         1 2 3 4 5

Important Note: Medicine is an ever-changing science undergoing continual development. Research and clinical experience are continually expanding our knowledge, in particular our knowledge of proper treatment and drug therapy. Insofar as this book mentions any dosage or application, readers may rest assured that the authors, editors, and publishers have made every effort to ensure that such references are in accordance with **the state of knowledge at the time of production of the book.**

Nevertheless, this does not involve, imply, or express any guarantee or responsibility on the part of the publishers in respect to any dosage instructions and forms of application stated in the book. **Every user is requested to examine carefully** the manufacturers' leaflets accompanying each drug and to check, if necessary in consultation with a physician or specialist, whether the dosage schedules mentioned therein or the contraindications stated by the manufacturers differ from the statements made in the present book. Such examination is particularly important with drugs that are either rarely used or have been newly released on the market. Every dosage schedule or every form of application used is entirely at the user's own risk and responsibility. The authors and publishers request every user to report to the publishers any discrepancies or inaccuracies noticed.

Some of the product names, patents, and registered designs referred to in this book are in fact registered trademarks or proprietary names even though specific reference to this fact is not always made in the text. Therefore, the appearance of a name without designation as proprietary is not to be construed as a representation by the publisher that it is in the public domain.

Learning
is finding out what you already know.

Doing
iis showing that you know it.

Teaching
is letting others know that they know it just as well as you do.

From *Illusions* by Richard Bach

Dedicated to our families

Petra, Florian and Julia

Ingrid, Janina and Raoul

Preface

In the study of medicine, *pathology* is the subject that concentrates on the mechanisms of a disease process and the morphologic changes in tissue that it causes. Therefore, it is only natural to attempt to render the material more accessible to students by making maximum use of illustrative images while keeping tedious theory to a minimum. In our approach to this book project, we opted for the *concept of a Thieme pocket atlas,* in which each topic is treated in a two-page spread that combines informative text and figures.

This pathology book focuses on *general pathology.* Aside from general pathology, the initial phase of the medical school curriculum customarily includes the basics of the pathology of organ systems and processes including the respiratory system, liver, gastrointestinal tract, excretory organs, nervous system, and endocrine system. The book covers these topics as patterns of injury that can affect more than one specific organ or tissue. As an integral whole, they affect life processes: metabolism and transport of substances, response to stimuli, preservation of the individual, cell growth and differentiation, and inheritance. We have also included numerous references to clinical findings. This was done to give the reader a better appreciation of our structuring of the subject of general pathology and to ensure that the book maintains a "medical" perspective. This approach uses general pathology to explain the processes occurring in the pathology of specific organs, and it uses the pathology of specific organs as examples to illustrate processes of general pathology. In our efforts to adequately address the diversity implied by such an understanding of pathology in a manner appropriate to an educational setting, we have proceeded as follows:

Chapter structure: Each of the 25 chapters begins with a "headline" that summarizes the content of the chapter in a single metaphoric sentence. This is followed by a *summary* in the style of a press release that gives readers both a concise overview of the goal of the specific chapter and a lively introduction to the topic. Completing the chapter is a *transition* to the next section.

Descriptive text: We have kept the text short in an effort to make the individual disease processes accessible at a glance without turning pages. Explanations and disease processes are presented in the form of *pathogenetic chain reactions,* in which these processes are presented as linear sequences of events. Wherever possible, we also provide the reader with *analogies* that illustrate the concept or serve as useful rules of thumb.

The medical thinking that leads to a clinical diagnosis is both algorithmic and associative. When one considers that most diagnoses are common but that the remaining rare diagnoses can apply in situations that initially appear to be clear-cut, it becomes clear that the physician must be familiar with these special cases as well. With this in mind, we have made an effort to briefly mention the *incidence* of clinically relevant processes and to point out the underlying pathogenetic principles for which they are *textbook examples.* As some of these principles occur in several disease processes, we have included cross references for recommended *recapitulation.*

The description of each disease process is divided into the sections *definition, pathogenesis,* and *morphology,* and is supplemented in applicable cases by the following additional passages:

Clinical presentation: Here the reader finds information on epidemiology, symptoms, and complications as they relate directly to the specific disease process.

Associated diseases: These entities follow the general pathologic principle discussed in the immediately preceding section. Chosen for their power of illustration, they represent examples that have a distinct effect on organs and tissues.

Sequelae: These are clinically distinct entities that are based on the general pathologic principle discussed in the immediately preceding section.

Note: This section includes illustrations, rules of thumb, and memory aids, some of which have been formulated by past instructors of pathology.

Prominent patients: Under this heading, we have attempted to break through the anonymity of the disease and give the disorder a very personal association. The purpose of this is to make it clear that the disease can affect any one of us and that it is not merely of clinical interest to the physician but represents a very human problem as well. This section also includes clinical records that illustrate the biologic extremes that can be reached.

Figures: We have devoted particular attention and great effort to the production and selection of images. Most of the images were created specifically for this atlas and entailed elaborate preparation of the specimens. In doing so, we paid special attention to several factors.

Normal tissue: Wherever possible, we have included the normal structures of the most important organs and tissues for the sake of comparison. Such a visual comparison makes a more lasting impression and conveys a better understanding of the altered structure than any verbal description.

Macrostructure and microstructure: Physicians who perform open or endoscopic surgery are routinely confronted with the macroscopic aspects of disease processes. For this reason, we have attached great importance to including both macroscopic and microscopic images of tissue changes. To illustrate histologic changes, we have used modern research and diagnostic techniques such as enzyme histochemical studies, immunohistochemical studies, and lectin histochemical studies; and with the aid of electron microscopy and molecular biology, we have expanded our coverage to include ultrastructural and supramolecular changes.

Diagrams and cartoons: Many concepts and disease processes cannot be suitably illustrated with histologic images. To facilitate an understanding of these concepts and processes, we have employed a concept that concentrates on representing the essential elements involved, wherever possible in the form a linear progression. To prevent the book from becoming overly tedious as a result of this objective presentation of information, we have taken the liberty of representing certain disease processes in the form of pathologic cartoons.

In this manner, we use a combination of text and images to examine those abnormal manifestations of life processes that lead to suffering. The purpose of pathology, literally "the study of suffering," is to teach one how to recognize a certain disease in its specific manifestation and how to comprehend its course so that the attending physician can act appropriately to relieve suffering. In this manner, pathology makes an important contribution to society as a whole. For a society that is oblivious to individual suffering is ruthless and inhuman. Moreover, the study of suffering can represent a gain for the individual as well. For it may well be that the only reason our soul is encased in a body is to allow it to experience that most important aspect of all creation: love.

Freiburg, spring 2004

Ursus-Nikolaus Riede

Acknowledgements

Here, I would like to express my thanks to all who have helped to make this book possible in its present form.
At Georg Thieme Verlag in Stuttgart, I thank Albrecht Hauff for his judicious management and Dr.-Jürgen Lüthje, Marianne Mauch, and Waltraud Haberberger for their meticulous and knowledgeable editing. I also extend my thanks to those colleagues who have assisted us by providing image material:

Prof. Dr. C. P. Adler, Patholog. Institut, Freiburg (359B-D)

Prof. Dr. R. Bässler, Patholog. Institut der Städt. Kliniken, Fulda (337A)

Prof. Dr. G. Bauer, Hygiene-Institut, Freiburg (129B-C)

Prof. Dr. K. A. Bienz, Hygiene-Institut, Basel (239D, 241B-C, 243A, 243D, 245A, 245D, 251E)

Prof. Dr. A. Böcking, Zytopatholog. Institut, Düsseldorf (375F)

Prof. Dr. N. Böhm, Patholog. Institut, Freiburg (17E, 25C-D, 45B, 65B-C, 65D-F, 93A-B, 101E-F, 289C-F, 325A-C, 383B, 383D, 383F)

Prof. Dr. B. Christ, Anat. Institut, Freiburg (297A-B)

Prof. Dr. H. Denk, Patholog. Institut, Graz (15B, 35E-F, 145C)

Prof. Dr. N. Freudenberg, Patholog. Institut, Freiburg (9D, 11D, 133F, 275D, 343A-B, 375D)

Prof. Dr. L. Hansen, Univ. Augenklinik, Freiburg (75D, 81F)

Dr. U. Hellerich, Patholog. Institut, Freiburg (119E)

Prof. Dr. E. Herbst, Patholog. Institut, Freiburg (179C)

Dr. C. Ihling, Patholog. Institut, Freiburg (173E, 183E, 391)

Prof. Dr. H. K. Koch, Patholog. Institut, Freiburg (83A-B, 249F)

Prof. Dr. G. Klöppel, Patholog. Institut, Kiel (79A-F, 121A-B, 121E, 187B, 187D)

Prof. Dr. G. Mall, Patholog. Institut, Darmstadt (117G)

Prof. Dr. H. P. Meister, Patholog. Institut, Städt. Krankenhaus München-Harlaching (351B)

Prof. Dr. M. Mihatsch, Patholog. Institut, Basel (139A, 191F, 373F)

Prof. Dr. C. Mittermayer, Abt. Pathologie, RWTH Aachen (217A, 397D, 407B)

PD Dr. H.-J. Müller, Univ.-Kinderklinik, Basel (17B-C, 55D, 67B, 113E, 123E-F, 291A, 291F-G, 325B, 325D)

Prof. Dr. H. Müntefering, H., Patholog. Institut, Mainz (301E, 303A, 301D-E, 305A, 301C)

Prof. Dr. A. Olah, Anatom. Institut, Bern (83D-E, 127A-D)

Prof. Dr. H. H. Peter, Abt. Rheumatologie, Univ.-Klinikum Freiburg (11B, 181A, 181C, 185A, 187A, 187C, 249E)

Prof. Dr. B. Rahn, AO-Forschungsinstitut, Davos (315A-C)

Prof. Dr. F. Rintelen, Univ.-Augenklinik, Basel (87D)

Prof. Dr. R. Rohrbach, Patholog. Institut, Freiburg (81A-B)

Prof. Dr. W. Saeger, Abt. Pathologie, Marienkrankenhaus Hamburg (389A)

Prof. Dr. H.-E. Schaefer, Patholog. Institut, Freiburg (19E, 45A, 49D, 75B, 75E, 83F-G, 87A, 89B, 89D-E, 91A-B, 99E, 101A, 101C, 103D, 181B, 187E, 191A-B, 219G, 243E, 247A-B, 249D, 251A, 257F, 259A, 263A-B, 263D, 269A, 271F, 275A, 275C, 277C, 277E, 279A, 281B, 283A, 283C, 285C, 319D, 333D, 365D, 401B)

Prof. Dr. W. Schlote, Neurolog. Institut, Frankfurt (25E-F, 93D-E, 253A, 369A-B)

Prof. Dr. R. Schuppli, Univ.-Hautklinik, Basel (81E, 89C-D, 115A, 177C, 213D, 247D, 255D, 263E, 263F, 275E, 385A, 427A)

Prof. Dr. M. A. Spycher, Patholog. Institut, Zürich (31C-D, 67A, 67C-D, 77A, 77D, 93C)

Prof. Dr. J. Staubesand, Anatom. Institut, Freiburg (149C, 405D, 407A)

Prof. Dr. B. Steinmann, Univ.-Kinderklinik, Zürich (39A, 49A)

Prof. Dr. W. Sterry, Univ.-Hautklinik, Charite, Berlin (169A, 173A, 177D-E, 181D, 251C, 251F, 367C-D, 401A)

Prof. Dr. M. Stolte, Patholog. Institut, Bayreuth (133C)

Dr. K. Technau, Patholog. Institut, Freiburg (409A-B, 411C, 421E)

Prof. Dr. J. Torhorst, Patholog. Institut, Basel (251G, 289A)

W. Villiger, Biozentrum, Basel (163C-D)

Prof. Dr. B. Volk, Neurozentrum, Freiburg (35A, 51E, 95D-E, 127F, 145E-F, 369D-F, 421C-D)

Prof. Dr. O. D. Wiestler, Neuropatholog. Institut, Bonn (35B, 51F, 115C-D, 193E-F)

Prof. Dr. C. Wittekind, Patholog. Institut, Leipzig (377A-D)

Prof. Dr. H. Wehner, Patholog. Inst., Kreiskrankenhaus Lahr (173C-D, 185D)

Prof. Dr. U. Wetterauer, Abt. Urologie, Univ.-Klinikum Freiburg (221A)

Prof. Dr. Z. Yoshi, Mikrobiol. Institut, Univ. Ube, Japan (255A-B, 259D, 259F, 261A-B, 263A, 263C, 273A, 275F)

Sources

243 C from: Carruthers GB. 400 Krankheitsbilder zur Schulung des diagnostischen Könnens. Weinheim: VCH; 1986
149 B, 405 D from: Zatouroff M. Farbatlas zur Blickdiagnostik in der Allgemeinmedizin. Schattauer 1977

Abbreviations

RES, RHS	Reticuloendothelial system
EvG	Elastica-van-Gieson stain
HE	Hematoxilin-Eosin stain
IF	Immune fluorescence
IH	Immune histochemistry
Iron stain	Prussian Blue stain
MGG	May-Gruenwald-Giemsa stain
PAS	periodic acid-Schiff's reaction
PNA	peanut agglutinin
SEM	scanning electron microscopy
Silver stain	Grocott's silver stain
TEM	transmission electron microscopy

Contents

3 Connective Tissue Lesions

4   Errors of Metabolism: Inorganic Compounds

5   Errors of Metabolism: Organic Compounds

6   Pigment Lesions

7   Sublethal Cell Damage

12   Immune Pathology

13 Pathology of Inflammation 194

14 Viral Infection

15 Bacterial Infection

16   Mycotic Infection

17   Protozoan Infection

18   Helminthic Infection

19   Hereditary Disorders

20   Congenital Malformations

21   Tissue Repair

22 Tumor Pathology

23   Generalized Circulatory Disorders

24   Localized Circulatory Disorders

25   Edema

1

Tracking Down Disease
Fundamentals of Pathology

──────── **Summary** ────────

Pathology (literally: the study of suffering) is the medical speciality that scientifically analyzes the causes, development, and forms of a disorder. Accordingly, the pathologist's duties include detecting and classifying a disorder in the tissue or cells of a living patient as well as determining the disease complex that has led to a patient's death. The pathologist does this by examining tissue specimens obtained from living patients (biopsy) or from dead patients (autopsy).

Pathology

Pathology is the branch of medicine that analyzes the causes, mechanisms of development, and morphologic manifestations of a disease using the methods of natural science. Nearly every disease is associated with dysfunction at the level of the organ, cell, or organelle. This allows the pathologist to identify functional damage and the cascade of disease processes on the basis of abnormal structural changes.

▬ Methods

General methods: The pathologist is able to identify the various forms of for example inflammation of an organ by analyzing biopsy material, whether in the form of needle aspiration or a specimen obtained endoscopically (by incision, forceps, or wedge biopsy). Analysis of 4 μm paraffin-embedded stained tissue sections (► B) determines whether a tumor is malignant or benign. These examinations require that an adequate amount of biopsy material has been obtained and sent to the pathologist (usually fixed in a 4% formaldehyde solution).

Examination of frozen sections: Biopsy material is sent to the pathologist as a fresh specimen during the surgical procedure. The pathologist then prepares frozen sections (► A) and within 5–10 minutes can verify or disprove clinical suspicion of malignancy. However, this quick fixation technique, with its greater slice thickness, produces less accurate results than conventional fixation.

Examination of crush preparation: Cerebral masses whose malignancy status is unknown are located and aspirated under stereotactic guidance. The needle biopsy obtained is flattened between two slides. Once the proper stain is applied, the cells contained in the specimen can be evaluated within a few minutes (► C, D).

Aspiration cytology: This technique permits quick morphologic diagnostic evaluation of a tumor. The affected organ, such as the prostate, or fluid-filled space is punctured with a fine needle, and the cells drawn out with a syringe are smeared on a slide (► E). The accuracy of this technique is quite high.

Exfoliative cytology: Here, cells obtained from the surfaces of tissues such as the cervix of the uterus (► F), or by centrifuging body fluids, are smeared on a slide.

> **Note:** *Tissue fixation for histology:* 4% formaldehyde solution buffered at pH 7.5.

> **Note:** *Tissue removal and diagnostic evaluation:* Specimens of excised tissue are often required to be submitted for histologic examination; failure to do so may constitute malpractice.

A **Mucinous carcinoma** (frozen section)
x 250

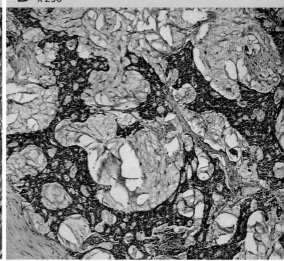

B **Mucinous carcinoma** (paraffin-embedded)
x 250

C **Pilocytic astrocytoma**
x 350 crush preparation toluidine blue

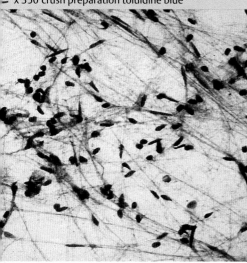

D **Anaplastic astrocytoma**
x 350 crush preparation toluidine blue

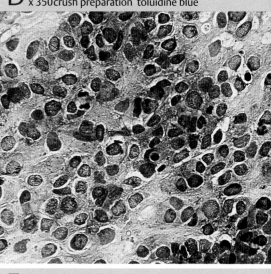

E **Mesothelioma cells** (MGG)
x 600

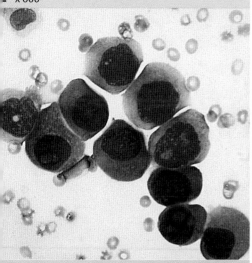

F **Cervical epithelial cells** (Papanicolaou smear)
x 600

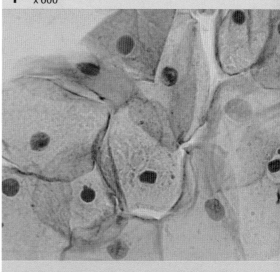

Disease

Disease is defined as a dysfunction of life processes that changes the entire body or its parts in such a manner that the affected person requires help for subjective, clinical, or social reasons.

■ Etiology

This involves the study of pathogens that cause disease and of developmental anomalies.

■ Causal Pathogenesis

This answers the question of why a certain pathogen causes disease in a certain individual. It describes the conditions under which disorders occur or, in other words, the interplay between the causes of disease and the body's susceptibility to disease. This involves several factors:

Environmental factors, which might include such factors as the causing size of quartz dust particles silicosis.

Disposition is the body's susceptibility to disease, without regard to its adaptability (see Chapter 7), and the affected individual's constitution.

Resistance is the body's ability to withstand the influence of disease-causing factors. It represents the interplay between unspecific immune mechanisms without the involvement of specific immune mechanisms (immunity; see Chapter 12).

■ Formal Pathogenesis

This describes the structural change observed during the clinical course of the disorder, which leads to the structural or functional damage specific to the disorder.

■ Clinical Course

Peracute disorders are fulminant and usually lead to death within several days.

Acute disorders are usually intense and last for a few days or weeks. Recuperation (recovery of normal health and function) is possible.

Subacute disorders are characterized by an insidious onset and a clinical course that lasts for weeks. Recuperation is often doubtful.

Chronic disorders are usually mild and progress in stages over a period of months:
— *Primary chronic disorders* begin without a manifest acute phase. The clinical course is episodic. Recuperation is not possible.
— *Secondary chronic disorders* occur subsequent to an acute inflammation that fails to heal because of complicating factors.
— *Recuperation* in these cases is characterized by structural damage and functional deficits that remain after the disease subsides. This results in restricted functional and social adaptability.

Recurrence is the resurgence of what is usually a chronic disorder after a period of time (see p. 350).

Remission is the temporary disappearance of the symptoms of the disorder (see p. 350).

Death (*exitus letalis* = lethal end).

Note: The WHO defines *health* as a condition of complete bodily, mental, and social well-being.

Signs of Death

The cessation of all vital processes can be clinically diagnosed by the following signs.

■ Equivocal Signs of Death

These signs include cardiac arrest, lack of pulse, cessation of breathing, areflexia, and decreasing body temperature. This is referred to as clinical death.

■ Brain Death

A patient is regarded as biologically dead where brain death has been diagnosed according to the following criteria:
- An isoelectric or 'flat' electroencephalogram for 24 hours.
- Two angiographic studies performed at an interval of 30 minutes demonstrating the absence of cerebral circulation.
- Irreversible absence of spontaneous respiration.
- Irreversible areflexia (lack of corneal and pupillary reflexes).

■ Unequivocal Signs of Death

Livores: After cardiac arrest, gravity causes the blood in the venous system to collect in the lowest parts of the body. This produces reddish violet skin spots that can be mobilized by applying local pressure.

Rigor mortis or postmortem rigidity begins 3–6 hours after death. According to Nysten's law, rigor mortis begins at the head and spreads toward the feet, later subsiding in the same manner. It occurs due to lack of ATP and the subsequent coagulation of actin and myosin filaments.

Autolysis or decomposition (p. 132): The failure of tissue respiration activates the intrinsic protease from lysosomes (p. 26) and extrinsic protease from intestinal bacteria, which digest the organic components of the body in the process of decomposition.

> **Note:** Reduced vital functions, such as can occur in barbiturate intoxication, can induce a state simulating death (apparent death).

Statistics

Average life expectancy is the time period in which 50% of a certain population group, such as women, have died.

Incidence is the number of new occurrences of a certain disease per year and per 100,000 population.

Prevalence is the number of persons per 100,000 inhabitants who suffer from a certain disease on a certain day.

Morbidity is number of persons per year and per 100,000 inhabitants who suffer from a certain disease.

Mortality is number of persons per year and per 100,000 inhabitants who die of a certain disease.

Lethality is the quotient obtained by dividing the number of persons who have died of a certain disease by the number of persons who have contracted the disease.

Autopsy

Synonym: postmortem examination

Definition: Examination of the organs of a dead body according to pathologic and anatomic criteria.

Official autopsies are required by law in certain cases involving sudden death from uncertain or unnatural causes, or in cases of death by suicide or by third parties. The procedure is ordered by the public prosecutor and usually performed by a medical examiner.

Epidemic autopsies should be performed in equivocal cases involving clinical suspicion of infectious disease.

Clinical autopsies are performed on patients who have died in hospitals. These procedures are for quality assurance and require the consent of the deceased's next of kin.

Insurance autopsies may be required by insurance companies in the following cases:
- Sudden death from uncertain or unnatural causes;
- Occupational exposure to certain pathogens.

These procedures are ordered by the insurer.

> **Note:** An insurance autopsy to resolve an insurance claim is almost never refused by the next of kin.

───────────────── **Summary** ─────────────────

Life is only possible in an organism where there is an orderly relationship among its constituent chemical elements. Such a relationship is created only by a spatial arrangement, i.e., a structure. The organism adapts the proportional relationship between the chemical elements to the specific requirements so that individual structural elements can neither be reduced in size nor enlarged without also changing their function. In a cell, this spatial arrangement corresponds to morphologically distinct compartments, the organelles of the cell, each of which has a defined function.

Nuclear Lesions

Physiology: The cell nucleus is surrounded by a double membrane containing selectively permeable nuclear pores. As the repository of genetic traits, it constantly controls the cell's overall function.

■ Forms of Nuclei

Interphase nucleus: This is characterized by a nucleolus containing RNA, loosely structured chromatin (euchromatin) and densely structured chromatin (heterochromatin).

Euchromatin is genetically active.
Heterochromatin is genetically inactive.

Mitotic nucleus: This is characterized by visible chromosomes.

■ Chromosomes

These are hierarchically arranged units in which the genetic material is packaged and transported. Genes are the basic units of heredity. They contain the information for a certain trait or function.

During the metaphase, the chromosomes consist of two strands or chromatids joined by a centromere (► A).

Structure of the chromosomes during metaphase:
— Short arm is **p** for "petit."
— Long arm is **q**.

Karyogram of the metaphase chromosomes: Chromosomes in a cell are arranged in a karyogram. This is a description of the chromosomes using a short formula according to these criteria:
— Total number of chromosomes
— Sex chromosome status
— Applicable aberrations.

DNA Repair Defects

The function of DNA and RNA may be compared to a modern data processing system. The software (program and base sequence) contains the instructions for copying the program (DNA replication), for repairing pro-

gram defects (DNA repair processes), and for using subprograms to create structural and functional proteins. The replication, transcription, and translation may be compared to the hardware (the computer itself).

DNA is subjected to damaging influences throughout the life of the body. This results in defective DNA duplicates, which normally can be restored by repair mechanisms. The defective segment is cut out of the DNA strand and the original base sequence is recreated with the aid of the portion of the DNA strand that is still intact. Congenital defects of the DNA repair system have devastating effects (see p. 290).

■ Xeroderma pigmentosum[1]

Textbook example of a DNA repair defect.

Definition: Rare, hereditary DNA repair derangement due to an endonuclease defect.

Pathogenetic chain reaction: Ultraviolet radiation causes DNA damage in the skin cells, which in turn causes increased DNA defects in skin cells. The sequelae include:
— Thinning of the skin (skin atrophy) triggers an adaptive reaction to ultraviolet radiation with excessive cornification and hyperpigmentation (► B, C);
— Mitotic dysfunction in the epidermis, resulting in skin tumors.

✚ Clinical Presentation: Patients will exhibit these lesions in adolescence:
– Dry, scaly skin (xeroderma) with a mottled pattern of hyperpigmentation (pigmentosum);
– Precursors of skin cancer (p. 85), later followed by multiple skin tumors such as basal cell carcinoma (p. 384), squamous cell carcinoma, and pigment cell cancers (malignant melanomas; p. 366).

Chromosome Abnormalities

See developmental anomalies (p. 294) and tumor development (p. 336).

───────────────

[1] Xeroderma pigmentosum (Greek and Latin): pigmented dry skin.

Structure of a chromosome
(schematic diagram)

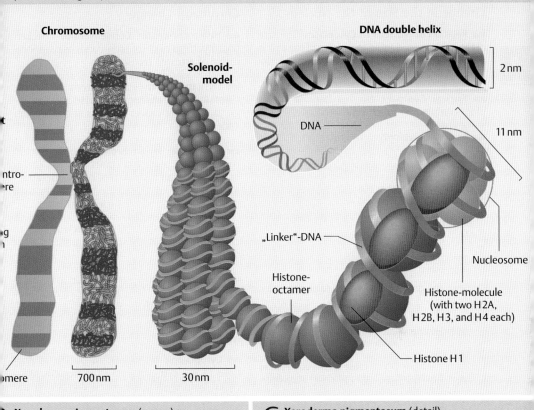

Chromosome

DNA double helix

Solenoid-
model

2 nm

DNA

11 nm

ntro-
re

„Linker"-DNA

Nucleosome

g

Histone-
octamer

Histone-molecule
(with two H2A,
H2B, H3, and H4 each)

Histone H1

mere

700 nm

30 nm

Xeroderma pigmentosum (survey)

Xeroderma pigmentosum (detail)

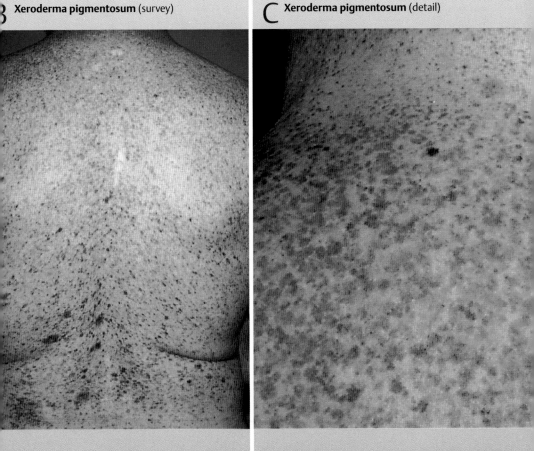

Change in the Size of the Nucleus

■ **Relation of Nucleus to Cytoplasm:** The size of the nucleus is adapted to the size of the cell. It also depends on the DNA content and on the functional state of the nucleus.

■ **Nuclear Euploidy:** Normal haploid or diploid complement of chromosomes.

■ **Nuclear Polyploidy:** Multiplied complement of chromosomes.

Most body cells contain diploid nuclei with a double complement of chromosomes. Proliferating cells double their DNA in the synthesis phase. Therefore, they temporarily become tetraploid and return to being diploid after mitosis (▶ A). Where mitosis fails to occur after the synthesis phase or it is followed by several additional synthesis phases, polyploid cell nuclei will result (▶ B). Haploid cell nuclei with half the complement of chromosomes are found only in spermiogenesis and oogenesis.

Nuclear polyploidy is a *morphologic sign* of a stress-induced adaptive reaction.

Examples:
— *Barbiturate abuse* causes increased metabolic activity in the liver, which in turn produces liver cell polyploidy.
— *Cardiac valvular defects* cause the myocardium to work harder, which in turn produces myocardial cell polyploidy.

■ **Nuclear Aneuploidy:** Deviation from the normal euploid complement of chromosomes in which individual chromosomes do not exist in their normal quantities.

Morphologic sequelae of nuclear aneuploidy (▶ C) include variability in the size of the nucleus (nuclear polymorphism) and chromatin content (nuclear polychromasia). Both are important criteria identifying a malignant tumor (p. 342).

> **Rule of thumb:**
> The larger the cell, the larger the nucleus.
> - A large cell nucleus indicates cellular activity.
> - A small cell nucleus indicates cellular inactivity.

> **Note:** Tumor malignancy criteria:
> - Nuclear polymorphism and nuclear polychromasia.
> - Proliferation, measured by mitosis count in the field of vision.
> - Dyskaryosis (see below).

Chromatin Change

■ **Heterochromatin Condensation:** Checkerboard pattern of chromatin condensation indicative of arrested transcription.

■ **Dyskaryosis:** Irregular pattern of heterochromatin condensation in coarse and fine aggregates giving cancer cells a salt-and-pepper appearance.

■ **Perinuclear Hyperchromatosis:** Chromatin condensation along the inner nuclear membrane. This is an early sign of cell death (apoptosis; p. 132), which later progresses to total chromatin clumping or nuclear pyknosis.

■ **Karyolysis:** Fading of the nucleus due to chromatin dissolution. This is a late sign of induced cell death.

■ **Karyorhexis:** Nuclear burst due to chromatin fragmentation. This is a late sign of programmed cell death.

Inclusions

■ **Cytoplasmic inclusions:** Migration of portions of the cytoplasm into the nucleus associated with dysfunctional cell division in the telophase causes a round lucency in the nucleus or a "frosted glass" nucleus.

Example: papillary thyroid carcinoma (▶ D).

■ **Paraplasmic inclusions:** Migration of portions of the paraplasm into the nucleus due to invagination of the nuclear membrane or dysfunctional telophase.

▥ **Glycogen inclusions:** following alcohol fixation cause nuclear defects (▶ E). They are signs of diabetic metabolism (p. 78).

▥ **Fatty inclusions** following fixation in paraffin cause lipid defects in the nucleus. They are typical of tumors in the form of fatty tissue, such as liposarcomas (p. 356).

▥ **Immunoglobulin inclusions** cause PAS-positive globules (Fahey-Dutcher bodies). They are typical of malignant lymphocytic tumors such as the lymphoplasmacytic lymphoma (p. 362).

▥ **Viral inclusions** usually consist of viral proteins arranged in para-crystalline configurations (▶ F).

A Nuclear diploidy (thyroid gland; Feulgen) x 400

B Nuclear polyploidy (thyroid gland; Feulgen) x 400

C Nuclear aneuploidy (tumor) (HE) x 800

D Frosted glass nucleus (thyroid tumor; MGG) x 800

E Nucleus with glycogen inclusion (HE) x 800

F Viral nuclear inclusions (HSV) (HE) x 300

Change in the Number of Nuclei

■ Polynuclear Cells

Definition: Physiologic and pathologic occurrence of two or more nuclei in a single cell.

Etiology: one of two mechanisms may be responsible.

Fusion of two or more cells into one large or giant cell may occur. This creates these types of giant polynuclear cells:
— *Resorptive giant cells (osteoclasts)* from fused histiocytes with resorptive capabilities;
— *Inflammatory giant cells* from fused histiocytes (epithelioid cells) with secretive capabilities that isolate a site of inflammation;
— *Placental syncytiotrophoblasts* from resorptive chorion cells;
— *Viral giant cells* from virus-infected cells that have merged by means of fusion peptide.

Mitotic dysfunction, in which normal mitotic division of the nucleus occurs but cytoplasmic division does not, can cause fusion. This may be seen in polynuclear giant cells following cytostasis in a tumor or in malignant tumors.

▦ Types of Giant Cells

Resorptive giant cells:
— Osteoclasts (histiocytic)
— Chondroclasts (histiocytic)
— Touton giant cells (histiocytic; p. 90)
— Syncytiotrophoblasts (chorial)
— Foreign-body giant cells (histiocytic)

Inflammatory giant cells:
— Langhans giant cell (orderly)
— Foreign-body giant cells (disorderly)

Viral giant cells:
— Warthin-Finkeldey giant cells (measles)
— Adenovirus giant cells
— Herpetic giant cells (herpes simplex)
— HIV giant cells (► A)

Tumor giant cells.

■ Anuclear Cells: These occur physiologically only as erythrocytes and thrombocytes. They are short-lived and do not undergo cell division.

Antinuclear Autoantibodies

Definition and pathogenesis: Some autoimmune diseases (p. 180) produce autoantibodies that attack certain of the body's own nuclear or nucleolar structures. These include:
— Double-stranded DNA (► B),
— Single-stranded DNA,
— Histone proteins,
— Nonhistone proteins,
— Centromere,
— DNA topoisomerase,
— RNA polymerase.

Nucleolar Change

Physiology: As the sites of ribosomal RNA transcription, the nucleoli are indicators of the level of cellular protein synthesis.

■ Inflammatory nucleoli: the prominent, round nucleoli in the activated cells of inflamed tissue.

■ Tumor nucleoli: the plump, enlarged, rough-edged, often eccentric nucleoli typical of cancer cells (► C, D). They are found in malignant tumor cells.

■ Giant nucleoli: exhibit excessive nucleolar enlargement almost to the size of lymphocyte nuclei.

Examples of giant nucleoli:
— *Cytomegalovirus infection* (p. 248): Cytomegalovirus is a DNA virus. Propagation of cytomegalovirus in the cell nucleus causes nuclear inclusions resembling nucleoli. These in turn result in cell enlargement and formation of a large viral pseudonucleus, creating cells that resemble an owl's eye (► E).
— *Hodgkin's lymphogranulomatosis* (p. 362) includes a group of malignant tumors of the lymphatic system with the following characteristics:
  — Hodgkin cells are mononuclear giant cells with large nucleoli.
  — Sternberg-Reed cells are mononuclear or binuclear giant cells with large nucleoli (► F).
  — Associated inflammatory infiltrate.

A **HIV-giant cells** (cell culture)
(HE) x 600

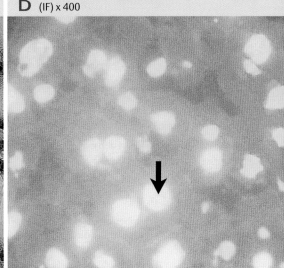

B **Antinuclear autoantibodies**
(IF) x 400

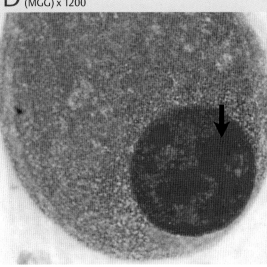

C **Tumor cell nucleoli**
(HE) x 600

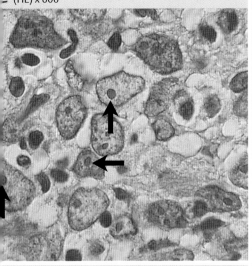

D **Tumor cell nucleoli**
(MGG) x 1200

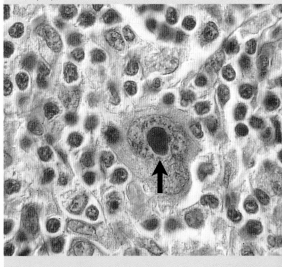

E **Cytomegaly giant cell nucleoli**
(IF; CMv) x 600

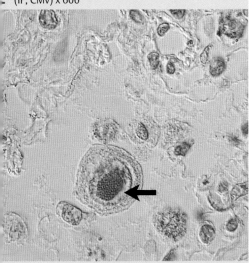

F **Tumor cell giant nucleoli**
(HE) x 600

Lesions of the Rough Endoplasmic Reticulum (RER)

Physiology: The cell's "protein factory," the rough endoplasmic reticulum or "RER" forms cisterns with exterior ribosomes attached their exteriors. The peptide chains manufactured by mRNA find their way into the cisternal lumina, where they are structured into proteins. Because of its high content of RNA and protein, the RER appears highly basophilic in stained histologic specimens. This basophilic fields are also referred to as ergastoplasm, and, in the ganglion cells, as Nissl fields or tigroid substance.

Quantitative Change

■ **Increase in the number of cisterns:** It occurs in all cells with high protein production and secretion, such as plasma cells.

■ **Decrease in the number of cisterns:** It characterizes inactive cells with reduced protein synthesis, such as the liver in undernourished patients (see p. 124).

Morphologic Change

■ **Fragmentation of the RER:** Fragmentation of the membrane system of the rough endoplasmic reticulum into small units is a sign of unspecific cell injury. These small units in turn change into tiny vesicles that are no longer recognizable under the light microscope.

■ **Formation of vacuoles in the RER:** Recognizable under the light microscope, this reversible cell injury (► A) is caused by interruption of energy metabolism in which the reaction chain involving Na⁺, K⁺-ATPase fails. This causes water to flow into the cell and the cisterns of the rough endoplasmic reticulum. Where accompanied by swelling of the smooth endoplasmic reticulum and mitochondria, it results in cytoplasmic degeneration with formation of vacuoles (see p. 68).

■ **Swelling of the RER:** Referred to in histologic contexts as "hydropic swelling," this irreversible cell injury is the final morphologic stage in the collapse of energy metabolism (p. 68) and is manifested in vesicular cytoplasmic vacuoles. It is the morphologic equivalent of what is known as accidental cell death (oncosis; p. 130).

■ **RER cistern collapse:** This is a consequence of a peroxidation injury to the membrane, such as CCl₄ intoxication (► B), and is the morphologic equivalent of the onset of programmed cell death (p. 128, 132).

Inclusions

■ **Amorphous inclusions:** Represent synthesis material that has accumulated in the lumen of the cisterns as a result of dysfunctional cellular synthesis or secretion processes (► C).

Examples:
— Genetic metabolic disorders.
— Drug-induced or toxic metabolic disorders.
— Tumor-induced metabolic disorders.

■ **Crystalline inclusions:** Are the consequence of delayed secretion in the presence of enzymopathy or in secreting tumors. In plasmocytoma (p. 364), a malignant plasma cell tumor, they consist of immunoglobulin chains (p. 160). In histologic contexts, these inclusions are called Russell bodies (► D).

■ **Particulate inclusions:** Consist of viral particles, such as cytomegalovirus.

Oncofetal Lesion

Definition: Deranged cisterns of the RER, which occur in this form only in fetal and tumor tissue (p. 340):

■ **Ribosome-layer complexes:** Are layered aggregates of RER cisterns with interposed rows of ribosomes.

■ **Annulated lamellae layers:** Are layered aggregates of perinuclear RER cisterns with nuclear pores (► F).

■ **Mitochondria-lamellar-layer complexes:** Are layered aggregates of longitudinally compressed mitochondria and RER cisterns.

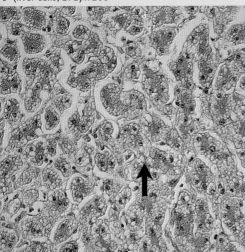

A Vacuolization of the RER
(liver cells, EvG) x 200

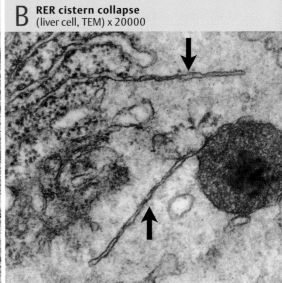

B RER cistern collapse
(liver cell, TEM) x 20000

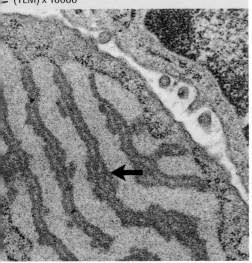

C Inclusion in the RER
(TEM) x 10000

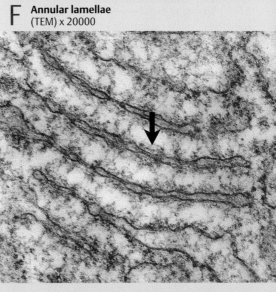

D Russell bodies
(HE) x 400

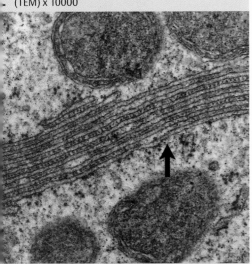

E Ribosome-lamellae complexes
(TEM) x 10000

F Annular lamellae
(TEM) x 20000

Lesions of the Smooth Endoplasmic Reticulum (SER)

Physiology: The smooth endoplasmic reticulum or "SER" forms a system of branching tubules that communicates with the rough endoplasmic reticulum. It contains demethylases, decarboxylases, deaminases, glucuronidases, and a multipurpose oxidase whose terminal oxidase is cytochrome P-450. Accordingly, the SER is able to split steroid bodies, and it can not only render drugs and toxins inactive but also facilitate their secretion. However, its multipurpose oxidase can also activate carcinogens.

Quantitative Change

■ Proliferation of SER

Definition: Increase in tubular structures of the smooth endoplasmic reticulum.

Morphology: As a consequence of proliferation of SER (► A), the affected cell increases in size and contains a large, homogeneous, slightly basophilic focus of cytoplasm set off from the cell membrane by a light halo. Such cells are often referred to "ground glass" cells (► B).

Proliferation of SER is the morphologic correlate of the following pathologic processes:
— **Enzyme induction:** Chronic exposure to toxic substances (as in barbiturate abuse) leads to an increase in the quantity of detoxifying SER enzymes and membranes.
  Result: The increased quantity of enzymes and membranes increases detoxification.

  Exception: Hypoactive hyperplastic SER is present in cholestasia, where cholate is retained in parenchymal liver cells (p. 110).
  Result: The increased quantity of membranes with fewer enzymes results in a loss of function.

— **Virus material production:** Hepatitis B (p. 248) results in intratubular formation of HBs antigen (surface antigen) with corresponding proliferation of the SER.

■ Atrophy of the SER

Definition: Shrinkage of the SER with reduction of reticular membranes.
Result: This reduces metabolism with a corresponding reduction in organ and tissue size (see general discussion of atrophy, p. 124).

  Exception: Protracted administration of fructose produces hyperactive hypoplastic SER.
  Result: This causes a paradoxical increase in enzymes despite the loss of membrane.

Morphologic Change

■ Formation of Vesicles in the SER

Definition and pathogenesis: Fragmentation of dilated tubules of the SER occurring in cytoplasmic degeneration with formation of vacuoles. This degeneration ranges from vesicle formation to vacuole formation. Vesicle formation is a nonspecific sign of cell injury (see p. 130).

■ "Cytoplasmic Nuclei"

Definition and pathogenesis: This is the histologic correlate of onion-like layered aggregations of SER (fingerprint degeneration; ► C). Cytoplasmic nuclei are a sign of blocked enzyme synthesis or decoupled cholesterol synthesis, such as is occasionally found in blocked or degenerative protein synthesis.

Inclusions

Pathogenesis: Inclusions are typical of:
— Lipoprotein synthesis disorders (which causes intratubular lipid accumulation, p. 88);
— Hepatitis B (which causes intratubular accumulation of filamentous viral shell proteins, ► D).

Disorders within the endoplasmic reticulum affect the primary synthesis products. These products remain within the cell because they have assembled abnormally and therefore lodge within the membrane labyrinth.

In contrast, disorders of the Golgi apparatus, where the synthesis products are prepared for secretion from the cell, always affect the secretion of substances into the lumen of a gland, the release of composite synthesis products into the bloodstream, or the discharge of connective-tissue components into the extracellular space. Disorders cause this sort of material to remain within the cells, impairing their function. The following examples of lesions of the Golgi apparatus illustrate this phenomenon.

Proliferation of SER (liver cell)
(TEM) x 10000 (M=mitochondrion)

B **Ground glass cells** (liver)
(HE) x 300

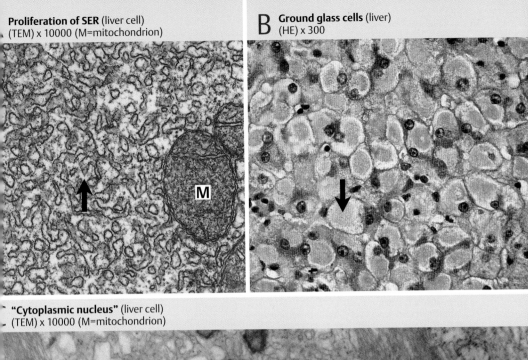

"Cytoplasmic nucleus" (liver cell)
(TEM) x 10000 (M=mitochondrion)

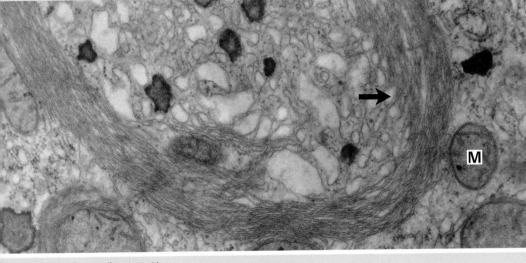

Inclusion in the SER (hepatitis B)
(TEM) x 20000

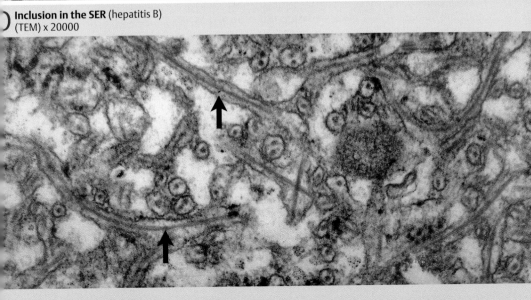

Golgi Lesions

Physiology: The Golgi apparatus consists of a layered aggregation of curved, flattened sacs. The function of this structure may be compared to the shipping department of a manufacturing company.

The prefabricated products assembled in the protein factory of the rough endoplasmic reticulum enter the Golgi apparatus through the "service door." What happens next depends on the mode of secretion of that particular cell.

— *Regulated secretion:* In cells with regulated secretion, such as pancreas cells, the products of the rough endoplasmic reticulum are initially stored in Golgi vacuoles (condensation vacuoles). The action of the Golgi apparatus's own glycosyltransferase and sulfatase enzymes creates complex compounds. Together with substrates, these compounds are then assembled into lipoproteins, glycoproteins, and proteoglycans in a process of protein modification. The addition of oligosaccharide groups to the cellular synthesis products addresses them after a fashion.

— *Unregulated secretion:* In cells with unregulated secretion, such as plasma cells, the prefabricated products of the rough endoplasmic reticulum are released directly into the extracellular space.

Atrophy of the Golgi Apparatus

General pathogenesis: Atrophy of the Golgi apparatus is the ultrastructural correlate of disturbed protein synthesis with or without an impairment of post-translation protein modification (see general discussion of atrophy, p. 124). It is therefore typical of the following disorders:

— Undifferentiated malignant tumors;
— Cells suffering from oxygen deprivation;
— Cells that lose their nuclei (such as erythroblasts).

Hypertrophy of the Golgi Apparatus

General pathogenesis: Hypertrophy of the Golgi apparatus is observed in every secreting cell that becomes polyploid. It also occurs where secretions are backed into the vacuoles of the Golgi apparatus. (See also general discussion of hypertrophy, p. 116.)

Golgi-associated disorders

Several disorders are attributable to disturbed secretion and therefore to dysfunction of the Golgi apparatus. This also alters the contents of the Golgi apparatus vacuoles.

■ Cholestasis

Pathogenesis (see also p. 110): Gall drainage disorder in which gall is backed up into the cisterns of the Golgi apparatus (► A).

■ Fatty Liver

Pathogenesis: Hereditary or acquired disorder of lipoprotein metabolism (p. 88). This causes lipoprotein component substances to accumulate in the cisterns of the Golgi apparatus, resulting in fatty liver (see also p. 84).

■ Achondroplasia

Synonym: chondrodystrophia fetalis.

Definition: Hereditary impairment of endochondral ossification with normal ligamentous ossification resulting in disproportionate short stature (dwarfism; ► B).

Pathogenesis: Hereditary defect of the receptor for fibroblast growth factor (FGFR-3), resulting in deficient regulation of chondrocyte proliferation and differentiation. The resulting impairment of proteoglycan synthesis causes proteoglycan to accumulate in the Golgi cisterns of the chondrocytes. Consequently, there is no zone of vesicular cartilage and no cartilage breakdown zone (► E1 and F). This results in the formation of a broad, shortened area of primary cancellous bone with delayed remodeling into secondary cancellous bone (► E2). The long cortical bones remain short and broad, with caps of epiphyseal cartilage (► D), resulting in dwarfism. However, ligamentous ossification proceeds normally; growth of the sides and top of the skull is normal, although the base of the skull remains small. This produces facial dysmorphia (facial deformity).

> **Note:** *Achondroplasia* characteristically produces a person of short stature (dwarf) with a large skull and short limbs, without mental retardation.

☺ **Prominent patients:** Circus clowns. Among other animals, the dachshund is an example.

■ Alveolar Proteinosis

Definition: Accumulation of surfactant[1] proteins within the alveoli; of uncertain etiology, leads to impaired breathing.

Pathogenesis: The disorder involves overproduction and reutilization of surfactant proteins, causing them to accumulate in the Golgi cisterns of the type II alveolar surface cells. This leads to accumulation of surfactant proteins in the alveoli with productive coughing. Further symptoms include impaired breathing and increased susceptibility to infection.

---

[1] Surfactant = **surf**ace **act**ive **agent**, the anti-adhesive agent of the alveoli of the lung.

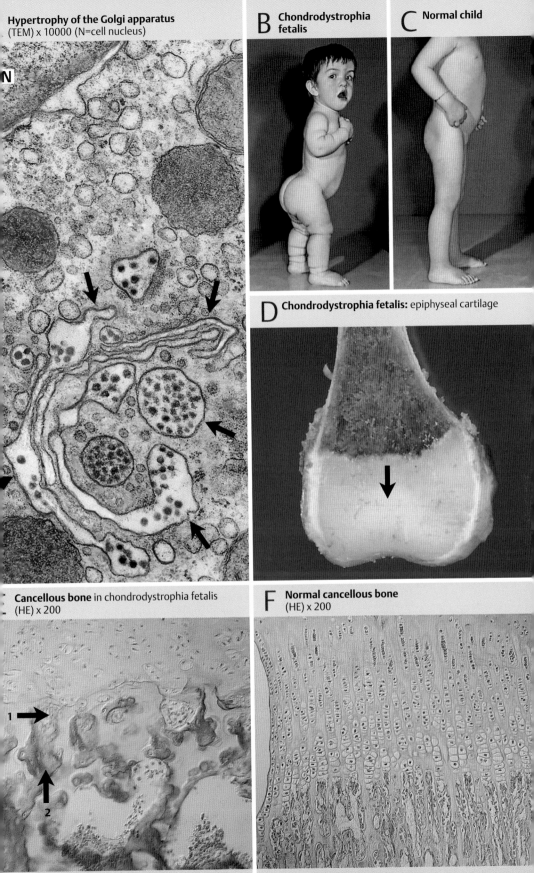

Hypertrophy of the Golgi apparatus
(TEM) x 10000 (N=cell nucleus)

N

B Chondrodystrophia fetalis

C Normal child

D Chondrodystrophia fetalis: epiphyseal cartilage

Cancellous bone in chondrodystrophia fetalis
(HE) x 200

1

2

F Normal cancellous bone
(HE) x 200

Mitochondrial Lesions

Physiology: The "powerhouses of the cell," the mitochondria provide energy-rich substrates that are vital for cell survival. These structures are filamentous or spherical and are surrounded by a double membrane. The inner membrane exhibits cristae or tubular invaginated structures at the supramolecular level to which oxysomes are attached. The mitochondrial matrix will be found to contain mitochondrial RNA and DNA, and calciosomes in the form of mitochondrial grana (p. 20). The matrix is the site where ß-oxidation, oxidative decarboxylation, the citrate cycle, and the urea cycle take place. The components of the respiration chain and oxidative phosphorylation are located in the inner membrane; the outer membrane contains the transferases for carbohydrate and fat metabolism.

Quantitative Change

Like bacteria, mitochondria can replicate themselves by dividing independently of cell division (► A), which leads to mitochondrial proliferation.

■ Mitochondrial Proliferation

This is a sign of adaptation to a prolonged high level of functional loading leading to a functional increase in a cell or tissue, such as in body building.

▥ Oncocytes[1] (= Hürthle cells)

Definition: Swollen cells with grainy, eosinophilic cytoplasm.

Pathogenesis: Mitochondrial DNA mutation disturbs ATP synthesis. This in turn causes compensatory mitochondrial proliferation. The consequence is that the cytoplasm becomes rich in mitochondria and swells, in a process referred to as oncocytic cytoplasm transformation (► B).

> **Note:** Oncocyte is a descriptive term for a cell rich in mitochondria.

> **Note:** An oncocyte is not a tumor cell.

> **Note:** Carcinomas of the salivary and thyroid glands may exhibit total or partial oncocytic transformation (oncocytic thyroid carcinoma, oncocytic salivary gland carcinoma).

▥ Oncocytoma

This is a *textbook example* of a tumor resulting from mitochondrial DNA mutation with dysfunctional cell respiration.

Occurrence: salivary gland, thyroid gland, and kidney.

Definition: Benign tumor composed of cells that have undergone oncocytic transformation. The tumor has a mahogany brown color due to its high cytochrome content (► B, C).

■ Mitochondrial Depletion

Where it is a consequence of increased destruction of mitochondria, mitochondrial depletion is the ultrastructural correlate of cell injury. Where it is the result of suppressed generation of mitochondria, it is a sign of immature or undifferentiated cells, and, for example, results in loss of muscular tissue in muscle atrophy (p. 124).

Morphologic Change

■ Megamitochondria

Pathogenesis: Megamitochondria occur in the presence of severe deficiencies (vitamin B complex deficiency or alcoholism; p. 144) as a result of defective mitochondrial division or fusion. They are *not* caused by toxic swelling.

■ Mitochondrial Swelling

Definition: Mitochondrial swelling is the ultrastructural correlate of the "turbid swelling" of parenchymal organs described by R. Virchow in 1852. It usually occurs together with generalized cytoplasmic degeneration with formation of vacuoles.

Macroscopic appearance of the organs: characterized by enlargement with a doughy, turbid cut surface.

Microscopic appearance of the cells: characterized by swelling with granular, light cytoplasm (► D).

Ultrastructural aspect: The swelling begins in response to the change in osmotic pressure with condensation of the matrix (► E) and swelling of the space between the cristae (crista type). This is followed by dissolution of the mitochondrial matrix and the mitochondrial cristae (matrix type).

---

[1] Oncocyte: from *onkos* (Greek), swelling.

Mitochondrial division
(TEM) x 10000 (M=mitochondria)

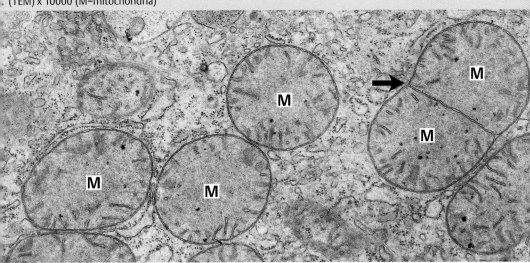

Oncocytes (excretory duct, parotid gland)
(HE) x 600

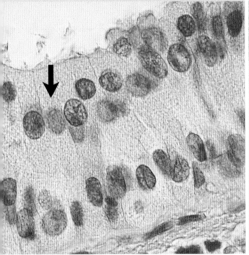

C **Oncocytoma** (thyroid)
(HE) x 600

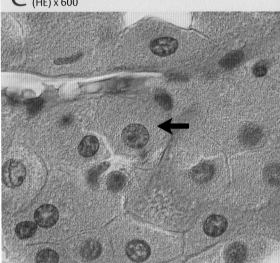

D **Turbid cellular swelling due to mitochondrial swelling** (HE) x 600

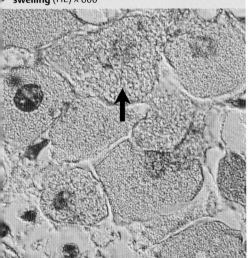

E **Mitochondrial swelling**
(TEM) x 10000

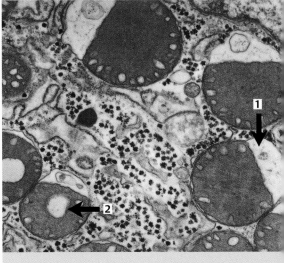

Structural Change in Mitochondrial DNA

Physiology: The mitochondria contain their own DNA (mitochondrial DNA) whose base coding differs from that of nuclear DNA. It is sufficient for coding several hydrophobic proteins of the mitochondrial cristae and subunits of the cytochrome oxidase.

The following variants of mitochondrial DNA occur in humans:
— *Catenated form* (chain-link form): It occurs in all cells.
— *Circular dimeric form* (figure-of-eight form): It occurs in malignant tumor cells, and oncocytoma. (An oncocyte is a cell with an overly large number of mitochondria.)

Mitochondrial DNA Mutations

■ Congenital Forms

Pathogenesis: Single-point mutations of mitochondrial DNA with maternal hereditary transmission.

Examples:
— Hereditary types of neuromyopathy (see below).
— Mitochondrial diabetes mellitus (p. 78).
— Neurologic symptoms such as ataxia and hearing disorders.

■ Acquired Forms

Occurrence: myocardial ischemia.

Pathogenesis: Following ischemia, toxic oxygen metabolites accumulate in the tissue during the reperfusion phase. This causes damage to mitochondrial DNA.

Changes in the Mitochondrial Cristae

■ Membrane proliferation: involves an increase in the number of cristae due to the following cellular adaptation mechanisms:

— *Proportional membrane and enzyme increase* (► A): This is caused by an increased functional load, such as athletic activity. The clinical result is an increased quantity of membranes and enzymes with an increase in function.

— *Disproportional membrane and enzyme increase* is indicative of poor adaptation to a deficiency in essential building blocks, such as riboflavin. The clinical result is an increased quantity of membranes with few enzymes. This sustains a reduced level of cell function in the presence of an extreme deficiency.

■ Membrane loss (► B): The mitochondrial cristae are indicator structures for energy metabolism. In lethal cell injury (p. 128) such as in oxygen deprivation, the loss of these cristae is attributable to membrane destruction.

Inclusions

Pathogenesis: Mitochondrial inclusions are attributable to dysfunctional mitochondrial membrane synthesis and/or accumulation of metabolites. The following variants occur:

■ Matrix inclusions are usually amorphous and lie in the mitochondrial matrix (► C). They occur most often in chronic ischemic disorders (p. 416).

■ Crista inclusions consist of deposits of enzyme-protein complexes and lie in the mitochondrial cristae between the crista membranes (► D, E). They are primarily typical of mitochondrial myopathy (muscle disorders involving loss of strength; p. 22).

■ Grana inclusions: Mitochondria are the main structures responsible for physiologic and orthotopic calcification because in their interior they contain small granular structures known as the mitochondrial grana, which are calciosomes. These structures bind excess intracellular calcium. They also store calcium, which is important for many cellular functions. Therefore it is not surprising that the mitochondria also play such a significant role in abnormal or heterotopic calcification (p. 134) and that the first calcium phosphate deposits occur in the mitochondrial grana.

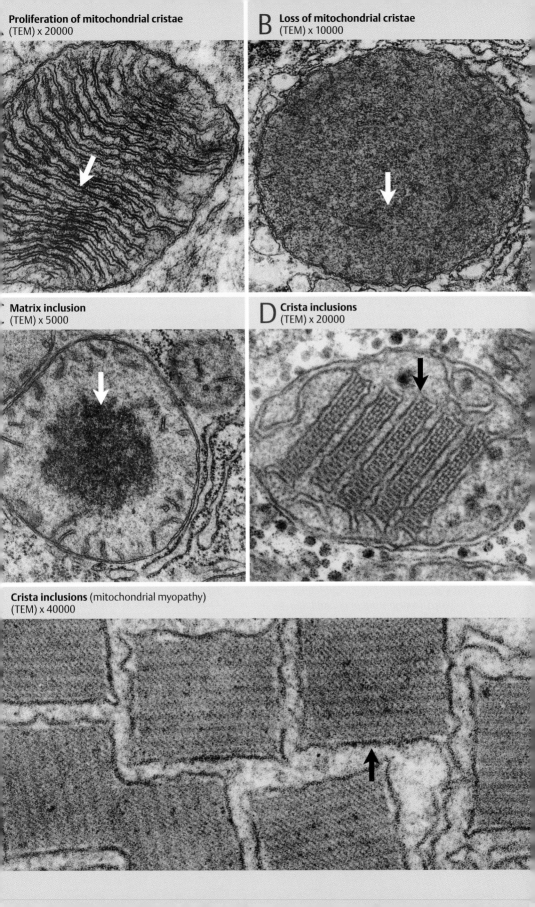

Proliferation of mitochondrial cristae
(TEM) x 20000

B **Loss of mitochondrial cristae**
(TEM) x 10000

Matrix inclusion
(TEM) x 5000

D **Crista inclusions**
(TEM) x 20000

Crista inclusions (mitochondrial myopathy)
(TEM) x 40000

Mitochondrial Disorders

General definition: Clinical syndromes in which an essential pathogenic process takes place in the mitochondria.

Mitochondrial Myopathies

Definition: Rare disorders affecting both the skeletal muscles and the brain and which are therefore known as mitochondrial encephalo-myopathies.

These disorders are attributable to the following processes:
— Mitochondrial substrate transport.
— Mitochondrial substrate utilization.
— Mitochondrial energy conservation.
— Mitochondrial energy transfer.
— Mitochondrial DNA (mutations).

Hypoxia

Textbook example of disorders involving or attributable to dysfunctional cell respiration.

Definition: Frequently encountered clinical syndrome due to disruption of the normal oxidative process of energy production (► A). Hypoxia is one possible cause of heart failure (see note).

■ Hypoxemic[1] Hypoxia (► B)

Pathogenesis: Oxygen content in the blood (hypoxemia) is decreased due to the following causes:
— Decreased partial pressure of oxygen in exterior air (high-altitude disease);
— Reduced supply of oxygen (ventilation disorder);
— Reduced pulmonary blood supply (perfusion disorder);
— Impaired pulmonary gas exchange (diffusion disorder);
— Impaired oxygen transport and uptake by the erythrocytes.

■ Ischemic[2] Hypoxia (► C)

Pathogenesis: Insufficient supply of arterial blood to tissue results in a lack of oxygen and oxidizable substrates. This in turn impairs the removal of metabolic waste products (primarily of CO_2) in tissue, causing tissue acidosis.

Sequelae:
— Acute ischemia causes necrosis (p. 74).
— Chronic ischemia causes fatty degeneration (p. 49) and fibrosis (p. 23).

■ Hyperglycemic Hypoxia (► D)

Pathogenic causes:
— *Maldigestion:* insufficient release of oxidizable substances such as glucose as a result of deficient nutrition or digestion (p. 82).
— *Malabsorption:* insufficient substrate uptake in the intestinal tract (p. 82).

■ Histotoxic Hypoxia (► E)

Pathogenic causes: Blockage of intracellular energy production due to impairment of these processes:
— Cellular substance uptake;
— Substrate oxidation;
— Electron transport chain (as in hydrogen cyanide poisoning);
— Coupling of oxidative phosphorylation and ATP formation (for example bacterial toxins).

> **Note:** Causes of heart failure include:
> – Destruction of myocardial cells;
> – Dysfunctional ß-adrenergic signal transduction (too little hormone, too few receptors):
> – Disturbance in the availability of intracellular calcium;
> – Hypoxia.

Mitochondrial Autoantibodies

Definition: Autoantibodies (p. 160) that react with mitochondrial components.

Examples: Autoantibodies reacting with mitochondrial components may be found in several types of self-destructive inflammation (autoimmune diseases, see p. 180).
— *Pseudo-lupus erythematosus* (self-reactive mitochondrial autoantibodies occur in 100% of all cases) creates a clinical syndrome resembling lupus erythematosus (p. 180) without nuclear antibodies (without involvement of the kidneys or central nervous system).
— *Primary biliary cirrhosis* (self-reactive mitochondrial autoantibodies occur in 98% of all cases) involves autoimmune inflammatory destruction of the bile ducts with progressive scarring that can develop into liver cirrhosis (p. 42).
— *Chronic aggressive hepatitis* of the lupoid type (self-reactive mitochondrial autoantibodies occur in 30% of all cases) involves autoimmune inflammatory destruction of the liver cells that can develop into liver cirrhosis (p. 42).
— *Lymphocytic Hashimoto thyroiditis* involves autoimmune lymphocytic destruction of the follicles, causing reduced thyroid function (p. 186).
— *Sjögren syndrome* involves autoimmune lymphocytic destruction of the tear and oral salivary glands with compensatory proliferation of the myoepithelial-like epithelial tissues of the acinar duct (a lymphoepithelial lesion). This causes a desiccation syndrome with a dry mouth and dry eyes (p. 184).

---

[1] Hypoxemia (Greek): blood with reduced oxygen.
[2] Ischemia: *ischo* (Greek), hold up + *haima* (Greek), blood.

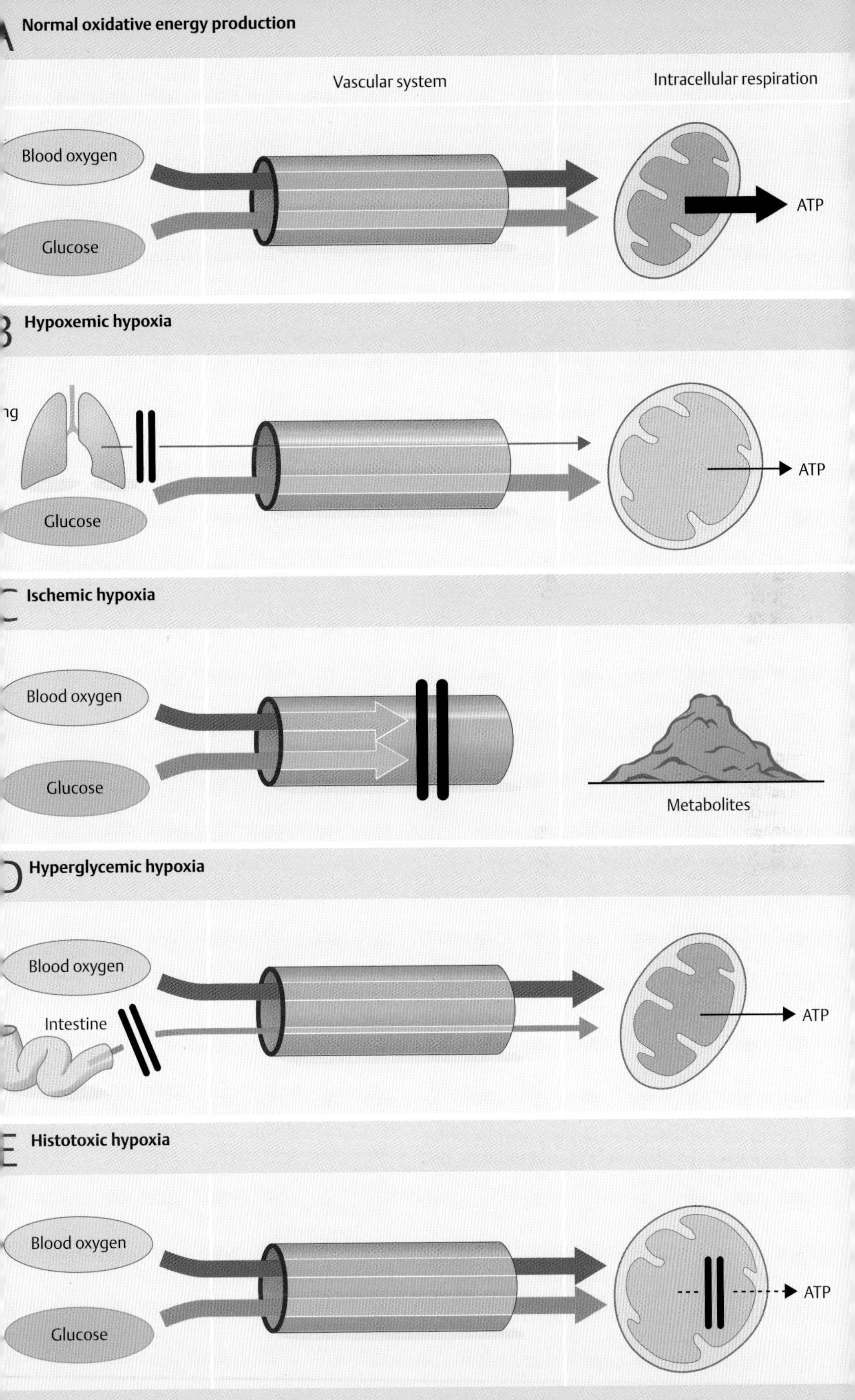

A Normal oxidative energy production

Vascular system | Intracellular respiration

Blood oxygen

Glucose

ATP

B Hypoxemic hypoxia

ng

Glucose

ATP

C Ischemic hypoxia

Blood oxygen

Glucose

Metabolites

D Hyperglycemic hypoxia

Blood oxygen

Intestine

ATP

E Histotoxic hypoxia

Blood oxygen

Glucose

ATP

Peroxisomal Lesions

Physiology: The peroxisomes are small organelles whose membranes are continuous with the rough endoplasmic reticulum (► A) and the SER (► B). They are removed by self-destruction or autophagy (see below).

Functions of the peroxisomes:
Fat metabolism:
— ß-oxidation of very long-chain fatty acids and of C_{12} dicarboxyl acids from the ω-oxidation.
— Phytanic acid α-hydroxylase breaks down the C_{20} branched-chain fatty acid from chlorophyll.
— Biosynthesis of ether phospholipids (plasmalogen), and therefore biosynthesis of membranes.
— 3-hydroxy-3-methylglutaryl-CoA-reductase, used in biosynthesis of cholesterol.
Breakdown of peroxide: Catalase breaks down H_2O_2.
— Carbohydrate metabolism:
— Reoxidation of NADH with L-α-hydroxy acid oxidase.
— Helps break down fructose with α-glycerophosphate dehydrogenase.
Bile acid biosynthesis: Conversion of trihydroxycoprostane acid in cholic acid.

Peroxisomal Diseases

General definition: Disorders due to primary disruption of one or more peroxisomal functions.

■ Acatalasemia

Definition and pathogenesis: Hereditary catalase instability causing shortages of available catalase in the liver and other organs.

> ✚ **Clinical presentation:** Rare autosomal recessive hereditary disease involving chronic gangrenous stomatitis (mouth rot).

■ Refsum Disease (see p. 86)

■ Cerebrohepatorenal Syndrome

Synonym: Zellweger Syndrome.

Definition: Hereditary peroxisomal defect with developmental anomaly syndrome.

Pathogenesis: A single-point mutation of the peroxisomal assembly factors prevents "final assembly" of the peroxisomal building blocks to functional organelles. This in turn disrupts the transport of electrons between succinate dehydrogenase flavoprotein and the coenzyme Q, causes deficient peroxisomal breakdown of fatty acids and phytanic acid, and results in deficient biosynthesis of plasmalogen and bile acid.

Morphology: Hepatocytes, renal tubules, and other organ cells lack peroxisomes containing catalase. The facial skull exhibits developmental anomalies (dysmorphia). Brain defects involving impaired myelin formation, and small convolutions of the brain (microgyria; ► C, D) are present, as is hepatomegaly (enlarged liver) with icterus (jaundice, see p. 108). This in turn causes liver cirrhosis (p. 42) and glomerular microcysts in the kidney.

> ✚ **Clinical presentation:** Autosomal recessive hereditary disease involving cerebral retardation with epilepsy, muscular hypotonia, spastic paralysis, deafness, and hepatic insufficiency. The disorder is rare and leads to death in infancy.

■ Adrenoleukodystrophy

Synonym: Familial Addison's disease.

Definition: Hereditary neural and metabolic disease.

Pathogenesis: A defective peroxisomal assembly factor (PEX-gene) results in a peroxisomal enzyme defect. This in turn impedes the breakdown of long-chain fatty acids and results in reduced plasmalogen formation in the brain and adrenal cortex, leading to storage of fatty acids.

Morphology: Diffuse neural and cerebral demyelinization process of the white matter (► E) that spares the subcortical pathways. The disorder is characterized by curved, plate-like lipid inclusions in scavenger cells of the brain (► F), Schwann cells, and cells of the adrenal cortex.

> ✚ **Clinical presentation:** This rare, X-chromosomal or autosomal recessive hereditary disorder manifests itself between the ages of five to ten years.
> – *CNS:* Demyelinization of the white matter leads to secondary degeneration of the cortical spinal pathways, causing paralysis and impaired vision.
> – *Adrenal cortex:* Cortical atrophy causes insufficiency of the adrenal cortex, which in turn manifests itself as Addison's disease (p. 112, 186).

■ Systemic Carnitine Deficiency

Definition: Peroxisomal disease involving lipid storage myopathy.

Pathogenesis: Peroxisomal carnitine acetyltransferase deficiency means that carnitine is unavailable as a carrier for long-chain fatty acids. This prevents ß-oxidation of long-chain fatty acids, resulting in fat storage in vacuoles in the musculature. This leads to muscle atrophy.

> ✚ **Clinical presentation:** Carnitine deficiency in skeletal muscle, blood serum, and liver leads to muscle weakness with exercise, paralysis of proximal and peripheral muscle groups, and episodic hepatic and cerebral dysfunction. The disorder is rare.

A Peroxisome and rough endoplasmic reticulum
(TEM) x 10000

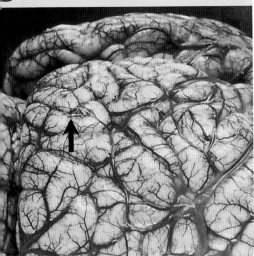

B Peroxisomes and smooth endoplasmic reticulum
(TEM) x 5000

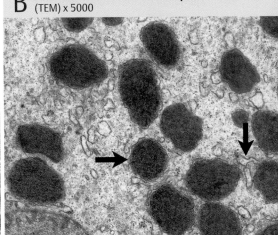

C Zellweger syndrome: microgyria

D Zellweger syndrome: microgyria

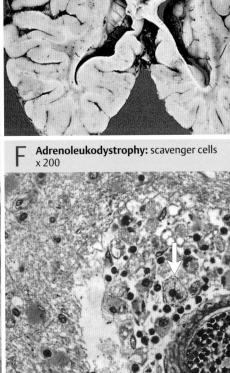

E Adrenoleukodystrophy: demyelinization
stain for myelin x 50

F Adrenoleukodystrophy: scavenger cells
x 200

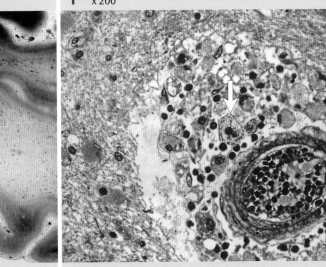

Lysosomal Lesions

Physiology of lysosome function:
— *Waste treatment plant:* This structure prevents the cell from becoming contaminated by breaking down harmful substances and bacteria in a process known as heterophagy.
— *Optimized operation:* The lysosomes also break down cellular components that have become ineffective in a process known as autophagy.
— *Garbage dump:* Telolysosomes dispose of cellular refuse.
— *Recycling:* These structures also reuse this cellular refuse.

Disturbances of the cellular disposal system lead to the following lysosomal disorders:
— *Storage disorders* in which waste removal and recycling is blocked.
— *Destabilizing disorders* in which the overflowing waste treatment plant produces local damage.
— *Stabilizing disorders* in which a work slowdown in refuse collection leads to cell contamination.

Lysosome activity may be divided in to the following phases and functional loops:

Prelysosomal Phase

▰ Heterophagy

Definition: Cellular uptake of foreign particulate material (phagocytosis) and the breakdown of that material.

Cellular uptake of foreign material is divided into three phases.

Recognition phase: The engulfing cell or phagocyte must first recognize the foreign material as such (▶ A, B). This requires "detection" proteins such as immunoglobulins (p. 160) and C3b complement factor (p. 162), which make the foreign material palatable for the phagocyte in a process known as opsonization. Now these particles can be detected by the phagocyte's receptors.

Uptake phase: After establishing contact with foreign material, the detection receptors concentrate in the phagocyte membrane at the site of contact (▶ C, D). This causes the material to better "adhere" to the membrane. The phagocyte forms tentacle-like cytoplasmic arms (▶ B) with which it encloses the foreign material. The ends of the tentacles fuse, and the pha-

gocyte envelops the foreign material together with the receptors in a digestion vacuole or phagocytic vacuole (▶ E). However, this uses up all of the receptors on the surface of the phagocyte. The phagocyte's heterophagic activity remains blocked until the receptors can release the foreign material and return to the surface of the cell.

Digestion phase: Contact with the foreign material stimulates the phagocyte. With its enzyme systems such as NADPH oxidase and NO synthase, it generates toxic oxygen compounds in the form of -OH and H_2O_2 and toxic nitrogen compounds in the form of NO. These compounds are transformed into HClO by means of myeloperoxidase and into peroxy nitrile by means of NO synthase. Both of these resulting compounds are bacteriotoxic; together with the hydrolases they concentrate in the lysosomal digestion vacuole. Digestion of the foreign material (such as a bacterium; ▶ F) begins, marking the beginning of the lysosomal phase p. 28).

▰ Autophagy

Autophagy is the process by which certain intracellular material is broken down. A damaged portion of cytoplasm is sequestered by a double membrane (rough endoplasmic reticulum cistern associated with the Golgi apparatus) so as to create a self-digestion vacuole known as an autophagic vacuole.

Note: *Phagocytes include:*
- Macrophages that give rise to histiocytes;
- Neutrophils or "microphages."

Note: *RHS block:*
In certain cases, such as in Shwartzmann-Sanarelli reaction and circulatory shock (p. 394), tiny fibrin clots develop in circulating blood. These clots are phagocytized, which uses up the appropriate receptors. This results in a temporary block of all macrophages of the reticulohistiocytic system (RHS block).

Note: Sudden generation of toxic oxygen metabolites by neutrophils and macrophages is also referred to as a "respiratory burst" reaction.

A Phagocytosis: recognition phase

B SEM x 1000

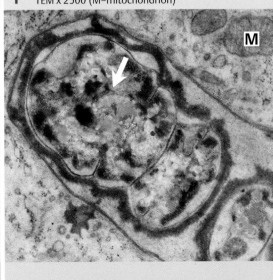

C Phagocytosis: uptake phase

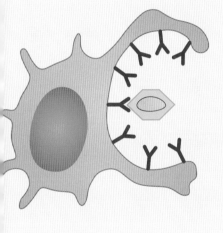

D TEM x 2000 (B=bacterium)

B

E Phagocytosis: digestion phase

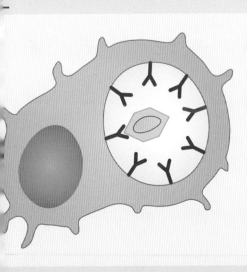

F TEM x 2500 (M=mitochondrion)

M

Lysosomal Phase

■ Heterophagy

The phagocytic vacuole and its contents (such as a gold particle; ► A) fuse with an intracellular hydrolase container (a primary lysosome) to release its digestive enzyme. This creates a heterophagosome, and the breakdown process begins.

■ Autophagy

The area of cytoplasm to be broken down is first enclosed in an autophagic vacuole (sequestration; ► B). As the vacuole then fuses with lysosomes (hydrolase containers), its inner membrane is dissolved and catabolic enzymes are introduced. The autophagosome becomes an autophagolysosome, and digestion begins.

Post-lysosomal Phase

Once breakdown of the material in the vacuole is complete, the autophagolysosomes and heterophagic phagolysosomes may remain in the cell in the postlysosomal phase as telolysosomes (residual bodies) that form lysosomal lipoid pigments, or they may be released into the extracellular space by exocytosis, the process of cellular defecation.

■ Lysosomal Lipid Pigments

Pathogenesis: In aging telolysosomes, an increasing accumulation of nondegradable substances will often lead to the formation of pigmented residual bodies. The intrinsic yellow and later brown color of these pigments is due to their content of fatty acids joined together by oxidation. On an ultrastructural level, these residual bodies consist of lipid droplets (►C1), structures with a myelin-like pattern (►C2), and amorphous granular material (►C3).

In terms of formal pathogenesis, the lysosomal lipid pigments may be divided into two main groups:

Lipofuscin:[1] Formation of lipid pigments increases with cell age. In older persons, hepatocytes in the central lobe and myocardial cells are characterized by abundant yellowish brown lipofuscin granules (► D; see also p. 114). This gives the tissue of aging organs a dark brown color (age-related atrophy, p. 124). L. Aschoff referred to lipofuscin in 1910 as "wear-and-tear pigment" because of its indication of cell age and its presence in telolysosomes.

Ceroid:[2] Increased lipid turnover in macrophages leads to formation of a lipid pigment with a coarse homogeneous appearance known as ceroid (► E). Ceroid stains red like the wax coatings of mycobacteria under a Ziehl-Neelsen stain (► F). Ceroid is typically observed in the liver in the resorption phase of acute viral hepatitis (p. 240) or in resorptive granulation tissue. Where there is simultaneous breakdown of hemoglobin, ceroid may also be mixed in with the ferrous hemosiderin pigment (p. 106).

> **Note:** Lipofuscin staining:
> – PAS reaction is negative.
> – Iron reaction is negative.

> **Note:** Ceroid and lipofuscin:
> – Ceroid ("clean-up pigment") occurs in macrophages as a result of heterophagy.
> – Lipofuscin ("aging pigment" or "wear-and-tear pigment") occurs in organ cells as a result of autophagy.

---

[1] Lipofuscin: *fuscus* (Latin), yellow
[2] Ceroid: *cera* (Latin), wax

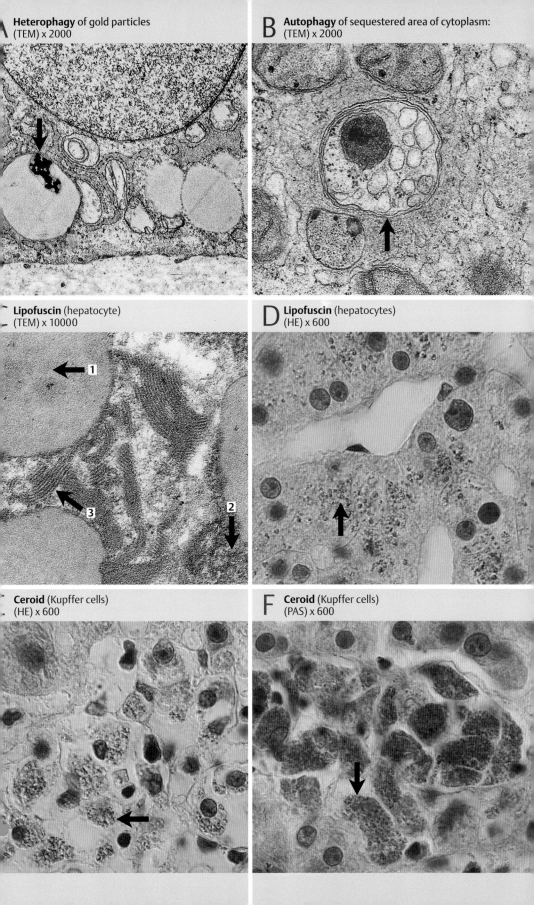

A **Heterophagy** of gold particles (TEM) x 2000

B **Autophagy** of sequestered area of cytoplasm: (TEM) x 2000

C **Lipofuscin** (hepatocyte) (TEM) x 10000

1
2
3

D **Lipofuscin** (hepatocytes) (HE) x 600

E **Ceroid** (Kupffer cells) (HE) x 600

F **Ceroid** (Kupffer cells) (PAS) x 600

Lysosomal Diseases

These are due to the following mechanisms:
— Delayed release of lysosomal enzymes;
— Increased release of lysosomal enzymes;
— Shortage of lysosomal enzymes.

■ Delayed Enzyme Release

▦ Chédiak-Higashi Syndrome

Definition: Rare hereditary lysosomal metabolic disorder characterized by leukocytes with giant granules, oculocutaneous albinism (p. 112), purulent infections, and hepatosplenomegaly.

Pathogenesis: Caused by mutation, this inherited autosomal recessive disorder is characterized by oversized primary lysosomes with aberrant fusion. The sequelae include:
— Giant granules (primary lysosomes) occur in granulocytes (lymphocytes and monocytes).
— Impaired formation of phagolysosomes interferes with phagocytosis. This in turn results in deficient immune response to infection; patients are susceptible to infection from pyogenic pathogens and have a reduced life expectancy.
— Impaired uptake of pigmented melanosomes results in a pigmentation block, leading to oculocutaneous albinism (p. 112, 196).

■ Increased Enzyme Release

Release without phagocytosis: This occurs in acute inflammation due to physical, bacterial, and viral pathogenic agents and in immune complexes complement activation (p. 162).

Release after phagocytosis: Many foreign bodies are phagocytized without damaging the phagocytes. Exceptions include crystalline substances such as quartz (p. 236), oxalate (p. 98), and urate (p. 102). Hydrogen bridges cause these substances to adhere the phagocyte membrane. Intrinsic cell motion causes the membrane to tear, releasing proteases and causing soft-tissue inflammation.

■ Lysosomal Enzyme Deficiency

Synonym: lysosomal storage diseases.

General definition: These hereditary diseases are characterized by intracellular storage of metabolic products that the lysosomes cannot to break down in what are known as storage lysosomes.

Depending on which lysosomal enzymes are present, metabolites of these substance groups may be stored as:
— Carbohydrates in glycogenosis;
— Lipids in gangliosidosis (p. 94) and other forms of sphingolipidosis (p. 92);
— Mucopolysaccharides in mucopolysaccharidosis (p. 66) and mucolipidosis (p. 66).

General causal pathogenesis: A mismatch between available lysosomal enzymes and those substances created during autophagy, or heterophagy, and normally broken down by hydrolysis, leads to accumulation of insoluble metabolite material. This material remains in the cell and is stored in vacuoles (storage lysosomes). The cytoplasm in the storage cells is transformed into vacuoles, and such storage cells accumulate in tissue.

The resulting cellular and tissue damage is attributable to one of these processes:
— Functional disruption of cell metabolism due to spatial constriction by the lysosomal storage material (▶ B, C, D).
— Cell death due to incompletely detoxified breakdown products.
— Secondary enzyme activation by the lysosomal storage material.
— Functional cell damage due to impaired recycling of intermediate metabolites.

The clinical result is the formation of enlarged, functionally ineffective storage organs (organomegaly).

General formal pathogenesis: The nature of the lysosomal storage product basically depends on the substrate specificity of the deficient enzyme:

1 enzyme acting on 1 substrate: The deficient enzyme normally attacks only one substance group; this means that the storage lysosomes (▶ A) will contain only one homogeneous substance, such as in Type 2 glycogenosis (p. 76).

1 enzyme acting on 2 substrates: The deficient enzyme normally attacks two substance groups, resulting in two types of storage lysosome (▶ A2). Depending on the organ cell, these will be accompanied by telolysosome vacuoles, as in Wolman disease.

1 enzyme acting on several substrates: The deficient enzyme normally attacks several substance groups, and the various substances will be stored in polymorphous lysosomes (▶ A3), as in GM$_1$ gangliosidosis (▶ D; p. 94).

A Lysosomal enzyme deficiency (storage diseases)

B Normal-hepatocyte
(TEM) x 5000 (N=nucleus, M=mitochondrion)

C Type IV mucolipidosis (hepatocyte)
(TEM) x 5000 (N=nucleus, M=mitochondrion

D GM$_1$ gangliosidosis (hepatocyte)
(TEM) x 5000 (N=nucleus, M=mitochondrion

Cytomembrane Lesions

Physiology: Together with the inner membrane system, the outer cell membrane regulates the exchange of substances between the various compartments of the cell. It separates the individual cells from adjacent cells and contains receptors that enable it to detect signal substances (ligands). The messages borne by these ligands are transmitted via an intracellular communication system to the nucleus, the executing organelle. The cytoskeleton, to which the cytomembrane is attached, aids in this process.

■ Apical Cell Edema

Definition and pathogenesis: Cell damage due to deficient energy metabolism, such as ischemia, causes failure of the fixation of the microtubule and/or pericellular microfilament system (p. 34). The result is a bubble-like evagination of the cell membrane due to cellular edema at the apex of the cell (► A). Following reperfusion and restoration of a sufficient supply of energy, the cell sequesters the apical bubble and temporarily becomes narrower (p. 69).

✚ **Clinical example:** In acute renal failure in circulatory shock, apical cellular edema occurs in the cells of the renal tubules, causing congestion of the tubules. This is followed by anuria or urine failure production, sequestration, flattening of epithelial cells, and "wide tubule" syndrome (► B).

■ Disrupted Communication

Pathogenesis: In tumor cells, the disappearance of the typical arrangement of oligosaccharides in the cell membrane (lectin[1] bonding sites), present in normal cells in the form of bloodgroup antigens and/or adhesion molecules, is indicative of their loss of cell specificity due to the change in their genetic makeup. This disrupts cell-to-cell and cell-to-matrix communication, with the result that tumor cells continue to divide despite contact with adjacent cells due to the loss of contact inhibition (p. 338, 344).

❗ **Note:** *Lectins* are glycoproteins, usually from plant seeds or invertebrates, that bond specifically to certain oligosaccharides.

Receptor Lesions

Physiology: The cell's various signal substances (ligands) are detected by specific receptor proteins (► C1). The receptors on the surface of the cell consist of extracellular, intramembranous, and intracellular components. The extracellular receptor component has the task of detecting signals.

Signal transmission often begins with the bonding of the ligand-receptor complex to *G-proteins* (► C2). These proteins dissociate from the receptor after exchanging the GDP bonded to them for GTP. Adenylate cyclase is attached to activate the substance, and cyclic AMP is formed. This substance in turn stimulates cytosolic protein kinase-C, which activates the effector protein by phosphorylation and triggers the specific cellular response. After the GTP is hydrolyzed by the G-protein, the G-protein dissociates from the adenylate cyclase and bonds to the receptor again.

The receptor enzyme itself can also be a *tyrosine kinase* (► C3). In this case, the ligand-receptor bond causes the receptor enzyme to phosphorylate itself and activate the effector protein.

In a few cell surface receptors, the receptor enzyme consists of a *phosphodiesterase* (► C4). This converts the phosphatidylinositol biphosphate to inositol triphosphate and diacylglycerol, resulting in accumulation of calcium within the cell.

Finally, there are also *receptors associated with calcium channels* (► C5). When they bond with ligands, these receptors open channels through the membrane that allow the passage of calcium.

■ Receptor dysfunction: Is due to one of the following processes:

— An atypical hormone occupies the receptor but fails to stimulate the effector.

— An antibody that acts like a hormone occupies the receptor and stimulates the effector.

— An excess of hormone A can suppress or enhance the receptor bond for hormone B.

— The number of receptors is no longer kept inversely proportional to the circulating quantity of hormone.

— The link between ligand bonding and activation of the effector fails.

— The ligand (hormone or growth factor) is formed by the same cell that expresses the respective receptors (autocrine selection; p. 321).

— A receptor mutation is present.

---

[1] Lectin: from *legere* (Latin), select

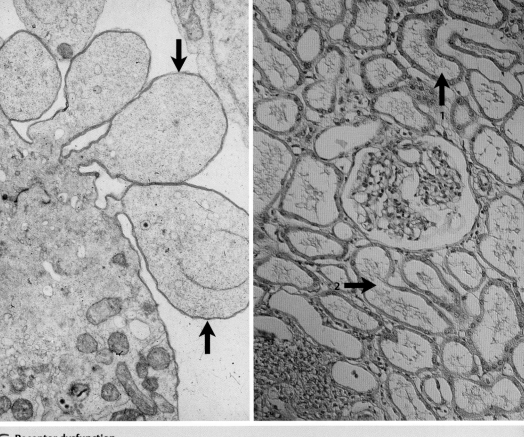

A Apical cell edema (renal tubulus) (TEM) x 5000

B Apical cell edema (Kidney) (HE) x 100

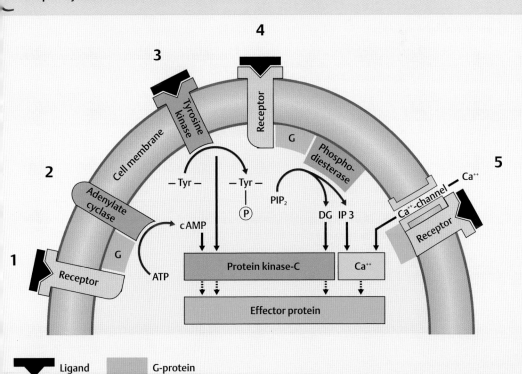

C Receptor dysfunction

4

3

Tyrosine kinase

Receptor

2

Cell membrane

Adenylate cyclase

G

— Tyr —   — Tyr —
                ⓟ

Phospho-diesterase

PIP₂

DG   IP 3

5

Ca⁺⁺

Ca⁺⁺-channel

Receptor

1

Receptor

G

ATP

cAMP

Protein kinase-C

Ca⁺⁺

Effector protein

◣ Ligand   G-protein

2

Cellular Pathology

Cytoskeletal Lesions

Physiology of the cytoskeleton:

Microtubules are spiral arrangements of globular proteins (tubulin) that form ultrastructural tubules. These structures aid in transmitting signals, providing structural support, and transporting substances.

Intermediate filaments are present in six different forms:
— *Keratin* is typically found in epithelial cells and is closely associated with desmosomes. It increases resistance to shear stress.
— *Desmin* is typically found in muscle cells and is closely associated with the Z bands and intercalated disks in muscle.
— *Vimentin* is typically found in mesenchymal cells and is closely associated with the cell nucleus, which it holds in place.
— *Neurofilaments* aid in intracellular fixation and signal transmission.
— *Glial filaments* aid in intracellular fixation and signal transmission.
— *Actin filaments* are 6 nm thick and usually lie beneath the cell membrane. They function as a sort of intracellular musculature. They attach to the same membrane molecules as do the fibronectin filaments outside.

Microtubular Lesions

■ Polymerization Block

Pathogenesis: Inhibited tubulin self-aggregation inhibits these processes:
— Mitosis;
— Discharge of secretions;
— Release of lysosomes.

Example: Colchicine therapy for acute gout (p. 102).

■ Microfilament Lesions

Paired Helical Filaments

Definition: These lesions appear as thickened coarse filaments resembling braids (► A2) in nerve cells. They are signs of a cytoskeletal lesion (► A1) and consist of hypophosphorylated neurofilaments, proteins associated with microtubules, and the stress protein ubiquitin.

Example: Alzheimer's disease (p. 126).

Lewy Bodies

Definition: Round, eosinophilic cytoplasmic inclusions of neurofilament material and the stress protein ubiquitin (► B).

Example: Parkinson's disease (p. 114).

Microfilament Retraction

Pathogenesis: Blockage of energy metabolism breaks the connection between the microfilaments and the rest of the cytoskeleton. This causes the cell membrane to bulge outward at these points (► C), causing an apical cell edema (p. 32).

Intermediate Filament Lesions

■ Actin Bodies

Definition: PAS-positive accumulation of actin filaments in myofibroblasts (► D).

Example: Infantile digital fibromatosis, a nodular tumorlike proliferation of myofibroblasts in children's knuckles.

■ Mallory Bodies

Pathogenesis: These bodies develop from cytoskeletal keratin with quantities of ubiquitin (stress protein) and often demarcate areas of damaged cytoplasm, whereby it is not clear whether they are a cause or an effect of damage. Where the cell membrane has been destroyed, they attract leukocytes, which gather around the Mallory bodies like jackals around a campfire.

Histology: These structures usually consist of perinuclear antler-shaped hyalin bodies (epithelial hyalin; ► E).

Ultrastructure: They consist of intermediate filaments (► F) with a ragged corpuscular structure.

Example: Alcoholic hepatitis (p. 144).

> **Note:** Mallory bodies are an equivocal sign of toxic liver damage from alcohol abuse.

The diseases discussed up to this point are attributable to enzyme deficiencies and functional derangements of certain cellular organelles. The following section examines diseases caused by aberrant synthesis or breakdown processes of the extracellular matrix. They represent dysfunctions of structural metabolism.

A Fibrils in Alzheimer's disease (Ag) x 200

B Lewy body (brain) (HE) x 200

C Microfilament retraction (Kidney tubulus) (TEM) x 3000

D Actin body (fibromatosis) (PAS) x 200 (N=nucleus)

E Mallory body (liver cell) (HE) x 600 (N=nucleus)

F Mallory body (liver cell) (TEM) x 2000

When Molecules Weaken
Connective Tissue Lesions

Summary

The extracellular matrix is composed of elastic collagen fibers and proteoglycans. It gives the tissue strength and pliability and influences the orientation and differentiation of the cells within the tissue.

▶ **Collagen:** The importance of this substance becomes clear in every lesion where its tensile strength is compromised. Such cases include structural defects in collagen molecules, abnormal collagen cross-linkage, abnormal composition of collagen chains, and uncontrolled collagenolysis. The most significant congenital disorders of collagen regeneration are included under Ehlers-Danlos syndrome.

▶ **Basement membrane:** Even minor molecular defects in the collagen components of this structure can cause defects such as impaired kidney function or weakening of the connections between the skin and subcutaneous tissue.

▶ **Microfibrils:** These consist primarily of fibrils. They are building blocks of the elastic fibers and help to stabilize cells on the basal membrane. Their range of functions becomes apparent in Marfan syndrome, which is due to a genetic defect in fibrillin. Patients are tall with long extremities and have fragile, weakened blood vessels and lax joints. The β-pleated fibrils also belong to the microfibrils. Accumulations of these structures in tissue are referred to as amyloid, and they impair organ function.

▶ **Elastin:** This macromolecule can undergo elastic deformation and is an important structural element in the skin and blood vessels. Accordingly, a congenital elastin deficiency will manifest itself in inflexibility of the skin, an elastin deformity in hyperelasticity of the skin, and unimpaired elastin lysis will result in vascular evagination.

▶ **Proteoglycans** (mucopolysaccharides): These substances are collagen-associated building blocks of cartilage and mucus. It is therefore no wonder that congenital defects involve deranged skeletal growth and excessive breakdown, such as occur in recurrent polychondritis, where tracheal collapse compromises the patient's airway. Mucopolysaccharidosis differs in that congenitally deficient breakdown causes proteoglycan cleavage products to accumulate in tissue until they deform certain parts of the skeleton and damage the brain.

Collagen Lesions

Physiology of collagen synthesis and breakdown:

Collagen biosynthesis: After the ribosomes read the mRNA matrix, procollagen α_1 and α_2 chains are formed, with one amino-terminal and one carboxy-terminal peptide each on one end.

The procollagen α chains enter the cisterns of the rough endoplasmic reticulum, where lysin hydroxylase hydroxylates their proline and lysine groups. Now the "right" procollagen chains for the respective tissue are selected according to the two terminal procollagen peptides and linked together by disulfide bridges. The hydroxyl lysine groups are then glycosylated. Hydrogen bridges then form on the hydroxy proline groups of the procollagen α chains so that three procollagen α chains each become wound together in a triple helix to form filamentous procollagen. This substance is then excreted into the extracellular space, where it must undergo further processing.

First, procollagen N-protease strips off the amino-terminal peptide and procollagen C-protease strips off the carboxy-terminal peptide from the actual collagen region of the procollagen. This gives the collagen molecules their fibril structure. The next step consists in end-to-end and side-to-side apposition of the collagen molecules. For this to occur, the hydroxylysine and lysine groups of the collagen must first be oxidized by copper-containing lysyl oxidase to aldehyde derivatives. This results in aldol condensation of the collagen molecule, in turn resulting in the cross-linkage that gives collagen its characteristic strength.

Collagenolysis: First, the inactive collagenase precursors must be activated and natural collagenolysis inhibitors such as α_2 macroglobulin and β_1 collagenase inhibitor. Cathepsin-D initially cleaves the collagen from the chelated proteoglycan and destroys the collagenase inhibitor, allowing the active collagenase to penetrate the base substance of the connective tissue and break down the collagen fibrils.

Types of Collagen

When its quaternary structure is intact, collagen exhibits its characteristic banding.

Type I Collagen (▶ A, B):
— Found in skin, tendons, bone, and dentin.
— Provides tensile strength.

Type II Collagen (▶ C, D):
— Found in hyaline cartilage.
— Provides compressive elasticity.

Type III Collagen (▶ E, F):
— Found in the skin, aorta, and uterus.
— Allows for tissue "gliding".

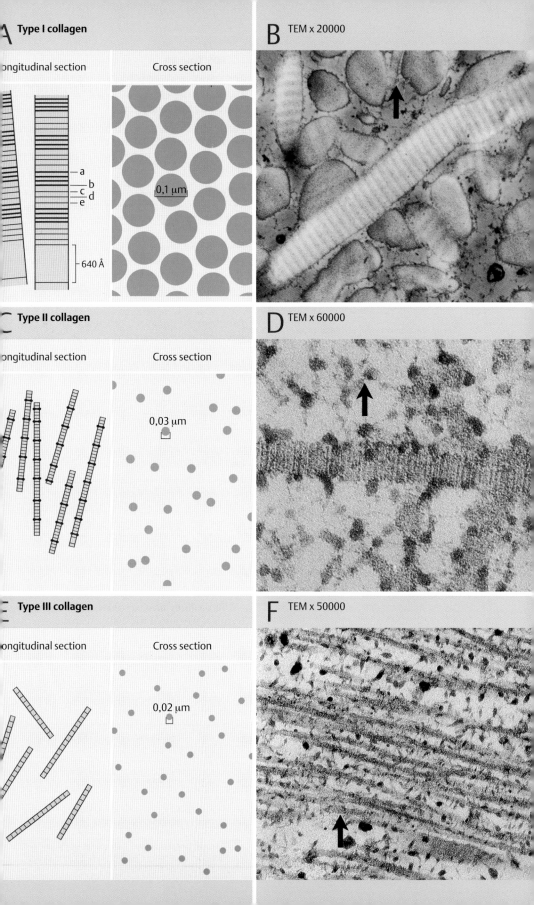

A Type I collagen

Longitudinal section   Cross section

a
b
c
d
e

640 Å

0,1 µm

B TEM x 20000

C Type II collagen

Longitudinal section   Cross section

0,03 µm

D TEM x 60000

E Type III collagen

Longitudinal section   Cross section

0,02 µm

F TEM x 50000

Biosynthesis Disorders

■ Ehlers-Danlos Syndrome (EDS)

Textbook example of a rare hereditary weakness of connective tissue in "rubber people."

▦ EDS Types I–III

Definition: Hereditary collagen disorder characterized by hyperelastic skin and hypermobile joints.

Pathogenesis: Abnormal transcription of the type I procollagen chains causes deranged fibrillogenesis. This in turn produces collagen fibrils whose cross section resembles a bear paw ("bear-paw" collagen; ▶ B).

✚ **Clinical presentation:** Autosomal dominant hereditary disorder whose severe form exhibits this triad of symptoms:
  – *"Rubber skin"* (▶ A): Large folds of skin can be lifted off the subcutaneous tissue; minor injuries produce skin tears (dermatorrhexis).
  – *"Rubber joints":* Joints are hypermobile and are easily dislocated due to lax ligaments.
  – *Childhood history of weak connective tissue:* Manifestations include inguinal hernia, intestinal diverticula, and rectal prolapse.

▦ EDS Type IV

Definition: Hereditary collagen disorder characterized by tissue tears.

Pathogenesis: A single-point mutation in the allele coded for the procollagen α_1 chain of type III collagen prevents formation of type III collagen. This results in fibroblasts of the skin, aorta, major vessels, hollow organs, and lungs.

✚ **Clinical presentation:** Autosomal dominant hereditary disorder in which tissue tears like wet toilet paper, characterized by this quartet of symptoms:
  – *Vulnerable skin* (dermatorrhexis).
  – *Aneurysm* (p. 62).
  – *Alveolar tearing* (spontaneous pneumothorax).
  – *Hollow organ ruptures* in the genital and intestinal regions.

▦ EDS Type V: See p. 54.

▦ EDS Type VI

Synonym: Oculoscoliotic EDS.

Definition: Hereditary collagen disorder characterized by fragility of the eyes and scoliosis of the spine.

Pathogenesis: Due to deficient activity of lysine hydroxylase, the procollagen contains hardly any hydroxy lysine for cross-linkage. This results in variably thin collagen fibrils of low tensile strength.

✚ **Clinical presentation:** Autosomal recessive hereditary disorder characterized by two symptoms:
  – *Scoliosis* (kyphoscoliosis).
  – *Vulnerable eyes* susceptible to retinal detachment and bulbar rupture.

▦ EDS Type VII

Synonym: Arthrochalasis multiplex congenita.

Definition: Hereditary collagen disorder characterized by unstable joints.

Pathogenesis: The amino-terminal peptides are missing in both procollagen chains of type I collagen. This results in mechanical instability of the joints.

✚ **Clinical presentation:** Autosomal dominant hereditary disorder leading to joint dislocation (usually the hip); the skin is rarely involved.

■ Scurvy

Definition: Connective-tissue disorder associated with vitamin C deficiency.

Vitamin C is a cofactor of proline hydroxylase that maintains that substance's enzyme iron in the bivalent form.

Pathogenesis: Vitamin C deficiency causes proline hydroxylase insufficiency. This interferes with glycosylation, which impairs collagen fibrillogenesis. Increased fragility of the vessels leads to hemorrhaging (p. 398).

✚ **Clinical presentation:** Patients may exhibit gingival bleeding, periodontal infection, skin hemorrhage (▶ C), joint hemorrhage, impaired wound healing, and anemia.

■ Osteogenesis Imperfecta

Textbook example of rare hereditary collagen insufficiency disorder.

Definition: Hereditary mechanical insufficiency of bone, ligament structures, sclera, and dentin.

Pathogenesis: Mutation of the procollagen α_1 chain of type I collagen. Morphology and clinical course of the disorder may vary depending on the site of the mutation.

▦ Tarda form involves a mutation in the N-terminal portion of the collagen chain.

✚ **Clinical presentation:** Autosomal dominant hereditary disorder characterized by a quartet of symptoms:
  – *Fragile bones:* Long cortical bones exhibit largely normal endochondral ossification. However, only frail cancellous trabeculae are formed, which are surrounded by persisting cartilage tissue (▶ D1) and uncalcified osteoid (▶ D2). Bone fails to develop into stable lamellar bone.
  – *Joint hypermobility.*
  – *Skin vulnerability.*
  – *Blue sclera* due to thinness of the tissue.
  – *Dentin* formation is often also impaired.

▦ Lethal form involves a mutation in the middle to C-terminal portion of the collagen chain.

✚ **Clinical presentation:** Autosomal dominant hereditary disorder whose early manifestations include intrauterine bone fractures.

A
"Rubber man", EDS type I

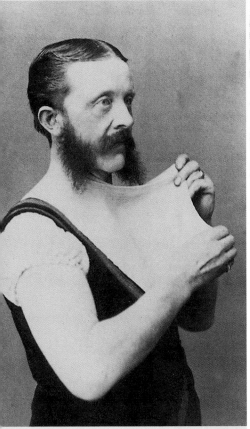

B
"Bear-paw" collagen (EDS-Type I)
(TEM) x 20000

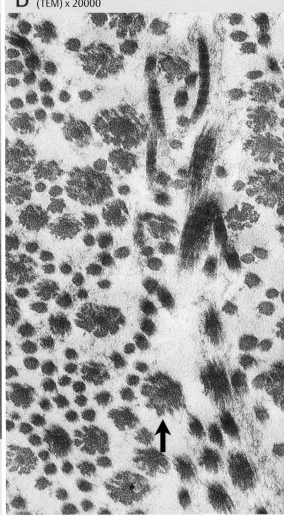

Scurvy skin

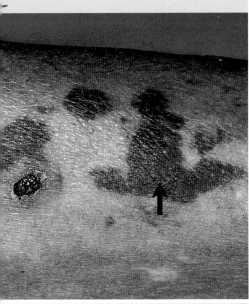

D
Osteogenesis imperfecta (bone)
(HE) x 200

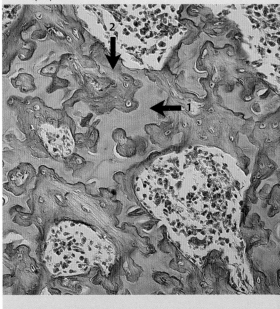

Fibrosis

General definition: Unusually high collagen fiber content per unit of tissue volume.

General pathogenesis: Inflammation, trauma, and stasis result in expression of growth factors (p. 296). This triggers proliferation and stimulation of fibroblasts and myofibroblasts, resulting in accelerated collagen synthesis with increased collagen cross-linkage. The resulting proliferation of hyaline fiber leads to abnormal tissue hardening and shrinkage of organs and tissues that can include stenosis, leading to impaired organ function.

Special forms of fibrosis:
— *Induration* is circumscribed or diffuse abnormal fibrotic hardening of a tissue or organ.
— *Sclerosis* is abnormal, occasionally systemic hardening of tissues and organs due to proliferation of widened collagen fibers.
— *Scarring* is a residual condition after wound healing.
— *Callus* is filling of hardened scar tissue around the periphery of tissue defects, as in a callous ulcer or fracture callus.
— *Cirrhosis* refers to progressive destructive fibrosis with shrinkage and hardening of an organ.

Sequelae of Fibrosis

■ Pulmonary Fibrosis

Definition: This is a pattern of reaction of the lungs to parenchymal damage in which lung tissue is replaced by tissue rich in collagen fiber.

With respect to causal pathogenesis and clinical presentation, several relevant forms of pulmonary fibrosis may be differentiated:

▦ Focal Pulmonary Fibrosis

Tuberculosis (p. 264):
— Fibrosis secondary to focal necrosis produces calluses, most frequently at the tip of the lung.
— Fibrosis secondary to advanced tissue disintegration with cavities formed by coughing up the disintegrated tissue occurs in cirrhotic pulmonary tuberculosis.

Silicosis: Exposure to quartz dust (p. 30) triggers a granulomatous inflammatory reaction (p. 236), producing diffuse nodular pulmonary fibrosis (► A, B).

▦ Congestion Fibrosis (diffuse fibrosis)

Early: Impaired blood flow to the left side of the heart (for example in mitral stenosis) causes vascular congestion upstream of the left heart. This in turn causes congestion in the capillaries of the alveolar walls. Blood serum is pressed out of the capillaries, resulting in alveolar edema (p. 424).

Result: red congestion induration.

Late: Alveolar macrophages express growth factors (p. 296) for fibrosis, causing reactive fibrosis of the alveolar walls (► C, D), alveolar macrophages phagocytize microhemorrhages and transform hemoglobin into ferrous brown hemosiderin (p. 106) around "heart defect" cells (► D2).

Result: brown congestion induration.

▦ Interstitial Pulmonary Fibrosis (diffuse fibrosis)

Usual Interstitial Pneumonia:

Definition: Fibrosis of the interstitial connective tissue of the alveolar walls secondary to inflammation from unknown causes.

Diffuse Alveolar Damage Syndrome:

Definition: This is a common pattern of reaction of the lung to alveolar damage due to physical, chemical, or microbial agents.

Early: Exudative alveolitis with damage to the alveolar epithelia. The resulting focal alveolar collapse stimulates alveolar macrophages; these macrophages express fibroblast growth factors, causing fibrosis.

Late: Fibrosing alveolitis with fibrosis of the collapsed alveoli and the pulmonary interstitium (► E; compare with C) causes replacement of the membranous alveolar epithelia by cubic alveolar epithelia (cubic epithelial transformation). The result is a grayish white fibrotic section through the lung (► F) with impaired oxygen diffusion.

✚ **Clinical presentation:** Adult respiratory distress syndrome (ARDS).

Complication: Respiration compresses the serofibrous exudate in the respiratory bronchioles to hyaline membranes (hyaline membrane disease). The remaining parenchyma becomes overinflated, leading to a honeycomb lung and death due to respiratory insufficiency.

❗ **Note:** Elastosis is the corresponding disease group to fibrosis with an overabundance of elastin fibers.

❗ **Note:** Fibrosis and scars tend to shrink; they represent replacement tissue.

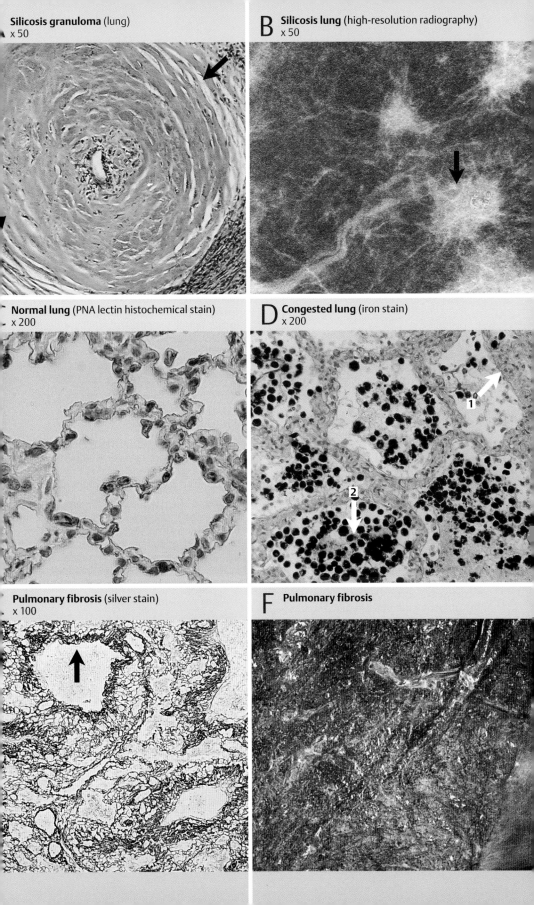

Silicosis granuloma (lung)
x 50

B Silicosis lung (high-resolution radiography)
x 50

Normal lung (PNA lectin histochemical stain)
x 200

D Congested lung (iron stain)
x 200

Pulmonary fibrosis (silver stain)
x 100

F Pulmonary fibrosis

Sequelae of Fibrosis (continued)

■ Cirrhosis of the Liver

Definition: Nodular remodeling of the liver due to necrosis, regeneration, and fibrotic tissue repair and destruction that impairs the vascular supply to the liver and the organ's function.

Etiologic forms of cirrhosis:
— *Alcoholic cirrhosis* is the type most frequently encountered in western industrialized countries (60% of all patients).
— *Posthepatitic cirrhosis* is the most common type throughout the world (20% of all patients in central Europe).
— *Metabolic cirrhosis* is the final stage of hereditary metabolic disease (hemochromatosis, p. 72; Wilson's disease, p. 74; α1-antitrypsin deficiency, p. 44).
— *Biliary cirrhosis* is the final stage of destructive bile duct inflammation (5% of all patients in central Europe).
— *Toxic cirrhosis* is the final stage of chronic exposure to chemicals.
— *Congestive cirrhosis* is the final stage of liver damage following chronic vascular congestion or occlusion of the hepatic vein (venous occlusive disease).
— *Cryptogenic cirrhosis* is cirrhosis of uncertain etiology (1% of all patients in central Europe).

Pathogenetic forms of cirrhosis:
— *Postnecrotic cirrhosis* is characterized by scarring linking massive areas of necrosis that extend from the portal regions to the central veins.
— *Posthepatitic cirrhosis* is characterized by scarring following chronic destructive inflammation of the liver parenchyma that slowly spreads from the portal regions throughout the lobe of the liver.
— *Biliary cirrhosis* is characterized by scarring that occurs in chronic destructive bile duct inflammation in which bile is released, destroying liver cells. The disease penetrates the liver lobe from the portal regions.

Formal pathogenesis: Cytokines released by inflamed cells transform the fat-storing Ito cells of the liver into myofibroblasts. This creates septa of connective tissue that cut apart the liver's normal lobular architecture like scissors (► B).
— *Active septa* proceed from granulation tissue (p. 224, 312) with histiocytic and lymphocytic infiltrate and follow the piece-meal necrosis. These areas of necrosis smoulder in the portal regions and then attack the hepatic lobe (► C).
— *Passive septa* are noninflammatory scar tissue that replaces collapsed necrotic liver parenchyma. These septa form bridges of scar tissue under the lobes (► D).

Morphologic forms of cirrhosis:

▓ Micronodular Cirrhosis

Synonyms: septal cirrhosis, Lannec's cirrhosis.

Etiologic types: metabolic, alcoholic, toxic, posthepatitic, biliary, and congestive.

Macroscopic appearance: The liver is hardened and usually reduced in size. A cross section will reveal nearly uniform parenchymal nodules with a maximum size of 5 mm (► D, E; compare with A).

Histology: The hepatic lobe is divided into segments by scarred septa of connective tissue (► C). Tissue regeneration proceeds from segments of the lobe, giving rise to nodules of regenerative tissue and creating pseudo-lobes. Once the noxious agent is eliminated, large nodules of regenerative tissue appear, and the condition progresses to macronodular cirrhosis. In the portal regions, the proliferating regenerative tissue usually includes the bile ducts as well.

▓ Macronodular Cirrhosis

Synonym: postnecrotic cirrhosis.

Etiologic types: metabolic, alcoholic, toxic, and posthepatitic.

Macroscopic appearance: The liver is hardened and usually reduced in size. A cross section will reveal irregular parenchymal nodules measuring 3 mm to 3 cm (► F; compare with A).

Histology: The parenchymal regions spared by the necrosis (in several hepatic lobes) are framed by scarred septa of connective tissue. The parenchyma of the liver regenerates, creating multilobular nodules of regenerative tissue. In the portal regions, the proliferating regenerative tissue usually includes the bile ducts as well.

✚ **Complications** of liver cirrhosis include:
– *Portal hypertension* (p. 392);
– *Ascites* (accumulation of serous fluid in the peritoneal cavity);
– *Hepatic coma* with flapping tremor leading to loss of consciousness;
– *Hepatic insufficiency* (icterus, propensity to hemorrhage, hepatic diabetes, and lactic acidosis);
– *Hepatocellular carcinoma* (p. 328, 332).

☺ **Prominent patient:** Ludwig van Beethoven, German composer (1770–1827).

❗ **Note:** Diagnostic modalities include ultrasound to evaluate whether cirrhosis is present and biopsy to evaluate the type of cirrhosis.

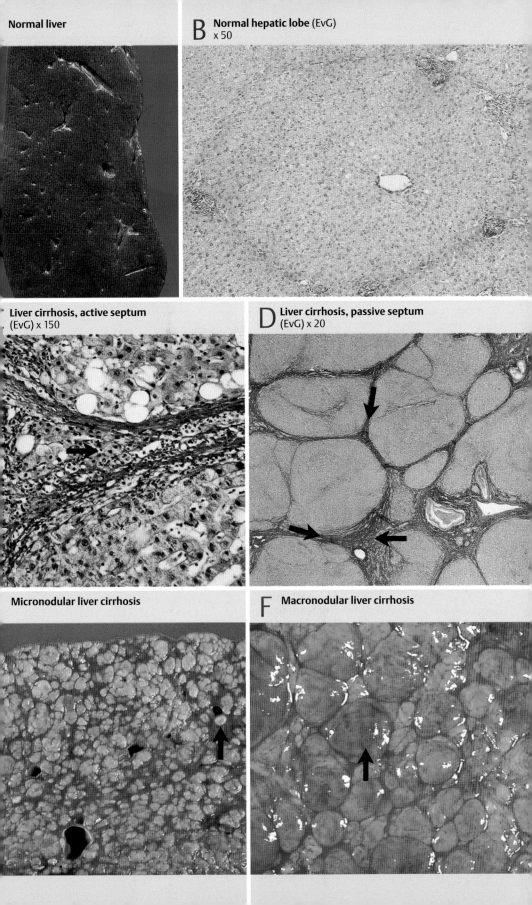

Normal liver

B **Normal hepatic lobe** (EvG) x 50

Liver cirrhosis, active septum (EvG) x 150

D **Liver cirrhosis, passive septum** (EvG) x 20

Micronodular liver cirrhosis

F **Macronodular liver cirrhosis**

Collagenolysis Disorders

■ α₁-Antitrypsin Deficiency

▦ Primary α₁-antitrypsin Deficiency

Textbook example of a systemic disease due to a defective proteinase inhibitor.

Definition: Hereditary defect of one of the main inhibitors of proteinase with liver cirrhosis, emphysema[1], and symptoms of Ehlers-Danlos syndrome (p. 38).

Pathogenesis: Single-point mutation of chromosome 14.

The genetic defect is associated with three alleles. They are referred to as M (medium), S (slow), and Z (zero) according to their electrophoretic migration speed. Persons with one normal (M) allele are asymptomatic.
- *M allele* → normal genetic product.
- *Z allele* → the glutamine in position 342 is replaced by lysine. The resulting incomplete glycosylation causes slower secretion of proteinase inhibitor, reducing enzyme activity to 10%.
- *S allele* → the glutamine in position 264 is replaced by valine, reducing enzyme activity to 60%.

In terms of formal pathogenesis, the following two mechanisms determine the clinical picture:
- *Inhibitor secretion disorder:* It involves retention of α₁-antitrypsin precursors in hepatocellular rough endoplasmic reticulum vacuoles (p. 12 and ► A). Histologic examination reveals diastasis-resistant PAS-positive spheres (reddish cytoplasmic inclusions; ► B). Stasis of secretion damages liver cells, which results in cirrhotic remodeling in the liver.
- *Enzyme inhibition disorder:* There is no inhibition of proteinases in tissue, causing unchecked destruction of collagen and elastin (p. 36, 54). This in turn results in proteolytic damage to the lungs and mesenchyme.

Morphologic characteristics:
- *Lung damage:* Unchecked proteolysis softens the alveolar support structures, weakening the alveolar wall. This causes diffuse overinflation of all of the alveoli in the lungs, resulting in *panacinar* emphysema. Compression of the alveolar capillaries due to stretching increases pulmonary vascular resistance, causing pulmonary hypertonia (p. 390). In the later stages, subpleural tears occur in the overstretched alveolar walls, creating a bubble-like pattern of overstretched lung tissue that progresses to bullous emphysema (► D; compare with C).
- *Mesenchymal damage* results in symptoms of Ehlers-Danlos syndrome (p. 38).

! **Note:** α₁-antitrypsin deficiency is diagnosed by analysis of fetal blood and amniocentesis. This lesion often shows a variable expression.

▦ Secondary α₁-antitrypsin Deficiency

Definition and pathogenesis: Acquired α₁-antitrypsin deficiency caused by absolute or relative loss of activity of the otherwise normal α₁-antitrypsin molecule due to the following mechanisms:
- *Oxidative damage* to the α₁-antitrypsin molecule from cigarette smoke and/or peroxide generated by phagocytes in inflammation (p. 26, 200);
- *Excess of protease* leading to a relative α₁-antitrypsin deficiency in lung damage from inhaled toxins (from industrial exhaust gases) or minerals (in miners).

! **Note:** Classification of emphysema:
The following forms are differentiated according to the affected section of the pulmonary acinus:
- *Centrilobular emphysema:* Inhaled toxins (other than cigarette smoke) cause chronic destructive bronchiolitis (small airway disease). This expands the proximal portions of the pulmonary acinus in the form of respiratory bronchioles (► E).
- *Panacinar emphysema:* In patients with a α₁-antitrypsin deficiency or Marfan syndrome (p. 48) or in cigarette smokers, the entire pulmonary acinus is expanded (► D). This leads to bullous emphysema, primarily in the subpleural portions of the lung (► F).
- *Paraseptal emphysema:* Chronic bronchitis (especially in smokers) leads to chronic coughing, in turn causing mechanical and proteolytic damage to the peripheral portions of the pulmonary acinus that are fused to the interlobular septa. Paraseptal emphysema is frequently observed in combination with other types of emphysema.
- *Emphysema from scarring:* Chronic inflammatory damage to the parenchyma of the lung leads to repair with scar tissue. Shrinkage of the scars creates irregular emphysema with large sclerotic areas of emphysema.

! **Note:** Special forms of emphysema:
- *Obstructive emphysema* involves a valve mechanism. The acute form (as in bronchial asthma, p. 168, or aspiration of a foreign body) is reversible; the chronic form is irreversible.
- *Compensatory emphysema* involves an increase in the air capacity of the remaining lung in response to pneumectomy.
- *Senile emphysema* is physiologic degeneration in old age.
- *Interstitial emphysema* occurs where air is pressed into the septal interstitium of the lung. A valve mechanism prevents the air for flowing out when the patient exhales. This can lead to mediastinal emphysema and subcutaneous emphysema.

---

[1] *Definition of emphysema* (in the strict sense): abnormal, persistent expansion of the respiratory portion of the lung distal to the terminal bronchiolus resulting from tissue destruction.

Retention of α_1-antitrypsin precursors in the RER
(hepatozyte) (TEM) 5000x

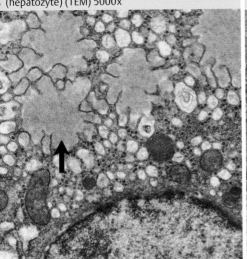

B **Retained α_1-antitrypsin in the liver**
(PAS) 300x

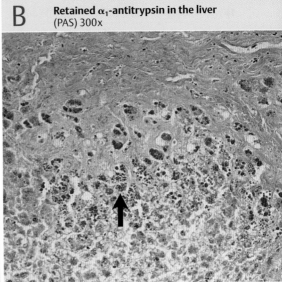

Normal lung
(high-resolution radiography) x 4

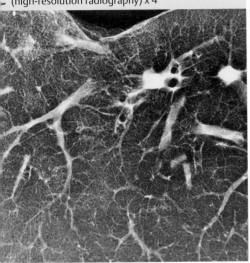

D **Panacinar emphysema**
(high-resolution radiography) x 4

Centrilobular emphysema

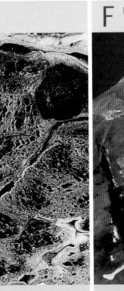

F **Bullous emphysema**

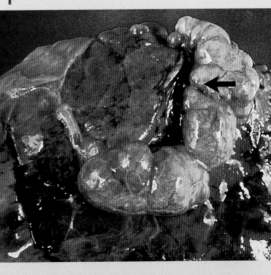

■ Fibrinoid Necrosis

General definition: Collagen changes associated with necrosis (p. 128) and/or inflammation (p. 196) in which the collagen fibers stain like fibrin.

With respect to causal pathogenesis, there are two relevant types of fibrinoid necrosis:

Swelling Fibrinoid

Pathogenesis: Collagenase (or acid) produces homogeneous swelling of collagen fibers, homogenizing the collagen.

Ultrastructure: The helical collagen strands split up into unwound collagen filaments (▶ A1 longitudinal view; A2 cross section).

Precipitation Fibrinoid

Synonym: immune deposit fibrinoid.

Pathogenesis: Deposits of immune complexes on collagen fibers (p. 162, 170) coat the collagen fibers so that from a histologic and chemical standpoint they appear like swelling fibrinoid (see p. 234).

Insudation

Synonym: necrotic fibrinoid.

Pathogenesis: Plasma components penetrate inflammatory or noninflammatory areas of damaged tissue adjacent to the surface of the body (such as the skin, mucous membranes, and walls of vascular structures). The swollen collagen fibers become permeated with plasma components, giving the fibers a homogeneous fibrin-like appearance (as in gastric ulcer, ▶ B; see also p. 218). Collagen homogenization occurs in vasculitis induced by chemotherapy (▶ C).

■ Collagen Hyalinization

General definition: There is no immune pathogenesis. Hyaline[1] is a homogeneous deposit or structural change in tissue. Under histologic examination it appears eosinophilic; macroscopically it appears as an area of whitish tissue.

Hyaline Connective Tissue

Definition: A hypocellular layer of homogenized broad collagen fibers that forms as a result of abnormal cross-linkage of collagen fibers in chronic infection and/or hemostasis. Macroscopically, it is characterized by a porcelain-white area of tissue (▶ D, E, F).

Examples:
— Pleura: pleural plaques (▶ D).
— Spleen: sugar-coated spleen (▶ E).
— Gallbladder: porcelain gallbladder (▶ F).

> **Note:** Non-collagen forms of hyaline:
>
> – *Vascular hyaline*: Intramural deposits of components of the basement membrane and plasma proteins in the walls of arterioles (vascular hyalinosis).
> – *Epithelial hyaline:*
>   – Deposits of intracellular secretion.
>   – Deposits of secretion in glands (such as thyroid follicles).

Collagen Vascular Diseases

Synonym: systemic autoimmune diseases.

General definition: Autoimmune diseases that involve formation of immune complex (p. 180) due to autoreactive antibodies (p. 180) and are associated with fibrinoid collagen necrosis and collagen deposits.

Forms of collagen vascular diseases include:
— Systemic lupus erythematosus (p. 180);
— Progressive systemic sclerosis (p. 182);
— Dermatomyositis (p. 182);
— Nodular panarteritis (p. 58);
— Sjögren's syndrome (p. 184);
— Wegener's granulomatosis (p. 184);
— Pseudo-lupus erythematosus;
— Combined connective tissue disease (Sharp's syndrome) with lupus erythematosus, scleroderma, and dermatomyositis;
— Rheumatic fever (p. 234);
— Rheumatoid arthritis (p. 184).

> **Rule of thumb:** In collagen vascular diseases, the collagen lesion is merely a spectacular secondary site of a systemic immune disorder.

Diseases may not only be caused by isolated collagen defects but also by isolated elastin defects. Before discussing those disorders, the next section will explore diseases that are attributable to deficiencies of the microfibrils, which represent another component of the extracellular matrix.

---

[1] Hyalin: from *hyalos* (Greek), glass.

Swelling fibrinoid
(TEM) x 2000

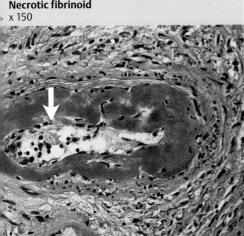

B Insudation
Goldner's trichrome stain) x 150

Necrotic fibrinoid
x 150

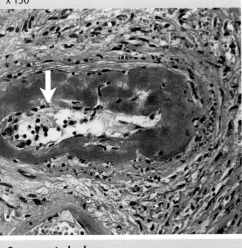

D Pleural plaque

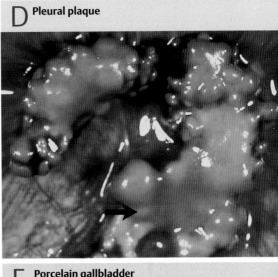

Sugar-coated spleen
(collagen hyalinization)

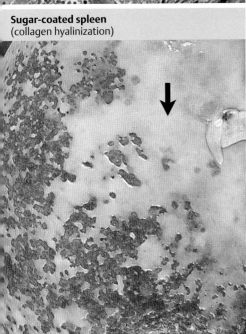

F Porcelain gallbladder
(collagen hyalinization)

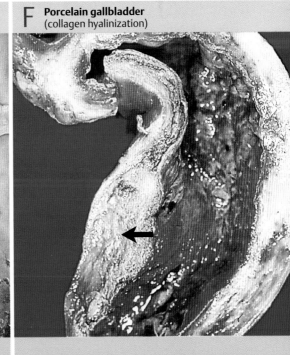

Microfibril Lesions

Physiology: The microfibrils are integral components of the elastic fibers. They occur in skin, tendons, cartilage, perichondrium, periosteum, muscle, kidneys, blood vessels, pleura, dura mater, and in the zonule fibers (the suspensory ligament of the lens of the eye). Their most important structural component is fibrillin, which is coded by the FBN1 and FBN2 genes and contains the epidermal growth factor (EGF) module that binds calcium. Calcium binding stabilizes the microfibrils; calcium loss causes them to disintegrate.

■ Marfan's Syndrome

Textbook example of a hereditary systemic disease caused by microfibril deficiency.

Definition: This is the most common hereditary group of connective tissue disorders. Manifestations vary in severity and include ocular, skeletal, cardiovascular, and dural lesions.

Pathogenesis: Defective FBN1 and FBN2 genes (usually in the calcium-binding EGF portion) cause the microfibrils to lose their mechanical strength, reducing the tensile strength of the tissue.

Primary morphologic criteria:

1. Skeletal lesions: The periosteum and perichondrium no longer provide support for bone growth, resulting in excessively long metacarpals and phalanges (► A).

The resulting symptoms include:
— *arachnodactyly;*
— *dolichostenomelia* (long, narrow extremities);
— *scoliosis* (abnormal spinal curvature);
— *pectus excavatum* (deeply depressed sternum);
— *flat foot* (pes planus) due to the medial deviation of the medial malleolus.

2. Cardiovascular lesions:
— *Aortic aneurysm* (p. 60, 62): The media of the aorta is thinned and atrophic. Its elastic fibers are thin, fragmented, and pushed apart by focal deposits of proteoglycan (► C). As a result, the aorta appears weakened (ectatic) and is susceptible to rupture. This means that the aortic rupture often occurs at several sites over time in the form of a recurrent dissecting aneurysm (► B). Fatal hemorrhage may result.
— *Aortic valve insufficiency.*
— *Mitral valve prolapse* may occasionally occur (p. 60).

3. Dural ectasia: This may occur in the lumbosacral region.

4. Dislocation of the lens: deficient zonule fibers may cause ectopia lentis, resulting in impaired vision.

Secondary morphologic criteria:

1. Pulmonary ectasia results in destructive emphysema (p. 44), which in turn leads to tearing of lung tissue and spontaneous pneumothorax.

2. Ectasia of the skin may be present with whitish scars (atrophic striations).

✚ **Clinical presentation**: This autosomal dominant hereditary disorder may be diagnosed before birth by amniocentesis. The following forms of Marfan syndrome may occur depending on the subtype and location of the defect in the FBN gene:
– *Neonatal Marfan syndrome:* primary criteria 1–4.
– *Isolated skeletal phenotype:* primary criterion 1.
– *Dominant ectopia lentis:* primary criterion 4.
– *MMASS phenotype* (myopia, mitral valve prolapse, aortic dilation; striae, and skeletal lesion).
– *Familial aortic aneurysm* (aortic dissection).
– *Congenital contractural arachnodactyly.*

☺ **Prominent patients:**
Abraham Lincoln (1809–1865), US President;
Nicolo Paganini (1782–1840), Italian violinist and composer. Paganini mastered the decimen technique, involving extremely wide fingering.

Amyloidosis

General Definitions

Amyloid[1] is a hyaline glycoprotein material with a microfibril structure that stains under Congo red dye. It is stored systemically or locally in the extracellular space, giving the respective tissue a glassy, wax-like appearance.

Amyloidoses represent a group of disorders of varying etiology that involve the deposit of amyloid in tissue. The following forms are differentiated according to the site:
— *Systemic amyloidoses* involve amyloid deposits in several organs and/or tissues.
— *Localized amyloidoses* involve amyloid deposits in one organ and/or tissue.

Examples:
— *Amyloidosis of the tongue* (► C): The amyloid stains brown under Lugol's solution and is deposited along the basement membrane.
— *Amyloidosis of the spleen* (► E): The amyloid deposits give the parenchyma of the organ a glassy, transparent appearance.

Note: Substances used for detecting amyloid:
– Lugol's solution normally detects starches (hence the name "amyloid").
– Amyloid is positive under Congo red.
– Amyloid shows green birefringence under polarized light.

Note: Amyloid is always located in extracellular space.

---

[1] Amyloid: from *amylon* (Greek), starch.

Arachnodactyly (Marfan syndrome)

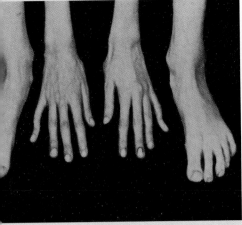

B Aortic aneurysm

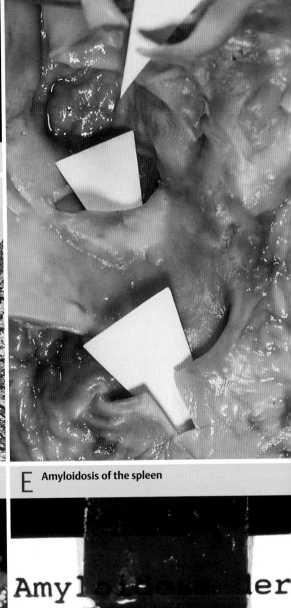

Aortic atrophy (EvG)
x 100

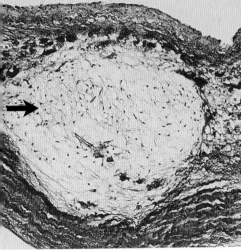

Amyloidosis of the tongue
(Lugol's solution)

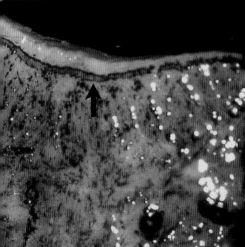

E Amyloidosis of the spleen

Amy

Structure of Amyloid

These components are common to all types of amyloid:

- *Fibril protein* with a β-pleated structure (β-pleated fibrils). This protein varies with the underlying disease and its name is used to identify the respective type of amyloid.
- *Amyloid P component* arises from SAP (serum amyloid P component, which is physiologic serum protein, a component of the glomerular basement membrane).
- *Heparan sulfate proteoglycanes* are proteoglycanes of the basement membrane type.

Types of Amyloid

■ AL Amyloid

Synonym: light-chain amyloid.

Pathogenesis: AL amyloid is the derivative of variable parts (p. 160) of the immunoglobulin light chains (λ chains more often than κ chains). An immune stimulus causes proliferation of a plasma cell clone, triggering formation of a monoclonal immunoglobulin with an excess of light chains (p. 160). The result is incomplete lysosomal breakdown of the immunoglobulin light chains in the macrophages, which in turn causes formation of λ and κ light chain fragments. These fragments condense to β-clumpy fibrils with a β-pleated sheet structure.

✚ **Manifestation** as systemic amyloidosis: see primary forms of amyloidosis (p. 52).

■ AA Amyloid

Synonym: amyloid A.

Pathogenesis: AA amyloid is the derivative of an HDL apolipoprotein (SAA = serum amyloid A precursor protein). In an inflammation, the acute-phase proteins are synthesized in the liver during the acute phase (p. 202). These include SAA, which is released into the serum and phagocytized by cells of the macrophage system. There, the lysosomes cleave off the amyloid-forming fragments. These fragments condense to β-clumpy fibrils with a β-pleated sheet structure.

✚ **Manifestation** as systemic amyloidosis: see secondary forms of amyloidosis (p. 52).

■ AF Amyloid

Synonym: familial amyloid.

Pathogenesis: AF amyloid is the derivative of transthyretin (the transport protein for thyroxin and retinol). A single-point mutation of transthyretin generates amyloid-forming fragments without prior proteolytic cleavage. These fragments condense to β-pleated fibrils with a β-clumpy sheet structure.

✚ **Manifestation** as local amyloidosis:
- *Kidney amyloidosis* (p. 52).
- *Predominant distal polyneuropathies:* Amyloid deposits cause nerve damage with sensory deficits and weakening of reflexes.
- *Hypertrophic cardiomyopathy* (p. 52, 116): Amyloid deposits between the muscle cells in the myocardium cause fatty hardening of the myocardium.

■ AE Amyloid

Synonym: endocrine amyloid.

Pathogenesis: AE amyloid comes from endocrine cells. Endocrine cells cause generation of abnormal peptides, which in turn result in incomplete proteolytic breakdown with residual amyloid fragments. These fragments condense to β-clumpy fibrils with a β-pleated sheet structure.

✚ **Manifestation** as local amyloidosis:
- *Islet amyloidosis:* Amyloid deposits in the islets of Langerhans in the pancreas displace the endocrine cells (► A, B), causing type II diabetes mellitus (p. 78).
- *Calcitonin amyloid:* The clumped configuration of cells in a C-cell thyroid carcinoma (► C1) form clumpy deposits of AE amyloid in the tumor stroma (► C2) and express calcitonin (► D).

■ AS Amyloid

Synonym: amyloid of aging.

Pathogenesis: AS amyloid is produced in abnormally aging brains. Mutation of a gene on chromosome 21 (which normally codes for a proteinase inhibitor) causes coding of an atypical β-amyloid precursor proteins (β-APP) These proteins condense to β-clumpy fibrils with a β-pleated sheet structure.

✚ **Manifestation** as local amyloidosis:
- *Alzheimer's disease* (p. 126) involves focal amyloid deposits in the brain known as "amyloid cores"(► E, F), some of which are surrounded by distended nerve endings with an abnormal cytoskeleton (p. 34).
- *Down's syndrome* (trisomy 21; p. 288).

Note: Peptide chains are stabilized in one of two ways:
- By an α-helix configuration of the peptide chains.
- By a β-pleated sheet structure of the peptide chains.

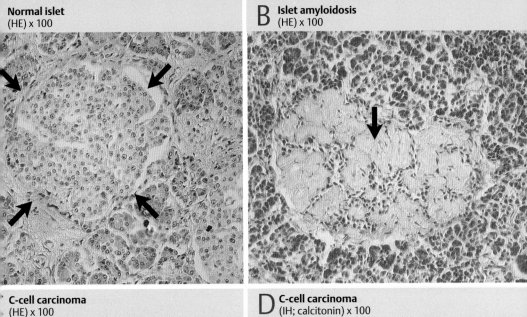

Normal islet
(HE) x 100

B Islet amyloidosis
(HE) x 100

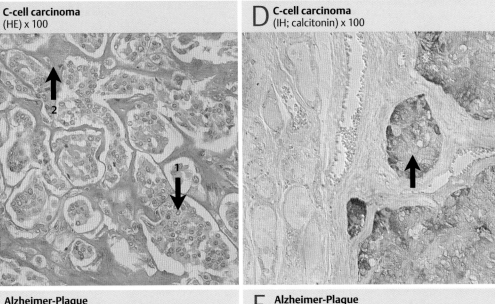

C-cell carcinoma
(HE) x 100

D C-cell carcinoma
(IH; calcitonin) x 100

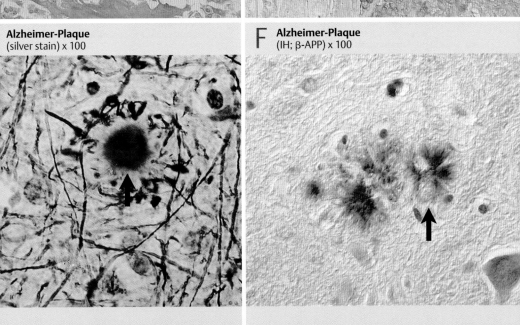

Alzheimer-Plaque
(silver stain) x 100

F Alzheimer-Plaque
(IH; β-APP) x 100

Classification of Amyloidosis

■ Systemic Amyloidosis

▥ Primary Amyloidosis

Synonym: atypical amyloidosis.

Pathogenesis: Primary amyloidoses occur in the absence of a discernible prior disorder or a discernible etiology.

This also includes the paramyloidoses. These disorders are characterized by generalized deposits of amyloid that occur in the setting of lymphoplasmacytic neoplasms. Deposition sites especially include mesenchymal organs less often affected in classic secondary amyloidosis: the tongue, skeletal musculature, and myocardium. The nerves, brain, skin, and lungs are affected less frequently.

▥ Secondary Amyloidosis

Synonym: reactive systemic amyloidosis.

Pathogenesis: Amyloidosis occurs secondary to:
— *Chronic infections* such as osteomyelitis and tuberculosis (p. 264);
— *Chronic autoimmune inflammations* such as rheumatoid arthritis (p. 234).

Morphology: The amyloid is deposited in the parenchymal organs such as the spleen, liver (► C, D), kidney (► E, F), adrenal gland, and bowel in one of two variations:
— *Sago spleen type* involves selective amyloid deposits in the splenic follicles (► A1), around the splenic arteries (► A2), or in the space of Disse in the liver (the renal glomeruli are largely spared).
— *Lardaceous spleen type* involves diffuse amyloid deposits in the connective tissue framework in the red pulp of the spleen (► B1), sparing the splenic follicles with their central splenic arterial branches (► B2), and in the renal glomeruli and arteries.

■ Localized Amyloidosis

Amyloidosis that is limited to a single organ or circumscribed area within organs. Locations and forms include:
— Brain: cerebral amyloidosis.
— Nerves: polyneuropathic amyloidosis.
— Heart: cardiomyopathic amyloidosis.
— Lung: respiratory-tract amyloidosis.
— Kidney: nephropathic amyloidosis.
— Eye: ocular amyloidosis.
— Endocrine system: AE amyloidosis.
— Skin: lichenoid cutaneous amyloidosis.

Note: Kidney involvement in amyloidosis:
- Primary amyloidosis: kidney involvement in less than 50% of all cases.
- Secondary amyloidosis: kidney involvement in over 75% of all cases.

Note: Diagnostic procedures in AL and AA amyloidosis include rectum biopsy that penetrates the submucosa.

✚ Clinical presentation of amyloidosis:

AL Amyloidosis

Initial symptoms:
- *Carpal tunnel syndrome* due to amyloid deposits in the transverse carpal ligament with secondary compressive neuropathy of the median nerve leading to atrophy of the muscles of the thenar eminence.
- *Macroglossia* with swallowing difficulties (dysphagia) due to amyloid deposits in the tongue.
- *Skin:* papillary lesions and purpura (punctate bleeding sites).
- *Joints:* Major joints exhibit arthritic symptoms.

Late symptoms:
- *Heart:* Heart failure not responding to treatment, occasionally accompanied by conduction disorders due to restrictive cardiomyopathy. Amyloid deposits in the myocardium impair its contractility and elasticity, producing reactive thickening of the myocardium (hypertrophy) with ventricular narrowing lacking mechanical efficiency.
- *Liver:* Hepatomegaly (enlargement of the liver) due to perisinusoidal amyloid deposits (► C, D). This causes atrophy of the hepatic cords with strikingly little functional impairment.
- *Small bowel:* Amyloid deposits in the submucosa and around the arteries cause obstructions, mucosal bleeding, and diarrhea where the autonomous nervous system is involved.
- *Nerves:* Peripheral neuropathy, usually associated with sensory deficits.
- *Lung:* Respiratory insufficiency is present only where there are diffuse amyloid deposits in the alveolar and extraalveolar interstitium (the bronchial wall).

AA Amyloidosis

- *Kidney:* Amyloid deposits occur in the mesangium and coils of the glomeruli (► E, F) and/or predominantly in the arterial branches (AA greater than 50%; AL 15%; AF 25%). This leads to impaired renal function in the form of a "nephrotic syndrome" characterized by:
  - Proteinuria;
  - Hypoproteinemia;
  - Hyperlipidemia;
  - Edemas, occurring primarily in the lower leg in adults and primarily in the eyelids in children.
- *Liver:* Hepatomegaly (enlargement of the liver) with negligible functional deficiency.
- *Small bowel:* Obstructions and mucosal bleeding.

The next section explores diseases primarily caused by dysfunctional synthesis or breakdown of the elastic fibers made of microfibrils. These diseases illustrate the functional spectrum of elastin.

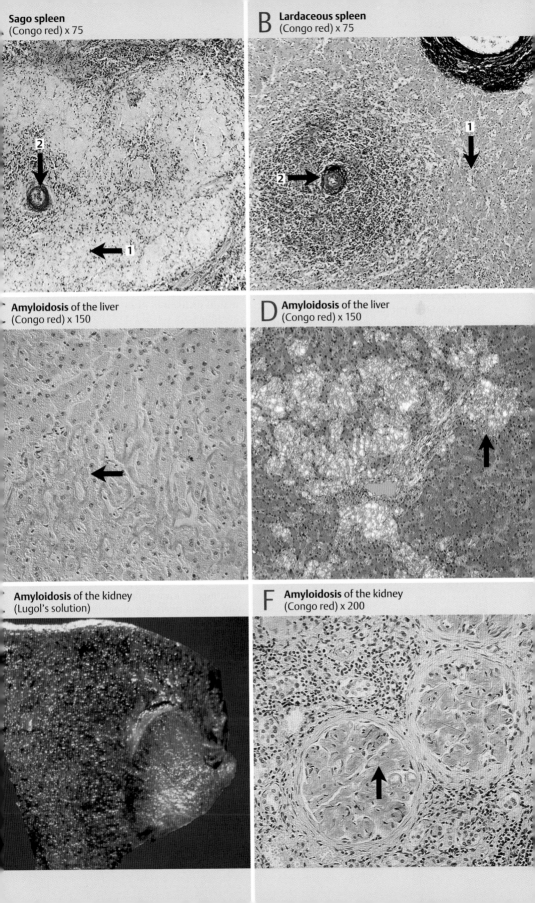

Sago spleen
(Congo red) x 75

B Lardaceous spleen
(Congo red) x 75

Amyloidosis of the liver
(Congo red) x 150

D Amyloidosis of the liver
(Congo red) x 150

Amyloidosis of the kidney
(Lugol's solution)

F Amyloidosis of the kidney
(Congo red) x 200

Elastin Lesions

Physiology of elastin synthesis and breakdown:

Elastin biosynthesis: This process is not yet fully understood. The myocytes of the vascular walls, fibrocytes of the subcutaneous tissue and the nuchal ligaments, and the chondrocytes of the elastic cartilage of the ear are "elastoblasts." These cells are able to synthesize fibrillin-containing microfibrils and elastin, the two components of elastin fibers. After it is secreted, the elastin bonds to the microfibrils and masks them. The elastin is then deaminized by a lysyl oxidase containing copper, and it cross-links to form elastin fibers.

Lysis of elastin: Pancreatic elastase is present in tissue as an inactive proelastase and must be activated by trypsin and/or enterokinase. Granulocyte elastase, a serine protease, is inhibited by specific inhibitors contained in blood (similarly to the inhibition of collagenase by α_1-antitrypsin). Macrophage elastase as a metallic protease has no such inhibitors.

Biosynthesis Disorders

■ Restrictive Dermopathy

Textbook example of an elastin deficiency disorder.

Definition: Hereditary elastin synthesis deficiency that leads to fetal hypokinesis and/or akinesis (lack of motion) and eventually to death.

Pathogenesis: Minimal formation of elastin fibers is accompanied by abnormally increased cross-linkage of collagen fibers.

✚ **Clinical presentation and morphology**: Extremely rare autosomal recessive hereditary disorder.
- The *skin* contains no elastin fibers (► A) and is therefore stiff and atrophic. This leads to contractures of the extremities and facial dysmorphia in which the mouth remains open (► B).
- The *lung* parenchyma fails to unfold, causing pulmonary hypoplasia that leads to respiratory insufficiency.

■ Senile Elastosis

Definition: Very common organ changes in the elderly due to deficient elastin synthesis (age-related changes in the skin, aorta, and lung; senile emphysema; and other disorders).

Pathogenesis: Decreasing quantity and increasing fragmentation of elastin fibers results in loss of tissue elasticity.

■ Trichopoliodystrophy

Synonym: kinky-hair disease, Menkes' disease.

Definition: Hereditary defect of copper metabolism manifested in kinky hair, cerebellar dysfunction, and scurvy symptoms (p. 74).

Pathogenesis: Copper is a cofactor of lysyl oxidase, which is important for the cross-linkage of collagen and elastin. This gene defect affects a copper ion-transporting P-type ATPase in the trans-Golgi membrane on chromosome Xq13. This ATPase carries the copper through the placental barrier, gastrointestinal tract, and the blood-brain barrier. It remains trapped before these barriers in those children so affected, and they suffer consequently from copper deficiency. This in turn causes abnormal elastin cross-linkage with an increased quantity of microfibrils and reduced elastin content. This manifests itself in kinky hair and tortuous cerebral vessels.

Histology: The elastica of the arteries is fragmented and frayed.

Macroscopic appearance: Blood vessels are tortuous with ectasia, aneurysms (p. 62), and ruptures.

✚ **Clinical presentation**: Rare disease exhibiting an X-linked inheritance pattern, characterized by kinky hair, cerebellar pathology, and scurvy symptoms. Incidence is 1:100 000.

■ Type V Ehlers-Danlos Syndrome

Definition: Hereditary elastin disorder with hypermobile joints and skin and aneurysms (see p. 38).

Pathogenesis: A lysyl oxidase deficiency and an unidentified elastase inhibitor combine to impair elastin and collagen synthesis.

Histology: Accumulations of very thin, immature elastin fibers are found the skin and arterial walls. These fibers are aligned like corkscrews along collagen fibers (► C).

✚ **Clinical presentation**: Rare, inherited X-linked recessive disease characterized by hypermobile and fragile skin, vascular ectasia, and hypermobile joints (► D).

❗ **Note:** *Ehlers-Danlos syndrome* is not a single disease entity. A variety of enzyme defects can lead to the main symptom of hypermobile skin.

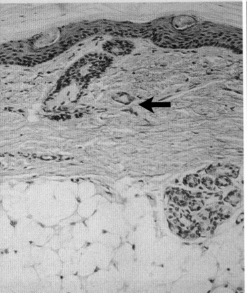

Restrictive Dermopathy (skin)
(Goldner's trichrome stain) x 150

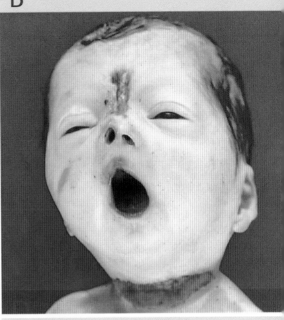

B **Restrictive Dermopathy**

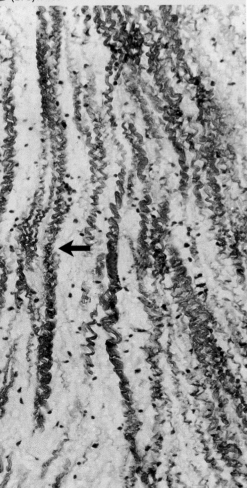

Type IV Ehlers-Danlos syndrome (collagen)
(EvG) x 400

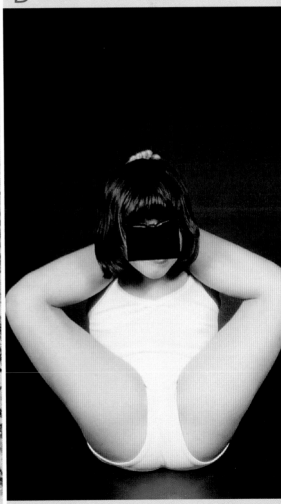

D **Type IV Ehlers-Danlos syndrome**

Elastosis

■ Actinic Elastosis

Definition: Common skin disorder due to ultraviolet radiation.

Pathogenesis: Radiation injury (p. 150) to the fibroblasts of the skin occurs especially in older persons in areas of the skin exposed to sunlight, such as the face, back of the neck, and the dorsum of the hand.

Histology: Atrophy of the epidermis is present (► A1). An assortment of thick, basophilic staining elastin fibers may be found in the superficial third of the skin (► A2). With increasing exposure to radiation, these fibers condense, fragment, and finally degenerate into amorphous clumps of material.

■ Pseudoxanthoma Elasticum

Synonym: Grönblad-Strandberg syndrome.

Definition: Hereditary systemic disorder of elastic connective tissue involving the skin and blood vessels.

Pathogenesis: The underlying defect consists of abnormal deposition of proteoglycan in elastin fibers, which decreases their elastin content. There is no collagen change.

Histology: Elastin fibers are fragmented, basophilic, and sausage-shaped (► B). From an ultrastructural perspective, they appear as a spheroid clump with a proteoglycan core containing deposits of calcium and magnesium salts.

✚ **Clinical presentation**: Rare autosomal recessive hereditary disorder with general symptoms of hypoelasticity that manifests itself between the ages of 20 and 40.
- The *skin* is lax with flexural creases and numerous yellowish plaques (hence the name pseudoxanthoma elasticum).
- The *retina* exhibits angioid streaks (variations in arterial diameter) and chorioretinitis (inflammation of the choroid and retina).
- The *gastrointestinal tract* is the site of bleeding.

Fibroelastosis

General pathogenesis: The disorder involves metabolic transformation of the myocytes of the vascular walls and/or endocardial myocytes due to a viral infection or overproduction of serotonin (see below and p. 202). This causes the myocytes to switch to synthesizing fiber, and they produce excessive quantities of elastic and collagen fibers together with clumps of proteoglycan.

Histology: Elastic fibers appear fragmented and frayed and are interwoven with collagen fibers in clumps of proteoglycan.

Macroscopic appearance: Cardiovascular tissue appears whitish gray and thickened.

Sequelae of Fibroelastosis

■ Intimal Fibroelastosis

Pathogenesis: The general response of the arterial wall to an abnormal hemodynamic or inflammatory stress is to stimulate the media myocytes adjacent to the intima. This triggers reactive formation of collagen and elastin fibers, which in turn produces reactive fibroelastosis of the intima (► C). The result is structural stabilization of the wall of the vessel.

■ Endocardial Fibroelastosis

Etiology: The causes of this disorder vary depending on the patient's age.
- *In children,* it may be due to intrauterine infection with mumps virus (p. 242) or possibly coxsackievirus.
- *In adults,* causes include carcinoid tumor of the small bowel (a malignant neuroendocrine tumor), resulting in the release of serotonin, which has a mitogenic effect on fibroblasts (p. 384).

Pathogenesis: Reactive proliferation of collagen and elastin fibers occurs as part of a repair process (► D). This causes whitish-gray endocardial thickening, reducing ventricular volume and leading to functional impairment of the heart and restrictive cardiomyopathy.

▐ **Note:** *Cardiomyopathy* is defined as a non-inflammatory myocardial disease of uncertain etiology.

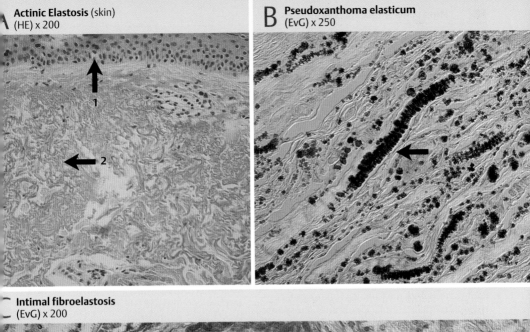

A Actinic Elastosis (skin)
(HE) x 200

B Pseudoxanthoma elasticum
(EvG) x 250

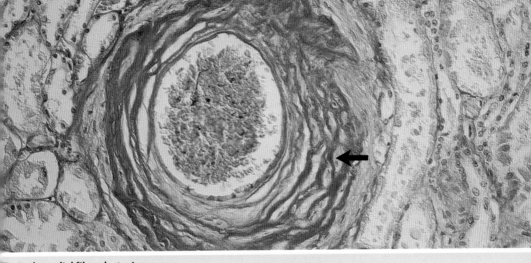

C Intimal fibroelastosis
(EvG) x 200

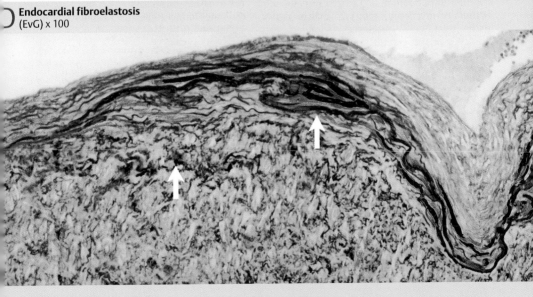

D Endocardial fibroelastosis
(EvG) x 100

Elastin Lysis Disorders

General pathogenesis: Inflammatory elastase hyperactivity or elastase inhibitor deficiency usually accompanied by simultaneous increase in collagen breakdown produces the histologic picture of rupture, fragmentation, or fraying of elastin fibers.

Note: Elastin fibers provide a necrosis-resistant, organic tissue structure.

Sequelae of Elastin Lysis Disorders

■ Polyarteritis nodosa

Synonyms: periarteritis nodosa, Kussmaul's disease.

Definition: Segmental inflammation of medium-sized arteries of various organs with palpable nodules resembling strings of pearls.

Pathogenesis and morphology: Unknown factors trigger an inflammatory autoimmune response with formation of immune complex (p. 162, 170). This activates the complement system (p. 162), resulting in intimal damage with fibrinoid necrosis. Thrombus (p. 404) covers the lesion, and the damaged area attracts neutrophils (p. 200). The proteolytic activity of the neutrophils softens the wall of the vessel and splits the elastin fibers (► A1). As the inflammation (► A2) spreads from the intima to the adventitia, it causes a circumscribed nodular evagination of the vascular wall (► B; hence the term *nodosa*), an inflammatory aneurysm. Granulation tissue fills the defect in the vessel wall (p. 224, 312). This tissue enters the vessel wall from the adventitia (hence the name periarteritis) and transforms the covered thrombus into scar tissue.

Result: vascular occlusion leading to tissue necrosis.

■ Temporal Arteritis

Definition: Systemic vascular inflammation with giant cells primarily involving the branches of the carotid artery, especially the temporal artery (hence the name temporal arteritis).

Pathogenesis: Unknown factors cause fragmentation of the elastica (► C1, D1), triggering an inflammatory autoimmune response with formation of immune complex (p. 162, 170). This leads to myocyte damage, and immune complex covers the elastica fragments. This process attracts lymphohistiocytic inflammatory cells and resorptive giant cells (p. 200). Giant cells (► C2, D2) crawl over the fragments of the elastica like snails on lettuce, producing worm-like inflammatory vascular indurations. In the later stages of the disorder, the inflamed portion of the vessel is sequestered by thrombus.

Result: headache and impaired vision that can progress to blindness.

■ Syphilitic Aortitis

Textbook example of an elastin lysis disease.

Definition: Chronic inflammation of the aorta in tertiary syphilis with destruction of the media progressing to aneurysm.

Pathogenesis and morphology: Exposure leads to infection with Treponema pallidum (p. 262), which causes syphilis. Primary syphilis is characterized by presence of a genital or anal chancre. This progresses to secondary syphilis with generalized inflammation and finally to tertiary syphilis with manifestations in various organ systems and granulomatous inflammatory reaction (p. 232).

One sequela is that the vessels supplying the media respond with inflammatory, fibrotic narrowing of the intima (syphilitic endarteritis obliterans). This compromises the vascular supply to the media. The myocytes of the media die off, and focal areas of destruction (► F) appear in the normally parallel elastin membrane systems (► E), giving the tissue a "moth-eaten" appearance. The defects fill with scar tissue, and the irregular shrinkage of this scar tissue gives the inner lining of the aorta a rough surface resembling the bark of a tree.

Result: Weakening of the vascular wall leads to syphilitic aneurysm (p. 62), especially in the aortic arch. Rupture of the aneurysm can result in fatal hemorrhage.

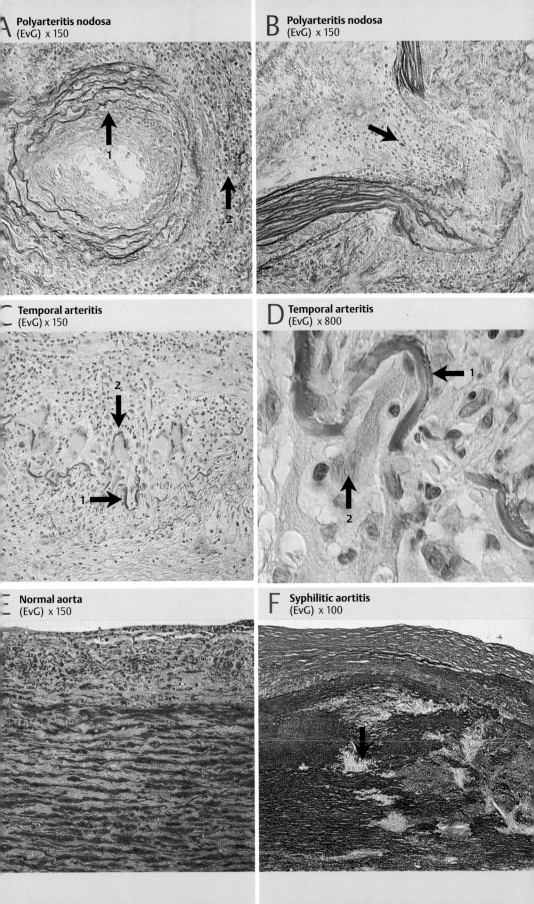

A Polyarteritis nodosa
(EvG) x 150

B Polyarteritis nodosa
(EvG) x 150

C Temporal arteritis
(EvG) x 150

D Temporal arteritis
(EvG) x 800

E Normal aorta
(EvG) x 150

F Syphilitic aortitis
(EvG) x 100

Proteoglycan Lesions

Physiology of proteoglycan synthesis and breakdown:

Proteoglycan biosynthesis: The process begins on the ribosomes of the rough endoplasmic reticulum, where the protein skeleton is synthesized. This substance is then conjugated with glycosaminoglycans in the Golgi apparatus (mucopolysaccharides) and secreted into the extracellular space. The proteoglycans are important in structuring the intracellular substance of connective and supporting tissue.

Lysis of proteoglycans: This process primarily occurs within the cell and requires that the proteoglycan be reabsorbed into the connective-tissue cell. Most of the enzymes that break down proteoglycan originate in the lysosomes. Among these are cathepsin B and D. There is minimal extracellular breakdown of proteoglycan. One reason for this is the presence of proteinase inhibitors in the extracellular space, which control the breakdown of proteoglycan.

Proteoglycan Complexing Disorders

Mucoid Degeneration

General pathogenesis: This is a common mesenchymal pattern of reaction involving the following chain of events: local mechanical stress causes abnormal reaction of connective-tissue cells. This may have several causes.
— Cell damage can cause focal apoptosis of connective-tissue cells (p. 128).
— Deficient composition of proteoglycan can impair collagen-proteoglycan complexing, resulting in mucoid transformation of the extracellular substance.

Result: tissue that is mechanically weak, which leads to structural weakening and rupture.

Sequelae of Mucoid Degeneration

■ Mucoid Meniscopathy

Pathogenesis: Meniscus injury due to overuse (for example in miners or soccer players) results in mucoid degeneration with formation of a hollow space filled with mucopolysaccharides (► A). This weakens the structure of the fibrocartilage tissue, precipitating a lateral tear in the meniscus.

> **Note:** Etiology of meniscus rupture:
> – Trauma produces a medial meniscus rupture.
> – Degeneration produces a lateral meniscus rupture.

■ Ganglion

Pathogenesis: Overuse results in mucoid degeneration, which in turn causes formation of a multiloculated cavity without an epithelial lining (► B1) in the tendon sheath or joint capsule (usually in the wrist). This cavity system is filled with watery mucopolysaccharides (► B2, partially dissected) and is also referred to as a hygroma (literally, a water sac).

■ Cystic Vascular Degeneration

General pathogenesis: Mucoid degeneration of the arteries and valves of the heart with destruction of the elastic fibers due to reservoirs of mucopolysaccharides.

▨ Dissecting Aortic Aneurysm

Synonyms: cystic medial necrosis, Erdheim's disease.

Definition: See aneurysm, p. 62.

Pathogenesis: The disorder is partially due to a fibrillin defect (p. 48). Mucoid degeneration produces intramural reservoirs of mucopolysaccharides (► C), resulting in cystic medial necrosis and defects in the elastica (► D).

Result: Weakness of the wall of the aorta leads to an aortic aneurysm. Rupture of the aneurysm can result in fatal hemorrhage.

▨ Cystic Degeneration of the Popliteal Artery

Pathogenesis: Mucoid degeneration produces intramural deposits of mucopolysaccharides in the adventitia of the artery. This results in cystic degeneration of the adventitia (► E1), leading to cystic medial necrosis. Together with reactive intimal fibrosis (► E2), this constricts the lumen of the artery. The disorder is rare.

Result: peripheral circulatory disruption.

■ Mitral Valve Prolapse Syndrome

Synonym: floppy mitral valve syndrome.

Pathogenesis: Due in part to a congenital fibrillin defect (p. 48), mucoid valvular degeneration produces an intramural accumulation of mucopolysaccharides in the valvular stroma. This diminishes the mitral valve's mechanical strength, causing the valve to "balloon" back into the atrium at the end of the systole (valve prolapse; ► F).

Result: mitral valve insufficiency. This is a common lesion.

> **Note:** Visualization of proteoglycan:
> – Epithelial mucus (acidic, neutral mucopolysaccharides): PAS reaction;
> – Nonepithelial mucus: Alcian blue.

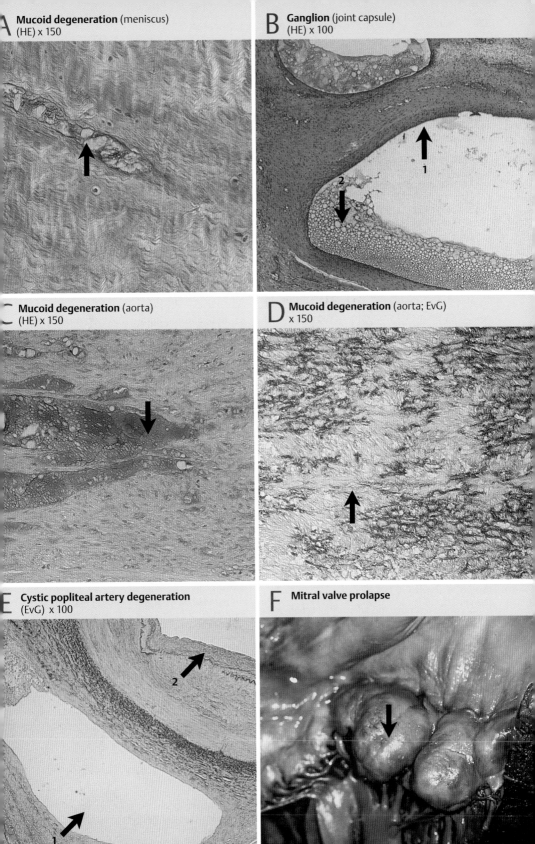

A Mucoid degeneration (meniscus)
(HE) x 150

B Ganglion (joint capsule)
(HE) x 100

C Mucoid degeneration (aorta)
(HE) x 150

D Mucoid degeneration (aorta; EvG)
x 150

E Cystic popliteal artery degeneration
(EvG) x 100

F Mitral valve prolapse

Sequelae of Mucoid Degeneration (Continued)

Dissecting Aneurysm

Definition: A circumscribed evagination of the wall of an artery due to dissection of the arterial wall in the direction flow because of a congenital or acquired intimal defect.

Factors in the causal pathogenesis of a dissecting aneurysm include:
- *Mucoid degeneration* (cystic medial necrosis).
  This is present in the following lesions:
  - Congenital vascular anomaly;
  - Congenital connective tissue disorder (p. 38, 48, 54);
  - Endocrine connective tissue disorder (hypothyroidism and abnormally elevated levels of progesterone or cortisol).

- *Hyperlipoproteinemia* (p. 88) resulting in atherosclerosis (p. 90).
- *Syphilitic aortitis* (p. 58).

Formal pathogenesis: The term "dissecting aneurysm" encompasses two processes:

Aneurysm: A bulge in the wall of an artery (see classification below).

Dissection: Mucoid degeneration of the arterial wall (usually in the aorta; see p. 60) increases the relative mobility of the individual layers. This increases the effect of shear forces from fluctuations in blood pressure, with these results:
- A primary, proximal intimal entry tear permits blood to enter wall of the vessel, splitting the wall into layers (► A2, C1). This forms a false lumen within the wall of the vessel (► A2, C2).
- A secondary, distal intimal exit tear then results, in which the false lumen reconnects with the physiologic lumen. The false lumen is only held together by a thin layer of residual media and adventitia, which expands outward to create the aneurysm. This produces eddy currents in the blood, precipitating parietal thrombi that adhere to the wall (► F; p. 404). An aneurysm rupture entails the risk of fatal hemorrhage.

✚ Clinical presentation: Patients report severe, gradually diminishing chest pain that tends to wander. The disorder is common; symptoms vary according to the vessel affected.
- Lumbar vessel involvement causes paraplegia.
- Renal artery involvement causes kidney failure.
- Intestinal arteries involvement causes ileus.
- Iliac vessels involvement causes claudication (lameness).

✚ Complication: A ruptured aneurysm leads to shock (p. 222) and eventually to fatal hemorrhage.

❗ Note: Location and etiology of aneurysms:
- Involvement of the ascending aorta and aortic arch (90% of all cases) is a manifestation of aortitis.
- Involvement of the abdominal aorta (10% of all cases) is a sequela of atherosclerosis.

❗ Note: Classification of aneurysms according to affected layers of the arterial wall:
- *True aneurysm:* It involves all three layers of the vascular wall (► A1, E, F).
- *Dissecting aneurysm:* It involves only part of the vascular wall (► A2, C).
- *False aneurysm:* It involves only the periadventitial tissue. It represents an endothelialized post-traumatic periarterial hematoma (► A3, D2) that lies adjacent to the original vascular lumen (► D; in this case, a vascular prosthesis).

❗ Note: Classification of aneurysms according to affected layers of the arterial wall:
- *Berry aneurysm:* It involves all layers of the wall in an expanded segment of a vessel measuring a few centimeters.
- *Fusiform aneurysm:* It involves expansion of an entire segment of a vessel gradually merging with the normal wall; all layers are involved (► B1).
- *Saccular aneurysm:* It involves a balloon-like expansion of an entire segment of a vessel (following a tear in the wall; ► B2).
- *Unilateral aneurysm:* It involves a one-sided expansion (following vascular injury or a tear in the wall; ► B3).
- *Serpentine aneurysm:* It involves several asymmetrical expansions in rapid succession, each on one side of the vessel (► B4).

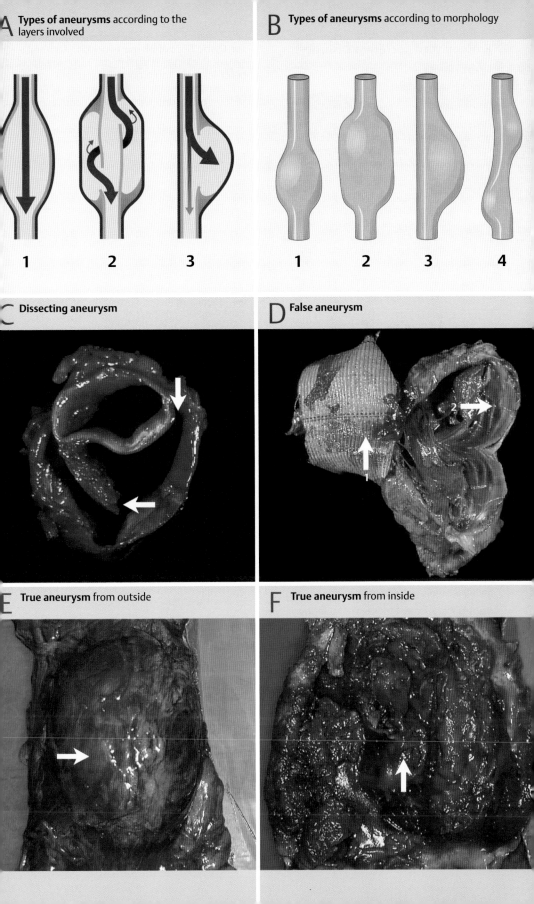

A Types of aneurysms according to the layers involved

1 **2** **3**

B Types of aneurysms according to morphology

1 **2** **3** **4**

C Dissecting aneurysm

D False aneurysm

E True aneurysm from outside

F True aneurysm from inside

Proteoglycan Secretion Disorders

Cystic Fibrosis

Synonym: mucoviscidosis.

Textbook example of an ion channel defect.

Definition: Hereditary defect of an anion channel that transports chloride ions. The defect results in dysfunctional exocrine secretion, creating excessively viscid mucus in the respiratory and digestive tracts. Accumulation of mucus in tissue results.

Causal pathogenesis: The disorder is caused by a single-point mutation of the **c**ystic **f**ibrosis **t**ransmembrane conductance **r**egulator (CFTR) protein, a membrane protein forming the chloride channel.

Formal pathogenesis: The CFTR protein is only formed by certain epithelial cells.

These primarily include:
— Crypt epithelia in the large and small bowel;
— Epithelia of the pancreatic ducts;
— Epithelia of the bile ducts in the liver;
— Ductal epithelia of the submucosal glands of the respiratory tree;
— Epithelia of the salivary, lacrimal, and sweat glands;
— Epithelia of the proximal tubules of the kidney;
— Lymphocytes and myocardial cells (function is not clear).

The lack of a choroid channel prevents normal reabsorption of Cl⁻, for example from sweat in the glandular lumen. This results in a high concentration of salt in secreted sweat (a clinical sign of the disease) and reduced Cl⁻ conductivity. It also causes secretion of viscid mucus by the submucosal glands of the respiratory tree (► A, C1, D), the sublingual glands, the intestinal mucosa (► B1), the pancreas (► E, F), and the bile ducts. This results in obstruction of the excretory duct by plugs of mucus and secretions.

Sequelae of Cystic Fibrosis

■ Bronchiectasis: Mucus accumulation in the goblet cells (► A) and glands, and ciliary hypomotility with defective mucociliary action, result in accumulation of secreted mucus. This leads to bronchitis, which in turn results in abnormal, irreversible expansion of the bronchi (► D; the lumen is partially filled with thickened whitish secretion). The result is persistent peribronchial inflammation.

Sequelae:
— *Peribronchial ectatic emphysema* results from overinflation of the alveoli (► C2) and leads to chronic obstructive pulmonary disease.
— *Reactive pulmonary fibrosis*, whose final stage is characterized by a honeycomb lung, leads to restrictive respiratory insufficiency.
— *Recurrent lung infection* (pneumonia) results from accumulation of mucus in the lung and leads to increased formation of asialoganglioside, which provides structures for bacteria such as *Pseudomonas aeruginosa* to adhere to.

■ Cystic fibrosis of the pancreas: Accumulation of thickened mucus in the excretory ducts (► E) leads to formation of pancreatic stones and expansion of the excretory duct (► F). Retention cysts form, which are accompanied by periductal resorptive inflammation. The excretory ducts become encased in scar tissue (► F2). This results in progressive atrophy of the exocrine acinar epithelia, with acinar metaplasia characterized by small cysts and replacement with fatty tissue.

Sequelae:
— *Destructive cystic fibrosis of the pancreas* (hence the name of the disorder) leads to insufficiency of the pancreas.
— *Secondary diabetes mellitus* (p. 78) occurs due to destruction of the islets of Langerhans.
— *Pulmonary fibrosis and inflammation* occur (see above).

■ Meconium ileus: Formation of an excessively viscid intestinal mucus leads to mucus obstruction in which the plug of mucus adheres to the crypts of the bowel like a network of roots (► B2). In the newborn, this leads to meconium ileus, obstruction of the bowel due to thickened meconium.

■ Liver cirrhosis: Maldigestion (p. 42) creates a protein deficiency, which leads to fatty changes in the liver in the form of retentive steatosis (p. 84). This results in a fatty liver with periportal fibrosis, which progresses to liver cirrhosis (p. 42) with portal vein hypertension (p. 392).

✚ Clinical presentation:
Cystic fibrosis is an autosomal recessive hereditary disorder; 5% of the population are heterozygotic carriers. Only homozygotic carriers develop the disease. Incidence of this disorder is approximately 1:2000. Symptoms include:
– Recurrent bronchopulmonary infections;
– Coughing up blood due to bronchial ectasia;
– Respiratory insufficiency due to pulmonary fibrosis;
– Maldigestion syndrome due to pancreatic insufficiency (p. 82);
– Dysfunctional sweat secretion associated with susceptibility to heat stroke (p. 146).

Note: Cystic fibrosis may be diagnosed before birth by amniocentesis.

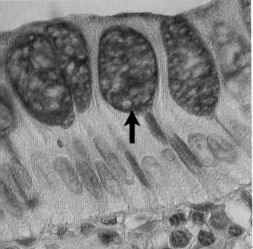

A **Mucus accumulation** in goblet cell of bronchi
(HE) x 200

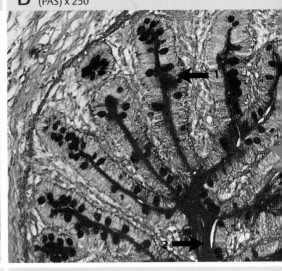

B **Mucus accumulation** in colon crypts
(PAS) x 250

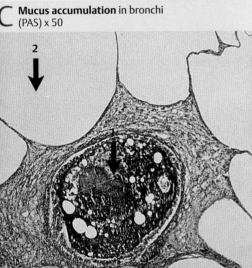

C **Mucus accumulation** in bronchi
(PAS) x 50

2

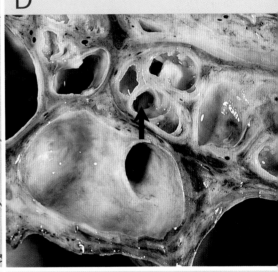

D **Bronchiectasis**

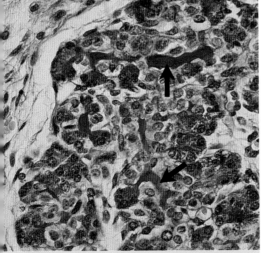

E **Mucus accumulation** in pancreas:
(19th week of gestation; PAS) x 60

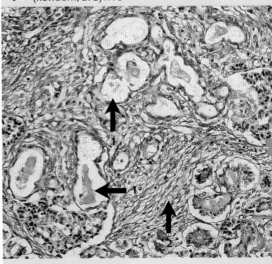

F **Cystic mucus accumulation** in pancreas
(newborn; EvG) x 75

Proteoglycan Lysis Deficiencies

Mucopolysaccharidoses

Textbook examples of lysosomal storage diseases associated with deformity syndromes.

General definition: Rare hereditary lysosomal disorder involving deficient metabolism of glycosaminoglycan in which mucopolysaccharide breakdown products are stored and excreted.

General pathogenesis: An autosomal recessive enzyme deficiency (except Hunter's syndrome) prevents complete metabolism of mucopolysaccharides. Metabolites are stored in lysosomes, creating a cytoplasmic vacuolization. When the lysosomal storage vacuoles are filled to capacity, mucopolysaccharide metabolites are excreted in the urine, which is how the diagnosis is made.

Mucopolysaccharide metabolites are stored in these cells:
— Chondrocytes;
— Fibrocytes;
— Media myocytes;
— Keratocytes (cornea);
— Hepatocytes (liver);
— Macrophages (organs of the reticuloendothelial system).

General morphology:
— *Gargoylism* occurs due to premature ossification of the skull sutures, leading to a heavy brow, depressed nose ridge, and protruding upper jaw (prognathy). The face resembles that of a gargoyle (► C, D).
— *Dwarfism* occurs due to retarded and abnormal bone growth. Patients have short stature, a hunchback, and clawed hands.
— *Hepatosplenomegaly* occurs due to storage of mucopolysaccharides in the reticuloendothelial system of the liver and spleen.
— *Cerebral degeneration* occurring due to storage of mucopolysaccharides in brain cells leads to dementia, inner-ear deafness, or spasticity.
— *Abnormal collagen cross-linkage* occurs as a result of defective mucopolysaccharide metabolism. This results in corneal opacification, premature arteriosclerosis, and aortic valve insufficiency.

> **Note:** The disorder is diagnosed by analyzing blood leukocytes to detect genetic carriers and before birth by amniocentesis.

The two best documented forms of mucopolysaccharidosis are described in the following section.

■ Hurler's Syndrome

Synonym: mucopolysaccharidosis I.

Definition: Hereditary mucopolysaccharide storage disorder due to deficient α-L-iduronidase with mucopolysacchariduria.

Morphologic characteristics: In contrast to normal cells, storage cells are characterized by honeycombed cytoplasm (► B) with PAS-positive material in lysosomal vacuoles. These storage lysosomes (p. 30) are large vacuoles containing fine granular material (► A).

> **✚ Clinical presentation and morphology:** Findings in Hurler's syndrome include:
> – Gargoylism (see above; ► C, D) with short stature, dementia, arteriosclerosis, aortic insufficiency, hepatosplenomegaly, and corneal opacification.
> – Mucopolysaccharides in the urine include dermatan and heparan sulphate.
>
> Maximum life expectancy is 10 years.

■ Hunter's Syndrome

Definition: Hereditary mucopolysaccharide storage disorder due to deficient α-L-iduronidase with mucopolysacchariduria.

> **✚ Clinical presentation and morphology:** Similar to Hurler's syndrome except without corneal opacification and with a milder clinical course. Mucopolysaccharides in the urine include dermatan and heparan sulfate.

Mucolipidoses

General definition: Very rare group of lysosomal storage disorders due to enzyme deficiencies in mucopolysaccharide metabolism without mucopolysacchariduria.

General pathogenesis: A defect in mucopolysaccharide metabolism results in intracellular accumulation of mucopolysaccharide metabolites and glycolipids (hence the name of the disorder).

General morphology:
— *Skeletal system:* short stature, dysostoses, and dysmorphia.
— *Myelin degeneration* leads to dementia and neurologic symptoms.
— *Hepatosplenomegaly* results from the lysosomal storage of mucopolysaccharide metabolites in the cells of the reticuloendothelial system of the liver and spleen. Storage lysosomes (for example in mucolipidosis IV) contain lipid material with a myelin-like configuration (► E, F).

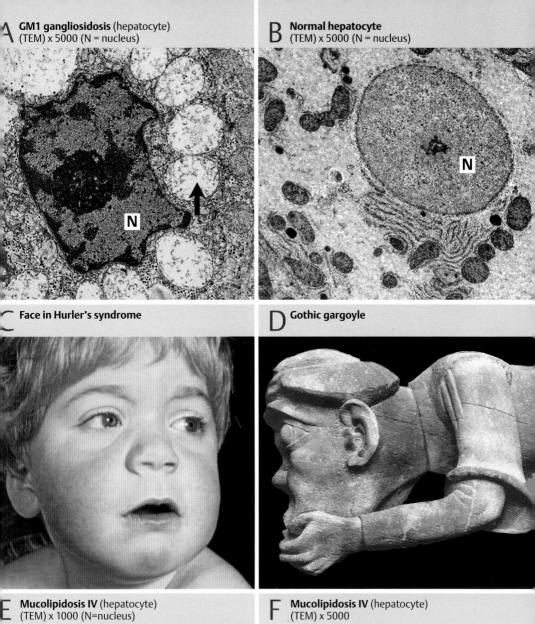

A **GM1 gangliosidosis** (hepatocyte)
(TEM) x 5000 (N = nucleus)

N

B **Normal hepatocyte**
(TEM) x 5000 (N = nucleus)

N

C Face in Hurler's syndrome

D Gothic gargoyle

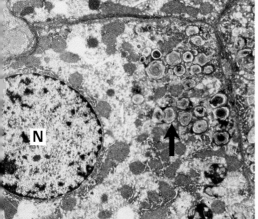

E **Mucolipidosis IV** (hepatocyte)
(TEM) x 1000 (N=nucleus)

N

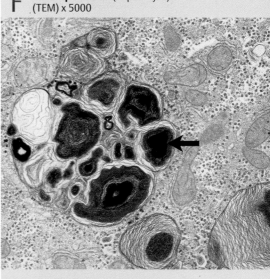

F **Mucolipidosis IV** (hepatocyte)
(TEM) x 5000

Serving Errors in Ion Ping-Pong

Errors of Metabolism: Inorganic Compounds

-------- **Summary** --------

Certain inorganic substances such as oxygen, calcium, iron, and copper play an important role in cellular metabolism or in transmitting signals within the cell. The appropriate transport proteins ensure that these substances are present in adequate quantities. Accumulations of ionized forms of these substances in tissue are as deadly as substance deficiencies and eventually result in cell death. Tissue dies within the living body (necrosis) but not without first sending out warning signals. These signals trigger an inflammatory reaction (p. 194) that helps to clear away the dead tissue. In this manner, inorganic substances may precipitate inflammation.

▶ **Oxygen:** The various forms of hypoxia probably represent the most crucial inorganic metabolic disorder. A variety of secondary lesions may be induced depending on the specific tissue's oxygen requirements and the duration of oxygen deprivation.

▶ **Calcium:** The most important disorders of calcium metabolism include hypocalcemia and hypercalcemia resulting from impaired intestinal absorption, renal excretion, and mobilization of skeletal calcium.

▶ **Iron:** An iron deficiency manifests itself in its most severe form as anemia. However, it also affects nearly all iron-dependent enzyme systems. Storage of toxic, ionized iron in various organ tissues is the pathogenetic basis of idiopathic hemochromatosis.

▶ **Copper:** Storage of excessive amounts of ionized copper plays an especially crucial role in Wilson's disease. This disorder manifests itself in lesions of the liver and basal ganglia of the brain.

Oxygen

Acute Generalized Hypoxia

Textbook example of common systemic disorders due to mitochondrial dysfunction.

Definition: Tissue injury resulting from oxygen deprivation. However, the severity of injury is not the same in every tissue.

The vulnerability and recovery time of any specific tissue are defined as follows:
— *Vulnerability* is the susceptibility to necrosis in hypoxic injury.
— *Recovery time* is the maximum duration of hypoxic impairment of energy metabolism that the decisive majority of cells required to maintain organ function will just barely survive.

Formal pathogenesis: At the subcellular level, it is primarily the mitochondria that are affected, which manifests itself in mitochondrial swelling with calcium deposits (p. 18, 20). Generalized hypoxia precipitates the following chain reaction: Hypoxia causes the cell to switch to anaerobic glycolysis. This causes rapid depletion of cellular ATP, increasing the level of intracellular lactic acid. This causes the Na^+–K^+ pump to fail, resulting in an influx of sodium, calcium, and water into the cell. Vacuolar degeneration of the cytoplasm (p. 12, 14) and/or apical cell edema then occur. This produces cellular swelling and nuclear pyknosis (p. 8)

Morphology: These histologic changes occur in the individual organs according to their specific vulnerability in the following order:
— *Brain:* Symmetrical pallidum necrosis[1] involving death of ganglion cells and necrosis in the subthalamic nuclei, substantia nigra, and Ammon's horn.
— *Heart:* Disseminated myocardial necrosis occurs, beginning in the papillary muscles and only then spreading into the inner layer of the left ventricle (the subendocardial region).
— *Liver:* perivenous necrosis occurs in the central portions of the lobes.

☺ **Clinical record:** Norwegian fisherman J. E. Rehdahl is on record as having survived the longest period of cardiac arrest with secondary hypoxia. On December 7, 1987, Rehdahl fell into icy seawater. His body temperature dropped to 24 °C, and cardiac arrest occurred. He was successfully resuscitated after 4 hours.

---

[1] Necrosis: *nekros* (Greek), death. Dead tissue in a living body with a more or less pronounced defensive reaction (p. aa129).

Acute Local Hypoxia

Pathogenesis: The degree of tissue injury frequently depends on the type, duration, and intensity of hypoxia; it also depends on whether re-perfusion occurs. During loss of blood supply (ischemia) DNA or RNA damage occurs, resulting in secondary synthesis of injurious peptides. However, the most severe damage is caused by reperfusion, during which xanthine oxidase plays a key role. This ubiquitous enzyme does not just catalyze the breakdown of purine, it also serves as an electron acceptor for oxygen, which is reduced to superoxide anion. This is in turn rendered innocuous by superoxide dismutase. During ischemia and reperfusion, non-radical forming xanthin dehydrogenase is "interconverted" into radical-forming xanthine oxidase, resulting in massive tissue damage. Because the parenchymal organ cells are more vulnerable to hypoxia than the mesenchymal cells of the organ stroma, necrosis in acute hypoxia may be limited to the parenchyma (partial necrosis). Involvement of both parenchyma and stroma is referred to as total necrosis. A region of necrotic tissue created by loss of blood supply is referred to as an infarction (p. 412).

Chronic Hypoxia

Pathogenesis: Three patterns of injury may occur, depending on the specific tissue and the duration of hypoxia. These types often occur in combination.

■ Fatty Degeneration (p. 84)

Morphology: This pattern of injury is characterized by intracellular accumulation of triglycerides. These are due primarily to reduced oxidation of fatty acids in the mitochondria (p. 22) and secondarily to impaired lipoprotein synthesis with delayed removal of lipids. The fatty degeneration always lies in the border area of a region of tissue supplied by two arterial branches. Therefore, the pattern of cellular fat deposition in large droplets manifests itself in a characteristic pattern of focal distribution.

— *Myocardium:* The fat droplets lie primarily in the region of the Z band and the mitochondria. This produces a tiger-striped pattern on the myocardium, visible on the papillary muscle with a transverse tiger-striped pattern extending to the insertion of the chorda tendinea (see p. 85 D).

— *Liver:* A pattern of perivenous fatty degeneration occurs in the central portions of the lobes with fat droplets surrounding the nuclei and the bile ducts.

— *Kidney:* The fatty degeneration occurs in the tubules, beginning in the basement membranes and epithelia of the proximal tubule and middle portion.

— *Meniscus:* The chronic compression leads to ischemic tissue injury. This produces fatty degeneration of the meniscal fibrocartilage with loss of the normal fibrous texture under polarized light, resulting in chronic degenerative meniscal changes (p. 60).

■ Organ Atrophy (p. 126)

Morphology: In temporary hypoxia, the mitochondria in the skeletal and cardiac musculature react with increased volume and proliferation of cristae (p. 20). Where hypoxia persists, the mass of the affected organ cells decreases. The cells become smaller and accumulate lipofuscin granules in their cytoplasm (p. 28). The result is brown discoloration and atrophy of the internal organs accompanied by interstitial tissue fibrosis (p. 40).

■ Interstitial Fibrosis

Morphology: In chronic hypoxia, connective tissue rich in collagen fiber compensates for the loss of parenchymal tissue due to atrophy especially in the brain and myocardium. This results in parenchymal fibrosis in these organs.

— *Myocardium:* The fibrosis of the myocardial interstitium reduces the strength of the heartbeat. This results in decreased perfusion of the myocardium, which in turn leads to additional fibrosis. The ventricular wall yields to internal pressure and dilates (dilated cardiomyopathy).

— *Brain:* The interstitial sclerosis is referred to as fibrous gliosis. This is an indirect sign of chronic hypoxic tissue injury.

Note: *Necrosis* refers to dead tissue in a living body with a more or less pronounced defensive reaction.

Calcium

Physiology: Calcium metabolism and phosphate metabolism are closely related. The kidney excretes calcium and phosphate in inversely proportional quantities.

Decrease in serum calcium concentration (▶ A1) leads to increased secretion of parathormone (▶ A2). This stimulates osteoclastic bone resorption (▶ A3) and renal reabsorption of calcium (▶ A4), which increases the calcium level. Parathormone simultaneously stimulates renal synthesis of 1,25-vitamin D_3 (▶ A5). This vitamin D_3 metabolite acts in synergy with parathormone to create the conditions required for adequate calcium uptake in the bowel (▶ A6).

Increase in serum calcium concentration (▶ A7) leads to an inverse regulatory mechanism that inhibits parathormone, releases 1,25-vitamin D_3, and stimulates the release of calcitonin (▶ A8). This reduces osteoclastic release of calcium (▶ A9).

Hypocalcemia

Definition: A decrease in the level of serum calcium below 2.2 mmol/l.

Etiologic factors include:
— Idiopathic, postoperative hypoparathyroidism;
— Pseudohypoparathyroidism;
— Malabsorption syndrome (p. 82);
— Vitamin D_3 deficiency due to renal insufficiency.

Morphology: The morphologic picture of hypocalcemia varies according to the specific etiology:
— *Ineffectiveness of parathormone* results in decreased osteoclastic and osteoblastic activity, which reduces bone turnover. This results in low-turnover osteoporosis (p. 126).
— *Vitamin D_3 deficiency:* a malabsorption syndrome (p. 82) due to renal insufficiency; causes compensatory activation of the parathyroid glands results in increased release of parathormone (secondary hyperparathyroidism). This causes excessively high bone turnover with intensive bone resorption in which osteoclasts drill tunnels in the trabeculae (dissecting bone resorption), producing resorption cysts. Production of uncalcified osteoid material is simultaneously increased, and broad osteoid halos containing osteoblasts form. These fibrous osteoid formations trigger reactive fibrosis around the trabeculae (endosteal fibrosis).

✚ **Clinical presentation:** The disorder is characterized by increased neuromuscular excitability (that may include tetanic spasms). Adynamia and muscular weakness are often present. Chronic cases exhibit mental retardation, basal ganglia calcification, cataract (lamellar cataract), skeletal and dental deformations, predisposition for *Candida* infection (p. 70).

Hypercalcemia

Definition: An increase in the level of serum calcium above 2.8 mmol/l.

Etiologic factors include:
— Osteolytic bone metastases;
— Parathormone-like substances excreted by tumor;
— Primary hyperparathyroidism.

Morphology: Endocrine-induced hypercalcemia leads to the following tissue changes:
— *Osteopenia* (decreased bone density): An excessive quantity of parathormone results in proliferation of osteoclasts that gnaw away at bone trabeculae in dissecting bone resorption. At the same time osteoblasts with uncalcified fibrous osteoid proliferate, causing fibrosis adjacent to the trabeculae. The result is an increase in the level of serum calcium.
— *Kidney calcifications* (p. 138) include kidney stones (nephrolithiasis) and metastatic calcification of the kidneys (nephrocalcinosis).
— *Gallstones* (cholelithiasis; p. 138) lead to cholecystitis.
— *Pancreatic stones* in excretory ducts of the pancreas lead to pancreatolithiasis and inflammation.
— *Salivary stones* in excretory ducts of the salivary glands lead to sialolithiasis and inflammation.
— *Gastric or duodenal ulcer* results from increased gastrin secretion (p. 218) induced by calcium or parathormone.
— *Corneal calcification* in the form of calcific band keratopathy.

✚ **Clinical presentation:** Hypercalciuria, hyposthenuria (inability of the kidneys to produce concentrated urine), metabolic alkalosis, exsiccosis desiccation (generalized drying out), shortened QT interval in the ECG with tachycardia.

❗ **Note:** Clinical presentation of hyperparathyroidism is best remembered with the phrase "bone, stone, and stomach ache," denoting osteopenia, urolithiasis and tissue calcification, and gastroduodenal ulcers.

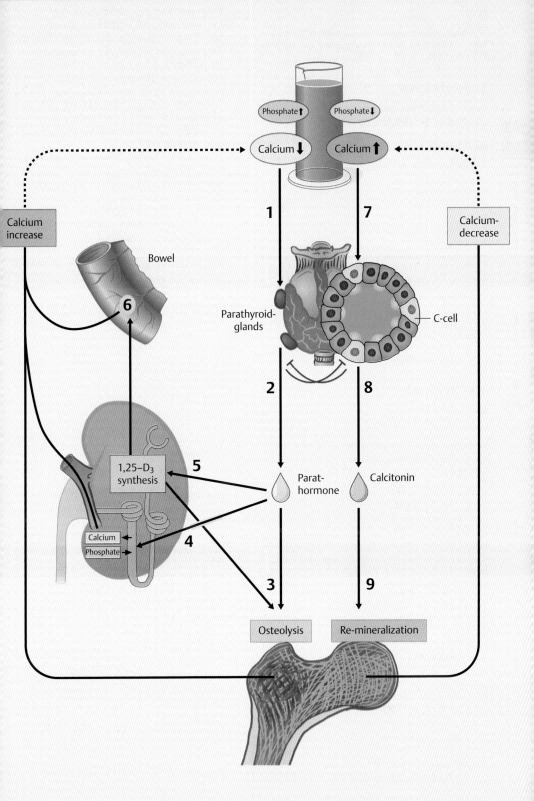

Iron

Physiology: The normal total iron content of the human body is about 3–4 g. Some 67% of this iron is in the form of hemoglobin.

Iron Deficiency

General definition and pathogenesis: Iron deficiency may be absolute or relative.

■ Absolute Iron Deficiency

Synonym: iron supply deficiency.

Etiologic factors:
— *Blood loss* (massive or chronic, p. 398).
— *Iron absorption disorder* in gastrointestinal diseases.

■ Relative Iron Deficiency

Etiologic factors:
— *Impaired iron transport:* A genetic defect results in a transferrin deficiency (congenital atransferrinemia). This disrupts the transport of iron in the blood and the uptake of iron in the erythroblasts facilitated by transferrin
— *Defective metabolism of absorbed iron:* In defective heme synthesis, the absorbed iron cannot be integrated into hemoglobin. This means that the normal supply of iron is not utilized, resulting in sideroachrestic anemia.

Iron Overload

■ Hemochromatosis

Synonym: von Recklinghausen-Applebaum disease.

Definition: Hereditary iron storage disease with systemic organ lesions due to increased iron absorption.

Pathogenesis: Failure of a control mechanism not yet fully understood results in a level of enteral iron absorption that is abnormally high in relation to the level of ferritin. In the early stages of the disease, increased quantities of iron are absorbed from the lumen of the small bowel. However, iron absorption may be subnormal in the later stages of the disease.

Morphologic characteristics:
— *Liver:* Early iron overloading results in storage of iron in the hepatocytes (► A, B) and bile duct epithelia. This causes brown discoloration of the parenchyma (► C) and leads to chronic liver damage and portal cirrhosis (p. 42) in the form of "pigment cirrhosis" (► D).
— *Myocardium:* The iron deposits in the myocardial cells produce toxic myocardial fibrosis that reduces the strength of the heartbeat. This in turn results in reactive myocardial thickening, leading to secondary cardiomyopathy.

— *Pancreas:* The iron deposits in the cells of the exocrine and endocrine glands (► G) cause toxic pluriglandular insufficiency. This results in progressive pancreatic fibrosis (pancreatic "cirrhosis") with brown discoloration of the parenchyma (giving the pancreas a rusty appearance; ► E, F) and secondary diabetes mellitus (p. 78). This disorder is referred to as "bronze diabetes" because of the accompanying bronze hyperpigmentation of the skin.
— *Joints:* Some patients develop chondrocalcinosis (cartilage calcification) from causes yet unknown. This leads to arthropathy in the fingers and hands.
— *Bone marrow:* The Medullar, plasma cell siderosis is a frequent hematologic finding.
— *Spleen:* No iron deposits.
— *Skin:* Inhibition of glutathione by free iron not bound by protein results in increased production of melanin (p. 112), giving the skin a brown color.

✚ **Clinical presentation:** Rarely beginning before the age of 30, and in women only after menopause due to iron loss in menstruation, this autosomal recessive hereditary disease exhibits variable penetrance. Incidence of the disorder is 1:500. It is associated with HLA-A3 (p. 164).
The diagnosis is made by determining blood ferritin and transferrin levels.

■ Secondary Siderosis (Hemosiderosis)

Definition: Increased iron deposits in tissue in the form of hemosiderin.

Pathogenesis: The disorder is due to one of the following mechanisms:
— **Iron overload** due to increased breakdown of hemoglobin (transfusion siderosis);
— **Defective iron utilization** due to defective heme or globin synthesis;
— **Nutritional or toxic liver damage** resulting from (a) alcohol abuse, in which iron is deposited in the spleen and liver (due to the increased iron content of fermented fruit juices) and/or (b) malnutrition (Bantu siderosis).

Morphology: In contrast to hemochromatosis, iron in hemosiderosis is initially absorbed by the cells of the macrophage system (reticuloendothelial system) and only later stored in parenchymal cells, leading to brown discoloration of the organs.

▼ **Rule of thumb:** Hemochromatosis is parenchymal siderosis; secondary siderosis is phagocytic siderosis.

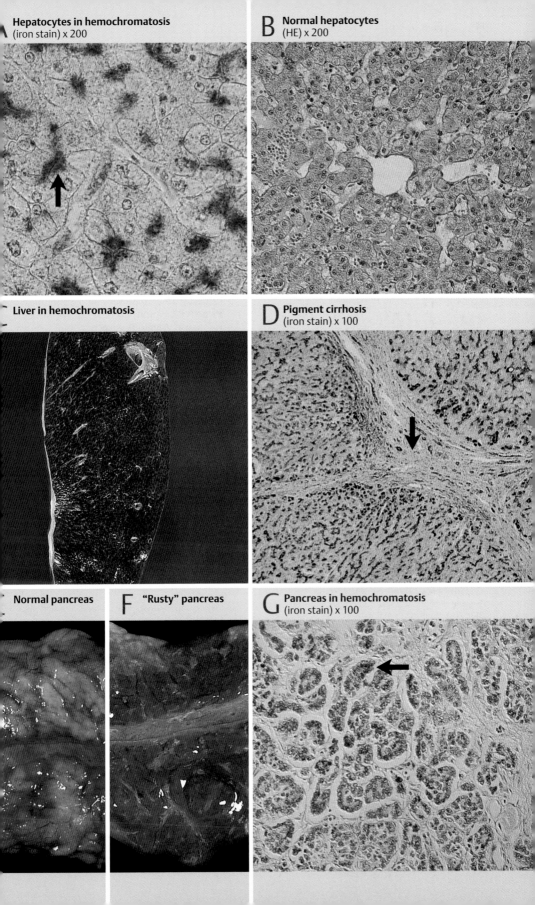

A Hepatocytes in hemochromatosis
(iron stain) x 200

B Normal hepatocytes
(HE) x 200

C Liver in hemochromatosis

D Pigment cirrhosis
(iron stain) x 100

E Normal pancreas

F "Rusty" pancreas

G Pancreas in hemochromatosis
(iron stain) x 100

Copper

Physiology: Copper is an important component in the copper enzymes, such as cytochrome-C oxidase. After being absorbed in serum, 95% of it is bound by a transport protein (ceruloplasmin) and the remaining 5% by albumin. Copper is primarily excreted in bile.

Copper Deficiency

■ Chronic Copper Deficiency

Pathogenesis: Chronic alimentary copper deficiency is rare in humans. It causes blood pancytopenia (deficiency of erythrocytes, leukocytes, and thrombocytes).

■ Trichopoliodystrophy

Synonym: kinky-hair disease, Menkes' syndrome.

Definition: Hereditary defect in copper distribution.

Pathogenesis: Defective copper transport ATPase produces low levels of copper in the liver, brain, skin, and blood vessels. Copper levels in the bowel, kidneys, muscles, and pancreas remain normal (p. 54).
The copper deficiency results in deficiency of the various copper enzymes in the affected organs. The copper enzymes are involved in electron transport in tissue respiration and in the synthesis of myelin, elastin, collagen, and keratin. Deficiency of these enzymes has several effects (p. 54).
- *Cerebellum:* The impaired differentiation of the Purkinje cells results in atrophy of the cerebellar cortex and cerebellar dysfunction (mental retardation).
- *Hair:* The keratin deformation results in kinky hair on the head.
- *Blood vessels:* They exhibit scurvy-like symptoms (p. 38) with vascular aneurysms (p. 62). This is accompanied by brittle bones.

Copper Overload

■ Wilson's Disease

Synonym: hepatolenticular degeneration.

Definition: Hereditary systemic copper toxicosis resulting from dysfunctional copper secretion in bile. This leads to damage of the liver and basal ganglia of the brain (degeneration of the lens nucleus).

Pathogenesis: This gene defect affects a copper ion-transporting P-type ATPase in the trans-Golgi membrane on chromosome 13. This ATPase carries the copper on the hepatocytic path of secretion to its incorporation in ceruloplasmin and to its excretion in the bile. This in turn selectively disturbs copper excretion in the gall capillaries, producing toxic ionized copper that is retained in the pericanalicular lysosomes

of the hepatocytes (▶ B). Later, this leads to storage of copper in other organs as well.

Morphology:
- *Liver:* Asymptomatic cases usually involve only minimal fatty degeneration. Symptomatic cases involve a feather-like pattern of vacuolar liver cell degeneration (▶ E, D1) leading to chronic liver inflammation (▶ D2) with progressive parenchymal destruction (▶ D2; chronic aggressive hepatitis). This later progresses to liver cirrhosis (▶ A).
- *Cerebral nuclei* (putamen, nucleus lentiformis, nucleus caudatus, substantia nigra): Ganglion cells accumulate copper. This causes degeneration, and narrowing of the striatum in particular, in the form of spongiform dystrophy (a spongy pattern of brain tissue damage) with proliferation of astrocytes and capillaries that disrupts the extrapyramidal system.
- *Kidney:* Copper deposits in the renal tubules results in the loss of the striated border of the tubules, causing tubular damage and glycosuria, aminoaciduria, and phosphate diabetes (Fanconi's syndrome, p. 100).
- *Cornea:* Patients exhibit a Kayser-Fleischer ring, a brownish-green ring-shaped pattern of copper deposits in the periphery of the cornea (▶ C).
- *Lens of the eye:* Copper storage produces a sunflower cataract.
- *Erythrocytes:* Hemolytic anemia (blood deficiency due to lysis of erythrocytes) is accompanied by icterus (jaundice; p. 108).
- *Bone tissue:* Symptoms include spontaneous fractures and osteomalacia (softening of bone).

✚ **Clinical presentation:** The incidence of the gene for this autosomal recessive hereditary disease is 1:500 in the total population. Only homozygous carriers develop symptoms; the incidence of the disease is 1:100 000.
- *Hepatopathy* includes chronic active hepatitis leading to liver cirrhosis; icterus results from hemolysis.
- *Nephropathy* includes Fanconi's syndrome.
- Ocular disorders include cataract and corneal ring.
- *Neuropathy* includes extrapyramidal symptoms.

The following chapter examines the organic substances that are most common in or crucial to an understanding of the pathologic biochemistry of the major metabolic disorders. Those attributable to a hereditary enzyme defect can be diagnosed before birth by amniocentesis.

Liver cirrhosis in Wilson's disease

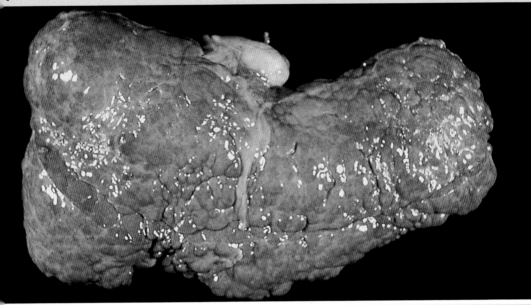

B Copper storage in the liver
(copper stain) x 300

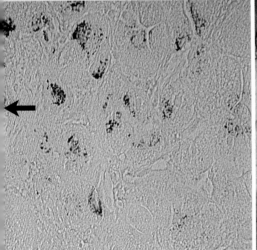

C Kayser-Fleischer corneal ring

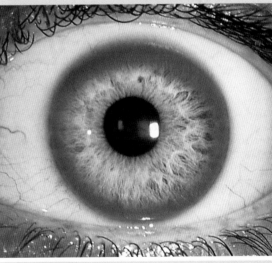

D Wilson's hepatitis
(HE) x 100

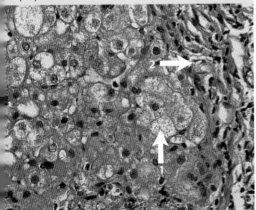

E Wilson's hepatitis
(HE) x 100

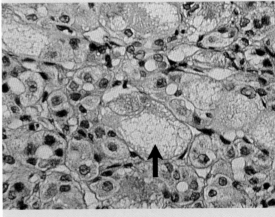

Errors of Metabolism: Organic Compounds

─────── **Summary** ───────

Organic molecules are structural materials and operating resources. Defective synthesis or breakdown causes accumulation of certain metabolites that can kill cells after first forming substances that trigger inflammation (p. 194).

▶ **Carbohydrates:** Usually of autosomal recessive inheritance, glycogenoses result from glycogen breakdown defects. Types I–III are characterized by hepatomegaly and/or muscle weakness. In the rare type IV, abnormal glycogen is stored in the liver due to a defective branching enzyme, causing destructive cirrhosis. The most common carbohydrate disorder is diabetes mellitus.

▶ **Lipids:** Fat absorption disorders belong to the group of malabsorption syndromes. The most frequent fat breakdown disorder is obesity; the most common fat transport disorder is hyperlipoproteinemia. It is usually complicated by arteriosclerosis. In sphingolipidosis, breakdown products are stored due to lysosomal enzyme defects.

▶ **Proteins:** Aside from proteinemia due to defects, it is primarily deficiencies of amino acid metabolism that are of pathologic and anatomic significance. Breakdown of amino acids leads to formation of ammonia, which is converted to urea. The purine bodies are broken down into uric acid. The most significant disorder of uric acid metabolism is gout.

Carbohydrates

Glycogenoses

General definition: Group of glycogen storage disorders due to a hereditary enzyme defect.

■ Type I Glycogenosis

Synonym: von Gierke disease.

Definition: Glycogenosis with liver and kidney enlargement.

Pathogenesis: A glucose-6-phosphatase defect renders liver cells and epithelia of the proximal renal tubule unable to synthesize glucose from stored glycogen, leading to accumulation of glucose-6-phosphatase. This primarily flows into anaerobic glycolysis, leading to increased lactic acid levels and lactic acidosis →
— *Hyperuricemia* results from inhibited renal excretion of uric acid (p. 102),
— *Hyperlipidemia* from mobilization of fat.

Morphology: The hepatic and tubular epithelia store glycogen in the cytoplasm (▶ A1) and nucleus (with glycogen defects; ▶ A2), which makes them resemble plant cells (▶ B).
This results in yellowish brown, enlarged liver (▶ C) and kidneys.

➕ **Clinical presentation:** The disorder manifests itself in infancy with hypoglycemia, impaired skeletal growth, hyperlipidemia, persistence of Bichat's protuberances, often a fat neck, hepatomegaly, renomegaly, and susceptibility to infection. Patients seldom live to adulthood.

■ Type II Glycogenosis

Synonym: Pompe disease.

Definition: Hereditary, generalized lysosomal glycogenosis with muscle weakness.

Pathogenesis: A defect in the acidic α(1,4)-glucosidase in lysosomes of the hepatic, cardiac, and skeletal muscle cells, and in the CNS and lymphocytes, blocks the lysosomal breakdown of glycogen, which accumulates in the lysosomes (▶ D), creating spider-like glycogen storage cells and cellular damage.

Morphology: Compensatory hypertrophy of cardiac, skeletal, and tongue musculature, resulting in abnormally enlarged heart and often a large, distended tongue.

➕ **Clinical presentation:** Muscle weakness, impaired peripheral reflexes, and cardiomegaly leading to heart failure; macroglossia. Most patients die in infancy.

■ Type III Glycogenosis

Synonym: Forbes disease.

Definition: Glycogenosis with cardiomegaly, hepatomegaly, and muscle weakness.

Pathogenesis: An amylo-1,6-glucosidase (debranching enzyme) defect in cardiac and skeletal muscles cells, hepatocytes, and enterocytes.

Morphology: Glycogen is stored in hepatocytes and myocytes (especially in the heart), causing cardiomegaly.

➕ **Clinical presentation:** Muscle weakness and heart failure. Patients survive to adulthood.

❗ **Note:** *Glycogenosis is diagnosed* by liver biopsy (type I) and muscle biopsy (types II and III).

❗ **Note:** Heart failure in an infant without a defect suggests glycogenosis.

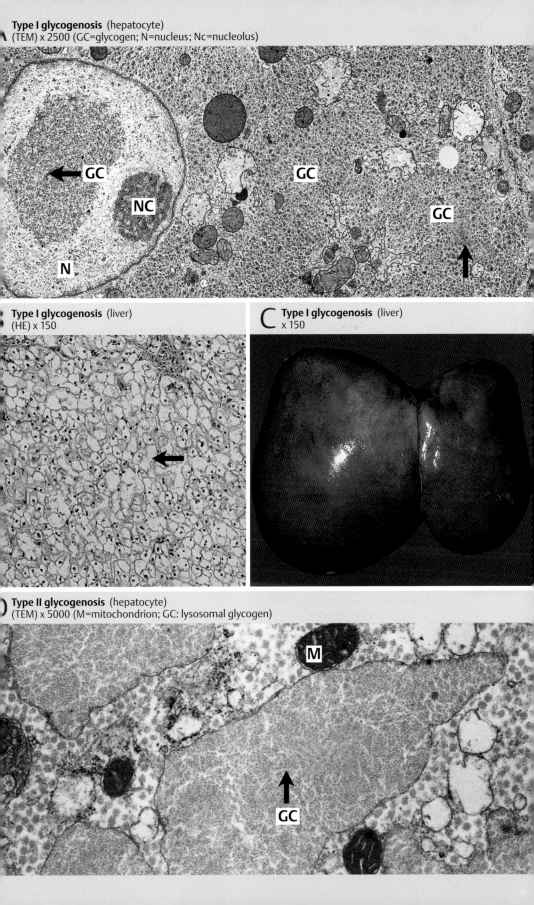

A Type I glycogenosis (hepatocyte)
(TEM) x 2500 (GC=glycogen; N=nucleus; Nc=nucleolus)

B Type I glycogenosis (liver)
(HE) x 150

C Type I glycogenosis (liver)
x 150

D Type II glycogenosis (hepatocyte)
(TEM) x 5000 (M=mitochondrion; GC: lysosomal glycogen)

Carbohydrate Malabsorption

■ Lactose Intolerance

Definition: Diarrhea from lactose incompatibility due to a hereditary or acquired lactase deficiency.

Pathogenesis: A lactase deficiency results in negligible enteral absorption of the non-hydrolyzed lactose. Large quantities of lactose (in diary foods) cause bacterial fermentation, formation of lactic acid and short-chain fatty acids, leading primarily to osmotic diarrhea.

Morphology: Intestinal histology is normal. Histochemical studies reveal no disaccharidase activity in the microvilli of the intestinal enterocytes.

✚ **Clinical presentation:** Lactase deficiency occurs in 5% of the Caucasian population and 40% of the eastern Asian population. Symptoms include diarrhea following consumption of dairy foods.

■ Saccharose-Isomaltose Intolerance

Definition: Rare disorder with diarrhea resulting from disaccharide intolerance due to lack of saccharase-isomaltase.

Pathogenesis: The enzyme deficiency causes osmotic diarrhea via a mechanism similar to that of lactose intolerance.

Glucose Synthesis Disorders

■ Fructose-1,6-Diphosphatase Deficiency

Definition: Hereditary deficiency of glucose synthesis with ketoacidosis.

Pathogenesis: An enzyme deficiency blocks glucose synthesis; the sole source of glucose is the breakdown of glycogen.

✚ **Clinical presentation:** Rare inherited autosomal recessive disorder. Hypoglycemia causes epileptic seizures with hyperventilation, ketosis, and lactic acidosis.

■ Hereditary Fructose Intolerance

Definition: Hereditary fructose intolerance with liver damage.

Pathogenesis: Reduced fructose-1-phosphate-aldolase activity.

✚ **Clinical presentation:** Rare inherited autosomal recessive disorder. Ingestion of fructose leads to hypoglycemia, vomiting, and coma. Patients develop an aversion to sweets and do not develop cavities. Prolonged alimentary exposure to fructose causes liver cirrhosis (p. 42).

Deficient Carbohydrate Metabolism

Diabetes Mellitus

Textbook example: the most significant disorder of glucose metabolism.

General definition: Chronic disorder of glucose metabolism with hyperglycemia, triggered by conditions associated with a relative or absolute insulin deficiency.

Primary diabetes mellitus (see below): Insulin deficiency due
— To islet damage from autoimmune inflammation (type I; p. 186) or
— Dysfunction of pancreatic insulin-producing cells (type II).

Secondary diabetes mellitus (see below): Insulin deficiency due
— To islet damage from pancreatic disease such as pancreatitis, hemochromatosis (p. 72), or cystic fibrosis (p. 64); or
— Overproduction of insulin antagonist hormones such as cortisone and somatotropic hormone (STH).

Pathogenesis of primary forms of diabetes mellitus:

■ Type I Diabetes Mellitus

Synonyms: juvenile-onset diabetes mellitus, insulin-dependent diabetes mellitus (IDDM).

Autoimmune lymphocytic insulitis in combination with genetic susceptibility (HLA-DR4 and/or DR3) leads to formation of autoimmune T-lymphocytes and islet-cell antibodies (p. 186). They destroy the β cells (► A) and leave the glucagon-forming cells intact (► B), causing insulin-dependent diabetes mellitus.

■ Type II Diabetes Mellitus

Synonyms: adult-onset diabetes mellitus, non-insulin-dependent diabetes mellitus (NIDDM).

Type IIa is without obesity; type IIb with obesity (p. 49).

Together with insulin, β cells form amylin (islet amyloid peptide), which condenses to AE amyloid (► C; see also p. 50), "smothering" the function of the islets. Peripheral organs and tissues in obese patients also exhibit insulin resistance due to the protein resistin, secreted by fat cells, leading to non-insulin-dependent diabetes mellitus. Immunohistochemical findings reveal normal counts of insulin-producing cells (► D) and glucagon-producing cells (► E).

 Prominent patient: Friedrich Dürrenmatt, Swiss author and stage producer.

❗ **Note:** *Diabetes is treated* with insulin (type I) or sulfonylurea (type II).

Type I diabetes mellitus: loss of β cells
(IH; insulin) x 200

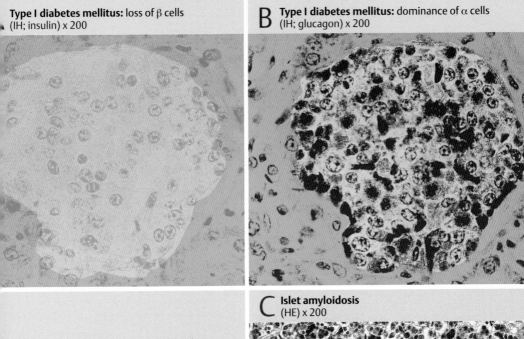

B **Type I diabetes mellitus:** dominance of α cells
(IH; glucagon) x 200

C **Islet amyloidosis**
(HE) x 200

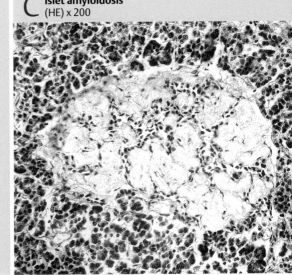

Type II diabetes mellitus: β cells
(IH; insulin) x 200

E **Type II diabetes mellitus:** α cells
(IH; glucagon) x 200

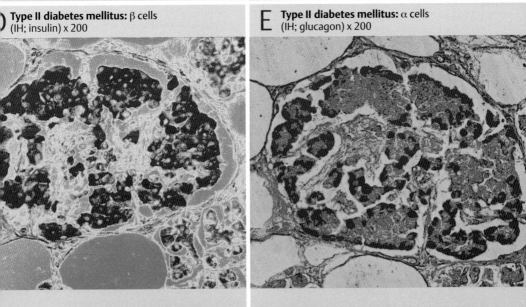

Diabetes Mellitus: Sequelae

▨ **Diabetic macroangiopathy** follows the pattern of atherosclerosis (p. 90).

✚ **Complications:**
- Coronary sclerosis can lead to myocardial infarction.
- Cerebral sclerosis can lead to cerebral infarction.
- Popliteal sclerosis can lead to gangrene (▶ E).

▨ **Diabetic microangiopathy:** Chronic increased glucose concentration leads to glycosylation of proteins, altering the structure and permeability of the microvascular basement membranes (▶ A, B).

✚ **Complications:**
- *Diabetic retinopathy* (a late complication): Capillary microaneurysms and arteriosclerosis cause microinfarctions (punctate hemorrhages; ▶ F). Proliferative retinitis leads to shrinkage of the vitreous body and retinal detachment.
- *Diabetic glomerulosclerosis* (Kimmelstiel-Wilson lesion): Deranged synthesis and breakdown of the glomerular basement membrane cause thickening of the membrane (▶ B). This causes diffuse and, later, nodular deposition of PAS-positive material in the mesangium (▶ C and D, respectively) and between the glomerular podocytes and basement membrane, leading to proteinuria and renal insufficiency.

▨ **Diabetic cataract:** Osmotic vacuolar degeneration of the epithelium of the lens creates lens opacities.

▨ **Diabetic liver:** Secondary glycogenosis (glycogen-induced nuclear defects; p. 8) occurs in relation to the level of blood glucose; simultaneous fatty degeneration (p. 85) correlates with obesity in type IIb diabetes.

▨ **Diabetic neuropathy:** After approximately 25 years of diabetes, 50 % of patients exhibit axonal and/or myelin degeneration leading to hyporeflexia and decreased deep sensation.

✚ **Complications:** diabetic microangiopathy and diabetic neuropathy lead to gangrene in the toes (▶ E).

▨ **Susceptibility to infection:** Immune defenses are impaired by "lame" granulocytes (due to deranged chemotaxis); patients suffer from purulent inflammations (furunculosis) and fungal infections (Candida mycosis; p. 270).

▨ **Diabetic embryopathy:** This occurs where the mother's diabetes is poorly controlled.

✚ **Sequelae of diabetic embryopathy:**
- *Giant babies* with a swollen, obese constitution due to reactive STH secretion.

- *Hyaline membrane disease:* Immature pulmonary epithelia and squamous alveolar cells lead to insufficient surfactant synthesis (which normally prevents alveolar adhesion).
  - The alveoli fail to expand and their walls adhere, with resulting atelectasis (incomplete expansion of the lung).
  - The increase in alveolar surface tension leads to excretion of fibrin into the alveolar ducts. This fibrin thickens to form hyaline membranes, causing respiratory insufficiency (infant respiratory distress syndrome).
- *Transient hypoglycemia:* The fetus reacts to maternal insulin deficiency with hyperplasia of the insulin-producing β cells, which enlarges and increases the number of fetal pancreatic islets. This increases the risk of postnatal hypoglycemic shock.

❗ **Note:** *Diabetes-specific syndromes* include
- Diabetic retinopathy and cataract,
- Diabetic nephropathy,
- Diabetic neuropathy, and
- Diabetic gangrene of the foot.

Galactosemia

Definition: Defect of galactose metabolizing enzyme with damage to the liver, brain, and lens of the eye.

Pathogenesis: Defective galactose-1-phosphate uridyltransferase prevents conversion of galactose to glucose. Galactose-1-phosphate (and its metabolite galactitol) accumulate in the liver, kidneys, brain, adrenal glands, lenses of the eyes, erythrocytes, and amniotic epithelium.

Morphologic organ manifestations:
- *Liver:* Galactose-1-phosphate and galactitol accumulation causes fatty degeneration with inflammatory destruction of hepatocytes (fatty liver hepatitis). Scarring (p. 42) progresses to liver cirrhosis (storage cirrhosis).
- *Kidney:* Galactose-1-phosphate and galactitol accumulation disrupts tubular transport, resulting in renal amino acidosis (Fanconi syndrome, p. 100).
- *Lens of the eye:* Galactose-1-phosphate and galactitol accumulation causes osmotic damage to the epithelium of the lens, leading to opacity. Galactosemic cataract is a late complication.
- *Brain:* Galactose-1-phosphate and galactitol accumulation causes damage to nerve cells. The resulting deranged myelinization leads to mental retardation.

✚ **Clinical presentation:** Prenatal diagnosis is made by amniocentesis. The inherited autosomal recessive disorder has an incidence of 1:20 000.
Symptoms include:
- Storage cirrhosis;
- Fanconi syndrome (p. 100);
- Cataract;
- Mental retardation.

Normal basement membrane (glomerulus)
(TEM) x 10 000

B **Diabetic basement membrane** (glomerulus)
(TEM) x 10 000

Diabetic glomerulosclerosis
(PAS) x 300

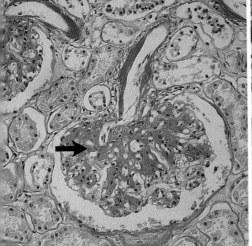

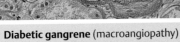

D **Diabetic glomerulosclerosis**
(PAS) x 300

Diabetic gangrene (macroangiopathy)

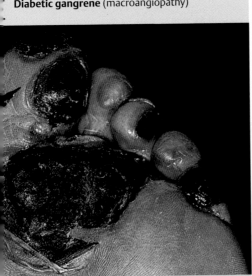

F **Diabetic retinopathy** (microangiopathy)

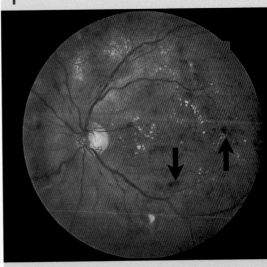

Lipids

Fat Uptake Disorders

Malabsorption Syndromes

General definition: Disorders involving (a) defective absorption of nutrients, especially neutral fats, from the intestinal lumen or (b) defective passage of these substances into the intestinal lymph system.

The following forms are differentiated according to the relevant cause:

— **Maldigestion** is defective intraluminal fat digestion due to one of these lesions:
 — *Hepatogenic* (biliary disorder): bile acid deficiency;
 — *Pancreatogenic* (pancreatopathy): lipase deficiency;
 — *Gastrogenic* (gastrectomy): lack of lipase activation.

— **Malabsorption** is defective transport of fat through the intestinal mucous membrane due to one of these lesions:
 — *Infectious:* tropical sprue, Whipple disease;
 — *Autoimmune:* gluten enteropathy (nontropical sprue);
 — *Enzymatic:* lactase deficiency causes diarrhea from fermentation;
 — *Dysproteinemic:* Abetalipoproteinemia (p. 86).

— **Impaired intestinal lymph drainage**
 — *Infectious:* Whipple disease.

Disorders Associated with Malabsorption

■ Gluten Enteropathy

Synonyms: celiac disease, celiac sprue, nontropical sprue.

Definition: Chronic inflammation of the bowel due to congenital hypersensitivity to gluten.[1] The disorder is referred to as celiac disease in children and sprue[2] in adults.

Pathogenesis: A genetic predisposition (HLA-DR3, HLA-B8) leads to formation of antibodies (p. 180) that attack the epithelial anchoring fibrils (reticulin) when the patient is exposed to gluten. The resulting chronic inflammation produces necrosis and separation of intestinal and dermal epithelial cells. The precise cause of this inflammatory bowel disease is still unclear.
— *Small bowel:* Damage to normal villi (► A) causes enterocytes to destroy themselves (p. 128, 132), with resulting atrophy of the villi (► B, C; see also p. 124).

— *Skin:* Separation of the epidermis occurs, producing cutaneous vesicles (dermatitis herpetiformis).

Morphology: lymphoplasmacytic inflammatory infiltrate in the mucosa of the small bowel (► C1) with destruction of the villi leads to atrophy of the villi ("flat" mucosa) and compensatory deepening (hyperplasia) of the crypts of the small bowel (► B, C2).

Histologic result: hyperplastic crypts with loss of villi (► B).

✚ Clinical presentation: malabsorption syndrome due to inadequate fat absorption. Symptoms:
- *Fatty stools* (steatorrhea) with deficiency of essential fats primarily leads to a deficiency in fat-soluble vitamins (especially vitamin D).
- *Osteomalacia:* Deficient absorption of vitamin D_1 prevents ossification of cancellous osteoid in bone tissue. This results in cancellous bone with broad osteoid borders (► D, E). Breakdown of bone by osteoclasts remains normal, resulting in bone softening and deformation.

■ Whipple Disease

Synonym: intestinal lipodystrophy.

Textbook example of a metabolic disorder caused by bacterial infection.

Definition: Intestinal disorder characterized by impaired lymphatic transport of fat as a result of bacterial infection, often accompanied by systemic symptoms.

Pathogenesis: An unknown genetic predisposition causes this immune defect. Whipple bacteria (Tropheryma whipplei) survive phagocytosis (► F) in bacterial infection. The resulting sickle-shaped bacteria accumulate in the histiocytes of the small bowel. These distended histiocytes prevent removal of chylous lymph, resulting in a malabsorption syndrome.

Morphology: Histiocytes distended with bacteria and fat accumulate in the intestinal mucosa and regional lymph nodes (► G) and prevent removal of fat.

✚ Clinical presentation: Rare malabsorption syndrome causing fatty stools (steatorrhea), weight loss, and enlarged lymph nodes; improves with antibiotic Therapy.

---

[1] Gluten = wheat protein
[2] Sprue: from *sprouw* (Dutch), vesicle (in dermatitis)

Normal intestinal villi (SEM) x 2000

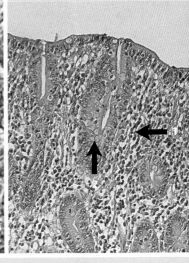

B **Hyperplastic crypts** (celiac disease) (REM) x 2000

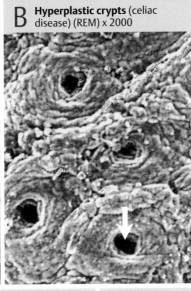

C **Small bowel in celiac disease** (PAS) x 300

D **Normal cancellous bone** (Goldner's trichrome stain) x 100

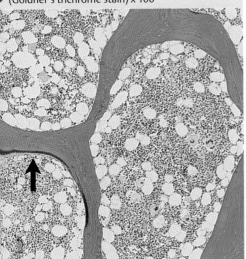

E **Cancellous bone in osteomalacia** (Goldner's trichrome stain) x 100

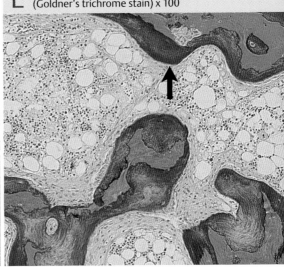

Tropheryma whipplei (TEM) x 10 000

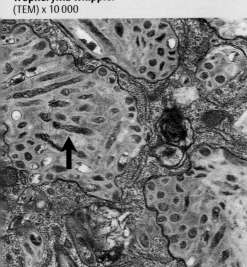

G **Small bowel in Whipple disease** (oil-red stain) x 50

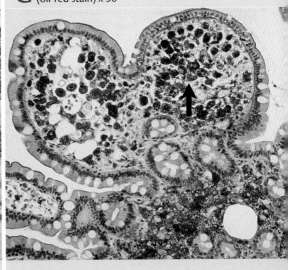

Fatty Degeneration

Synonyms: fatty change, steatosis.

Definition: Conditions characterized by abnormal storage of fat due to a mismatch between the supply of and demand for fat.

■ Dietary Steatosis

Increased intestinal uptake of fats and carbohydrates overloads the fat transport and catabolism system, resulting in deposit of large droplets of fat in the epithelia of the central portions of the hepatic lobes (► A) or the renal tubules (► B).

Culinary example: pâté de foie gras (goose liver pâté).

■ Transport Steatosis

Etiologic factors:
— **Endocrine factors** include increased fat mobilization due to (a) release of adrenaline, STH, or ACTH, or (b) insulin deficiency.
— **Nutritional factors** include hypolipoproteinemia and defective fat transport due to starvation, malnutrition, or kwashiorkor (disease caused by protein-deficient diet). This results in increased fat removal, with fat storage in the central portions of the hepatic lobes.

■ Absorptive Steatosis

Etiologic factors:
— **Removal of necrotic tissue:** Focal encephalomalacia with myelin sheath destruction, chronic abscess (p. 226) with leukocyte destruction, and fatty tissue necrosis (p. 132) induce histiocytes to phagocytize fats, transforming these cells to foam cells (► C).
— **Hypercholesteremia** (p. 88) leads to increased phagocytosis of lipids or cholesterol and storage of these substances in vacuoles. This transforms the histiocytes into foam cells and the microglial cells into fat granule storage cells.

■ Retention Steatosis

Etiologic factors:
— **Hypoxia** causes oxidation of fatty acids. This in turn causes (a) fatty degeneration in the central portions of the hepatic lobes, and (b) nodular fatty degeneration of the myocardium (tiger-striped pattern of fatty myocardial deposits ► D; see also p. 69).
— **Enzyme deficiency:** Lack of fat-metabolizing enzymes (carnitine deficiency).
— **Intoxication:** Cell damage (such as from alcohol) produces deposits of small droplets of fat in the hepatocytes of the central portions of the lobes (► E).

> **Note:** The location of the fatty changes in the liver is independent of their etiology.

Disorders of Fat Catabolism

■ Starvation

Definition: p. 124.

Pathogenesis and morphology: Starvation leads to catabolism of fat deposits, which in turn transforms adipose tissue into reticular connective tissue. This results in water retention (gelatinous degeneration of adipose tissue); vascular structures lie in gelatinous connective tissue (► F).

■ Obesity

Textbook example of a common disorder exhibiting polygenic inheritance and popularly oversimplified as gluttony.

General definition: Abnormal increase in the mass of body fat in excess of 20% over normal body weight.
— **Primary obesity** is abnormally high body weight in the absence of a recognizable underlying disorder. Location of fat deposits are gender-specific: on the hips, upper arms, thighs, and buttocks in women, and on the anterior abdominal wall, back, and back of the neck in men.
— **Secondary obesity** results from endocrine, cerebral, and psychological disorders.

Pathogenesis of primary obesity: Leptin, the fat cell protein hormone and product of the "obesity gene," reduces food intake and increases overall energy consumption. In obese people, binding of leptin to leptin receptors in the hypothalamus is partially impaired, and the satiety center of the hypothalamus is not restrained. This results in increased hunger and elevated levels of serum leptin. Adipocytes produce a further hormone, resistin. In the obese there is greater propagation thereof, effecting a resistance to insulin in fat and skeletal muscle tissue, which leads to fat accumulation and weight gain. This illustrates the connection between obesity and diabetes mellitus Type II.

> **Note:** Normal body weight (in kilograms) is given by the length of the body (in cm) minus 100.

■ Ketonemia

Definition: Common disruption of the acid-base equilibrium and electrolyte equilibrium by "flooding" with ketone bodies from increased fat catabolism.

Pathogenesis: Hunger and diabetes mellitus lead to mobilization of fatty acids, producing ketonemia.

> **+ Complication:** The ketone bodies (acetone, acetoacetate, and β-hydroxy butyrate) are broken down in peripheral tissue as normal metabolic breakdown products. Normally they are only present in the blood in low concentrations. Ketonemia (a common metabolic disorder) causes metabolic ketoacidosis, which disrupts the acid-base equilibrium and produces ketonuria, disrupting the elimination of electrolytes.

Dietary liver steatosis
(HE) x 200

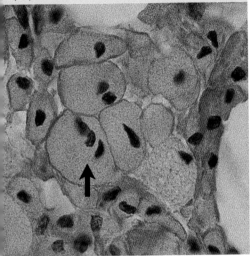

B **Steatosis** of the renal tubules
(oil-red stain) x 150 (G=glomerulus)

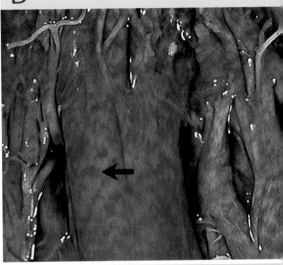

Foam cells (histiocytes)
(HE) x 200

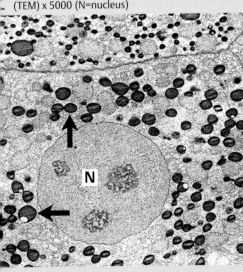

D **Tiger-stripped pattern** of fatty myocardial deposits

Toxic fatty degeneration of the liver
(TEM) x 5000 (N=nucleus)

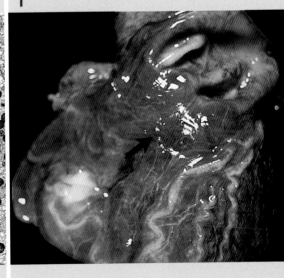

F **Gelatinous degeneration** of the epicardium

■ Phytanic Acid Storage Disease

Synonym: Refsum disease.

Definition: Neurologic disorder due to a peroxisomal enzyme defect resulting in storage of branched chain fatty acids (of the same type as phytanic acid) in myelin.

Pathogenesis: A defect in peroxisomal phytanic acid α-hydroxylase causes storage of phytanic acid from chlorophyll in blood, tissues, and ganglia and Schwann cells. Phytanic acid is incorporated into myelin, causing disintegration of the myelin sheath that leads to ganglion cell necrosis in the anterior horns of the spinal cord, cerebellum, and brain stem.

Histology: Abnormal compensatory Schwann-cell proliferation causes thickening of the peripheral nerves like the layers of an onion (demyelinating polyneuropathy). Lipid-laden macrophages cause fibrous thickening of the leptomeninges.

✚ **Clinical presentation:** Rare inherited autosomal recessive disorder characterized by chronic polyneuropathy, cerebellar ataxia (poor coordination with stumbling gait), night blindness, atypical retinitis pigmentosa (see note).

■ Propionic Acidemia

Definition: Rare hereditary propionyl coenzyme A carboxylase defect with propionic acidemia.

Pathogenesis: Because of the enzyme defect, branched fatty and amino acids are only broken down to propionyl-CoA carboxylase. This successively causes propionic acidemia, propionic aciduria (partially as sodium salt), and electrolyte loss.

■ Methylmalonic Aciduria

Definition: Rare hereditary methylmalonyl coenzyme A mutase defect with ketoacidosis.

Pathogenesis: Because of the enzyme defect, isomerization of l-methylmalonyl-CoA to succinyl-CoA fails to occur, leading to methylmalonic acidemia and aciduria.

Hypolipoproteinemia Disorders

General definition: Hereditary disorders of apolipoprotein synthesis with reduced serum levels of the respective lipoprotein.

General pathogenesis: A genetic defect impairs the synthesis of apolipoprotein A or B. Depending on the type of hypolipoproteinemia, this either compromises removal of absorbed fats and cholesterol or the cholesterol remains in place and is stored in phagocytes.

■ Abetalipoproteinemia

Synonym: Bassen-Kornzweig syndrome.

Definition and pathogenesis: Hereditary defect of β lipoprotein synthesis blocks synthesis of apolipoprotein B. Sequelae of β lipoprotein deficiency include:
— **Hypolipidemia:** Absorbed enteral triglycerides and cholesterol are not removed, resulting in storage of lipids in the enterocytes (▶ A, B).
— **Impaired membrane synthesis:** Lack of lipids disrupts myelinization and membrane synthesis, causing erythrocytes to develop spiny projections and producing acanthocytosis (▶ C).

✚ **Clinical presentation and morphology:** Very rare disorder, usually with autosomal recessive inheritance. In autosomal dominant hereditary hypobetalipoproteinemia, synthesis of β lipoproteins is only depressed. However, the same symptoms occur as in abetalipoproteinemia.
– *Malabsorption syndrome:* Fats are absorbed by intestinal enterocytes but cannot be transported from there. This leads to fatty degeneration of the enterocytes progressing up to the tips of the villi (▶ A, B), and the enterocytes do not absorb any more fat.
– *Steatorrhea* occurs as a result. Fat remains in the stool, and a general deficiency of fat-soluble vitamins (especially D and E) results.
– *Demyelination* due to lipid deficiency (especially of vitamin E) causes neurologic symptoms and retinitis pigmentosa (▶ D).

■ Analphalipoproteinemia

Synonym: Tangier disease.

Definition and pathogenesis: Hereditary absence of high density lipoprotein (HDL) in blood plasma impairs export of cholesterol from macrophages in the liver. Phagocytes of the reticuloendothelial system store primarily cholesterol oleate in vacuoles, which transforms them into foam cells.

✚ **Clinical presentation and morphology:** Very rare inherited autosomal recessive disorder.
– *Blood levels* of cholesterol, phospholipids, and triglycerides, are elevated. HDL is almost totally absent in homozygous carriers.
– *Cholesterol oleate* storage occurs in the tonsils in children, causing yellow discoloration. In adults, it is stored in the spleen (causing splenomegaly with anemia due to hypersplenism), liver, bone marrow, and Schwann cells (causing neuropathy).

❗ **Note:** *Retinitis pigmentosa* is a group of hereditary metabolic lesions with retinal degeneration and primarily peripheral deposits of dark brown pigment (▶ D) leading to night blindness, tunnel vision, and blindness.

A **Abetalipoproteinemia** at an early stage: (enterocyte) TEM x 3500

B **Abetalipoproteinemia** at a late stage: (enterocyte)

C **Acanthocyte** (REM) x 3000

D **Retinitis pigmentosa**

Hyperlipoproteinemia Disorders

General definition: Disorder of fat metabolism in which one or more serum lipid fractions are increased. Most of these disorders are quite common.

- *Primary forms* involve genetic defects (prenatal diagnosis is made by amniocentesis);
- *Secondary forms* occur with diabetes mellitus, alcoholism (p. 144), obesity (p. 84), primary biliary liver cirrhosis (p. 22), nephrotic syndrome, and hypothyroidism (p. 186).

■ Type I Hyperlipoproteinemia

Definition: Hyperchylomicronemia and hypertriglyceridemia without increased risk of atherosclerosis, caused by an autosomal recessive genetic defect of lipoprotein lipase.

Pathogenesis: This lipase defect reduces the rate at which chylomicrons are broken down (► A). This delays the removal of triglycerides from the blood.

✚ Clinical presentation and morphology: Rare disorder.
- *Eruptive xanthomas* (see p. 90): skin lesions on the lateral extremities (► E), buttocks, and back.
- *Hepatosplenomegaly* results from accumulations of histiocytic foam cells.
- *Lipemia retinalis:* lipid deposits in the retina.
- *Recurrent pancreatitis* occurs following ingestion of fat (p. 132, 216).

■ Type II Hyperlipoproteinemia

Definition: Hypercholesterolemia due to deficiency of low density lipoprotein (LDL) receptors with formation of xanthomas and early atherosclerosis.

Pathogenesis: Primarily fibroblasts and myocytes vascular walls lack receptors for LDL (► C). Therefore, they do not absorb cholesterol but cover their demand for cholesterol by synthesizing their own, resulting in hypercholesterolemia.

✚ Clinical presentation and morphology: Common disorder. Symptoms include:
- *Tuberous xanthomas* (see below) in juveniles (extremities, shoulders, back, and tendons);
- *Xanthelasma,* fatty deposits in the eyelid;
- *Arcus senilis,* yellow corneal ring from lipid deposits.
- *Atherosclerosis,* leading to cardiovascular complications.

■ Type III Hyperlipoproteinemia

Definition: Disorder of fat metabolism resulting from a genetic defect of apolipoprotein E with xanthomas and increased risk of atherosclerosis.

Pathogenesis: Defective apolipoprotein E reduces the binding affinity for LDL receptors in the liver cells. This blocks endocytic absorption of very low density lipoprotein (VLDL) and chylomi-

crons, resulting in accumulation of abnormal VLDL in the blood (dysbetalipoproteinemia).

✚ Clinical presentation and morphology: Common disorder. Symptoms include:
- *Flat xanthomas* (see p. 90), skin lesions (volar folds);
- *Tuberous xanthomas* (see p. 90), raised skin lesions (fingers, elbows, tendons; ► F);
- *Atherosclerosis,* leading to cardiovascular complications.

■ Type IV Hyperlipoproteinemia

Definition: Hypertriglyceridemia caused by deficient breakdown of VLDL with an increased risk of atherosclerosis.

Pathogenesis: Two forms exist. The *autosomal dominant hereditary form* involves a defect in breakdown of VLDL (increases with ingestion of carbohydrates); the *symptomatic form* involves secondary hyperlipoproteinemia.

✚ Clinical presentation and morphology: Common disorder. Symptoms include *atherosclerosis,* leading to cardiovascular complications in adults. Xanthoma and pancreatitis are absent.

■ Type V Hyperlipoproteinemia

Definition and pathogenesis: Hyperchylomicronemia of unknown etiology with a high risk of atherosclerosis and myocardial infarction in the presence of high levels of VLDL (► B) and slightly elevated serum cholesterol. The disorder is rare.

■ Familial LCAT Deficiency

Definition: Hereditary defect of lecithin cholesterol acyltransferase (LCAT) with tendency toward hemolysis.

LCAT catalyzes esterification of fatty acids from lecithin. Therefore, blood cholesterol is only present in the lipoprotein-bound form (most of this is esterified with fatty acid).

Pathogenesis: The enzyme defect reduces the level of serum cholesterol and HDL (► D), increasing plasma triglycerides. This produces membranes of endothelial cells and erythrocytes with defective lipid components (excess unesterified cholesterol).

✚ Clinical presentation and morphology: Very common disorder.
- *Anemia:* Membrane defects in the erythrocytes result in formation of flattened erythrocytes and tendency toward hemolysis, producing normochromic anemia.
- *Nephropathy:* Membrane defects in the endothelial cells result in subepithelial lipid deposits in the glomeruli, causing proteinuria and hypertension (p. 386).
- *Arterial disease:* Membrane defects in the endothelial cells result in calcifying arteriosclerosis of the kidney as early as the fourth decade of life.

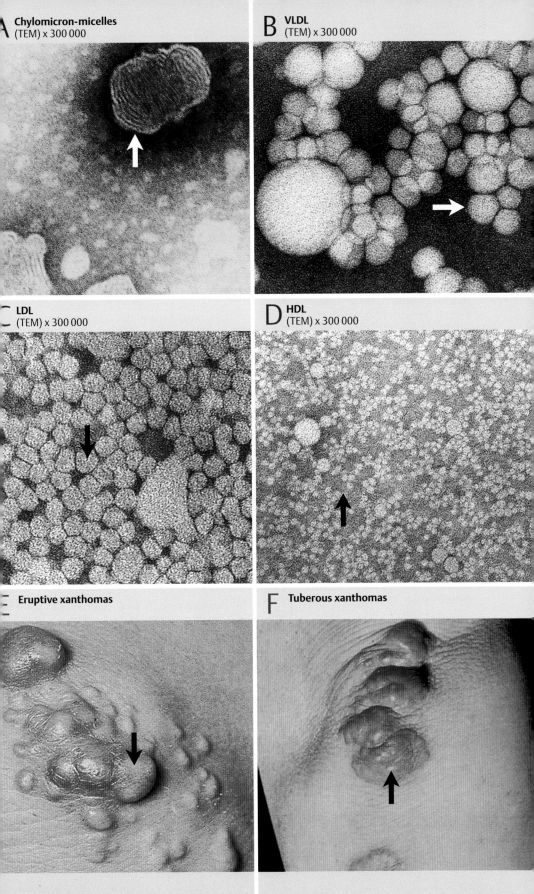

A Chylomicron-micelles
(TEM) x 300 000

B VLDL
(TEM) x 300 000

C LDL
(TEM) x 300 000

D HDL
(TEM) x 300 000

E Eruptive xanthomas

F Tuberous xanthomas

Sequelae of Hyperlipoproteinemia

> **Note:** Lipoprotein transport route: HDL and LDL pass through the endothelial barrier and enter the media. There they are phagocytized by myocytes. HDL absorbs cholesterol from the respective storage cells and transports it to the liver where it is metabolized.

■ Atherosclerosis

Textbook example: **the number one** epidemic disease.

Definition: Arterial disease that spreads from the intima to the media with focal lipid accumulations (*athero-*), diffuse *sclerosis,* characterized by chronic inflammation.

Risk factors:
— *Hyperlipidemia,* especially with types II and IV hyperlipoproteinemia with increased LDL, which transports fat to the periphery.
— *Hypertension* leads to vascular damage (p. 388).
— *Cigarette smoking* leads to carbon monoxide tissue ischemia. Mutagens contained in smoke cause proliferation of media myocytes. Substances contained in smoke activate factor VIII, resulting in formation of clots (p. 402) in the vessel wall.
— *Gender:* Premenopausal women have lower LDL levels than men. However, smoking and oral contraceptives cancel out this advantage.

Pathogenesis is multifactorial; there may be an association with Chlamydia. The disease develops as follows:
— **Lipid plaque** (fatty streaks): With a lot of LDL in the blood and vessel wall, LDL remains in the subintimal space where it ages and oxidizes. Macrophages "smell" the oxidized LDL via scavenger receptors and phagocytize it, which transforms them to lipophages. These cells accumulate in the subintima for lipid phagocytosis (▶ A: lipophages dyed red; ▶ B: lipids dyed red). The result is a lipid plaque (yellowish raised focal lesion on the intima of the artery).
— **Atherosclerotic plaque:** Lipophages cannot digest cholesterol. This means that cholesterol crystallizes out, and these cells are destroyed by the perforin of the cytotoxic T-lymphocytes present. The lipid plaque in the subintima becomes a grave for lipophages, consisting of a fatty pool (Greek *athyrea,* pap) with cholesterol crystals (atheroma). The surviving lipophages excrete proinflammatory substances (endothelin-1 and interleukin-1), stimulating the intimal media myocytes to form collagen fibers to stabilize the wall of the vessel. The endothelia are also stimulated to the same effect; their platelet-activating factor attracts thrombocytes, which continue the fibrotic change with their platelet-derived growth factor (PDGF).

The result is a *stable plaque* (▶ D; compare with C).

The inflammatory reaction triggered by the macrophages and lymphocytes results in focal destruction of the endothelium; the result is an occlusive thrombus (p. 406).
— **Atherosclerotic ulcer:** The myocytes in the fibrotic covering of the atheroma gradually succumb to apoptosis. Macrophages release metalloproteinases, which loosen the sclerotic wall of the plaque. The result is an unstable plaque.

The plaque tears, and bleeding into the plaque occurs. The resulting rapid swelling of the plaque increases the risk of stenosis and platelet aggregation. This activates plasmin, resulting in formation of thrombin and blood clots in and on the wall of the vessel. Platelets release PDGF, causing proliferation of myofibroblasts and reparative sclerosis. Where this does not succeed, the plaque ruptures.

The result is an atherosclerotic ulcer (▶ E), leading to occlusive thrombus.

✚ Complications:
– *Vascular occlusion* leads to infarction (p. 414).
– *Cholesterol embolism* may occur due to emptying of the contents of the atheroma into the vascular lumen (p. 412).
– *Atherosclerotic aneurysm* (especially in the abdominal aorta) may occur due to weakening of the arterial wall, with the risk of rupture.

■ Xanthoma

Definition: An accumulation of fat-storing macrophages in tissue that simulates a tumor and occurs in hyperlipoproteinemia.

Macroscopic *types of xanthoma* include the
— *Planar* or flat type (volar folds),
— *Tuberous* or nodular type (in the elbow, knee, and finger; p. 88 ▶ F), and the
— *Eruptive* type (p. 88 ▶ E). The latter come and go according to the lipid level.

Morphology: yellowish focal lesions (Greek *xanthos,* yellow) of lipophages (▶ F1) with foamy cytoplasm. Some of these fuse to Touton giant cells (▶ F2). When necrosis of the lipophages occurs, cholesterol drains into the tissue, precipitating a foreign-body inflammation (p. 236).

> **Note:** *Touton giant cells* are multinuclear cells with foamy cytoplasm and a ring of nuclei along the periphery of the cell (▶ G).

A Atherosclerosis (acid phosphatase) x 50

B Atherosclerosis (oil-red stain) x 50

C Normal aorta

D Atherosclerotic aorta

E Atherosclerotic ulcer

F Xanthoma (HE) x 200

G Touton giant cell (EvG) x 200

Sphingolipidoses

General definition: Rare hereditary disorder of lysosomal sphingolipid catabolism.

Most importantly, sphingolipids are components of the myelin sheaths. Accordingly, sphingolipidoses manifest themselves as (a) neuronal disorders and (b) visceromegaly (enlargement of internal organs) due to storage in the reticuloendothelial system.

■ Gaucher's Disease

Synonym: cerebroside lipidosis, glucosylcerebroside lipidosis.

Definition: Storage disease due to deficiency of glucocerebrosidase of varying severity, especially in phagocytes.

Pathogenesis: Activity of lysosomal glucocerebrosidase in the phagocytes, endothelial cells, and nerve cells is reduced or absent. Consequently, phagocytized cell membranes (erythrocyte membranes in particular) can only be incompletely catabolized. This results in storage of cerebroside in digestive vacuoles (▶ A, B), creating Gaucher cells. Similar vacuoles may be found in nerve cells and vascular epithelia.

Morphology: Measuring up to 30 μm, Gaucher cells typically exhibit cytoplasm that resembles crumpled tissue paper (▶ C).
- *Storage organs* include the liver (▶ D), spleen, and lymph nodes, producing hepatosplenomegaly and enlarged lymph nodes.
- *Bones:* Bone-marrow lesions in the adult form lead to osteoporosis and pancytopenia with "Erlenmeyer flask" flaring of the distal femur.
- *Brain:* Gaucher cells accumulate perivascularly and in the Virchow-Robin's spaces. The destruction of the ganglion cells is apparently induced secondarily-perhaps by the toxic storage material. Causing cell death, demyelination, and brain damage (dentate nucleus of the cerebellum, thalamus, and cerebral cortex)

+ Clinical presentation: This varies depending on the age of manifestation:
- *Type II* (acute infantile neuropathic form): cranial nerve failure and extrapyramidal symptoms.
- *Type III* (subacute infantile neuropathic form).
- *Type I* (chronic adult form without neuropathy): osteoporosis (p. 126), thrombocytopenic bleeding (p. 400).

■ Sphingomyelin Lipidosis

Synonym: Niemann-Pick's disease.

Definition: Storage disease due to defective sphingomyelinase isoenzyme with visceral and/or neurologic symptoms.

Pathogenesis: This varies depending on the type of the disorder. In *type I,* sphingomyelinase is absent in the cells of the reticuloendothelial system, glial cells, and ganglion cells, resulting in lysosomal storage of sphingomyelin and cholesterol as osmophilic lamellar corpuscles. The resulting storage cells (Pick cells) appear as foam cells. In *type II,* there are no known enzyme defects.

Morphology (Type I): Changes resembling those in Tay-Sachs disease (p. 94) occur, accompanied by the following lesions:
- *Storage organs:* Hepatosplenomegaly characterized by a yellowish white appearance of the cross section and nests of storage cells of "sea-blue" histiocytes.
- *Brain:* Ballooning of the ganglion cells due to storage of sudanophilic material, leading to neurologic degeneration, causing increased consistency and atrophy of the white matter.

+ Clinical presentation: Autosomal recessive hereditary disorder whose symptoms vary according to the age of manifestation.
- *Type A* occurs in neonates, causing cramps, ophthalmoplegia (paralysis of the eye muscles) and is fatal.
- *Type B* occurs in adults and causes hepatosplenomegaly.

■ Krabbe's Disease

Synonym: globoid cell leukodystrophy.

Definition: Storage disease resulting from galactosylceramidase deficiency with rapid destruction of the white matter of the brain.

Pathogenesis: Deficiency of lysosomal β-galactosidase, the specific enzyme for galactosylceramide, results in formation of giant storage cells in the form of multinuclear globoid cells with spherical vacuoles (▶ E). The resulting myelin destruction leads to degeneration of the white matter of the brain (globoid cell leukodystrophy).

Morphology: Symmetrical demyelination (▶ F) of the cerebrum and cerebellum (leukodystrophy) is accompanied by diffuse sclerosis. This causes severe shrinkage of the white matter, producing gray discoloration and often rubbery tissue changes.

+ Clinical presentation: Autosomal recessive hereditary disorder characterized by
- *Spasticity* (simultaneous stimulation of flexors and extensors),
- *Ataxia* (inability to coordinate muscular activity, producing disturbed motion and posture),
- *Decerebration* (cortical brain defect).

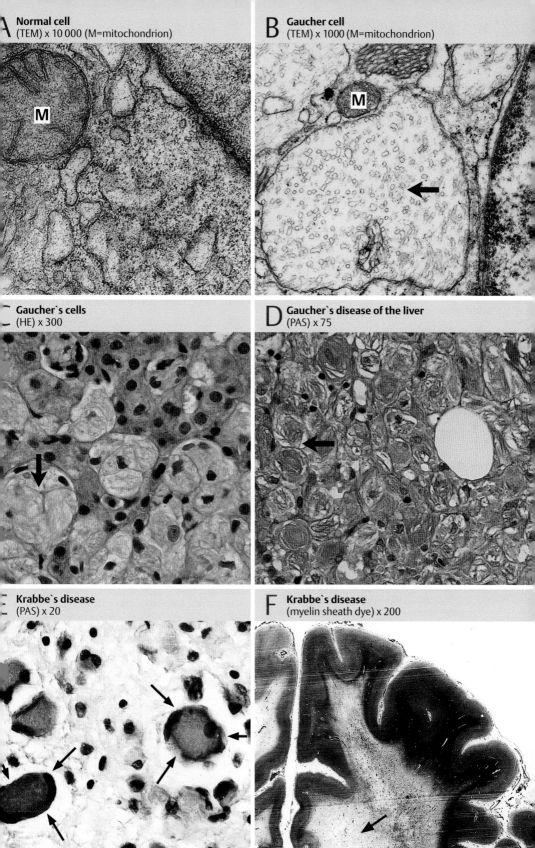

A Normal cell
(TEM) x 10 000 (M=mitochondrion)

B Gaucher cell
(TEM) x 1000 (M=mitochondrion)

C Gaucher`s cells
(HE) x 300

D Gaucher`s disease of the liver
(PAS) x 75

E Krabbe`s disease
(PAS) x 20

F Krabbe`s disease
(myelin sheath dye) x 200

■ Metachromatic Leukodystrophy

Definition: Lysosomal storage disease resulting from deficient cerebroside sulfatase enzymes causing damage to the brain-stem and basal ganglion cells.

Pathogenesis: Deficiency of lysosomal cerebroside sulfatase enzymes (especially arylsulfatase A) blocks catabolism of the cerebroside sulfates, resulting in storage of cerebroside sulfate in lysosomes of oligodendroglia, Schwann, and nerve cells (primarily basal ganglia and brain stem).

Morphology: The medulla oblongata is grayish white due to demyelination with diffuse hardening or rubbery honeycombing. Histologic examination reveals scavenger cells with PAS-positive storage granules (metachromasia). These are lysosomes with clumps of myelin-like material (► A).

✚ **Clinical presentation:** Very rare inherited autosomal recessive disorder. Symptoms include hypotonic spasticity and sulfatide in the urine. Diagnosis is made by sural nerve biopsy.

■ Fabry Disease

Synonyms: diffuse angiokeratoma, glycolipid lipidosis.

Definition: Lysosomal storage disease with formation of angiokeratomas.

Pathogenesis: Defective α-galactosidase A (ceramide trihexosidase) in endothelia and fibroblasts (in the skin, liver, kidneys, and bowel) leads to storage of ceramide trihexoside, creating "mulberry cells."

✚ **Clinical presentation and morphology:** Very rare X-linked recessive hereditary disorder.
– *Skin* symptoms include angiokeratomas, dark red spots measuring 1–2 mm with capillary proliferation under thickened epidermis, some with hyperkeratosis due to lysosomal storage of glycolipids in the form of myelin-like tubular structures (► B) in endothelium and pericytes of subepidermal capillaries.
– *Kidney* symptoms include storage of glycolipids in the glomerular and tubule epithelia, causing renal insufficiency.
– *Fundus of the eye:* It exhibits phlebectasia, leading to impaired vision.
– *Cardiac* symptoms include heart failure.

■ Type I GM₂ Gangliosidosis

General definition: Lysosomal diseases involving storage of neuronal gangliosides.

▦ Tay-Sachs Disease

Synonym: infantile GM_2 gangliosidosis.

Definition: Rare ganglioside storage disease causing blindness and dementia.

Pathogenesis: A defect of β-acetyl galactosidase causes lysosomal storage of GM_2 ganglioside in glial and ganglion cells, causing cell death. Substances are not stored by the macrophage system.

Morphology: The brain may be abnormally large and/or atrophic with narrowing of the cortex (especially with atrophy of the cerebellar cortex). Myelin-like lipid material with an ultrastructure resembling the layers of an onion is stored in nerve cells (► C, D), causing vacuolar degeneration (► E) and destruction of ganglion cells especially in the neocortex with proliferation of astrocytes and fibrous gliosis (p. 69).

✚ **Clinical presentation:** Very rare inherited autosomal recessive disorder.
– *Demyelination* of the white matter and spinal cord is accompanied by axon destruction, leading to dementia.
– *Retinopathy* is present, with neuron destruction leading to blindness and retinal thinning that produces a cherry red spot.

⁞ **Note:** Tay-Sachs disease is *diagnosed* by fundus examination; prenatal diagnosis is made by amniocentesis.

■ GM₁ Gangliosidosis

Definition: Rare storage disease caused by deficient β-galactosidase, which helps catabolize glycosamine glycan.

Pathogenesis: An enzyme defect causes cytoplasmic storage of (a) GM_1-gangliosides in ganglion cells of the gray matter of the brain and (b) acidic proteoglycans in histiocytes, transforming the storage cells into foam cells.

✚ **Clinical presentation and morphology:** Autosomal recessive hereditary disorder.
– *Neuropathy* includes psychomotor dysfunction with spastic quadriplegia, ataxia, and convulsions.
– *Retinopathy* occurs as in Tay-Sachs disease.
– *Renomegaly and hepatosplenomegaly* occur due to proteoglycan storage.
– *Bone deformation* in the form of dysostosis multiplex occurs. This involves growth deformation of the skull and spine with thickening of the ribs, shoulder blades, and long cortical bones.
  – *Type I,* primarily characterized by retinopathy and neuropathy, leads to death in infancy.
  – *Type II,* usually without retinopathy but with visceromegaly, leads to death by about age 10.

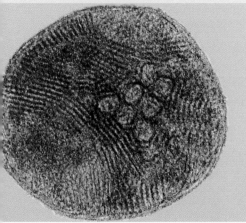

A Metachromatic leukodystrophy
(TEM) x 2000

B Fabry disease
(TEM) x 60 000

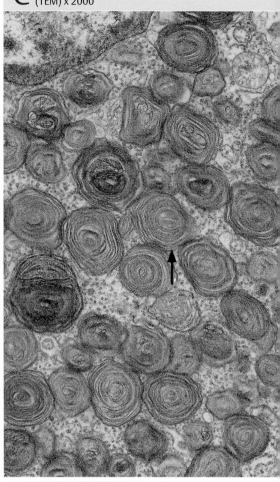

C Tay-Sachs disease
(TEM) x 2000

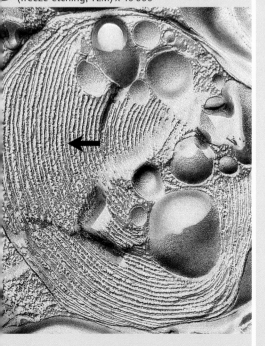

D Tay-Sachs disease
(freeze-etching, TEM) x 40 000

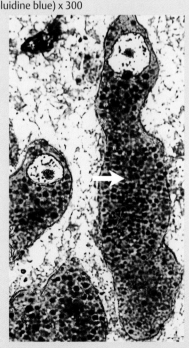

E Tay-Sachs disease
(toluidine blue) x 300

Proteins

Defective Serum Proteins

Definition: Disorders due to a genetic inability to properly synthesize specific plasma proteins.

These include:
— *Analbuminemia,* serum albumin deficiency (1% or normal) with increased risk of edema;
— *Immunoglobulin deficiency;*
— *Complement factor deficiency;*
— α_1-*antitrypsin deficiency;*
— *Serum hemoglobin deficiencies;*
— *Clotting factor deficiency, afibrinogenemia;*
— *Hyperlipoproteinemia;*
— *Absence of serum lipoproteins.*

Disorders of Amino Acid Metabolism

General definition: Disorders due to enzymatic disruption of amino acid metabolism.

The following section examines disorders of amino acid metabolism that are either frequently encountered or whose early detection is important to avoid late sequelae.

■ Phenylketonuria

Synonym: phenylpyruvic oligophrenia.

Definition: Hereditary disorder of phenylalanine. Left untreated, it can lead to mental retardation (oligophrenia).

Pathogenesis: Due to a defect in hepatic phenylalanine hydroxylase, phenylalanine is not hydroxylated to form tyrosine, and neurotransmitter synthesis is impaired. Some of the metabolites that accumulate at the enzyme block undergo transamination and are oxidized at an atypical location.

+ Clinical presentation and morphology: Quite common disorder exhibiting autosomal recessive inheritance.
– *Decreased pigmentation* of hair, skin, and pupils due to competitive inhibition by phenylalanine of the tyrosinase involved in melanin synthesis (p. 112).
– *Brain damage* (in the absence of dietary treatment) with reduced myelination of the central and peripheral nervous system, occasionally accompanied by axon destruction and glial proliferation. This results in loose, spongy brain tissue (spongiform dystrophy) that causes mental retardation or oligophrenia (hence the name) and susceptibility to convulsions.
– *Skin* is characterized by a mouse-like body odor due to excretion of indoleacetic acid in sweat.

! Note:
– *Prenatal diagnosis* of phenylketonuria is made by amniocentesis;
– *Postnatal early diagnosis* is made by the Guthrie test.

■ Albinism

Definition: Very rare group of diseases with lack of pigmentation in the skin, hair, and/or eyes due to genetically blocked melanin synthesis.

Etiology varies according to the specific type.

— *Ocular albinism* is characterized by lack of pigmentation in the eyes only; the etiology is not clear.
— *Oculocutaneous albinism* involves lack of pigmentation in the skin, hair, and eyes (p. 112).
  — In *type I oculocutaneous albinism,* absence of tyrosinase completely blocks melanin synthesis.
  — In *type II oculocutaneous albinism,* tyrosinase is present but missing in the melanocytes due to deficient transport, also resulting in blocked melanin synthesis.

+ Clinical presentation: Prenatal diagnosis is made by amniocentesis. Extreme photosensitivity leads to radiation tumors of the skin (p. 150); patients are photophobic.

■ Alkaptonuria[1]

Synonym: ochronosis.

Textbook example of an inborn error of metabolism.

Definition: Hereditary disorder of homogentisic acid catabolism with mesenchymal damage from brownish-black pigment deposits.

Pathogenesis: A homogentisic acid dioxygenase deficiency blocks renal excretion of homogentisic acid. This acid oxidizes in the air (primarily in the alkali range, hence the name) to a brownish-black quinonoid pigment. In the body, a polymeric quinonoid pigment is formed by p-diphenol oxidase. This pigment diffuses into tissue rich in collagen fibers such as cartilage (► A). Pigment deposits (► B1) on collagen fibrils (► B2) result in dark brown tissue discoloration and degeneration of connective tissue.

Morphology: Cartilage tissue with patches of dark brown pigment (► C) leads to loss of articular cartilage, with resulting arthritis and joint stiffening (p. 114). The intervertebral disks (► E, F), tendons, aorta (► D), heart valves, and sclerae also exhibit brown discoloration.

+ Clinical presentation: Inherited autosomal recessive disorder occurring with greater frequency where intermarriage is prevalent. Diagnosis by inspection is made on finding black urine spots in the underwear.

---

[1] Alkaptonuria: alkali-hapto from Arabic *al-kalii,* calcined ash + Greek *haptein,* fasten + Greek *uron,* urine.

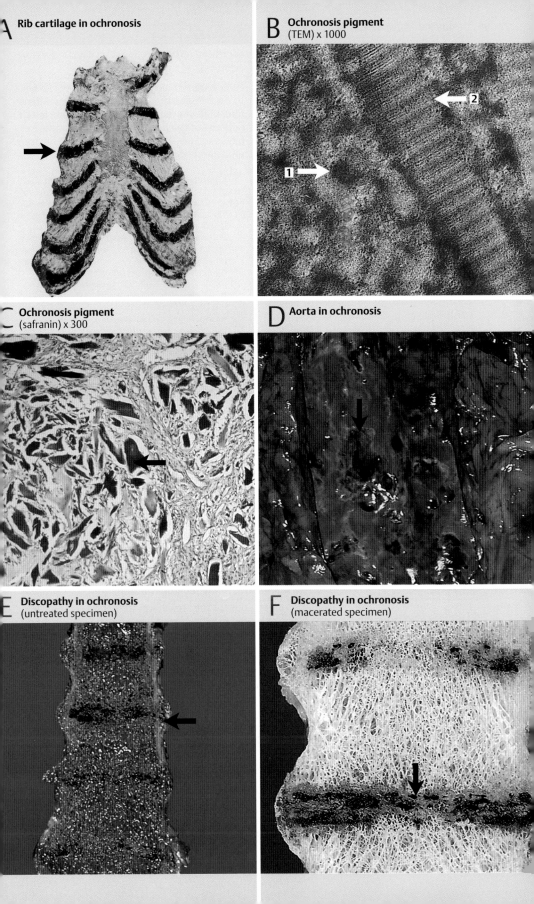

A Rib cartilage in ochronosis

B Ochronosis pigment
(TEM) × 1000

C Ochronosis pigment
(safranin) × 300

D Aorta in ochronosis

E Discopathy in ochronosis
(untreated specimen)

F Discopathy in ochronosis
(macerated specimen)

■ **Maple Syrup Urine Disease**

Synonym: branched chain ketonuria.

Definition: Genetically heterogeneous group of disorders (five different phenotypes) due to deranged metabolism of branched chain amino acids.

Pathogenesis: Reduced oxidative decarboxylation of the branched chain amino acids (valine, leucine, and isoleucine) following transamination or oxidative deamination results in accumulation of these amino acids and their α-keto and α-hydroxy acids. It also causes massive metabolic acidosis, which blocks other enzymes. This disrupts the transport of numerous monoamino monocarboxylic acids in the renal tubules and bowel.

✚ **Clinical presentation and morphology:**
– *Brain:* Impaired myelination causes astrocytosis and spongiform degeneration of the white matter. This in turn results in impaired cerebral motor function with susceptibility to convulsions and mental status changes.
– *Urine* smells like maple syrup or sweet soup seasonings.
– *Skin:* Impaired intestinal absorption produces a grayish-white mottling of the skin such as in pellagra.

❗ **Note:** *Pellagra* is a grayish-white and brownish mottled skin change resulting from a nicotinic acid deficiency.

■ **Primary Hyperoxaluria**

Synonym: oxalosis.

Definition: Group of diseases with hereditary enzyme defects of glycine metabolism which lead to urinary tract calculi due to increased renal excretion of oxalate.

Two types are differentiated according to the respective enzyme defect:

Type I primary hyperoxaluria: This is based upon a mutation of that chaperone* responsible for the "installation" of functionally-efficient alanine-glyoxalate-aminotransferase into the peroxisomes. The enzyme is instead built into the mitochondria, and the transanimation of glyoxalate to glycine is blocked. The result is the production of oxalate, which appears with glycolate in the urine (glycolic aciduria).

Type II primary hyperoxaluria: Deficient d-glycerate dehydrogenase causes accumulation of β-hydroxy pyruvate. This leads to reduction of this substance by lactate dehydrogenase to l-glycerate and in excretion in the urine. This reduction process is enzymatically coupled with the oxidation of glyoxylate to oxalate, resulting in creased renal excretion of oxalate (l-glycerate aciduria).

Pathogenesis: Calcium oxalate is poorly soluble in neutral and slightly alkali pH ranges. Therefore, high concentrations of oxalate precipitate deposits of calcium oxalate crystals in the kidney, skeletal system, bone marrow, myocardium, and testes.

✚ **Clinical presentation and morphology:** The most significant consequences of crystallized oxalate occur in the interstitial tissue of the kidney (► A, B).
– *Stones* (oxalate stones) due to oxaluria lead to pyelonephritis (p. 214).
– *Damage to the tubules:* Absorption and crystallization of oxalate (► D) damages the epithelia of the proximal tubules (► C1) leading to subsequent thickening of the basement membrane (► C2).
– *Foreign-body inflammation:* Deposits of double refractive rosette-shaped oxalate crystals (► E) in the interstitium and vascular walls cause chronic foreign-body inflammation (p. 236) with absorptive multinuclear giant cells (► E2). This leads to tubular and interstitial inflammation of the renal parenchyma (pyelonephritis), in turn causing inflammatory parenchymal shrinkage leading to renal insufficiency.
– *Extrarenal organ manifestations:* Oxalate deposits in the myocardium, joints, and bone marrow lead to chronic inflammation and myocarditis, and metabolic arthritis with joint stiffness.

■ **Type I Homocystinuria**

Definition: Hereditary metabolic disorder of mesenchymal tissue producing the clinical triad of ectopia lentis, long limbs, and cardiovascular lesions.

Homocystinuria belongs to the group of disorders of sulfurous amino acid metabolism.

Pathogenesis: A presumably multifactorial cystathionine synthetase deficiency leads to accumulation of homocystine and methionine. Cystine and cysteine must be obtained exogenously. The resulting formation of enzyme-blocking homocystine metabolites damages mesenchymal and vascular tissues by disrupting biosynthesis of collagen and elastin and also causes brain damage.

✚ **Clinical presentation and morphology:** Common inherited autosomal recessive disorder.
– *Eyes:* ocular pathology with subluxation of the lens.
– *Arteries:* Myocyte atrophy, fragmentation of the elastica, and endothelial necrosis with recurrent thrombi (p. 406) lead to peripheral circulatory disruption.
– *Skeletal system:* Osteoporosis (p. 126) and symptoms resembling Marfan's syndrome are present.
– *Brain:* Reduced myelination leads to mental retardation.

---

* chaperone: the protein responsible for the pleating and transport of a protein to its intracellular destination.

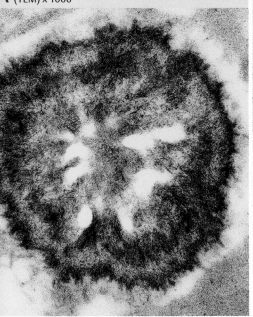

A Crystallized oxalate
(TEM) x 1000

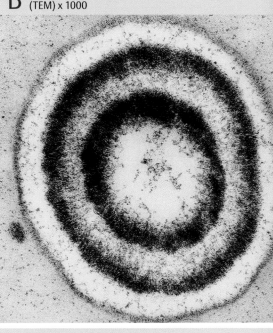

B Crystallized oxalate
(TEM) x 1000

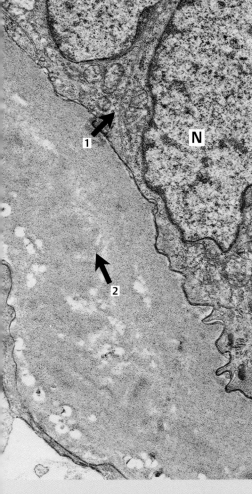

C Renal tubulus in oxalosis
(TEM) x 300 (N=nucleus)

N

1

2

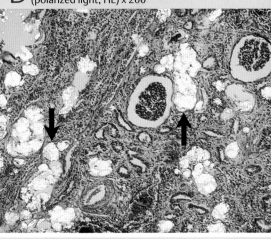

D Kidney in oxalosis
(polarized light, HE) x 200

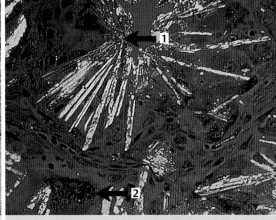

E Kidney in oxalosis
(polarized light, HE) x 400

1

2

▪ Cystinuria

Definition: Hereditary disorder of the renal tubules with urolithiasis due to deficient cystine transport.

Cystinuria belongs to the group of disorders of sulfurous amino acid metabolism.

Pathogenesis: A mutation in the gene of a membrane transport protein for dibasic amino acids causes reduced reabsorption of cystine (and lysine, arginine, and ornithine) in the kidney. As these amino acids are absorbed primarily in the intestinal tract, no deficiency symptom develops. This results in urine that is supersaturated with cystine. The cystine crystallizes (► A) and forms cystine stones, leading to nephrolithiasis and/or urinary tract cystolithiasis (p. 138). This in turn leads to crystalline deposits in the interstitium and an inflammatory foreign-body reaction with enlargement of the interstitium and tubules.

✚ Clinical presentation: Tubular and interstitial parenchymal inflammation (pyelonephritis) leads to inflammatory parenchymal shrinkage and eventually to renal insufficiency.

▪ Cystinosis

Synonym: Cystine storage disease.

Definition: Lysosomal storage disease with Fanconi syndrome (see note).

Cystinosis belongs to the group of disorders of sulfurous amino acid metabolism.

Pathogenesis: Based on a mutation of the CTNS-gene's defective carrier protein, which ensures the transport of the "sulphurated amino acid" cystine through the lysosome membrane. Due to this dysfunction many body cells, especially granulocytes, contain abnormally high concentrations of cystine in their lysosomes (► C1). This leads to storage of crystals (► C2, D) and deposits of L-cystine crystals in the interstitium.

Morphology: Hexagonal deposits of cystine crystals occur in the kidney, cornea, and organs of the macrophage system (► B). In the kidney, the hexagonal deposits of cystine crystals primarily lie in interstitial histiocytes. This successively leads to an inflammatory foreign-body reaction (p. 236), tubular and interstitial parenchymal inflammation (pyelonephritis), and parenchymal shrinkage. Only isolated crystalline deposits occur in the epithelium of the proximal tubule, podocytes, mesangium cells, and vascular epithelia. A "swan-neck deformity" of the proximal tubules with flattened epithelia is typically present. The crystalline deposits are discernible upon macroscopic examination of a cross section (► E) and plain tissue specimen of the spleen (► F).

✚ Clinical presentation: Inherited autosomal recessive disorder.

– *Nephropathy:* Impaired reabsorption of glucose, phosphate, and amino acids in the proximal renal tubule manifests itself in the form of Fanconi syndrome with amino aciduria (amino acid diabetes), phosphaturia, and glucosuria.

– *Osteopathy:* Nephropathy leads to secondary hyperparathyroidism with vitamin D refractory rachitis, an enchondral ossification disorder with impaired mineralization and cartilage resorption. This results in widening of the growth plates and dwarfism.

– *Corneal symptoms:* Cystine crystals in the cornea cause opacification that leads to visual impairment and photophobia.

❗ Note: Fanconi syndrome:
Definition: A group of transport disorders of the renal tubules with amino aciduria, phosphaturia, glucosuria, and uricosuria.
Occurence:
– In hereditary tubular disorders such as
  – Cystinosis,
  – Glycogenosis,
  – Galactosemia,
  – Wilson disease, and
  – Coproporphyrinuria;
– It also occurs in acquired tubular disorders such as
  – the effects of tubular toxins (mercury, lead, and decayed tetracycline) and
  – Paraprotein nephrosis.

Urea Synthesis Disorders

General pathogenesis: Breakdown of amino acids in the body releases ammonia. A cytotoxin for many types of cells (especially ganglion cells and astrocytes), ammonia must be catabolized by enzymes to nontoxic urea, which can be readily excreted. This detoxification process involves five liver enzymes:
— Carbamyl phosphate synthase;
— Ornithine carbamyl transferase;
— Arginine succinate synthase;
— Arginine succinate lyase;
— Arginase.

Each of these enzymes can be impaired in its activity by a rare genetic defect, thereby blocking urea synthesis.

General morphology: All cases examined to date exhibit ganglion cell death with glial proliferation and spongiosis.

✚ General clinical presentation:
– *Blood:* It exhibits a greatly increased level of ammonia.
– *Brain* symptoms include mental and physical developmental disorders and neurologic symptoms.

A Cystinuria
(polarized light) x 350

B Liver in cystinosis
(polarized light) x 50

C Histiocyte in cystinosis (cross-section)
(TEM) x 8000

D Histiocyte in cystinosis (longitudinal section)
(TEM) x 8000

E Spleen in cystinosis (cross section)

F Spleen in cystinosis
(crush preparation; polarized light x 25)

Nucleotides

Hyperuricemia

General definition: Group of disorders with high serum uric acid levels due to impaired purine metabolism (gout).

■ Primary Gout

General definition: Familial disorders of purine metabolism with clinical symptoms resulting from urate deposits in tissue.

The following forms of primary gout are differentiated according to the age of the patient:

▨ Infantile Gout

Synonym: Lesch-Nyhan syndrome.

Definition: Hereditary defect of hypoxanthine guanine phosphoribosyltransferase with renal and cerebral symptoms.

Pathogenesis: A hypoxanthine deficiency due to the above-mentioned enzyme defect causes reactive disinhibition of purine synthesis, leading to hyperuricemia.

> ✚ **Clinical presentation and morphology:** Rare X-linked recessive hereditary disorder affecting males only.
> – *Kidney* symptoms include gout nephropathy (see below).
> – *Brain* symptoms occur without visible lesions.
>   – These include impaired cerebral motor function with spastic quadriplegia (upper and lower extremities are affected) and athetosis (exaggerated movements with abrupt change of muscle tone).
>   – Mental status changes include belligerence and self-mutilation.

▨ Adult Gout

Definition: A non-variable defect of purine metabolism manifests itself in gout symptoms that occur in adulthood.

Pathogenesis is usually multifactorial. A hereditary predisposition is present in the form of
— Impaired renal excretion of uric acid or
— Increased uric acid synthesis. The latter may be due to either (a) increased endogenous activity of purine base recycling enzymes with secondary disinhibition of uric acid synthesis or (b) uptake of exogenous purine bases from ingested foods.

The resulting hyperuricemia leads to crystallization of uric acid, which is phagocytized by neutrophils. The uric acid damages their lysosomal membranes, causing release of proteases that set in motion a variety of mediators that mutually intensify the inflammatory reaction.

These include: factor XII; kallikrein and kinin systems; complement system. These factors produce painful inflammatory attacks.

> �ⓘ **Note:** Gout attacks do not occur without neutrophils.

■ Sequelae of Adult Gout

▨ Gouty Arthritis

Definition: Acute episodic joint inflammation induced by deposits of urate crystals.

Pathogenesis: Deposits of water-soluble, negatively birefringent, fan-shaped urate crystals (► A, B1) form in the connective tissue of the lower extremity, most commonly in the synovia of the metatarsophalangeal joint of the great toe (► A). Resembling pumice in cross section, the nodular aggregations of these crystals induce a foreign-body inflammation (► B3; p. 236) with giant cells (► B2), producing what are referred to as tophi. Urate deposits in the articular cartilage and in chondral bone later come to resemble a coat of plaster (► C) in their macroscopic appearance. Late sequelae include inflammatory destruction of cartilage and bone, and tophi that break through the skin and spill their viscous contents.

> ✚ **Clinical presentation:** Sudden onset of painful erythema and swelling in only one joint (► E) with asymptomatic intervals lasting for years. Affected sites include, in descending order of frequency, the great toe (podagra), knee (gonagra), and fingers (chiragra).

> ⓘ **Note:** *Pseudogout* is a joint disorder simulating gout that is caused by deposits of calcium pyrophosphate crystals.

▨ Chronic Urate Nephropathy

Synonym: gouty nephropathy.

Definition: Destructive tubular and interstitial nephritis due to urate deposits.

Pathogenesis: Urate deposits in the collecting tubules and intertubular stroma produce grayish yellow papillary stripes (urate infarctions; ► D). Sequelae include:
— *Foreign-body inflammation with giant cells* leads to destructive tubular and interstitial inflammation (pyelonephritis) with parenchymal shrinkage and renal insufficiency.
— *Reactive proliferation of the mesangium* leads to gouty glomerular hyalinization, which causes hypertension (p. 388). Urate stones occur in 20% of all cases (p. 138).

■ Secondary Gout

Definition: Late sequela of another known metabolic disorder, such as a
— *Glucose-6-phosphatase deficiency* (von Gierke disease; p. 75) with inhibition of excretion of uric acid or
— *Cellular disintegration* with formation of excessive amounts of uric acid. This latter condition can occur in: leukemia; hemolytic anemia; tumor chemotherapy; chronic renal insufficiency leading to reduced excretion of uric acid.

A Gouty tophus
(HE) x 75

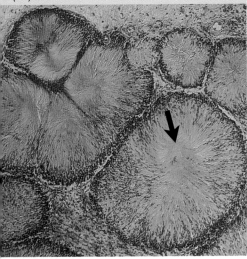

B Gouty tophus
(HE) (polarized light) x 150

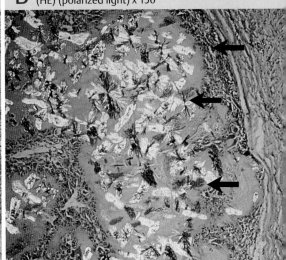

Gouty joint

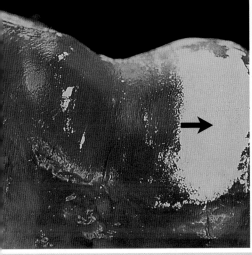

D Gouty nephropathy

Podagra

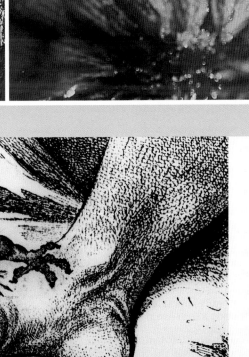

6 Pigment Lesions

Summary

Pigments are substances whose intrinsic color makes them recognizable in living tissue. They are either synthesized within the body itself (endogenous pigments) or are introduced into the body (exogenous pigments). They may be inert and, ignored by the body, lie on or within tissue. Alternatively, they may act on the body as foreign or poisonous substances, eliciting an inflammatory reaction (p. 194).

▶ **Exogenous pigments** in the form of cosmetic allergens or local discoloration around metallic implants are of secondary importance in a clinical setting.

▶ **Endogenous pigments** have important biologic functions. Disorders of their synthesis or breakdown can have far-reaching consequences, as the most important of these substances either catalyze several steps in metabolism or certain steps in sensory physiology. Due to their intrinsic color, their absence or overabundance is a sign of tissue damage. The following groups of pigments are differentiated according to their origin:

— **Hematogenous pigments** may contain iron. They can be associated with defective porphyrin synthesis (porphyria), which is accompanied by photodermatosis, liver damage, and occasionally anemia. They can also be associated with blockage of some stage of the metabolism and excretion of bilirubin. The bilirubin accumulation in blood manifests itself clinically as jaundice (icterus). The hematogenous pigments also include the malaria pigment.

— **Tyrosine derivative pigments** in the form of cutaneous melanin act as a natural sunscreen. Neuromelanin defects lead to neurologic and sensory deficits such as Parkinson's disease, retinitis pigmentosa (blindness), and Waardenburg syndrome (inner ear deafness).

— **Lipogenous pigments** only have potential pathologic significance in the form of visual purple (rhodopsin), whereas lipofuscin and ceroid are color indicators of tissue damage.

Exogenous Pigments

Cosmetic Pigments

Tattooing (▶ A, B) introduces carbon, ink, or cinnabar (red mercuric sulfide) into the skin. These substances are phagocytized, resulting in deposits in connective tissue and transport of substances to the nearest lymph node.

Occupational Toxin Pigments

▬ **Anthracosis:** Nodular black discoloration of the lungs (▶ C, D) with inhaled carbon dust (coal dust or cigarette smoke). The substances are phagocytized by alveolar macrophages and removed via the lymph vessels. The condition is common.

The same process occurs with the ferrous dusts inhaled by workers at steel and/or ceramics factories.

▬ **Plumbism:** Chronic lead poisoning (p. 142) causes this condition. Pathogens stimulating decomposition in the pockets of the gums (periodontitis) transform lead into lead sulfide, producing a halo-like deposits in the gingiva.

▬ **Chalcosis:** Exhaust gases containing copper and dusts from the copper processing industry cause green discoloration of the hair. The disorder is rare.

Iatrogenic Pigments

▬ **Argyria:** Long-term administration of medications containing silver leads to gray tissue discoloration. The disorder is rare.

▬ **Amalgam:** Chronic abrasion of mercury-containing tooth fillings produces grayish blue mucosal discoloration (▶ E) with metal deposits in the mucosal stroma (▶ F). This disorder is common.

▬ **Tetracycline:** Integration of the substance in bone and teeth in children leads to irreversible yellow discoloration.

▬ **Carotene:** Overfeeding the newborn with carrots leads to storage of carotene, causing yellowish-orange discoloration of the skin and fatty tissue.

Ingestion of cosmetics containing beta carotene to change the color tone of the skin can have the same effect.

Skin tattoo

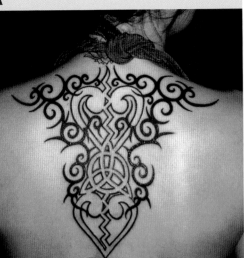

B Skin tattoo

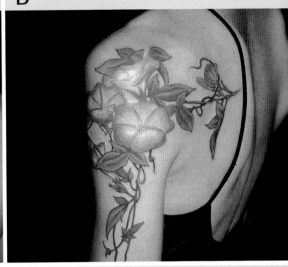

Lung in anthracosis

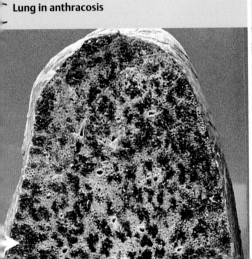

D Lung in anthracosis
(HE) x 100

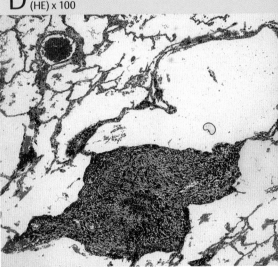

Gingiva in amalgam carrier

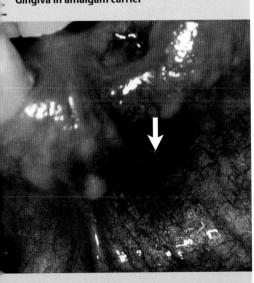

F Gingiva in amalgam carrier
(HE) x 150

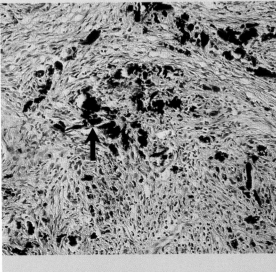

Endogenous Pigments

Hematogenous Pigments

Porphyria

General definition: This group of diseases involves atypical types of porphyria and alternating skin, liver, and blood damage due to defective porphyrin synthesis. Primary porphyria result from congenital enzyme defects, secondary porphyria from toxic enzyme blockages.

General pathogenesis: Atypical metabolites of heme synthesis (porphyrin) are created. Some of these are excreted in the stool and in urine. Symptoms depend on the type of porphyrin involved and may include red discoloration; there are intralysomal porphyrin deposits erythroblasts, and in epidermal, cartilaginons and bone cells, and liver cells → brown discoloration.

■ Congenital Erythropoietic Porphyria

Definition: Prototype of a congenital porphyria, also called Günther's disease.

Morphology:
— *Skin:* Exposure to light creates peroxide radicals from stored porphyrins. These damage epidermal cells, leading to photodermatosis that begins with bullous lesions and separation of the epidermis above the basement membrane (varicelliform hydroa; ► B). These lesions heal with scarring, accompanied by hyperpigmentation and hypertrichosis (facial hair).
— *Bone and cartilage:* Porphyrin storage leads to cell damage and tissue destruction with deformities of the face (nose), hands, and outer ears (► A).
— *Teeth:* Porphyrin storage and the action of ultraviolet light cause red teeth (erythrodontia).
— *Blood:* Erythroblasts laden with atypical porphyrins result in reduced osmotic resistance. This in turn leads to hemolytic anemia, usually with normal coloration and erythrocytes (cardinal clinical symptom).
— *Liver:* Catalase, which catalyzes hydrogen peroxide, is greatly reduced among hepatic porphyrins. This causes liver cell damage with fatty degeneration and focal cell necrosis (p. 128) and in turn aggressive hepatitis. This leads to portal fibrosis and, in some cases, liver cirrhosis (p. 42). Iron cannot be incorporated into heme and is stored in the liver (hepatic siderosis).

✚ **Clinical presentation:** Symptoms presented by Count Dracula and the werewolf well illustrate congenital erythropoietic porphyria.

Note: The *"Dracula syndrome"* includes daytime sleep (photophobia), "bloody" teeth (erythrodontia), and deathly paleness (anemia). The *"werewolf syndrome"* includes facial hair (hypertrichosis), "bloody" teeth (erythrodontia), and missing nose and fingers (mutilation).

Hemoglobin Breakdown Pigments

Hematoidin:
Definition: Nonferrous, reddish brown pigment containing pyrrole (indirect bilirubin).

Pathogenesis: Macrophages are unable to approach erythrocytes in the center of a hemorrhage. The resulting disintegration of hemoglobin results in the release of iron and crystallization of residual material containing pyrrole rings (► C). The disorder takes three weeks to develop.

Note: Where hemoglobin is broken down, green *biliverdin* and then yellow *bilirubin* are created. This color change may be observed in hematomas.

Hemosiderin:
Definition: Ferrous, yellowish brown pigment that is free of pyrrole (siderin).

Pathogenesis: Requiring 2 days to develop, the substance forms only in living cells that also store the phagocytized iron in this form, i.e., cells of the reticuloendothelial system. This produces brown discoloration in the storage tissue (► D, E).

Note: Hemosiderin is a product of living cells.

Hematin:
Definition: Blackish-brown pigment.

Pathogenesis: The substance develops in an upper gastrointestinal hemorrhage when the hemoglobin comes into contact with hydrochloric acid (► F). Therefore vomited blood is black (hematemesis).

Hematozoidin:
Definition: Brownish-gray malarial pigment (partially crystallized hematin).

Pathogenesis: The substance is formed by the living malaria pathogen (Plasmodium; p. 278) in erythrocyte parasitism and is stored in cells of the reticuloendothelial system (► G).

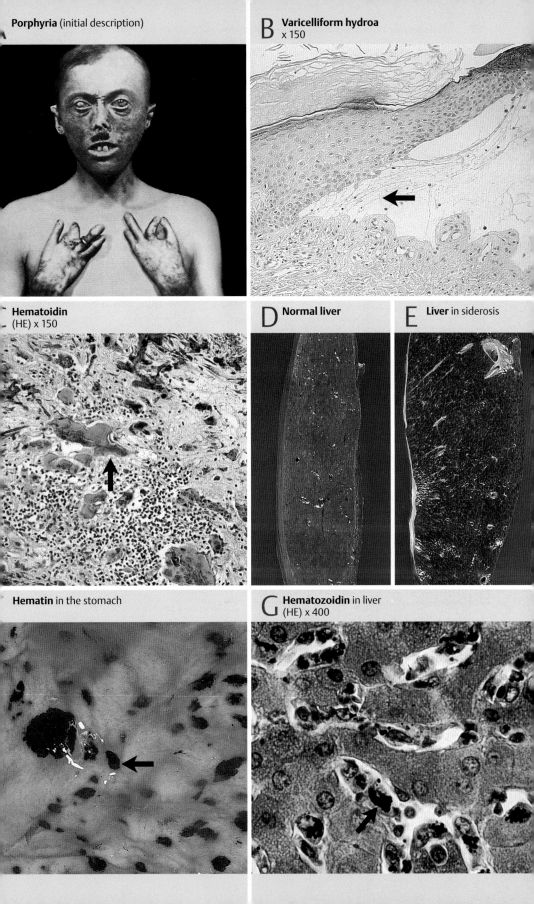

A Porphyria (initial description)

B Varicelliform hydroa
x 150

C Hematoidin
(HE) x 150

D Normal liver

E Liver in siderosis

F Hematin in the stomach

G Hematozoidin in liver
(HE) x 400

Hyperbilirubinemia

General definition: The cardinal symptom is jaundice with yellow discoloration of the skin (► A), sclera, soft palate, and internal organs (► E, F).

General etiologic factors of hyperbilirubinemia may be isolated or occur in combination and include:
— An oversupply of bilirubin to the cells;
— A defect in the transport or uptake of bilirubin in the liver cells;
— Defective bilirubin conjugation in the liver;
— Defective excretion of conjugated bilirubin from the liver cells into the biliary canaliculi;
— Intrahepatic or extrahepatic cholestasis (p. 110).

The following section describes the most important types of hyperbilirubinemia together with the physiologic sequence of bilirubin catabolism.

Bilirubin catabolism (beginning): Catabolism of the heme from hemoglobin, myoglobin, and cytochromes yields bilirubin. This process is increased in all disorders involving hemolysis or myolysis (hemolytic jaundice). It begins in the cells of the reticuloendothelial system in which hemoxygenase oxidizes the heme to biliverdin. In another step, biliverdin reductase reduces the biliverdin to bilirubin. This bilirubin is practically insoluble (indirect bilirubin) and is excreted by cells of the reticuloendothelial system into the bloodstream, where each albumin molecule binds two bilirubin molecules.

■ Excessive Bilirubin Production

▦ Hemolysis

Pathogenesis: Etiologic factors:
— *Hemolysis* (erythrocyte disintegration) involves massive premature destruction of erythrocytes due to membrane, enzyme, or hemoglobin defects, or due to mechanical, toxic, immunologic, or microbial damage. The resulting increased breakdown of erythrocytes in the spleen causes spent erythrocytes to accumulate in the sinus (► C); the sinus epithelia contain iron due to the phagocytosis of erythrocytes (► D).
— *Breakdown of hematomas* from bleeding into tissue results in extravascular erythrocyte destruction, which produces increased quantities of bilirubin (► B).

Result: The liver's capacity for glucuronidation is exceeded, as is often its capacity to transport glucuronidated bilirubin. This results in hyperbilirubinemia.

▦ Primary Shunt Hyperbilirubinemia

Synonym: chronic unconjugated hyperbilirubinemia without hemolysis.

Definition: Hereditary disorder of bilirubin metabolism prior to actual heme catabolism.

Pathogenesis: A defect of erythropoiesis with inefficient integration of hemoglobin causes premature destruction of abnormal erythroblasts. This results in the breakdown of heme shortly before synthesis.

✚ Clinical presentation: This very rare autosomal recessive disorder usually manifests itself at puberty. Symptoms include varying jaundice with unconjugated hyperbilirubinemia and signs of compensated hemolysis.

Bilirubin catabolism (continued): The bilirubin albumin gets into the liver, where a carrier system actively transports it into the hepatocytes. In the cytosol, bilirubin binds to the binding proteins ligandin, Y protein and Z protein.

■ Defective Bilirubin Uptake

▦ Gilbert Syndrome

Definition and pathogenesis: Hereditary hyperbilirubinemia due to defective bilirubin uptake into the hepatocytes from blood and reduced activity of bilirubin uridine diphosphate glucuronyl transferase.

Morphology: Liver histology reveals no pathologic findings.

✚ Clinical presentation: This rare disorder is characterized by episodic onset of unconjugated hyperbilirubinemia. Stress can trigger episodes of jaundice.

Bilirubin catabolism (continued): Bilirubin is conjugated (i.e., glucuronidated) in the smooth endoplasmic reticulum of the liver cells by the action of glucuronyl transferase. This makes bilirubin soluble in water compatible with bile (direct bilirubin).

■ Defective Bilirubin Conjugation

▦ Crigler-Najjar Syndrome

Definition and pathogenesis: Hereditary deficiency of bilirubin uridine diphosphate glucuronyl transferase.

✚ Clinical presentation: This is a rare autosomal recessive disorder. Complete absence of the enzyme manifests itself as kernicterus (bilirubin encephalopathy) and leads to death in neonates.

▦ Neonatal Jaundice

Definition and pathogenesis: Underdeveloped enzyme leads to a relative deficiency of bilirubin uridine diphosphate glucuronyl transferase due to transient hyperbilirubinemia on the second through fifth day after birth. The disorder is common.

❗ Note: In *subclinical hyperbilirubinemia,* serum bilirubin 1.0 mg/dl; in *jaundice,* serum bilirubin 2.0 mg/dl.

❗ Note: The definition of *cholestasis* varies according to specialty:
– Morphology: bile retention in the bile ducts.
– Physiology: impaired bile drainage.
– Clinical presentation: retention of substances normally eliminated with the bile.

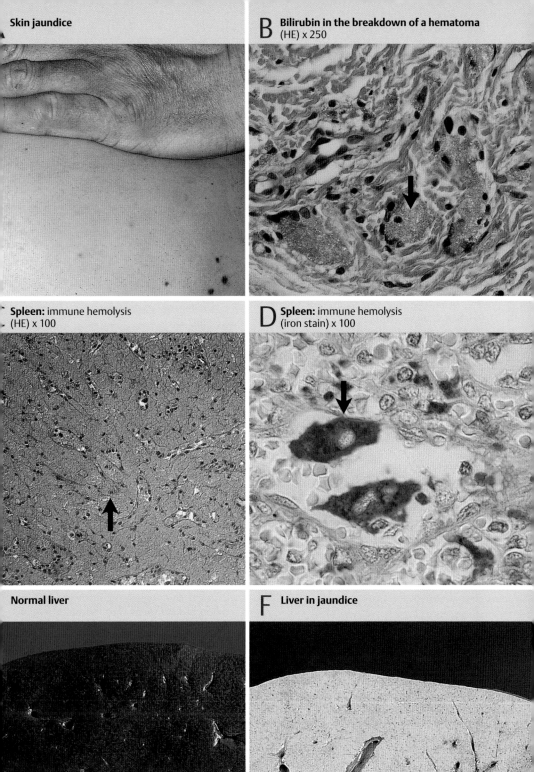

A | **Skin jaundice**

B | **Bilirubin in the breakdown of a hematoma** (HE) x 250

C | **Spleen: immune hemolysis** (HE) x 100

D | **Spleen: immune hemolysis** (iron stain) x 100

E | **Normal liver**

F | **Liver in jaundice**

6

Pigment Lesions

Bilirubin catabolism (continued): The bilirubin glucuronide (direct bilirubin) is excreted into the biliary canaliculi by a system of active transport whose excretion capacity is low compared with the capacity for glucuronidation.

■ Defective Bilirubin Excretion

▦ Dubin-Johnson Syndrome

Definition: A hereditary excretion defect of the liver for bilirubin and other organic anions. This syndrome is caused by an autosomal recessive mutation of the canalicular conjugate export pump (MRP-2 protein) for bilirubin and related anions. Result: bilirubin is conjugated in SER, then regurgitated back into the blood, as the necessary transport protein system is deficient (= microsomal conjugated bilirubinemia). This is accompanied by an excretion disorder of catecholamine metabolites. The complexing of the latter yields a brownish-black pigment (= atypical adrenochrome) which is deposited together with lipofuscin in telolysosomes around the biliary ducts.
Result: The liver parenchyma reveals grayish-black discoloration (► A).

✚ **Clinical presentation:** This rare inherited autosomal recessive disorder exhibits variable penetration. Jaundice of varying severity is present. Symptoms are minimal. Patients tend to develop gallstones and generally have normal life expectancy.

▦ Rotor Syndrome

Definition and pathogenesis: This hereditary bilirubin excretion defect results in chronically fluctuating, direct hyperbilirubinemia as in Dubin-Johnson syndrome but without liver discoloration.

✚ **Clinical presentation:** Rare inherited autosomal recessive disorder exhibiting fluctuating jaundice. Symptoms are minimal, and patients generally have normal life expectancy.

Bilirubin catabolism (end): The bilirubin glucuronide in the bile passes through the bile ducts and enters the bowel.

▦ Hepatocellular Jaundice

Pathogenesis: Defective excretion of bilirubin in the diseased liver, in which conjugated bilirubin is presumably regurgitated from the liver cells into the blood plasma by a yet unknown mechanism.

▦ Intralobular Intrahepatic Cholestasis

Pathogenesis: Defective hepatocellular excretion of bilirubin. Causes include:
— Toxic cholestasis;
— Hepatitic cholestasis;
— Gestational cholestasis;
— Postoperative cholestasis;
— Cholestasis due to venostasis.

Morphology resembles the mechanical forms of jaundice (extralobular intrahepatic cholestasis and extrahepatic cholestasis).

▦ Extralobular Intrahepatic Cholestasis

Pathogenesis: Destructive cholangitis or cirrhotic liver changes (p. 42) destroy the intrahepatic bile drainage routes. This in turn disrupts the intrahepatic passage of bile, resulting in intrahepatic obstructive jaundice.

▦ Extrahepatic Cholestasis

Pathogenesis: Gallstones (p. 138), tumors, inflammatory strictures, or biliary tract deformities result in the mechanical blockage of bile excretion, resulting in occlusive jaundice.

Morphology: Greenish cylinders of bile (bile thrombi), occasionally resembling antlers, are observed in expanded intracellular canaliculi. This is accompanied by droplets of bile in the hepatic epithelia, progressing from the center to periphery of the lobes. Extrahepatic obstructive jaundice leads to accumulation of bile in the periphery of the lobes, with bile excretion from the ductuli. This has several repercussions:
— Greenish discoloration of the liver parenchyma (► C) occurs.
— Damage to the hepatic and biliary epithelia successively results in hepatocyte degeneration (ballooning, p. 12; ► B2), bile infarction and necrosis, phagocytosis of the excreted bile droplets by astrocytes, infiltration of histiocytes into the portal regions, and elimination of the necrotic tissue.
— Ductuli from interrupted biliary ducts proliferate into the portal regions.

✚ **Clinical complications** of cholestasis:
– *Secondary biliary liver cirrhosis:* Persistent cholestasis causes cell necrosis to spread from the portal region to the central vein (portal vein necrosis). This causes cirrhotic liver changes, producing a hardened, green liver with a nodular cross section (► D).
– *Cholemic nephrosis:* Accumulation of bile pigment in the lumens of the renal tubules leads to formation of greenish yellow tubule excretions, resulting in cylinders of bile (► E) and green discoloration of the renal parenchyma (► F, G).

❗ **Note:** Bile cylinders in renal tubules are the result, not the cause, of kidney failure due to previous liver damage.

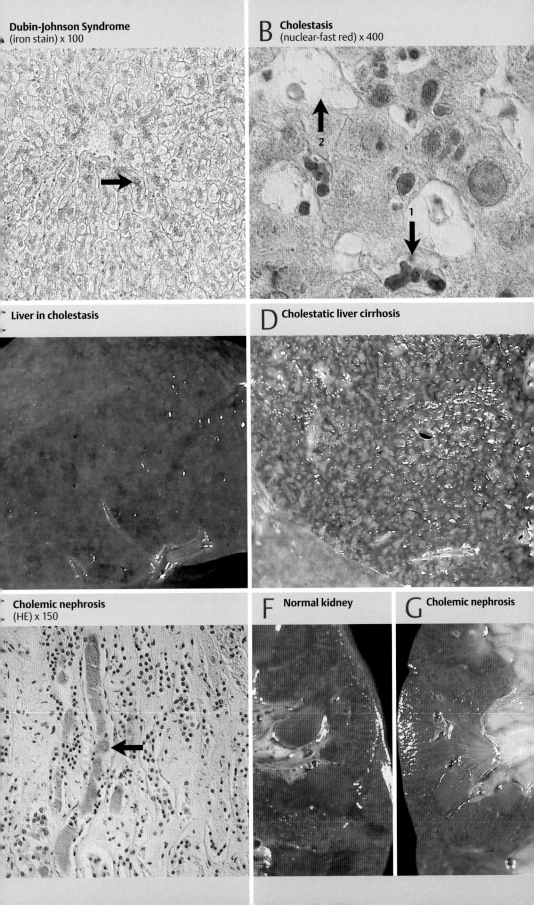

Dubin-Johnson Syndrome
(iron stain) x 100

B **Cholestasis**
(nuclear-fast red) x 400

Liver in cholestasis

D **Cholestatic liver cirrhosis**

Cholemic nephrosis
(HE) x 150

F **Normal kidney**

G **Cholemic nephrosis**

Tyrosine-Derivative Pigments

Cutaneous Melanin

Physiology: Melanin is a brownish-black pigment. It is generated in the form of small granules in normal melanocytes and in melanoma cells (▶ B; p. 366).

The following section examines the most important melanin disorders together with the physiologic process of melanin formation (melanogenesis).

Melanogenesis (beginning): Melanin formation begins in the melanoblasts of the neural crest. Beginning in the eighth week of pregnancy, they form families of cells that migrate in a mosaic-like pattern initially into the epidermis and later into the hair follicles.

■ Vitiligo

Definition: Rare, focal absence of skin pigmentation (zebra effect).

Pathogenesis: The genetically determined death of certain melanoblasts (apoptosis p. 128, 132) leads to areas devoid of melanoblasts.

Melanogenesis (continued ▶ A): Melanoblasts differentiate in the skin into melanocytes. Requirements for melanogenesis include:
— Ribosomal synthesis of tyrosinase, which is controlled by a gene in the albino locus.
— Transport of tyrosinase into the cisterns of the rough endoplasmic reticulum (▶ A1).
— Active membrane transport of tyrosine into the melanocytes (▶ A2).

The tyrosinase enters the Golgi apparatus (▶ A3) and is packaged together with the tyrosine in melanosomes (▶ A4). There the melanin is synthesized. Synthesis is controlled by tyrosinase (phenol oxidase); the sequence is tyrosine to dopa to dopaquinone to indole quinone to polymerization and protein binding.

■ Albinism *(pathogenesis p. 96)*

✚ **Clinical presentation:** Extreme sensitivity to sunlight leads to skin tumors induced by ultraviolet radiation (p. 150), impaired vision, and photophobia. Prenatal diagnosis is made by amniocentesis.

Melanogenesis (continued): This process can be inhibited or stimulated according to the cell cycle. In the G1 phase, tyrosinase activation (ACTH and estrogens) results in increased melanin synthesis. In the G2 phase, melanotropin (MSH) stimulates melanin synthesis. Inhibitors of the tyrosinase system include melatonin (epiphyseal hormone), phenylalanine, and glutathione.

■ Hemochromatosis (p. 72)

Inactivation of glutathione by non-protein-bound iron leads to disinhibition of the tyrosinase system and increased melanin synthesis. The result is brown skin.

■ Addison's Disease

Definition: This common disorder involves an adrenal cortex insufficiency syndrome with glucocorticoid deficiency (hypocorticism).

Etiologic forms of Addison's disease:
— *Primary or adrenal forms* involve hereditary (metabolic disorder or deformity), inflammatory (autoimmune or tuberculous), neoplastic, circulatory, or necrotic damage to the adrenal cortex.
— *Secondary or hypophyseal forms* involve hereditary (brain deformity), necrotic, or neoplastic hypophyseal damage.

▦ Primary forms:

Damage to the adrenal cortex lowers the level of glucocorticoids, androgens, and aldosterone, resulting in reactive overproduction of ACTH and MSH. This stimulates the melanocytes, which increase melanin synthesis.

✚ **Clinical presentation:** "Brown Addison" patients present with brown skin especially around the mouth, hypotension, adynamia, desiccation, and sparse pubic hair.

☺ **Prominent patient:** John F. Kennedy (1917–1963), 35th President of the United States.

▦ Secondary forms: Hypophyseal damage

lowers the level of ACTH and MSH. This depresses the level of glucocorticoids but not the level of aldosterone, which is regulated by the renin-angiotensin system. The resulting MSH deficiency means that melanocytes are not stimulated, blocking melanin synthesis.

✚ **Clinical presentation:** "White Addison" patients present with pale skin and hypotension.

■ Phenylketonuria (p. 96)

Phenylalanine hydroxylase deficiency leads to increased levels of serum phenylalanine, causing competitive inhibition of tyrosinase. This blocks melanin synthesis, causing hypopigmentation of skin, hair, and eyes.

Melanogenesis (end): The melanosomes are transported into the melanocytes in the basement membrane keratinocytes, where they pigment the skin either in an aggregated configuration in whites (▶ A5, D) or in a dispersed configuration in blacks (▶ A6, E).

Schematic diagram: melanogenesis

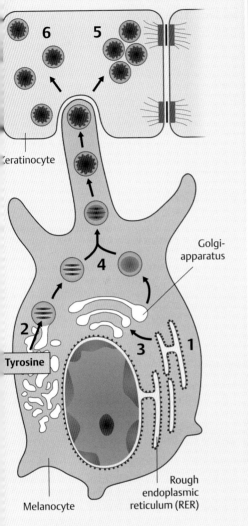

Keratinocyte

6 **5**

4

Golgi-apparatus

2

Tyrosine

3 **1**

Melanocyte

Rough endoplasmic reticulum (RER)

C **Albino patient** (and parents)

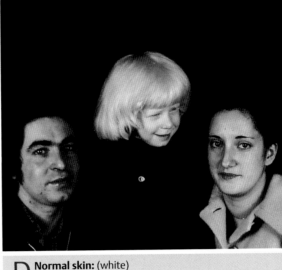

D **Normal skin:** (white)
(HE) x 100

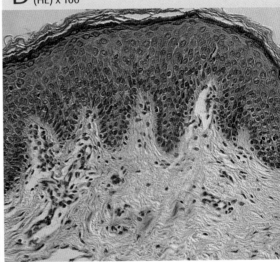

Malignant melanoma
(HE) x 400

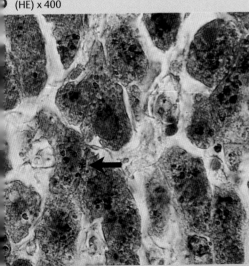

E **Normal skin:** (black)
(HE) x 100

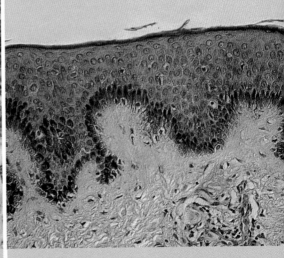

■ Melasma

Synonym: "mask of pregnancy."

Pathogenesis: Large quantities of estrogen, from oral contraceptives or during pregnancy, stimulate the melanocytes and produce a mask-like, usually reversible pattern of pigmentation around the mouth (► A).

Neuromelanin

Neuromelanin has an important function in stimulus transmission in catecholaminergic nerve cell systems. The following disorders of the brain and sensory organs are associated with a loss of neuromelanin:

— *Retinitis pigmentosa* (p. 94) leads to blindness.
— *Waardenburg syndrome:* A complex deformity syndrome involving lateral displacement of the medial margin of the eye; inner ear deafness (depigmentation of the vascular stria); pigmentation disorders of the iris, skin, and hair; and a nose shaped like parrot's beak.
— *Parkinson's disease.*

■ Parkinson's Disease

Definition: Generalized neurodegenerative disorder with defective neuromelanin synthesis and extrapyramidal symptoms.

Pathogenesis: The action of an unknown neurotoxin and/or DNA mutation cause apoptosis (p. 128, 132) of dopaminergic nerve cells containing neuromelanin, primarily in the cortical region of the substantia nigra whose axons extend to the lenticular nucleus. This causes a transmitter imbalance, with an excess of cholinergic stimuli and a deficiency of dopaminergic stimuli. The substantia nigra becomes pale (► C, D), and the released neuromelanin spreads throughout what used to be the zona nigra. This triggers pigment phagocytosis by glial cells. Cytoskeletal derangement in the nerves cells produce Lewy bodies (p. 34).

✚ **Clinical presentation:** Common hereditary or acquired disorder with a classic triad of symptoms including *tremor* (involuntary shaking), *rigor* (increased muscle tone), and *akinesis* (decrease in or lack of motion).
Early stages: Mental status changes and rigidity of the extremities.
Late stages: Partial or total loss of facial expression, drooling, loss of loud voice, propulsive and retropulsive motions (patient falls backward when attempting to stop a backward motion).

☺ **Prominent patients:**
Muhammed Ali: world heavyweight boxing champion.
Adolf Hitler (1889–1945), Austrian-born Chancellor and *Führer* of Germany.

Non-Melanin Pigments

■ Brown Colon

Pathogenesis: Chronic constipation treated with repeated use of laxatives containing anthraquinone leads to lysosomal accumulation of yellowish-brown granules in the histiocytes of the large bowel via an unknown mechanism. This pigment of fecal origin contains tyrosine and fat.

Morphology: Histiocytes with PAS-positive pigment granules in the mucosa of the colon (► E) cause brown discoloration of the mucosa of the colon (► F).

■ Alkaptonuria (p. 96)

The pigment in this disorder is derived from tyrosine. Irreversible pigment deposits in connective tissue result in dark brown tissue discoloration and degeneration of connective tissue. Hyaline joint cartilage is transformed into fibrous cartilage, resulting in mechanical abrasion of the articular cartilage and compensatory thickening of the subchondral bone (osteosclerosis). This leads to stiffening of the joints (p. 96).

Lipogenic Pigments

Lipochrome pigments:
Definition: Pigments that are ingested with food in the form of beta carotene (precursor is lycopin) and give fatty tissue the color of an egg yolk (such as the corpus luteum).

Rhodopsin:
Synonym: visual purple.

Definition: Vitamin A protein complex that helps control the vision process.

✚ **Clinical presentation:** Rhodopsin deficiency causes night blindness.

Lipofuscin (p. 28):
Definition: Autophagic, golden yellow, iron-negative, age-related pigment in parenchymal cells (► B).

Ceroid (p. 28):
Definition: Heterophagic, yellow "cellular debris" pigment in the cells of the reticuloendothelial system.

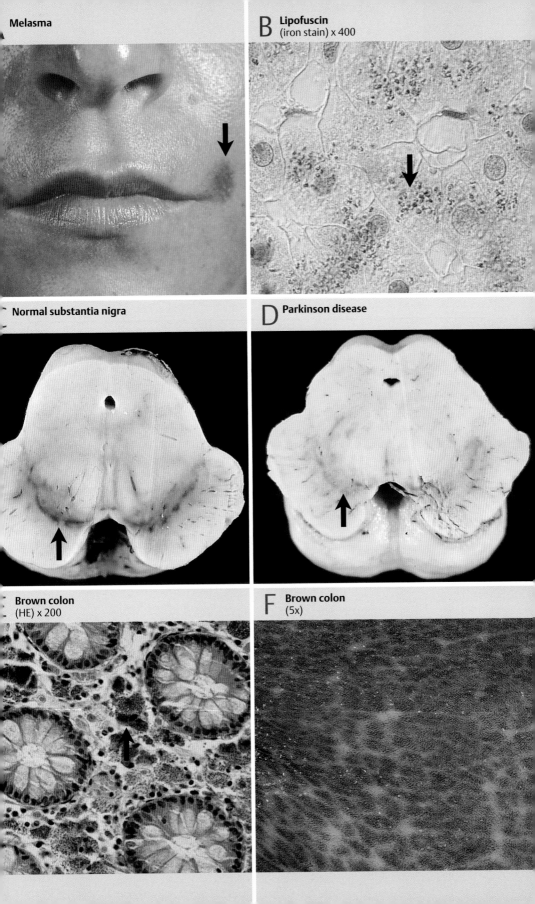

A Melasma

B Lipofuscin
(iron stain) x 400

C Normal substantia nigra

D Parkinson disease

E Brown colon
(HE) x 200

F Brown colon
(5x)

Summary

The cell responds to injuries that fail to destroy it with either increased or decreased function. This response results from changes in its metabolism of structural and functional substances and may include cell proliferation. This also applies to the term dystrophy, which harkens back to the time before biochemistry and refers to the development of weakened structures originally attributed to nutritional deficiencies, and to the term degeneration, referring to transformation of a tissue into one of lesser quality.

▶ **Adaptive response with increased function** (hypertrophy and hyperplasia): Hypertrophy results when functional internal cellular structures increase, causing the volume of the organ to increase. In hyperplasia, the expansion of the organ is also due to an increase in the number of cells. Cellular proliferation in these cases continues to follow the normal pattern of cell division and maturation. However, it is not always possible to draw a clear histologic distinction between this type of proliferation and the autonomous cell growth of a tumor.

▶ **Adaptive response with decreased function** (atrophy): This response initially manifests itself as atrophy in which a reduction in only the structural components of the cells occurs (simple atrophy). Later the total number of cells in the organ also decreases (numeric atrophy). The reduction in the quantity of cells is effected by the programmed death of individual cells.

Hypertrophy

Definition: Organ or cell enlargement caused by an increase in volume of the individual organ cells with proliferation of their functional substance.

Pathogenesis: A stimulus inducing increased function activates proto-oncogenes (p. 157). The resulting expression of transcription factors increases the synthesis of RNA and proteins and later DNA as well (causing nuclear polyploidy). This accelerates intracellular growth processes and proliferation of organelles (p. 12, 15, 18) while growth inhibitors simultaneously prevent mitosis. The limiting factor for organ function is density of capillaries in the tissue, which does not increase proportionally.

> ! **Note:** All physiologic hypertrophies are reversible once the triggering stimulus is removed.

Types of Hypertrophy

— *Compensatory hypertrophy* results from the increased workload on an organ. Examples include weight training, which produces hypertrophy of skeletal muscle, and aortic valvular stenosis, which produces hypertrophy of the left ventricle (▶ A, B; see p. 388).
— *Endocrinal hypertrophy* results from increased functional load. For example, pregnancy increases the estrogen level, causing hypertrophy of the uterus.

Diseases Associated with Hypertrophy

▬ Hypertrophic Cardiomyopathy

Synonym: idiopathic hypertrophic subaortic stenosis.

Definition: This usually hereditary (noninflammatory) defect in the metabolism of structural substances by the myocardium results in decreased function with compensatory myocardial hypertrophy.

Pathogenesis of the obstructive forms: A genetic defect in the β-myosin heavy chain results in synthesis of abnormal myosin. The myofibrils (▶ F, G) and myocardial cells (▶ C, E) are not properly aligned, resulting in disrupted texture with the myocytes aligned in a star-shaped pattern (▶ E).

Reduced stroke volume results in abnormal myocardial hypertrophy (▶ D), especially upstream of the aortic valve.

▬ Congenital Hypertrophic Pyloric Stenosis

Synonym: pyloric spasm.

Definition: Congenital pyloric stenosis.

Pathogenesis: Defective NO-synthase in the smooth pyloric musculature means that NO is not available to relax the muscle. This results in increased muscle tone and a firm ovoid mass of hypertrophic pyloric muscle that blocks the passage of food from the stomach to the duodenum.

> ✚ **Clinical presentation:** The disorder affects boys five times more often than girls and occurs in about 0.3% of all live births. Symptoms include projectile vomiting shortly after feeding.

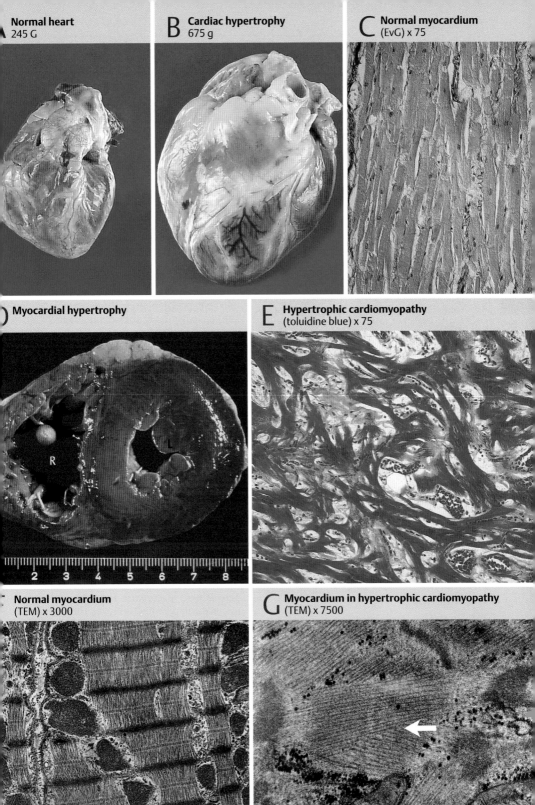

A Normal heart
245 G

B Cardiac hypertrophy
675 g

C Normal myocardium
(EvG) x 75

D Myocardial hypertrophy

R

L

E Hypertrophic cardiomyopathy
(toluidine blue) x 75

Normal myocardium
(TEM) x 3000

G Myocardium in hypertrophic cardiomyopathy
(TEM) x 7500

Hyperplasia

Definition: Enlargement of an organ resulting from proliferation of parenchymal cells.

Pathogenesis: Increased load on the tissue causes cellular hypertrophy. When the critical cell mass is exceeded, proto-oncogenes (p. 157) are activated and factors triggering mitosis (mitogenes) are expressed. This results in cell proliferation. The limiting factor for organ function is density of capillaries in the tissue, which does not increase proportionally.

Types of Hyperplasia

Several types are distinguished according to their pathogenesis:

— *Overload hyperplasia* results from chronic loads placed on an organ.
— *Regenerative hyperplasia* results from structural and functional compensation of tissue damage in organs capable of regeneration.
— *Hyperregenerative hyperplasia* results from permanent damage that triggers excessive regeneration.
— *Endocrinal hyperplasia* may result from three causes. Deficiency of a substrate may result in decreased hormone synthesis and compensatory hyperplasia of the hormone-synthesizing organ. The endocrine feedback mechanism may be deranged. An increased hormone supply may cause hyperplasia of the endocrine effector organ.

Note: Hyperplasia is only clinically significant where it is associated with a functional impairment.

Diseases Associated with Hyperplasia

■ Endometrial Hyperplasia

Definition: Hyperplasia of the endometrium due to an oversupply of endogenous or exogenous estrogens.

Pathogenesis: Hyperestrogenism leads to growth and proliferation of the endometrial glands with resulting irregular thickening of the endometrium (▶ A) with numerous glands distended by cysts (glandular cystic hyperplasia; ▶ C). Persistent hyperestrogenism leads to glandular proliferation; the glands move closer together (in what is known as a back-to-back position), and the glandular epithelium becomes stratified (adenomatous hyperplasia; ▶ C). Mucosal necrosis (p. 128) and bleeding occur (rejection response) when the critical mucosa height is exceeded.

＋ Clinical presentation and complications: Common in older women, this lesion is characterized by metrorrhagia (uterine bleeding) and can progress into malignancy.

Note: *Menorrhagia* refers to heavy menstrual bleeding; *metrorrhagia* refers to bleeding outside the normal cycle.

Note: *Endometrial hyperplasia* is hormonal glandular hyperplasia.

■ Prostatic Hyperplasia

Synonym: Benign prostatic hypertrophy or hyperplasia.

Definition: Benign nodular enlargement of the prostate due to hormonal imbalance.

Pathogenesis: Increased activity of the 5α-reductase in the prostatic stroma, for reasons yet unknown, causes dihydrotestosterone, androstenediol, and 17β-estradiol to accumulate in tissue. The resulting imbalance between estrogen and testosterone leads to expression of fibroblast growth factors (FGF, TGF, and EGF) and to expression of proto-oncogenes. The resulting activation of transcription factor causes stromal proliferation with activation of the smooth muscle cells. Hyperplasia begins in the superior and central region of the gland in the form of a nodule that protrudes into the urinary bladder (a "central lobe"; ▶ B1). This produces capsule-like compression of the peripheral and inferior portions of the gland, resulting in compression of the urethra and difficulty in urination.

Morphologic result: Diffuse, semi-nodular proliferation of actin-containing smooth musculature (▶ E) with mild glandular proliferation (▶ D). The resulting impairment of secretion triggers cystic transformation of the gland. The secretion thickens to form stratified psammoma bodies, in turn producing calcification, prostate stones, black dots on the cross-section of the prostate (giving it a snuff-like appearance), and reactive prostatitis.

Macroscopic appearance: The lobes of the prostate are enlarged and nodular. Their yellowish cross section is penetrated with very fine pores, and a milky secretion is present.

＋ Clinical presentation and complications: Common in older men, this lesion is characterized by difficulties in urination. Sequelae include:
Bladder trabeculae (▶ B2): Compensatory hyperplasia of the musculature of the urinary bladder creates a trabecular relief of the inside of the urinary bladder with evaginations of the wall between the hypertrophic muscle bundles that primarily consist of mucosal and submucosal tissue.
Hydronephrosis: Urinary retention gradually leads to a sac-like widening of the renal pelvis with loss of parenchyma in response to increased pressure, especially in the cortical region. This transforms the kidney into a urine-filled "water bag" (hydronephrosis) and leads to renal insufficiency.

Note: *Prostatic hyperplasia* is hormonal stromal hyperplasia.

A Glandular endometrial hyperplasia

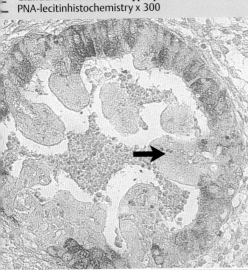

B Prostatic hyperplasia (bladder trabeculation)

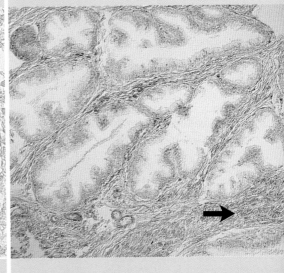

Glandular-cystic endometrial hyperplasia
(HE) x 50

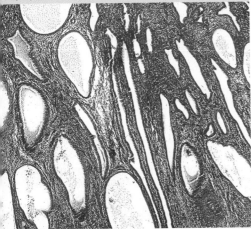

D Prostatic hyperplasia
(HE) x 250

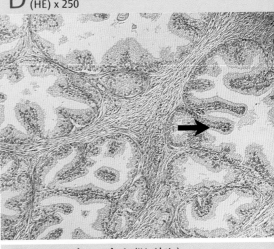

E Glandular endometrial hyperplasia
PNA-lecitinhistochemistry x 300

F Prostatic hyperplasia (IH, Aktin)
x 300

Endocrinal Hyperplasia

General definition: Disorders resulting from endocrine dysfunction (p. 117) that are associated with hyperplasia.

■ Thyroid Hyperplasia

General definition: Regulative hyperplasia of the thyroid follicle with visible and/or palpable thyroid enlargement.

> **Note:** Every non-neoplastic thyroid enlargement is referred to as a goiter.

> **Note:** Goiters are termed endemic where they occur in >10% of a population and sporadic where they occur in <10% of a population.

Euthyroid Goiter

Synonyms: diffuse nontoxic goiter, simple goiter.

Textbook example of the commonest endocrine disorder.

Definition: Goiter with sufficient thyroid hormone synthesis in the presence of iodine deficiency.

Pathogenesis: Relative or absolute iodine deficiency due to exogenous or endogenous causes leads to expression of growth factors (EGF). This in turn causes compensatory thyroid cell proliferation and hyperplasia of thyroid follicular cells.

Morphology: Thyroid enlargement is initially diffuse (diffuse goiter) and later nodular (nodular goiter; ► A) with storage of colloid (► C1). This causes follicular enlargement with a lining of flattened thyroid cells (► C2). Later involution and dystrophic calcification occur (colloid goiter).

Graves Disease

Textbook example of hyperplasia due to endocrine dysfunction.

Definition: Goiter with diffuse thyroid hyperfunction due to TSH receptor dysfunction.

Pathogenesis: IgG autoantibodies (p. 96) are formed that bind to the TSH receptors. The most important activates adenylate cyclase, resulting in continuous stimulation of thyroid cells and overproduction of T_3 and T_4. Another antibody triggers thyroid cell proliferation, resulting in excessive thyroid growth.

Morphology: Thyroid cell proliferation and hypertrophy produce cushion-like or papillary enlargement of the follicular cells ("Sanderson cushion"; ► D1). Activation of the thyroid cells results in colloid absorption into vacuoles in the periphery of the follicle (absorption vacuoles; ► D2).

Macroscopic appearance: Diffuse goiter (► B).

✚ **Clinical presentation:** The disorder is more common in geographic regions with sporadic goiter. *Clinical symptoms* include the **triad of Merseburg:**
- Goiter,
- Exophthalmos (protruding eyeballs),
- Tachycardia.
  Other symptoms include pretibial edema, weight loss, warm, moist skin, and heavy sweating.

> **Note:** The clinical picture of Graves disease is best characterized by the catchphrase "The *heart races* (tachycardia), the *eye rolls* (exophthalmos), and the *neck rumbles* (buzzing sounds due to hyperemia superficial to the goiter)."

Hypothyroid Goiter

Definition: Form of goiter occurring in thyroid function due to a hereditary defect in an enzyme involved in thyroid hormone synthesis.

Pathogenesis: The enzyme defect causes a hormone deficit in the periphery. This leads to pituitary release of TSH, causing continuous proliferation of thyroid cells (in the absence of endocrine stimulation).

Morphology: The goiter is initially diffuse and later becomes nodular with colloid-deficient thyroid follicles lined with non-stimulated thyroid cells.

✚ **Clinical presentation:** This rare disorder is characterized by metabolic depression, doughy skin, myxedema, and hyporeflexia.

■ Parathyroid Hyperplasia

Definition: Diffuse and/or nodular hyperplasia of all four glands (primarily involving the central cells or clear cells). The following forms are differentiated according to their etiology:

Primary hyperplasia is rare. In 70% of all cases, the cause is unknown; the remaining 30% occur as part of type I multiple endocrine neoplasia syndrome.

Secondary hyperplasia is common. Chronic renal insufficiency leads to hypocalcemia. The disorder involves defective synthesis of vitamin D precursors (25-cholecalciferol).

Morphology: In the commonest form of primary hyperparathyroidism, the glands are asymmetrically enlarged (► E) and weigh several grams. Nodular proliferations of central cells in solid, occasionally follicular configurations (► F) displace the stromal fat cells, resulting in an absence of fatty tissue in the glands.

✚ **Clinical presentation:** This depends on the etiology.
- *Primary hyperplasia* leads to primary hyperparathyroidism (p. 39).
- *Secondary hyperplasia* leads to secondary hyperparathyroidism (p. 39) and to hypercalcemia, resulting in metastatic soft-tissue calcifications (p. 136).

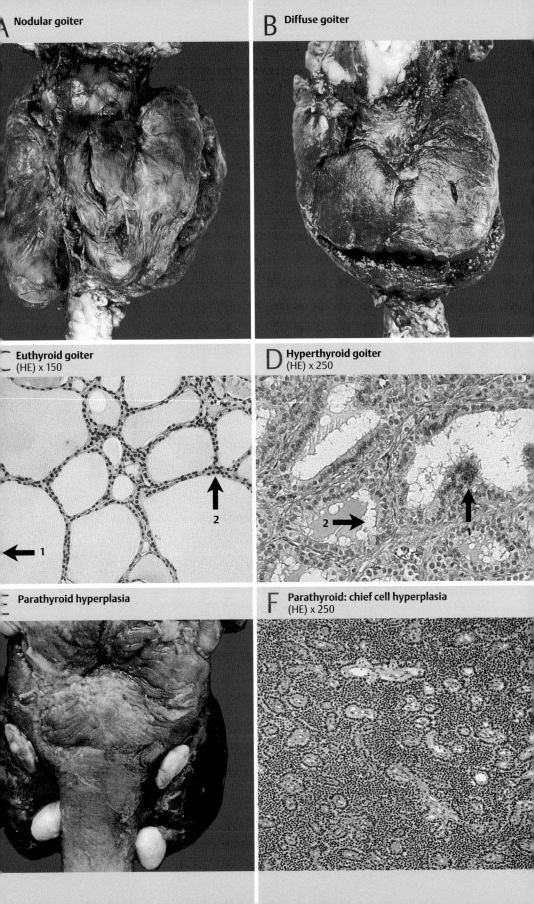

A Nodular goiter

B Diffuse goiter

C Euthyroid goiter
(HE) x 150

D Hyperthyroid goiter
(HE) x 250

E Parathyroid hyperplasia

F Parathyroid: chief cell hyperplasia
(HE) x 250

Hyperplasia of the Adrenal Cortex

General definition: Hyperplasia associated with hyperfunction of the adrenal cortex (hypercorticism) in which the weight of both cortexes exceeds 15 g.

Etiologic forms of hyperplasia: Depending on which type of cell of the adrenal cortex is involved, overproduction of a different hormone will result:
— *Glomerulosa cell* involvement causes hyperaldosteronism.
— *Fasciculata reticularis cell* involvement can cause hypercortisolism (Cushing syndrome).
— *Fasciculata reticularis cell* involvement can also cause adrenogenital syndrome.

Depending on the causative mechanism of the respective cellular proliferation, primary and secondary forms of the disorder are differentiated.
— *Primary forms* involve autonomous growth leading to tumor (adenoma).
— *Secondary forms* involve a response to a higher-order releasing hormone or adaptive growth in response to a deficiency signal, both of which lead to hyperplasia.

Adrenal Cortex Hyperfunction Syndrome

■ Hyperaldosteronism

Primary form: Adrenal cortex adenoma (Conn syndrome) in the form of a yellowish nodule of tissue in the adrenal cortex (► A1). The nodule is separated from the rest of the adrenal cortex by a capsule (► A2) and consists of clear, fatty cells (► B). A rare disorder, this Clear-cell adenoma is associated with aldosterone overproduction.
Secondary form: Stimuli external to adrenal cortex such as angiotensin II, sodium withdrawal, addition of potassium, or ACTH stimulates the adrenal cortex, resulting in synthesis of aldosterone.

✚ **Clinical presentation:** Symptoms include arterial hypertension (p. 388), hypopotassemia, proteinuria, muscle weakness, polyuria, and paresthesia (sensation of "crawling ants").

■ Hypercortisolism

Synonym: Cushing syndrome.

Primary hypothalamic-pituitary form (Cushing syndrome): An adenoma in the anterior lobe of the hypophysis leads to continuous ACTH synthesis with continuous stimulation of the adrenal cortex, leading to fasciculata reticularis hyperplasia.

Primary adrenal form: Usually a yellowish-brown tumor is present (► C1) proceeding from the adrenal cortex (► C2) and consisting of compact cells (► D1) and cells with clear cytoplasm (► D2). This mixed-cell adenoma suppresses corticotropic pituitary function, resulting in atrophy of the healthy adrenal cortex (► C2).

Paraneoplastic form (ectopic ACTH syndrome): A tumor external to the adrenal cortex and pituitary gland, such as a small-cell bronchogenic carcinoma (p. 378), produces ACTH peptides.

Iatrogenic form: The disorder can occur as a side effect of glucocorticoid or ACTH therapy.

✚ **Clinical presentation** of hypercortisolism:
– *Skeleton:* cortisone osteoporosis (p. 67).
– *Musculature:* Muscular atrophy produces thin, bird-like legs.
– *Blood:* Lymphocytic and eosinophilic deficiency.
– *Skin:* Atrophic thinning leads to formation of yellowish-white striae.
– *Fatty tissue* accumulates on the trunk.
– *Circulatory system:* arterial hypertension (p. 386).
– *Metabolism:* secondary diabetes mellitus.
– *Stomach:* Increased susceptibility to peptic ulcer.

❗ **Note:** Side effects of corticosteroid include osteoporosis (p. 126), impaired wound healing (p. 312), susceptibility to infection, and suppression of the adrenal glands.

■ Adrenogenital Syndrome

Textbook example of impaired sexual differentiation due to enzyme dysfunction.

Pathogenesis: This hereditary enzyme defect of steroid hormone synthesis involves a defect in 21-hydroxylase in 90% of all cases and a defect in 11-hydroxylase in 5%.

The resulting congenital adrenal hyperplasia leads to synthesis of hormone precursors with androgenic effects. Occasionally, hormone precursors with the effects of aldosterone or ACTH are produced.

✚ **Clinical presentation:** The disorder is rare. The possible existence of acquired forms of adrenogenital syndrome is being discussed. Symptoms of adrenogenital syndrome vary with gender:
– *Girls:* Virilization of the genitals involving clitoral hypertrophy (► E), a male pattern of pubic hair growth, and fusion of the labia occurs in the presence of normal female internal reproductive organs, resulting in female pseudohermaphroditism. Precocious puberty also occurs.
– *Boys:* Increased scrotal skin pigmentation and precocious puberty (► F) occur.
– *Boys and girls:* Initial acceleration of growth results in premature closure of the epiphyseal growth plates. This results in arrested growth and subnormal stature.

A Clear-cell adenoma of the adrenal cortex

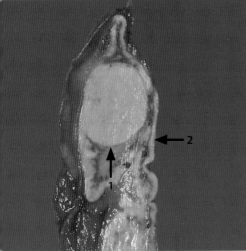

B Clear-cell adenoma of the adrenal cortex
(HE) x 200

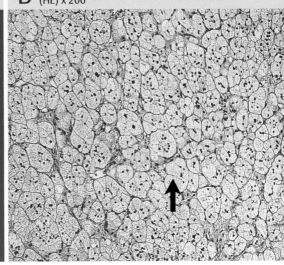

Mixed-cell adenoma of the adrenal cortex

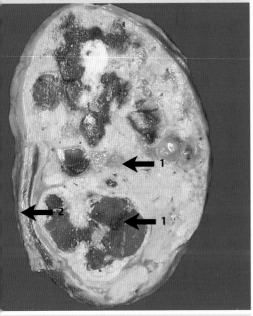

D Mixed-cell adenoma of the adrenal cortex
(HE) x 200

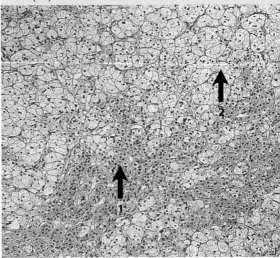

Adrenogenital syndrome:
virilization

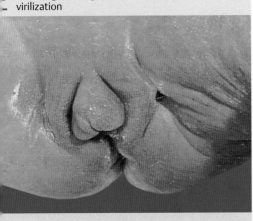

F Adrenogenital syndrome: precocious puberty
(3-year-old boy)

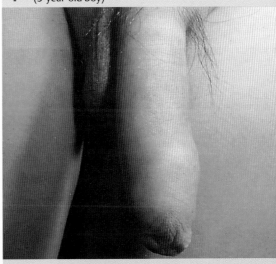

Atrophy

Definition: Diminished size of an organ or tissue shrinkage of the parenchymal cells. *Simple atrophy* refers to diminished organ size resulting from a reduction in cell volume; *numeric atrophy* refers to diminished organ size resulting from a reduction in the total number of cells in the organ as well as a reduction in their volume.

Pathogenesis: Atrophy is the correlate of cellular adaption to reduced activity, decreased workload, decreased blood supply, inadequate nutrition, and reduced neural and/or endocrine stimulation.

Atrophy proceeds according to the following two patterns.

— *Autophagic cell destruction* (p. 26) causes loss of functional substance. This in turn precipitates a loss of cell volume and simple atrophy. Where the noxious agent persists,
— *apoptosis* (p. 128) leads to a decrease in the number of cells and numeric atrophy.

Types of Atrophy

The following types are differentiated according to pathogenesis:

— *Involutional atrophy:* Regression of organs that temporarily formed during embryonic development, such as the ductus arteriosus, or that are temporarily enlarged during some stage of life, such as the lactating breast.
— *Atrophy of disuse:* Loss of workload results in regression. In bedridden or paralyzed patients, for example, muscular atrophy with proliferation of fatty tissue (► A1, B1) between the atrophied muscle fibers(► A2,B2).
— *Trophoneurotic atrophy:* Peripheral or central nervous vascular impairment reduces the blood supply to the tissue. Tabes dorsalis (syphilitic spinal cord atrophy) leads to perforating ulcer of the foot.
— *Vascular atrophy* results from a mismatch between workload and vascular supply. For example, occlusion of the portal artery causes atrophy of the hepatic lobe.
— *Compressive atrophy* is a mechanical overload. For example, a pulsating aneurysm may cause vertebral atrophy; overinflation of the lung may increase pressure on the diaphragm and create compression furrows in the liver.
— *Endocrine atrophy:* Lack of a releasing hormone eliminates the stimulus to produce hormone in the endocrine effector organ, which then atrophies. In thyroid inactivity, the lack of FSH causes follicular atrophy. The absorption vacuoles, which indicate activity in an active thyroid gland, are absent (► C, D1), and colloid accumulates in the follicles (► D2).

Disorders Associated with Generalized Atrophy

▬ Senile Atrophy

Definition: The sum of all changes during the course of life, which occur in every human as a function of time.

Etiologic mechanisms:
— *Molecular DNA aging:* Congenital defects (p. 6) or acquired defects in the DNA repair system result in catastrophic DNA errors.
— *Telomere erosion:* The chromosomes consistently lose genetic material from their telomere portion as a result of mitosis in a process known as telomere erosion. Once a certain threshold value has been exceeded, the ends of the chromosomes become "sticky" and fuse together. This molecular damage attracts the attention of "genome watchdog proteins." If the cell does not succeed in repairing the chromosome damage, the cell death program is initiated (p. 128, 132).

Morphology: Age-related reduction in functional substance leads to organ atrophy with brown discoloration from lipofuscin accumulation (which in physiologic aging only becomes apparent after the age of 70) and fibrous proliferation.

☺ **Biologic record:** The longest officially confirmed human life to date has been that Shigechiyo Izumi of Japan, who lived to the age of 120 years and 237 days.

> **❗ Note:** There are two exceptions to the cell aging.
> – *Regenerative tissue cells* (p. 309) contain telomerase, the "immortality enzyme" that leads to complete repair of the loss of telomere material, preventing aging and effectively making the cell immortal.
> – *Cancer cells* also contain active telomerase.

▬ Atrophy Due to Inanition (Cachexia)

Etiologic factors include inadequate nutrient intake and insufficient nutrient uptake.

Pathogenesis: An adult in a state of normal nutrition has sufficient energy reserves for at least 40–50 days. In fasting or starvation, the glycogen in the liver is consumed on the first day. Following this, fat deposits are consumed (such as in the greater omentum; ► E, F), leading to emaciation. Later, the body's protein reserves are consumed, leading to reduced protein synthesis. The resulting hypoproteinemia (primarily hypoalbuminemia) induces apoptosis (p. 128) and leads to numeric atrophy of the hemopoietic and lymphopoietic system.

✚ Clinical presentation: This disorder is common in developing countries. Symptoms include nutritional edema, anemia, and susceptibility to infection. Death occurs in a hypoglycemic coma with keto-acidosis.

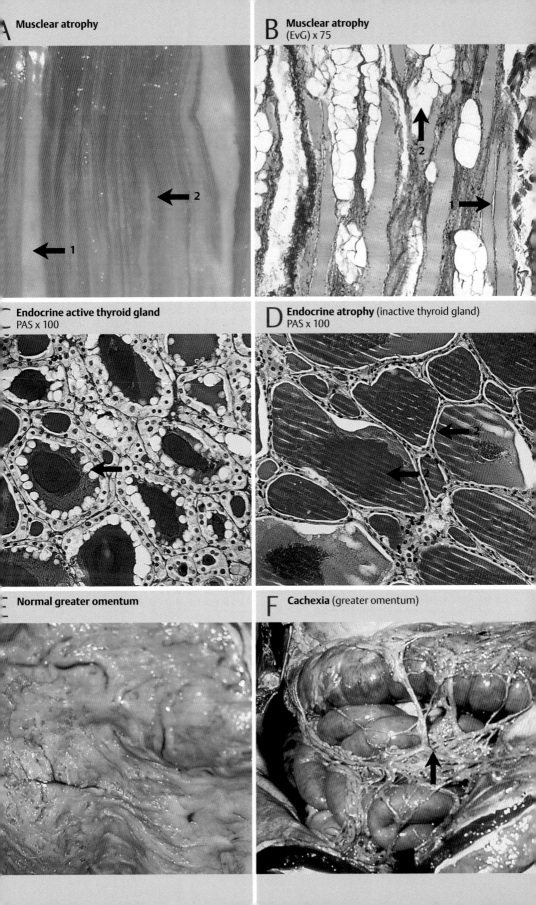

A Musclear atrophy

B Musclear atrophy (EvG) x 75

C Endocrine active thyroid gland
PAS x 100

D Endocrine atrophy (inactive thyroid gland)
PAS x 100

E Normal greater omentum

F Cachexia (greater omentum)

Disorders Associated with Organ Atrophy

■ Osteoporosis

Textbook example of bone atrophy.

Definition: Any loss of bone substance exceeding age-related physiologic values.

Etiologic forms of osteoporosis:
— *Primary osteoporosis* is due to uncertain causes. It occurs more often in women than men and may be related to postmenopausal estrogen deficiency.
— *Secondary osteoporosis* is due to hormonal causes, such as hypercorticism and hyperthyroidism, or to biomechanical causes, such as inactivity.

Both forms trigger apoptosis (p. 128) that leads to numeric atrophy.

Pathogenetic principle: Excessive bone resorption and/or impaired new bone formation.

The result is a persistent systemic negative balance of bone remodeling. Osteoclastic areas of bone resorption on the surface of the cancellous bone are no longer filled with new bone substance due to the inactivity of the osteoblasts. This results in trabecular atrophy; Bone becomes porous and brittle, hence the name osteoporosis.

Morphology (primary osteoporosis): loss and thinning of the trabeculae (trabecular atrophy; ► A2, B2) produces a rarified pattern of cancellous trabeculae (► C, D), later progressing to narrowing of the cortex. The lack of osteoid formation is indicative of the inactivity of the osteoblasts, and the osteoid halos are largely absent (► A1, B1).

✚ **Clinical presentation:** This very common disorder is characterized by spontaneous fractures and compression fractures of the superior vertebral end plates, especially in the thoracic and lumbar spine, producing typical "fish vertebra" deformities. Anterior subsidence produces wedge-shaped vertebrae. This vertebral subsidence also reduces body height.

■ Alzheimer's Disease

Textbook example of brain atrophy.

Definition: Premature abnormal aging of the brain within the scope of degenerative neurologic disease with loss of higher intellectual function.

Pathogenesis: An unknown defect in the structural metabolism of the ganglion cells causes the formation of AS amyloid (known as A4 amyloid; p. 50), whereby the gene for the amyloid precursor protein locus is located on chromosome 21.

For this reason, Alzheimer's disease regularly occurs in trisomy 21.

The result is the Alzheimer triad:
— *Alzheimer plaque:* especially in the associative cortical regions, frontal lobe, and hippocampus; concentric amyloid deposits in the neuropil[1] of the ganglion cells with subsequent degenerative cytoskeletal damage in the adjacent neurons and astrocyte processes (p. 34).

This is accompanied by further sequelae of cytoskeletal damage.

— *Alzheimer fibrils:* paired helical filaments (p. 34) form and accumulate together with the stress protein ubiquitin and the microtubule-associated protein tau in the damaged neuron processes.
— *Amyloid angiopathy* (angiopathy that stains under Congo red dye): amyloid deposits in the cerebral blood vessels.

Morphology: Cortical atrophy of the frontal, parietal, and temporal lobes of the brain exhibiting the Alzheimer triad of microscopic findings:

✚ **Clinical presentation:** Common disorder producing progressive dementia with progressive loss of memory, cognitive faculties, and speech.

☺ **Prominent patient:** Ronald Reagan, former US President.

■ Pick's Disease

Definition: Premature abnormal aging of the brain within the scope of degenerative neurologic disease with behavioral changes and dementia.

Pathogenesis: A defect in the structural metabolism of the ganglion cells leads to cytoskeletal damage in the form of neuron filament tangles containing the stress protein ubiquitin (Pick bodies). This in turn produces spongiform encephalopathy that triggers apoptosis (p. 128), leading to numeric cortical atrophy in the region of the frontal and temporal lobes (► E, F).

✚ **Clinical presentation:** Rare disorder producing behavioral changes, inhibition, progressive loss of motivation and speech, and dementia.

☺ **Prominent patient:** Maurice Ravel (1875–1937), French composer.

❗ **Note:** In the presence of atrophy, the body attempts to compensate for the loss of tissue volume with filler material.
— Cerebral atrophy therefore produces hydrocephaly *ex vacuo,*
— renal atrophy produces lipomatosis of the renal hilum,
— muscle atrophy produces proliferation of fatty tissue.

---

[1] Neuropil = web of ganglion cell processes.

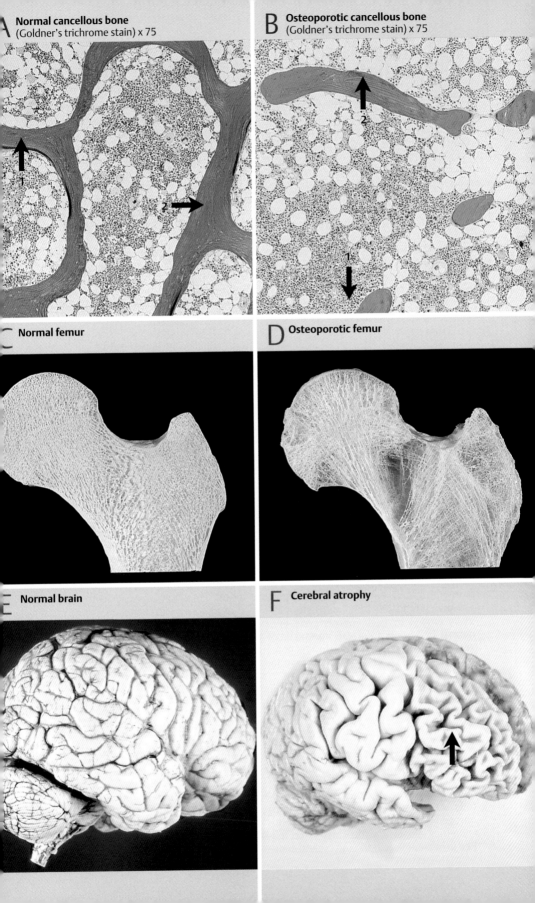

A Normal cancellous bone
(Goldner's trichrome stain) x 75

B Osteoporotic cancellous bone
(Goldner's trichrome stain) x 75

C Normal femur

D Osteoporotic femur

E Normal brain

F Cerebral atrophy

8 Cell Death as Last Resort
Lethal Cell Injury

Summary

The death of cells and tissue from lethal cell injury occurs either according to an internal program or as a result of external forces. The dead tissue manifests itself as necrosis. This tissue can be repaired via the mechanism of inflammation (p. 194). Tissue in a dead organism dissociates itself by means of enzyme action and decomposition (autolysis).

▶ **Programmed selective cell death** (apoptosis): cell death occurs as a result of a killing process either initiated by the cell itself (programmed *cell suicide*) or triggered by adjacent cells (programmed *cell fratricide*). The result is shrinkage and necrosis. Derangements of the process of apoptosis can lead to deformities and tumors.

▶ **Accidental cell death** (oncosis): the effects of exogenous or endogenous noxious agents severely injure the cell. Its response to these attacks is seen in the associated adaptive processes that give cell death, in the form of necrosis, its characteristic histologic appearance. Two types of necrosis are distinguished according to their causative mechanism.

— **Coagulative necrosis** is characterized by predominance of protein denaturation and dehydration;

— **Liquefactive necrosis** is characterized by predominance of hydrolytic breakdown.

Apoptosis

Definition: In this genetically mediated programmed cell destruction, cells die, shrink, and disintegrate in the absence of any reactive inflammation.

Programmed Cell Death

General pathogenesis: occurs in 3 phases:

■ **Commitment phase:**

referred to as such in that a cell that "decides" to destroy itself reacts to the following **trigger signals** (these factors can initiate the apoptosis mechanism):

— *Number of mitoses:* cells in embryonic tissue have a "mitosis counting" gene which introduces the cell death program once a certain number of mitoses has been reached. In postnatal tissues not possessing telomerase, the chromosomal telomeres are minimally eroded by each mitosis cycle until normal DNS replication can no longer be guaranteed. At this point, the "genome guardian protein" p53 clears the way for apoptosis.

— *Cell age:* once cells have reached a certain age their cell death program is triggered. This is particularly the case for erythropoiesis, endochondral ossification, and molting tissue.

— *Function-sustaining signal substance loss,* i.e., hormones or growth factors: when their threshold level falls in those tissues dependent on them, the relationship of antiapoptotic bcl-2 proteins (the B-cell lymphoma oncogene) is shifted, inducing the mitochondrial apoptosis path. This is exemplified in involution atrophy and cyclical endometrial rejection.

— *Cell communication:* When cells lose their cadherin-mediated cell-to-cell communication, or their integrin-mediated anchorage in the extracellular matrix, the "focal adhesion kinase" is deactivated in the non-tumorous cells, DNA is blocked, and apoptosis begins.

— *Contact-less cytotoxic lymphocytes:* As these cells track down foreign cells, they also express Fas-ligand (FS7-associated surface antigen = CD95) and thereby bind onto thier Fas receptors. Apoptosis begins. Alternatively, they can secrete the pore-forming protein perforin, with which they "inject" serin-protease granzyme-B into the target cell; they then activate the cysteine aspartate-protein-cleaving enzyme system (CASPASE). Apoptosis begins.

— *Noxins:* Heat, radiation, and/or cytostatics cause DNA damage, whereby the p53 genomic guardian protein clears the way for apoptosis. Nitrogen and oxygen radicals can directly trigger the mitochondrial pathway of apoptosis by oxidative stress.

● **Signaling paths:** Triggering signals can engage the cellular execution mechanism indirectly with the aid of receptors (the transmembrane-signaling, or death receptor path), or directly in cytoplasm (the intracellular-signalling or mitochondrial path).

● **Controlling mechanisms:** There are two mechanisms controlling the actual initiation of programmed cell death: for one, specific adaptor proteins (like FADD = Fas-associated protein with death domain) are interposed, "flipping" the cell death program switch, effectively condemning the cell to death; the other mechanism involves proteins such as those in the bcl-2 family, which dock onto the death program's

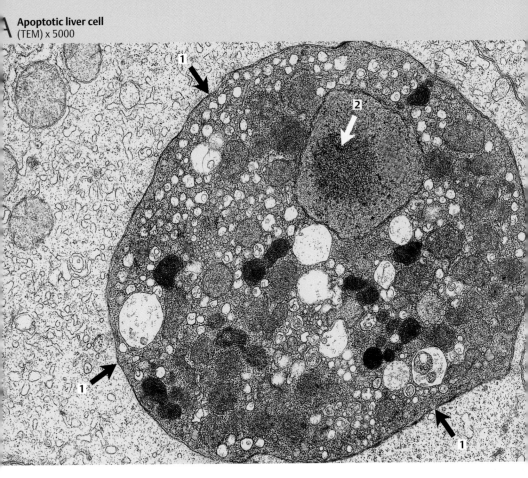

Apaf-1-type activator proteins, thereby preventing the activation of the "igniting enzyme" (Initiator-CASPASE), which would then trigger the "death enzyme" (execution-CASPASE).

■ Execution phase:

In this phase, programmed cell death progresses until the cell is irreversably damaged. The core element in programmed cell death's efficacy is the system of cell death proteases in the form of CASPASEs. The program is activated by two cascades:

- **Death-receptor path.** It begins by the binding of certain death signals, such as the cytokine TNF (tumor necrosis factor), or the soluble Fas-ligand (FasL/CD95L), formed by immune cells, to the death receptors on the cell such as TNFR-1 or Fas. These receptors then associate with adaptor proteins (TRADD, FADD) in the cell, which bear a "death-effector-domain" with which they bond to homologous CASPASE sites. This is the first CASPASE cascade step that "exe-

cutes" the cell. The suppressor gene p53 furthers apoptosis by depositing CD95 on the cell membrane surface. A "rash" activation of the cell receptor path is halted by a series of inhibitor proteins that intervene at various levels of the CASPASE cascade. This is the mechanism several viruses use to prevent the elimination of infected cells by lymphocytes.

- **Mitochondrial path:** begins with the release of mitochondrial apoptosis factor (= AIF) and/or the cytochrome -c from damaged mitochondria; both trigger the CASPASE cascade. This path is activated by a series of inhibitors (primarily bcl-2). It prevents the release of cytochrome -c and AIF.

- **Targets of executing CASPASEs:** these enzymes attack at the following death substrata, among others:
- *Focal adhesion kinase:* Its inactivation triggers the loss of the cell's cytoskeletal cell-to-cell cohesion.

Accidental Cell Death

Synonym: oncosis.

Definition: Irreversibly impaired metabolism (generally oxidative metabolism) brings about the death of the cell with subsequent vacuolar swelling of the cell and reactive inflammation in the absence of programmed cell death.

The *morphologic result* is necrosis.

> ! Note: Cell death and necrosis are not identical. A once-living cell submerged and fixed in formaldehyde is chemically dead, although from a structural standpoint it remains intact and "animate."

Necrosis

General definition: Generic term for the sum of all morphologic phenomena occurring in the wake of partial or total cell or tissue death in a living body.

Focal Cytoplasmic Necrosis

Definition and pathogenesis: Not every lethal cellular injury leads to necrosis of the entire cell. Often the cell is able to sequester the site of the irreversible injury (▶ A2) in a membrane (▶ A1) in the process of autophagy (p. 28), separating it from the intact cytoplasm.

Coagulative Necrosis

Definition: This terms refers to the macroscopic transformation of a completely dead area of tissue into a yellowish, dry, mortar-like mass as a result of the protein precipitation (▶ B, splenic infarction).

General causal pathogenesis: Accidental cell death can be initiated by the following mechanisms, regardless of etiogenicity/eflogenic factor/elicitor:

— *ATP deficiency* as caused by hypoxia (ischemia), leads to the cessation of cellular calcium homeostasis and membrane function.
— *Impairment of calcium homeostasis* by ischemia or toxins leads to calcium influx into the cell and later to the activation of phospholipases, proteases, ATPases, and endonucleases to damage of the cytoskeleton, cell membrane and DNS.
— *Toxic oxygen metabolites:* when their removal by vitamin E, glutathion, and superoxide dismutase fails, they damage the cell membrane and cell enzymes together with DNS.
— *Cytomembrane damage* as caused by ATP deficiency, physical or chemical toxins, microbe toxins, complement factors, and lymphocyte perforin, leads to a permeability disorder.

Morphology: Foci of coagulative necrosis are initially swollen. They exhibit diminished transparency and their tissue delineation is indistinct; the cytoplasm of the affected cells shows increased eosinophilia (▶ C). The consistency of the tissue gradually increases. The tissue appears "cooked" and assumes a clay-like yellowish color. Necrotic tissue releases inflammatory substances (cytokines such as interleukin-2). These lead to inflammation of the injured area, attracting proteolytic scavenger cells. Their action softens the necrotic area, increasing the risk of rupture. A capillary-rich reparative mesenchyma of granulation tissue forms (p. 224, 312), creating a dark red halo around the necrotic focus (a "hemorrhagic marginal zone"; ▶ E). Later, the necrotic area is transformed into a whitish yellow mass of tissue in which the original histologic structures are only barely recognizable (▶ D).

Special Forms of Coagulative Necrosis

Dry gangrene: corresponds to the summation of the effects of structure-preserving coagulative necrosis and desiccation. The tissue is mummified and appears burned (▶ F).

Scab necrosis: In coagulative necrosis of the skin and/or mucous membranes, water evaporation and exudation of fibrin produce a dirty whitish plaque that can be wiped off.

Caseation: This form of coagulative necrosis is typical of tuberculosis (p. 264) and is characterized by an abundance of dead granulocytes, producing necrotic tissue that is rich in lipids resembling crumbly cottage cheese.

Zenker degeneration (waxy degeneration): This refers to necrosis of skeletal muscle in infectious diseases with high fevers (such as typhoid fever, p. 260). The musculature becomes opaque and waxy, tears easily, and loses its cross-striation.

A Focal cytoplasmic necrosis
(TEM) × 5000

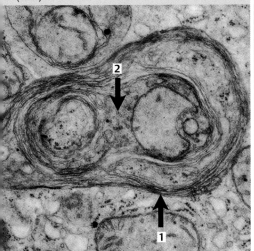

B Coagulative necrosis (spleen)

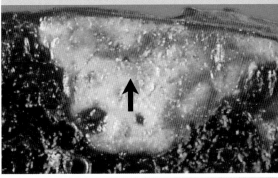

C Coagulative necrosis (muscle)
(HE) × 200

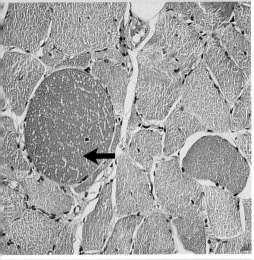

D Coagulative necrosis (spleen)
(HE) × 100

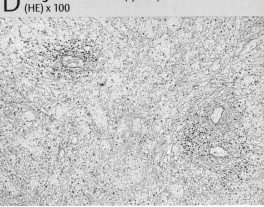

E Bone necrosis

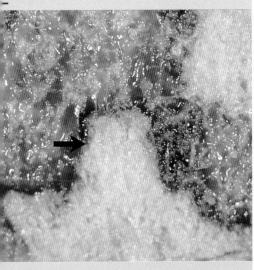

F Gangrene of the foot

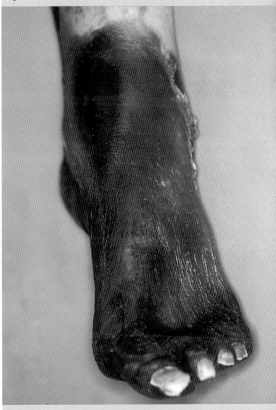

Liquefactive Necrosis

Definition: This terms refers to macroscopic soft, mushy transformation of an area of dead tissue due to rapid enzymatic dissolution or an alkali burn.

Pathogenetic chain reaction: The affected tissue contains proteins that are nearly noncoagulable, or massive quantities of proteases. This results in a primary hydrolytic pattern of tissue breakdown.

After initial swelling, the necrotic tissue is rapidly dissolved by enzymatic action, producing focal softening (malacia). The tissue acquires a mushy, greasy consistency (► A2, C), later progressing to liquefaction of the necrotic area that leaves a large defect after it is absorbed. If the lesion includes vascular structures, bleeding into the tissue will result, producing what is known as hemorrhagic necrosis (► A1; see also p. 216).

Special Forms of Liquefactive Necrosis

Simple fat necrosis: This results from hypoxic necrosis or mechanical injury to fat cells. The fat liquefies at body temperature and is released as an oily mass, resulting in formation of oil cysts.

Lipolytic fat necrosis: This disorder is due to acute pancreatitis (p. 216; ► A, C). The resulting damage to the exocrine pancreatic cells releases pancreatic lipase and trypsin. This causes hydrolysis of triglycerides within and around the pancreatic fatty tissue (► A2, C) or in the more remote fatty tissue (extending into the mesentery and retroperitoneal tissue) without phagocytic involvement. This in turn results in nodular foci of fatty tissue necrosis. The fatty acids that are released bind calcium. This causes local precipitation of insoluble calcium fat soaps (► E), forming macroscopic droplet-like necrotic foci like wax on a candle.

Shrinking Necrosis

Definition: This is a histologic and ultrastructural term for selective necrosis in the same type of differentiated cell in a tissue due to internally programmed cell death (apoptosis), characterized by shrinkage and bursting of the dead cells.

Morphology: This form of necrosis is never accompanied by demarcating inflammation; it occurs in individual cells or in groups of differentiated cells of the same type.

Proceeds according to a characteristic pattern:
— *Peripheral nuclear chromatin condensation:* Activation of endonuclease produces a crescent-shaped pattern of chromatin condensation under the nuclear membrane (► B1); the contacts with other cells are dissolved, and the cell assumes a spherical shape (► B2).
— *Formation of cytoplasmic blebs:* at several points along the surface of the cell (► D).
— *Formation of apoptotic bodies:* The cell rapidly disintegrates into a number of fragments with structurally intact organelles (► F). The nucleus shows a karyorhexis (p. 8).
— *Sequestration of the apoptotic bodies:* The apoptotic bodies are either sloughed off into the lumen of the gland, or they are phagocytosed by adjacent cells and/or macrophages.

> **Rule of thumb for necrosis:**
> – *Coagulative necrosis* is structured mass necrosis.
> – *Liquefactive necrosis* is unstructured mass necrosis.
> – *Apoptosis* is necrosis in individual cells or in groups of differentiated cells of the same type.

Autolysis

Definition: This is a morphologic term for tissue and cells that have died together with the entire body or with a part that has been separated from the rest of the body, such as an amputated leg.

Pathogenesis: The body is no longer able to respond to systemic damage with sequestration, phagocytosis, or reparative actions. It dissolves itself with its own catabolic (usually lysosomal) enzymes in a process of autolysis. The action of anaerobic bacteria, which enter the body after death or were present during life and spread from the inner organs such as the intestinal lumen or through the skin, transform this into a secondary process of decomposition. The organs then disintegrate, for example in postmortem gastromalacia or softening of the stomach walls.

In autolysis, the tissue of the dead body disintegrates in a process of decomposition. However, the living body attempts to sequester the necrotic sites. This will be discussed in the following section.

A Liquefactive necrosis of the pancreas

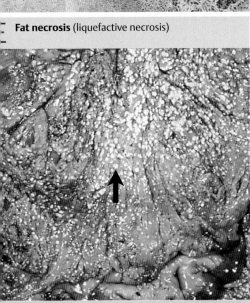

B Apoptosis
(TEM) x 5000

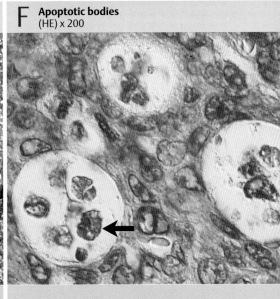

C Liquefactive necrosis of the pancreas
(HE) x 75

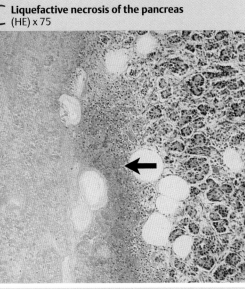

D Apoptosis
(cell culture phase contrast) x 75

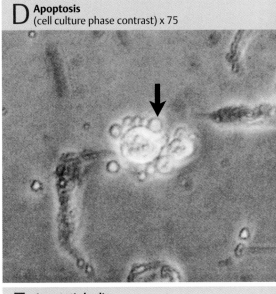

E Fat necrosis (liquefactive necrosis)

F Apoptotic bodies
(HE) x 200

When the Rest Calcifies or petrifies
Calcification and Stone Disorders

Summary

▶ *Heterotopic calcification:* calcium salts deposited in tissues that do not physiologically calcify are referred to as heterotopic calcification. With respect to causal pathogenesis, two forms are differentiated.

Dystrophic calcification: a catastrophic inflammatory or ischemic event can cause degenerative or necrotic material to accumulate in tissue in quantities that exceed the capability of the macrophages to eliminate it. The body employs a special pattern of response to cope with these situations. First, the accumulated material is impregnated with calcium salts. Occasionally, multinucleated giant cells will "nibble" at these deposits because they regard them as foreign material (foreign body inflammatory reaction). In other cases, such calcium foci are transformed into bone.

Metastatic calcification: occasionally, more calcium may be leached from the bone than the body can process. The body's initial response is by the mitochondria, which store part of the calcium. However, especially in the tissues that normally produce acidic valences, calcium phosphate continues to be precipitated in the cells until they are essentially buried in calcification.

▶ *Stone disorders:* in a few excretory organs, such as the liver and kidneys, metabolic disorders lead to accumulation of certain salt-forming metabolites in the excretory products. Where inflammation or hypercalcemia occurs in the presence of this underlying condition, stones will form. Remnants of dead cells act as seed crystals in such cases, much like the foreign bodies used to produce pearls. Similarly, stasis of pancreatic secretion can produce pancreatic stones and stasis of prostatic secretion can lead to prostatic stones. Such situations usually produce an inflammatory reaction (p. 194) and pain.

Calcification

Dystrophic Calcification

Definition: localized calcium deposits in necrotic or degenerative tissue with normal systemic calcium and phosphate metabolism. This disorder is common.

In terms of *formal pathogenesis,* dystrophic calcification of necrotic tissue develops differently from that of degenerative tissue.

Degenerative Calcification

Classic animal model *(calciphylaxis syndrome):* Local administration of an inductor (such as $KMnO_4$) after inducing hypercalcemia leads to controllable tissue calcification in many locations.

Pathogenesis: A noxious agent triggers apoptosis (p. 128), releasing telolysosomes (p. 28) and vesicular cell membrane derivatives in the form of matrix vesicles (▶ A, B1). These bodies contain ATPase and pyrophosphatase and lead to extracellular accumulation of phosphate, producing deposits of calcium apatite crystals or calcification (▶ B2).

> **Note:** *Degenerative calcification* is apoptotic calcification without the aid of the mitochondria.

Disorders Associated with Degenerative Calcification

■ **Calcinosis cutis:** Local inflammatory sclerosing of the skin resulting in focal skin calcifications (▶ C1, D1) beneath the epidermis (▶ C2) with an inflammatory foreign-body reaction (p. 236) with resorptive giant cells (▶ D2). The disorder is quite rare.

■ **Myositis ossificans** (heterotopic ossification): Trauma causing bleeding, which produces local inflammatory sclerosis of the necrotic musculature. This in turn leads to calcification and ossification. The disorder is rare.

■ **Valvular calcific degeneration:** Inflammatory or degenerative valvular damage leads to calcification and/or ossification of the cardiac valves, producing valvular stenosis. This disorder is common.

■ **Mönckeberg medial calcific sclerosis:** Abnormal hemodynamic stress results in damage to the elastica, producing calcifications of the elastica in the shape of plates or rings (▶ E). This progresses to calcification of the media (without inflammation) and heterotopic ossification. The artery has a macroscopic appearance resembling the neck of a goose (▶ F). The disorder is quite common.

> **Note:** Under hematoxylin and eosin stain, calcium has a grainy and dark blue appearance; under von Kossa stain it appears black.

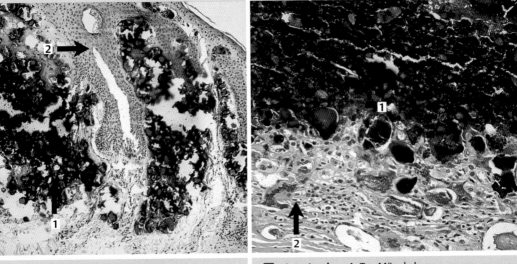

A Matrix vesicles
(freeze-etching, TEM) x 2000

B Matrix vesicles
(TEM) x 2000

Calcinosis cutis (survey)
(HE) x 50

D Calcinosis cutis (detail)
(HE) x 200

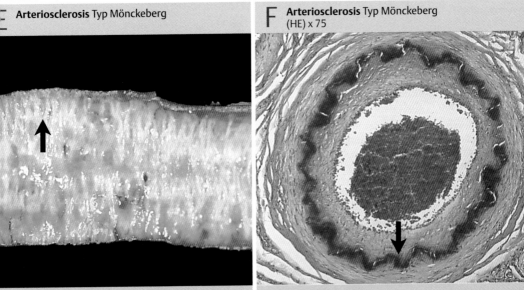

E Arteriosclerosis Typ Mönckeberg

F Arteriosclerosis Typ Mönckeberg
(HE) x 75

Necrotic Calcification

Classic animal model *(calcergy syndrome):* Local administration of an inductor (e.g., $KMnO_4$) without having induced hypercalcemia leads to localized tissue calcification, such as skin calcification (▶ A).

Pathogenesis (based on the model of infarction calcification). Ischemia in the tissue halts mitochondrial production of ATP. This in turns brings the transport of calcium through the cell membrane to a standstill as it depends on ATP. If the tissue is re-perfused, Ca^{2+} and H_2O flow into the cell and into the mitochondria. The mitochondria trap the Ca^{2+}. Calcium and phosphate accumulate in the mitochondrial grana (p. 20) until the mitochondria burst, resulting in calcification of the rest of the cytoplasm.

This process occurs in:
— *Foci of tubercular caseous necrosis,* where the foci calcify;
— *Muscle calcification,* where the infarction calcifies following re-perfusion (▶ C, D);
— *Lithopedion* ("stone child"), where a dead retained fetus calcifies;
— *Phlebolith* ("venous stone"), calcified thrombus;

> **Note:** Necrotic calcification occurs with the aid of the mitochondria or apoptotic calcification.

Metastatic Calcification

Classic animal model *(hypercalcemia syndrome):* Administration of a sensitizing agent (such as vitamin D_3 or parathormone) leads to uncontrollable calcification at many sites in the body without prior administration of an inductor.

Etiologic factors in hypercalcemia include:
— *Bone mineralization syndrome:* osteoporosis due to inactivity, hyperparathyroidism, osteolytic metastases, and paraneoplasia;
— *Hypervitaminosis D;*
— *Sarcoidosis* (p. 230) due to macrophage synthesis of 1-25-hydroxyl vitamin D_3;
— *Addison's disease:* absence of vitamin D antagonists;
— *Milk-alkali syndrome* due to excessive consumption of calcium with gastric hyperacidity;
— *Reduced calcium excretion* due to administration of thiazide diuretics.

Pathogenesis: A condition involving prolonged leaching of calcium salts from bone leads to hypercalcemia (see below) in a concentration exceeding the serum solubility of calcium. This causes precipitation of calcium phosphate in other organs and tissues, or metastatic calcification.

In terms of *formal pathogenesis,* the calcium concentrating function of the mitochondria (p. 20) is the most important factor.

This process occurs primarily in tissue that produces acidic valences, resulting in a tendency toward alkalinity:
— *Lung* (CO_2): pulmonary calcinosis (▶ B);
— *Kidney* (urate): renal calcinosis (▶ E);
— *Body of the stomach* (hydrochloric acid): gastric calcinosis;
— *Myocardium:* myocardial calcinosis;
— *Cornea:* calcific band keratopathy.

Disorders Associated with Metastatic Calcification

These are rare disorders because the underlying disease must go untreated for a long time before its complete clinical syndrome can develop.

▬ Pulmonary Calcinosis

Diffuse, often focal calcification of the walls of the pulmonary vessels, especially of the connective-tissue framework of the alveolar wall (▶ B) leads to reactive fibrosis of the alveolar wall and stiffening of the pulmonary parenchyma.

Result: respiratory insufficiency.

▬ Renal calcinosis: Calcium accumulates in the epithelium of the renal tubules, forming strips of calcification. This calcification causes the necrotic tubular epithelium to be sloughed off. This cast-off tissue forms cylindrical plugs of calcium in the tubules, creating strips of calcification (▶ E1) in the medullary interstitium between the tubules (▶ E2). Exacerbating this is the calcification of the vascular walls.

Result: progressive kidney failure.

▬ Gastric calcinosis: Calcification of the gastric fundus (with strips of mucosal calcification) and submucosal vessels disrupts gastric secretions. This results in chronic reactive inflammation of the gastric mucosa.

Result: chronic gastritis.

▬ Myocardial calcinosis: Strips of calcification in individual groups of myocardial cells (▶ F) lead to reactive myocardial fibrosis. This damages the structure of the myocardium. The muscular pump responds with compensatory myocardial hypertrophy, i.e., secondary metabolic cardiomyopathy.

Result: heart failure.

In several hollow organs with excretory function, necrosis or abnormal composition of the secreted substances can result in formation of stones. These conditions will be examined in the following section.

9

Calcification and Stone Disorders

Calcergy syndrome

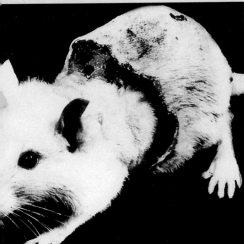

B **Pulmonary calcinosis**
(HE) x 75

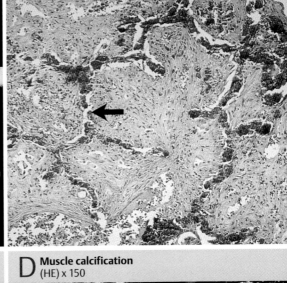

Muscle calcification
(HE) x 50

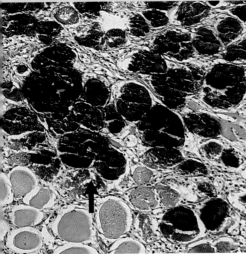

D **Muscle calcification**
(HE) x 150

Renal calcinosis
(EvG) x 35

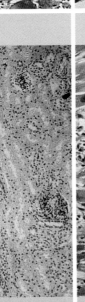

F **Myocardial calcinosis**
(HE) x 50

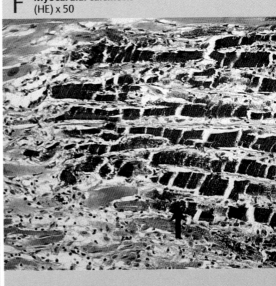

Stone Disorders

▪ Urolithiasis

Definition: Formation of concretions of component substances of urine in the lumen and/or terminal sacs of the excretory urinary tract.

Etiologic factors:
— *Salt concentration in urine* due to dehydration (perspiration) or concentration of metabolites in the blood (hyperuricemia, hypercalcemia, hyperoxaluria, or cystinuria).
— *Deficiency of complexing agents* such as magnesium.
— *High pH* (due to bacterial urease) causes formation of magnesium ammonium phosphate calculi. In hypercalcemia, calcium phosphate calculi are formed.
— *Low pH* causes formation of urate and cystine urinary calculi.
— *Natural inhibitors of stone formation:* may also be absent.
— *Nucleation factors* such as cellular detritus, necrotic sequestered papillae, thrombi, and bacteria.

Morphology:
— **Calcium oxalate calculi** are hard, brownish-black, small, mulberry-shaped, and radiopaque.
— **Calcium phosphate calculi** are brittle, grayish-white, 5–10 mm in size, and radiopaque.
— **Magnesium ammonium phosphate calculi** are crumbly, pale yellow, antler-shaped, 3–5 cm in size, and radiolucent.
— **Urate calculi** are soft or hard, yellowish-brown, oval, 3–5 cm in size, and radiolucent.
— **Cystine calculi** are crystalline with a pattern of radial leaves, yellowish-green, 3–5 cm in size, and radiolucent.

✚ **Clinical presentation:** Urinary calculi occur more often in men than in women. Symptoms vary according to the size of the stone.

Small calculi pass through the ureter, triggering colicky pain. Possible sequelae include stasis of the urine causing distension of the urinary tract with compressive atrophy of the renal parenchyma (hydroureter and hydronephrosis). This may lead to bacterial inflammation of the urinary tract (ureteritis) with rising inflammation spreading to the renal pelvis and tubules (purulent pyelonephritis). The urinary calculus may injure the urothelium, resulting in hematuria.

Large calculi remain lodged in the renal pelvis (► A), where they may cause injury, leading to hematuria and pyelonephritis.

☺ **Prominent patient:** Ludwig van Beethoven (1770–1827), German composer.

▪ Cholelithiasis

Definition: Formation of concretions of component biliary substances in the gallbladder (cholecystolithiasis) and/or bile ducts (choledocholithiasis).

Etiologic factors:
— *Concentration of precipitating substances:* Supersaturation of cholesterol leads to reduced cholesterol synthesis due to (a) hypersecretion of cholesterol (in obesity, senile diabetes mellitus, type IV hyperlipoproteinemia, and multiple pregnancy) and (b) hypersecretion of bile acid (in liver cirrhosis). Supersaturation of bilirubin leads to increased synthesis of conjugated bilirubin due to (a) bacterial β-glucuronidase, (b) release of Ca^{2+} from necrotic bile ducts, and (c) destruction of erythrocytes.
— *Delayed emptying of the gallbladder* leads to thickening of the bile and bacterial inflammation.
— *Nucleation factors* such as cell detritus and mucin.

Morphology:
— **Cholesterol gallstones** are metabolic calculi. They are large, smooth, yellowish, and radiolucent. Their cross-section (► B) has a radial pattern.
— **Cholesterol pigment gallstones** are metabolic calculi. These may be solitary monolithic stones (► C), multifaceted (► E), or mulberry-shaped. Their cross section shows a pattern of layered rings of yellow, brownish black, and white material (► C). The stones are radiolucent.
— **Black pigment gallstones** are hemolytic calculi. They are small, mulberry-shaped, multiple, black (► D), and radiolucent.
— **Brown pigment gallstones** are cholangitis calculi. They are ellipsoid-to-cylindrical, crumbly, and earthy.

✚ **Clinical presentation:** Gallstones are very common and occur more often in women than in men. Symptoms vary according to the size of the stone.

Small calculi pass through bile ducts, triggering colicky pain and obstructing the flow of bile. Possible sequelae include:
– Cholangitis and obstructive jaundice (cholestasis) can lead to cholangitic liver cirrhosis, which in turn can cause acute pancreatitis (where the hepatic duct and pancreatic duct have a common mouth).
– Cholecystitis can lead to chronic scarring and shrinking of the gallbladder.

Large calculi remain in the gallbladder, causing inflammation leading to cholecystolithiasis. The gallstone presses against the gallbladder wall, resulting in ulcerous cholecystitis, compressive necrosis, and gallbladder perforation. Possible sequelae include:
– Penetration and emptying of the bile into the abdominal cavity (cholascos), resulting in biliary peritonitis.
– Penetration into an adjacent organ, creating a biliary digestive fistula.
– Penetration and passage of bile into the small bowel, causing bowel obstruction and ileus.

❗ **Note:** *Risk factors* for cholelithiasis include the five Fs: fat, female, fair, forty, and fertile.

Therapeutic principle: Therapeutic infestation with stone lice of the species *Petrophaga lorioti* (► F).

A Renal pelvic stone

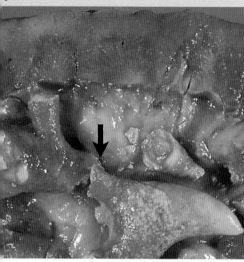

B Cholesterol stone

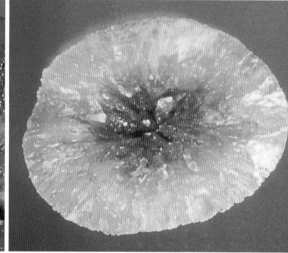

C Cholesterol pigment stone

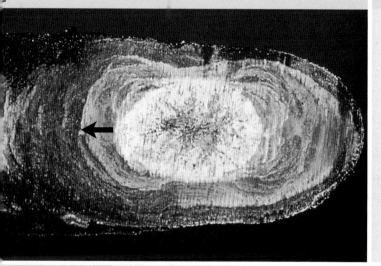

D black pigment gall stone

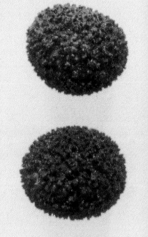

E Pigment gallstones

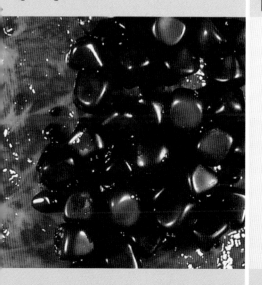

F Stone louse: Petrophaga lorioti

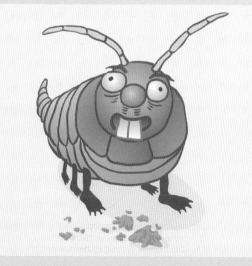

10 Chemical Cell Injury

When Poisons Mix With Life Processes

Summary

A toxin's potential for injury essentially depends on the degree of its absorption, accumulation, and duration of action at the site. Once in the body, hydrophilic toxins in particular develop their injurious effect by binding to certain cell structures. Lipophilic substances primarily accumulate in fatty tissues. Of the myriad possible mechanisms of action of toxic foreign substances, effects on enzymes are the most severe. Other toxins develop their injurious effects by altering hemoglobin so that it can no longer transport oxygen. A large group of toxins and therapeutic drugs inhibit the neurohumoral transmission of stimuli or interfere with the genetic or immune system. After interacting with such toxins, cells of the affected tissue attempt to break down the toxin by enzymatic action or to flood the region with bodily fluids (secretions or exudates) to dilute it at the site of the injury. Cells only lose this battle where the toxin is present in large quantities.

▶ **Medications** can injure erythrocytes, leukocytes, or thrombocytes to produce anemia, leukocyte deficiency, or punctate hemorrhaging. In the skin, they primarily produce exanthemas. They can also produce damage to liver cells similar to that occurring in hepatitis or cause damage to the renal tubules or glomeruli.

▶ **Environmental toxins** occur in a wide variety of forms. This section will limit itself to a discussion of the most important and/or hazardous of these. The most common intoxications with gaseous agents include inhalation of carbon monoxide, which interferes with oxygen-hemoglobin bonding, and inhalation of exhaust gases containing lead, which primarily causes anemia and neurologic damage. Asbestos, once used commonly in industry without any precautions, has since "taken its revenge" in the form of a toxic dust causing mesotheliomas in patients with sufficient exposure.

▶ **Alimentary toxins** may produce intoxications that are rare but distinctive in their molecular pathology, such as poisoning by the mushroom Amanita phalloides. Far more common, ethyl alcohol is not only an addictive substance but also a severe organic toxin for the liver, brain, and embryo.

Drug-Induced Disorders

Drug-Induced Damage to Blood Cells

Pathogenesis: Medications can damage blood cells via several different mechanisms:
— Direct toxic damage to mature blood cells (hemolysis);
— Direct damage to mature blood cells through a hypersensitivity reaction (p. 170);
— Direct damage to certain blood cells in the bone marrow (as in aplastic anemia);
— Indirect damage to blood cells due to a pre-existing metabolic defect in these cells (such as a glucose-6-phosphate dehydrogenase deficiency of the erythrocytes). (Treating this deficiency with the antimalaria agent primaquine causes hemolytic anemia.)

✚ **Clinical presentation and morphology:** The disorder is characterized by *agranulocytosis* (severe leukocyte deficiency), *anemia* (severe erythrocyte deficiency), and *thrombocytopenia* (severe platelet deficiency).

Drug-Induced Skin Disease

Pathogenesis: Undesirable side effects of medications most frequently manifest themselves in the skin. The severest types of drug-induced skin damage are generally attributable to hypersensitivity reactions (p. 166).

✚ **Clinical examples:**
— *Exanthema* is caused by a type I hypersensitivity reaction. Histamines are released, causing an itching exudative inflammation (p. 196).
— *Fixed drug-induced exanthema* results from a few drugs such as barbiturates. Use of these drugs induces erythema at a certain site on the skin, which returns at the same site every time the drug is used.
— *Urticaria* is caused by a type III hypersensitivity reaction (p. 170). This produces allergic vascular inflammation with severe itching in the skin (leukocytoclastic vasculitis) accompanied by hives. This can lead to vesicular skin eruptions in the epidermis (Lyell syndrome).[1]
— *Contact dermatitis* is caused by medications or noxious agents that act like haptens. These substances cause a type IV hypersensitivity reaction, often in combination with type I (p. 166).

---

[1] Lyell syndrome: vesicular separation of the irreversibly damaged epidermis in thermal damage to the skin; also known as toxic epidermal necrolysis.

Drug-Induced Liver Disease

Pathogenesis: Many medications can cause liver damage.

Predictable liver toxins consistently damage the liver in *all* patients, causing (a) direct dose-dependent cell injury or (b) indirect injury due to impaired metabolism. Such toxins may act in four ways.

— *Hepatocytotoxic:*
Damage to liver cells and tissue follows the pattern of acute viral hepatitis (with tuberculostatic agents) or severe chronic hepatitis (with halothane).
— *Cholangiopathic:*
The function of the intrahepatic bile ducts is compromised, leading to cholestasis (with chlorpromazine).
— *Phlebotoxic:*
Damage to the hepatic veins (such as from contraceptive steroids) leads to thrombotic venous occlusion, later progressing to venous occlusive disease.
— *Hepatofibrotic:*
Fibrotic transformation of the periportal liver (such as from vinyl chloride) leads to portal hypertension (p. 392).

Unpredictable liver toxins cause liver damage that is *dose-dependent* and occurs only in patients who already suffer from (a) an allergic hypersensitivity reaction and/or (b) abnormal metabolism. These liver toxins produce are hepatotoxic and/or cholangiopathic (cholestasis).

Drug-Induced Kidney Disease

Pathogenesis: Many medications or their metabolites that are normally eliminated with the urine cause kidney damage in one or more of the following ways:

— *Tubular-toxic:*
Kidney toxins (such as gentamicin) selectively destroy the tubular epithelium. The resulting tubular necrosis leads to diffusion of the noxious agent throughout the medullary interstitium, damaging the proteoglycan-containing extracellular matrix. This results in destructive interstitial nephritis with subsequent scarring.
— *Glomerular-toxic:*
Damage to the loops of the glomerulus (such as from penicillamine) leads to inflammation of the glomerulus, interfering with secondary urine production and causing hematuria, proteinuria, and hypertension.
— *Vascular-toxic:*
The toxin (such as a sulfonamide) triggers a hypersensitivity reaction (type I, III, or IV), resulting in allergic vascular inflammation (angiitis).
— *Erythrocyte-toxic:*
Primary damage to the erythrocytes (such as from rifampicin) triggers hemolysis. This leads to occlusion of the renal tubules with congealed hemoglobin, causing kidney (chromoprotein nephrosis).[1]

Drug-Induced Lung Disease

Pathogenesis: Some medications cause lung damage in one or more of the following ways.
— *Allergotoxic:*
The reaction occurs in the lung and/or pleura. The medication causes (a) a toxic pulmonary edema (diffuse alveolar damage syndrome) with exudation from an edema into the alveolar interstitium (p. 40), or (b) eosinophilic pneumonia, or (c) inflammatory pleuropulmonary fibrosis.
— *Alveocytotoxic:*
Direct damage to the alveolar epithelia (such as from busulfan) causes fibrotic inflammation in the alveolar interstitium. This in turn leads to excessive compensatory alveolar cell regeneration (membranous alveolar cells become cubic and polyploid), causing chronic inflammation in the interstitial tissue of the lung. This progresses to chronic interstitial pneumonia, resulting in pulmonary insufficiency (p. 40).
— *Bronchiolotoxic:*
Direct damage to the bronchial epithelia (such as from bleomycin) causes destructive fibrotic inflammation of the alveolar parenchyma of the lung. The respiratory bronchioli become obstructed, resulting in mucus retention and chronic inflammation of the lung. This produces a syndrome of obliterating bronchiolitis with organizing pneumonia.
— *Arteriotoxic:*
Direct damage to the pulmonary arteries (such as from amphetamines) causes obstructive fibrosis of the pulmonary arteries, leading to pulmonary hypertension (p. 392).
— *Phlebotoxic:*
Direct damage to the pulmonary veins (such as from bleomycin) leads to thrombotic obstructive fibrosis of the pulmonary veins, later progressing to venous occlusive disease.

Drug-Induced Neurologic Disorders

Pathogenesis: Certain medications damage the central nervous system and/or peripheral nervous system in one or more of the following ways.
— **Impairment of the CSF-brain barrier**
results in a toxic cerebral edema (such as in barbiturate intoxication).
— **Necrosis of the cerebral cortex**
may occur in barbiturate intoxication.
— **Necrotizing leucencephalopathy**
— **Impaired breakdown of ganglioside**
(such as from chloroquine) causes damage to ganglion cells (storage dystrophy).
— **Toxic nerve cell injury**
(such as from vincristine) causes neuronal polyneuropathy.
— **Toxic Schwann cell injury**
destroys the myelin, resulting in demyelinating polyneuropathy. The reparative reaction of the Schwann cells with repeated remyelination results in an onion-like pattern of Schwann cell proliferation and thickening of the nerves.

---

[1] Nephrosis and nephrotic syndrome are generic terms for kidney disease with 1) proteinuria, 2) hypoproteinemia or dysproteinemia, 3) hyperlipidemia and hypercholesteremia, and 4) edema (primarily eyelid edema).

Diseases from Environmental Factors

Carbon Monoxide Poisoning

Pathogenesis: Carbon monoxide poisoning results in formation of carboxyhemoglobin, which is unable to bind oxygen and only slowly releases the carbon monoxide.

Sequelae

■ **Severe carbon monoxide poisoning** causes death from asphyxiation.

■ **Acute carbon monoxide poisoning** manifests itself only in patients surviving longer than three days. It produces necrosis in the basal ganglia and gray matter of the cortex and damage to embryos.

Lead Poisoning

Pathogenesis: Lead absorbed by the gastrointestinal tract accumulates in the skeleton, where it displaces calcium. From there, the lead is only gradually released to form accumulations in other organ tissues.

Sequelae

■ **Metaphyseal lead lines** appear in the growing skeleton. Lead impairs osteoclastic bone remodeling and remains in bone for many years.

■ **Acquired porphyria:** Lead blocks urine synthesizing enzymes containing sulfhydryl (α-aminolevulinic acid dehydrogenase and coproporphyrin-III-decarboxylase), leading to a deficiency in heme-containing cytochromes and porphyrinuria.

■ **Anemia:** Lead impairs ferrochelatase, preventing the breakdown of iron into heme. This results in hypochromic sideroachrestic anemia (anemia characterized by heme deficiency and lack of iron metabolism).

■ **Erythrocyte disease:** Lead causes condensation of ribosomes, leading to basophilic mottling in erythrocytes and their precursors.

■ **Lead nephropathy:** Lead causes dysfunction of the renal tubules leading to Fanconi syndrome (p. 100).

■ **Lead encephalopathy:** Accumulation of lead primarily in the gray matter of the cerebral cortex and the basal ganglia results in ganglion cell necrosis and demyelination leading to dementia.

■ **Polyneuropathy:** Lead causes segmental demyelination and axon degeneration. This causes peroneal nerve palsy in children and radial nerve palsy in adults.

☺ **Prominent patients:** The patricians of the Roman empire suffered poisoning from their lead water pipes.

Asbestosis

Definition: Disorder caused by asbestos fibers, generally as a result of occupational exposure.

Pathogenesis: Asbestos fibers inhaled in the form of dust particles are phagocytosed by macrophages and alveolar cells. They are transported by the lymph system (a) into the pulmonary interstitium, where they activate fibroblasts, (b) into the pleural mesothelia, and (c) via sputum to the intestinal tract and via lymph into the peritoneal mesothelia. After phagocytosis, the macrophages envelop the asbestos fibers with a ferrite-protein mixture, producing club-shaped asbestos bodies (▶ A, B). The phagocytes release cytokines and growth factors, leading to inflammatory fibrosis of the lung and pleura.

The precise mechanism of asbestos' carcinogenic effect is not known. It acts as a co-carcinogen in combination with cigarette smoke.

Sequelae

■ **Pneumoconiosis** (asbestos lung) involves fibrosis of the pulmonary interstitium.

■ **Pleural plaques:** The pleura (the lateral wall of the chest) is transformed into a solid cartilage-like fibrous plate that interferes with breathing.

■ **Malignant mesotheliomas:** malignant pulpy tumors that extend as diffuse plates of tissue into the pleural and peritoneal spaces (▶ C, D). They rarely metastasize.

Histologic subtypes are classified according to their primary components:

— *Epithelial mesothelioma:* with polymorphous proliferative mesothelial cells, forming slit-like structures within in a fibrous stroma (▶ E).
— *Sarcomatous mesothelioma:* with polymorphous proliferative fibroblast-like mesothelial cells and a fibrous or fascial pattern of growth (▶ F).

Note: *Immunohistochemical findings in mesothelioma:* cells express cytokeratin and vimentin and calretinin without expressing of CEA.

Note: *Asbestos* is a generic term for heat-resistant hydrated silicates reduced to fibrous form by mechanical processing. These materials are used in the manufacture of cement, textiles, insulation, rubber tires, and brake lining.

10

Chemical Cell Injury

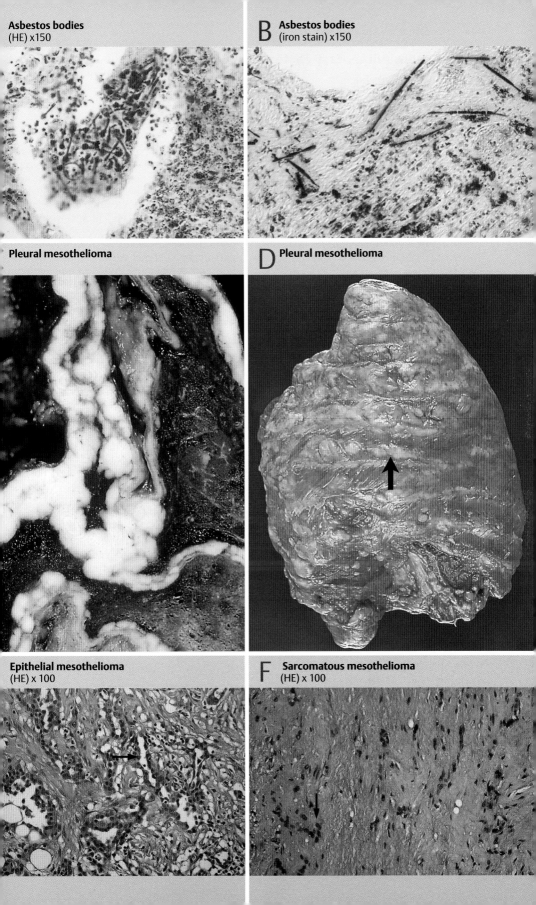

Asbestos bodies
(HE) x150

B **Asbestos bodies**
(iron stain) x150

Pleural mesothelioma

D **Pleural mesothelioma**

Epithelial mesothelioma
(HE) x 100

F **Sarcomatous mesothelioma**
(HE) x 100

Disease from Alimentary Factors

■ α-Amanitine Poisoning

Pathogenesis: Ingestion of mushrooms of the species Amanita phalloides results in the poison selectively binding to hepatocyte nuclei. This inhibits RNA polymerase B, blocking RNA transcription and protein synthesis and causing cytotoxicity.

Morphologic signs of poisoning include the following.

In the *liver,* fatty cytoplasmic degeneration and hydropic swelling (p. 12) occur, leading to necrosis in the central portions of the lobes. This causes jaundice (p. 108) and eventually liver failure.

In the *endothelium,* endothelial necrosis leads to disseminated intravascular coagulation (p. 402).

> **Note:** Poisonous mushrooms of the species *Amanita phalloides* may be mistaken for edible mushrooms. The primary toxin is α-amanitine (an octapeptide). The quantity of toxin contained in a single mushroom can be fatal.

■ Alcoholism

Textbook example of disease from drug addiction.

Definition: Disease from addiction to ethyl alcohol.

Alcohol metabolism: Ethyl alcohol is absorbed in the upper gastrointestinal tract. This means that alcohol is quickly transported to every tissue. The level of alcohol catabolism in the liver is a constant 100 mg per hour and kg of body weight. Alcohol is catabolized by ethyl alcohol dehydrogenase in cytosol, the catalase of the peroxisomes, and the ethanol oxidizing system of the smooth endoplasmic reticulum to acetaldehyde. This product is further oxidized to acetyl coenzyme A, which together with $NADH_2$ (produced in quantity) is used in fat synthesis. Finally, the acetyl coenzyme A is broken down in muscle tissue into CO_2 and H_2O in the citrate cycle.

Pathogenesis: The toxicity of ethyl alcohol is due to the following mechanisms. *Acetaldehyde* is a toxic ethyl alcohol metabolite that inhibits protein synthesis in ribosomes and mitochondria, damaging the cell. *Hypovitaminosis* results from the alcoholic's "liquid nutrition." This leads to chronic protein and vitamin deficiency, especially of the vitamin B complex.

☺ **Prominent patient:** Ernest Hemingway (1899–1961), American author and Nobel prize winner.

Sequelae of Alcoholism

■ Alcoholic Fatty Degeneration of the Liver

Pathogenesis: Ethyl alcohol leads to reduced oxidation of fatty acids, in turn leading to delayed release of lipids by the liver and inhibition of VLDL formation. This causes hyperlipidemia and globular fatty degeneration of the liver cells in the central portions of the lobes (affecting over 50% of all cells). This produces the distinctive yellow liver at laparoscopy (▶ A, B) and causes alcoholic hepatitis.

■ Alcoholic Hepatitis

Pathogenesis: Ethyl alcohol damages the cytoskeleton, resulting in the formation of Mallory bodies (▶ C1; see also p. 34) and liver cell necrosis, which attracts neutrophils (▶ C2). The neutrophils surround the Mallory bodies like jackals around a campfire, creating fibrous tissue to replace the necrosis. The "chicken-wire" fibrosis surrounds the hepatocytes in the central portions of the lobes. Necrosis of the bile duct epithelia occurs with reactive inflammation and regenerative bile-duct proliferation. Iron deposits in the reticuloendothelial system also occur.

■ Alcoholic Liver Cirrhosis

Pathogenesis: Ethyl alcohol causes progressive destruction of hepatocytes and bile ducts, leading to repair with fibrous scarring. This progressive fibrotic transformation of the hepatic parenchyma into small nodules leads to cirrhosis (▶ D).

■ Megaloblastic Anemia

Pathogenesis: Ethyl alcohol causes folic acid deficiency. This in turn interferes with erythrocyte maturation, producing abnormally large, nucleated erythrocyte precursors (megaloblasts) in the blood.

■ Wernicke-Korsakoff Syndrome

Pathogenesis: Ethyl alcohol causes thiamine deficiency (vitamin B_1). This in turn causes brain damage with recurrent bleeding. Sequelae include deposits of hemosiderin in tissue, leading to brown discoloration of the brain tissue, especially in the mamillary bodies (▶ E, F), and spongiform tissue dystrophy, primarily in the mamillary bodies, hypothalamus, inferior quadrigeminal region, aqueduct region, and the nuclei of the oculomotor nerve.

✚ **Clinical presentation:** Patients present with somnolence (sleepiness), loss of memory, ataxia (gait disturbances), and ocular muscle palsy.

■ Cardiomyopathy

Pathogenesis: Ethyl alcohol causes hypovitaminosis B_1 and B_6. This disrupts mitochondrial enzyme synthesis, impairing cell respiration and causing heart muscle disease. The myocardium responds with compensatory dilatative thickening of the heart wall (see p. 116) accompanied by finely nodular fibrosis and fatty degeneration.

> **Note:** *Alcohol* "spikes the liver but spares the vessel." There is hardly any atherosclerosis due to increased HDL.

Normal liver

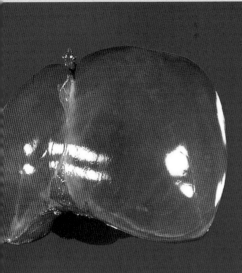

B **Liver with fatty degeneration**

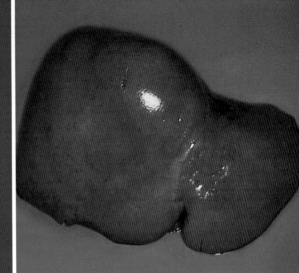

Mallory bodies (liver)
(Goldner's trichrome) x 120

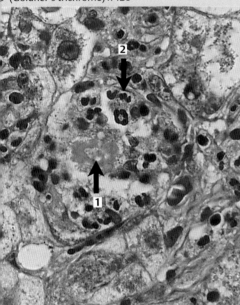

D **Alcoholic cirrhosis**

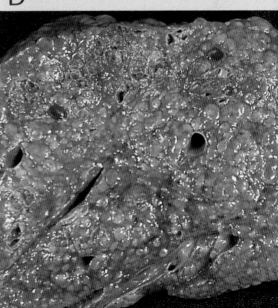

Mamillary body hemorrhage
(HE) x 3

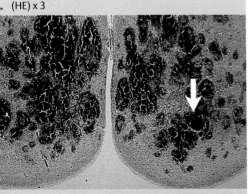

F **Mamillary body siderosis**

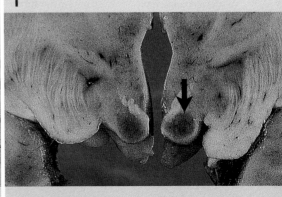

11

Surviving The Molecular Bombardment
Physical Cell Injury

Summary

Physical cell injuries can produce systemic and local tissue lesions. In addition to injuries produced by mechanical force (discussed in the section on wound healing), cell injuries from physical agents include thermal, electrical, and radiation injuries. In these injuries, the extent to which capillary structures are compromised largely determines the severity of the resulting tissue lesion. This defect in thermoregulation, following the longterm effect of high temperatures (without adequate heat dissipation), manifests itself as an inflammatory reaction in the early phases of the injury (p. 194) and as fibrotic sclerosis in its late phases.

Thermal Injury

Heat-Induced Injuries

■ Heat Stroke

Etiology: Elevated ambient temperature in combination with high humidity and/or inability to dissipate heat as a result of muscular exertion (such as extreme sports), unsuitable clothing or obesity, or deficient physical adaptability.

Pathogenesis: Acute risk of mortality is present where body temperature approaches the 41 °C threshold (approximately 106 °F). Endothelial injury is the pivotal lesion. It leads to disseminated intravascular coagulation (p. 402), which in turn triggers circulatory shock (p. 392).

Morphology: Microthrombi in the minor vessels of the brain lead to punctate ring hemorrhages around the minor vessels (purpura cerebri) and destruction of ganglion cells. Similar tissue damage occurs in the liver, heart, and kidneys with apoptosis.

☺ **Clinical record:** At 46.5 °C (115.7 °F), 52-year-old W. Jones of Atlanta, Georgia, holds the clinical record for the highest body temperature survived.

■ Burns

Definition: Injury due to acute local hyperthermia.

Pathogenesis: Cell injury occurs at exposure to temperatures exceeding 65 °C (149 °F), at which temperature protein denaturation occurs. This causes coagulative necrosis, resulting in formation of toxic proteins ("burn toxins") that damage capillary structures and generate inflammation mediators (p. 202). *Local effects* of this include an exudative inflammatory reaction (p. 196); *systemic effects* include burn shock with gastroduodenal stress ulcer (generally a peptic stomach ulcer; p. 217) and kidney failure.

Morphology: A skin burn can be present in the following degrees of severity.

— *First-degree burn* (*thermal erythema*) causes vasodilatation, resulting in hyperemia with erythema. The injury heals completely.
— *Second-degree burn* (*blistering*) exhibits thermally induced disruption of microcirculation with increased permeability (p. 198). This leads to exudation of blood serum in an inflammatory reaction, resulting in epithelial separation in the form of blisters (subepidermal blistering; ► A). Destruction of the epithelial blisters leads to ulceration in which the dermis is intact (► B). The injury can heal completely.
— *Third-degree burn* (*scabbing*) exhibits dark brown necrosis that can vary in depth and may be accompanied by areas of less severe injury (► C). The dead tissue is sloughed off, often leaving behind areas of ulceration. As the injury heals, it scars and contracts severely, resulting in keloid formation (p. 312) and contracture (► D).
— *Fourth-degree burn* (*charred tissue*) results from extremely high heat that chars tissue. The injury heals like a third-degree burn.

> ❗ **Note:** The surface area involved in a burn is a more important prognostic criterion than the degree of the burn. Surface area is determined by the rule of nines (► E).

> ❗ **Note:** Death in the *early* phase after a burn injury results from hypovolemic shock and burn shock; death in the *late* phase (after one week) results from uremia due to kidney damage.

☺ **Prominent "patients":**
Prisoners of Buchenwald concentration camp in 1943 were subjected to burn experiments to test the preparation Echinacin manufactured by Madaus. Civilian victims of napalm bombs (► D) during the Vietnam war (1964–1973).

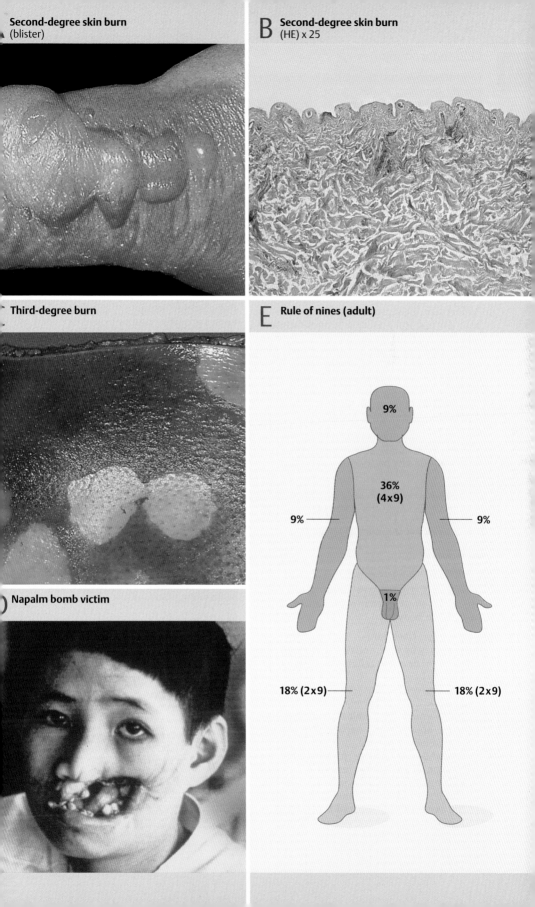

Second-degree skin burn
(blister)

B **Second-degree skin burn**
(HE) x 25

Third-degree burn

E **Rule of nines (adult)**

9%

36%
(4x9)

9%   9%

1%

18% (2x9)   18% (2x9)

Napalm bomb victim

Cold-Induced Injuries

General pathogenesis: The human body requires a body temperature of at least 35 °C (95 °F). Where body temperature falls below 25 °C (77 °F), all biological processes slow down. This delays the dissociation of oxygen from hemoglobin and increases the solubility of CO_2 in plasma. The reduced consumption of glucose in tissue leads to loss of consciousness and cardiac arrest. Where temperature continues to fall below freezing, water crystallizes out of tissue fluids. This increases the pressure of the remaining tissue fluid, causing the cell to burst.

■ Hypothermia

Definition: Injury due to a mismatch between heat production and heat loss resulting in a drop in body temperature.

Pathogenesis: Heat production can be disrupted by lack of physical activity or by previous disorders that have decreased the body's defenses against cold. The result is a drop in body temperature. A drop in body temperature below 25 °C (77 °F) causes heart and circulatory system failure with vascular thrombosis (p. 404). This leads to organ infarction (p. 414) and/or failure of the respiratory center.

☺ **Clinical record:** Two-year-old M. Troke who had fallen into a snow bank in Milwaukee, Wisconsin, holds the clinical record for the lowest body temperature survived at 16 °C (60.8 °F).

☺ **Prominent "patients":** Many Jews died of hypothermia in ice water baths in Nazi Germany, in experiments conducted by doctors to determine survival time as a function of ambient temperature.

■ Frostbite

Synonyms: cold injury, local hypothermia.

Pathogenesis: Local tissue freezing can occur where the effect of cold is limited to certain areas of the body.

Morphology: Like burns, several degrees of frostbite may be differentiated whose full clinical picture develops after the tissue is rewarmed.

— **First-degree frostbite** *(cold erythema):* The blood vessels remain dilated after the tissue is rewarmed. The result is that the injured tissue areas remain hyperemic for a prolonged period of time.

— **Second-degree frostbite** *(frost blisters):* Restoration of circulation results in alterative inflammation with exudation (p. 196). This leads to a high volume of fluid within the tissue, causing separation of the epidermis from underlying tissue in blisters.

— **Third-degree frostbite** *(freezing gangrene):* Irreversible paralysis of vascular structures is accompanied by stasis and thrombosis. This leads to freezing gangrene of the skin and deeper tissues, producing a burn-like injury in the affected limb (▶ A, B).

— **Fourth-degree frostbite** *(completely frozen tissue):* This results in complete destruction of tissue.

Sequelae of Cold Injuries

General pathogenesis: The following severe changes typically occur in the blood vessels of tissue affected by cold injuries.

■ Endangiitis obliterans

Definition: Reactive inflammatory vascular stenosis with intimal fibrosis.

Pathogenesis: Transient cold injury to the tissue causes apoptotic death of the endothelial cells (▶ C1) that may expose the subintima (▶ C2). This triggers aggregation of thrombocytes on the subintima, resulting in a reactive inflammatory and stenosing thickening of the intima in veins and arteries. This narrowing of the vascular lumina reduces the volume of blood flowing through the affected area, producing sensitivity to cold and Raynaud syndrome.

■ Raynaud Syndrome

Definition: Cold disrupts the peripheral regulation of blood flow. When the patient is later exposed to cold, a symmetrical paling of the digits (the thumb is spared) may be observed with a "tricolor phenomenon" as a result of deficient vascular supply.

! **Note:** *Tricolor phenomenon* is characterized by *white* (initial paleness with paresthesia), then *blue* (cyanosis due to venostasis), and finally *red* (hyperemia due to vasodilatation).

! **Note:**
– *Raynaud's disease* (primary Raynaud's phenomenon) involves impaired acral blood supply due to vascular cramps originating in the central nervous system.
– *Secondary Raynaud's syndrome* (Raynaud's phenomenon) involves impaired acral blood supply due to primary vascular injury.

! **Note:** *Signs of death from freezing* include:
– Livid skin discoloration (without livores);
– Erosion of the gastric mucosa;
– Strips of hemorrhaging in the iliopsoas;
– Acetonemia.

Freezing gangrene

B **Freezing gangrene**

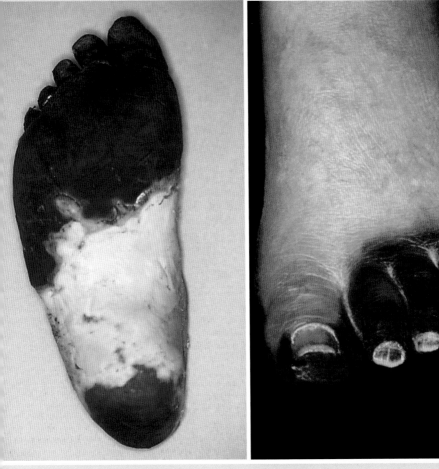

Endothelium following exposure to cold
(TEM) x 3000

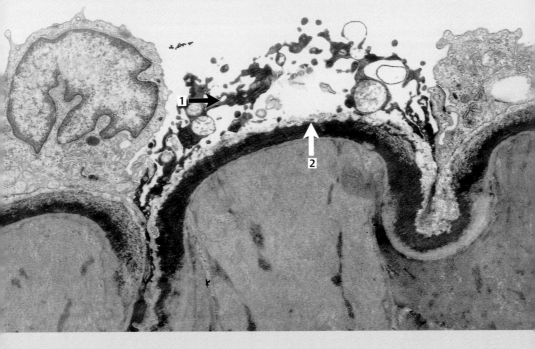

Electrical Injuries

Pathogenesis: Injuries involving electrical current are classified in four ranges of current intensity:

— *Current range I* (9–25 mA): This current causes spasms of skeletal, respiratory, and cardiac muscle that will result in cessation of breathing if the electrical contact is not interrupted in time. Electricity in this current range does not produce histologic damage, and the heart is not directly involved.
— *Current range II* (25–80 mA): The heart is involved to the extent that passage of current disrupts stimulus generation and conduction. Permanent late sequelae in the ECG are rare.
— *Current range III* (80 mA): This current causes death by inducing ventricular fibrillation.
— *Current range IV* (voltages exceeding 1000 V, i.e., high voltage, and currents exceeding 3–8 A): These currents produce burns, from the heat of the electrical arc, muscle contractions, and cardiac arrest.

Morphologic characteristics:
— **Electrical burns** at the entry and/or exit points (usually on the hands) are produced in accidents involving current ranges II and III.
Macroscopic appearance: Small, grayish white skin lesions with a central depression are observed. High-voltage accidents produce larger electrical burns with necrosis (▶ A).
Histologic examination reveals coagulative necrosis (p. 130) of the epidermis at this site with fascicular distended nuclei in the epithelial cells. In the marginal regions they are aligned toward the center of coagulation.
— **Myolysis** (disintegration of muscle) releases myoglobin into the blood, which then obstructs the renal tubules and causes kidney failure in the form of chromoprotein nephrosis (p. 141).
— **Cardiovascular shock** occurs, causing kidney failure.

Radiation Injury

Microwaves and Infrared Radiation

Pathogenesis: Microwaves and infrared radiation penetrate tissue and causes their atoms and molecules to vibrate. The heat generated causes protein denaturation and water evaporation.

> **Note:** Infrared radiation only penetrates the skin to a depth of about 5–10 mm. The heat damage from microwaves is more severe than from infrared radiation.

Visible Light and Ultraviolet Radiation

Pathogenesis:
— **Direct effects of radiation:** When the skin absorbs radiation from the shortwave ultraviolet range, the incident quantum energy exceeds the bonding energy of the molecules of the skin. This causes ionization, in which electrons are released from their bonds.
— **Indirect effects of radiation:** Ionization creates highly active radicals. These diffuse or are transported into surrounding tissues, where they trigger oxidative reactions. This absorption of light radiation is followed by non-light-dependent reactions such as dissociation, dehydration, and decarboxylation. These reactions affect the function of the affected molecules.

Sequelae of Light Radiation

■ **Acute photodermatosis:** Ultraviolet radiation overtaxes the skin's natural light protection mechanism. This produces DNA damage and acute exudative inflammation (p. 204) with bullous lesions and separation of the epidermis (sunburn).

■ **Chronic photodermatosis:** Where the skin's natural light protection mechanism is chronically overtaxed over a period of decades, irreversible ultraviolet damage leading to other complications will appear following a latency period of several years.

✚ **Complications:**
– *Solar elastosis* (actinic elastosis, p. 56).
– *Telangiectasia:* permanent dilation of the small veins of the skin, resulting in a visible cutaneous vascular network.
– *Actinic keratosis* (a precancerous condition; p. 340): As a result of permanent DNA damage, the epidermal epithelium exhibits nuclear polymorphism (▶ B1) and nuclear polychromasia accompanied by excessive formation of keratinized corneal scales (parakeratosis; ▶ B2). However, these changes do not penetrate the basement membrane (▶ B3).

Laser Radiation

Definition and pathogenesis: Laser radiation consists of emission-induced, coherently amplified, highly focused electromagnetic light waves. The beam can be used as a "radiation scalpel." Necrosis occurs to a depth of 100 μm in the tissue surrounding the laser channel (▶ C).

Example: Patients with inoperable coronary artery disease that does not respond to treatment may be treated by transmyocardial laser revascularization. A laser is used to "drill" numerous channels through the myocardium (▶ D) to improve its blood supply.

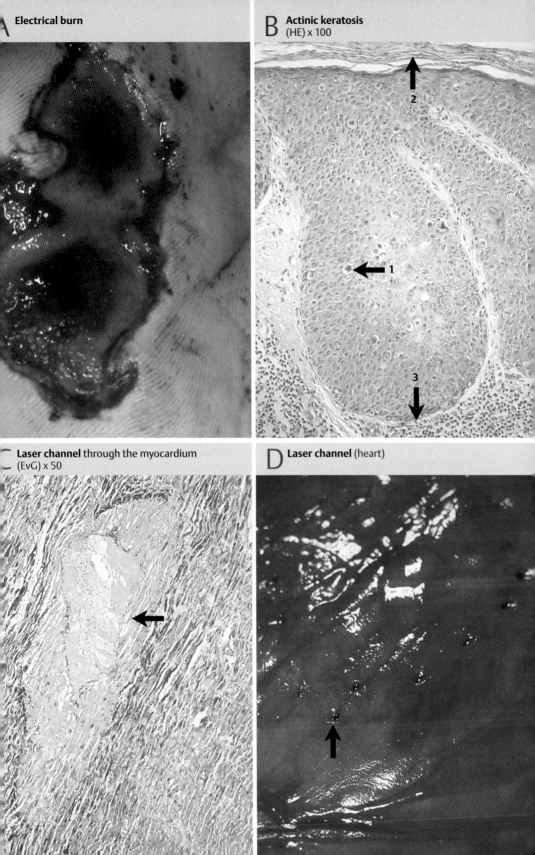

A Electrical burn

B Actinic keratosis
(HE) x 100

1
2
3

C Laser channel through the myocardium
(EvG) x 50

D Laser channel (heart)

Ionizing Radiation

Physiology: Radiation is migration of energy through space. In particulate radiation, this migration is caused by charged particles. *Particulate radiation* includes electrons (beta particles), protons, alpha particles (helium nuclei), neutrons, pi mesons, and heavy ions. The kinetic energy of particulate radiation is determined by the mass of the particles, their electric charge, and their velocity.

As they pass through matter, the particles change their direction and lose energy. Radiation in the form of waves as X-rays and gamma rays, which lack mass or electric charge, loses it energy in tissue through less random collisions with molecules. Similarly, electrically charged particles such as beta particles also lose energy through decelerating collisions with electrons in the irradiated tissue. Referred to as bremsstrahlung (braking radiation), this decelerating radiation produces linear traces on radiographic images (▶ A: thorium deposit in tissue, A1, with radiographic traces, A2; p. 334).

A collision can knock an orbiting electron completely out of the electron cloud surrounding the nucleus of the atom, or it can displace the electron into a new orbit. This causes an atom that was previously neutral to become electrically unstable, a process referred to as ionization. This occurs within 10^{-13} seconds and triggers radiolysis of the water in the cell to form aggressive radicals within a period of 10^{-9} seconds. Within a few seconds, these radicals react with the water in the cell to form peroxide, in turn causing the radiolysis products to react with DNA, RNA, and the membrane and enzyme lipids.

Sensitivity of cells to radiation depends on several factors.
— *Degree of differentiation* of the cells.
— *Phase in the cell cycle:* Radiation of cells in the G2 phase generally leads to impairment of mitosis, whereas it often leads to cell death in the M, G2, or early S phase.
— *Recovery period:* Where the entire radiation dose is divided into several separate fractions, the cell can have an opportunity to recover.

> **Note:** The relationship of nucleus to cytoplasm and the quantity of organelles give a rough indication of the degree of differentiation of a cell.

Sequelae of Radiation

General pathogenesis: Depending on which phase of the cycle the cell is in at the time, ionizing radiation may produce the following injuries:
— *Cells in the G0 phase* exhibit chromatin damage that leads to apoptosis (p. 128, 132), causing the nucleus to disintegrate into fragments (karyorrhexis; ▶ B).
— *Cells in the S phase* exhibit DNA and/or chromosome damage. This can cause (a) mutations leading to malignant transformation or (b) cell death in the form of apoptosis in the subsequent mitosis.

— *Cells in the M phase* exhibit destruction of the mitotic spindle. DNA synthesis is spared. However, this leads to formation of polyploid and/or multinucleate giant cells.

> **Note:** The *principle of radiation tissue damage* is that ionizing radiation triggers "damage" inflammation (alterative inflammation) that begins as exudative inflammation and ends as scarring and sclerosis.

◼ Radiation Vasculitis

▨ Capillary Injury

— *Early phase:* The endothelium in irradiated tissue often responds with swelling only after 10 days at the earliest. Massive radiation injury (<60 Gy) causes endothelial apoptosis within a few days, leading to hemorrhage (p. 398) that progresses to thrombotic vascular occlusion. Regenerating endothelial cells are multinucleate and/or polyploid (p. 8).

The ***result*** is radiation capillary necrosis.

— *Late phase:* Permanent capillary proliferation into the irradiated area (radiation telangiectasia) or focal capillary proliferation (capillary aneurysm) leads to increased vulnerability of the blood vessels and increased propensity to hemorrhage.

The ***result*** is radiation telangiectasia (▶ D).

▨ Arterial Injury

— *Early phase:* Endothelial damage (▶ C1) leads to increased vascular permeability, causing plasma to seep into the intima. This produces intimal swelling (▶ C2) and thrombus (p. 404) on the endothelial defect (▶ C3) with reactive inflammation and isolated myocyte apoptosis (▶ C4). The endothelium regenerates within a period of weeks (p. 310).

The ***result*** is a radiation-induced intimal lesion.

— *Late phase:* The regenerative capacity of the tissue is exhausted, resulting in disseminated apoptotic myocyte necrosis (▶ C5). This results in tears in the elastica interna (▶ C6), allowing plasma and fibrinogen to seep into the wall of the vessel (▶ C7). This in turn triggers an alterative inflammatory reaction, successively leading to scarring and sclerotic transformation of the intimal seepage (▶ C8).

The ***result*** is radiation-induced vascular sclerosis (▶ E).

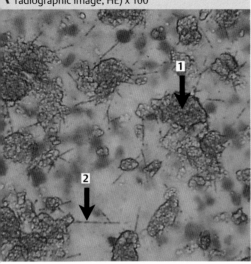

A **Thorium deposits** (bremsstrahlung traces in radiographic image; HE) x 100

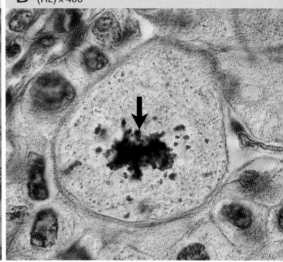

B **Radiation karyorrhexis** (HE) x 400

C **Radiation-induced vasculopathy**

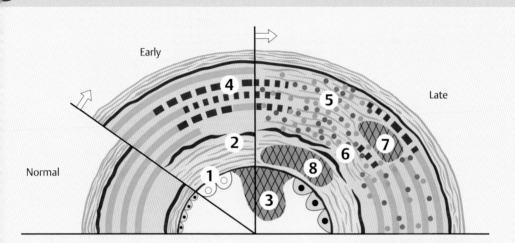

Early

Late

Normal

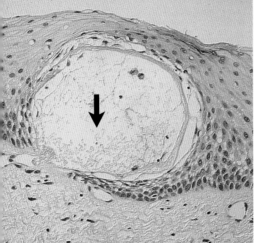

D **Radiation telangiectasia** (skin) (HE) x 50

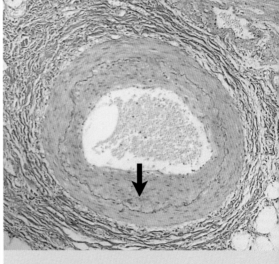

E **Radiation-induced vascular sclerosis** (EvG) x 50

■ **Radiation Dermatitis**

— *Early phase:* Only the basal cells (► A1) and appendages of the skin are sensitive to radiation. The resulting damage to the basal cells leads to loss of contact between cells in the spinous layer of the epidermis (acantholysis; ► A2). This in turn leads to focal necrosis (p. 132) and radiation ulcer. This is accompanied by radiation vasculitis leading to exudative inflammation (p. 196) and edema (► A3, p. 424).

The *result* is radiation-induced cutaneous edema and ulcer.

— *Late phase:* Skin telangiectasia is accompanied by strangely shaped polyploid "radiation fibroblasts" resembling cancer cells (pseudosarcoma; ► B), causing atrophic sclerosis of the skin and cutaneous appendages.

The *result* is radiation sclerosis of the skin.

■ **Radiation Enteritis**

— *Early phase:* Radiation sensitivity of the enterocytes leads to apoptotic epithelial necrosis and/or hydropic epithelial swelling. This is complicated by vascular damage, producing submucosal edema. This develops successively into acute erosive enteritis, progressive necrosis, and ulcerous enteritis.

The *result* is radiation enteritis.

— *Late phase:* Associated radiation-induced vascular disease delays the healing of the ulcerations, resulting in formation of fistulas that heal with scarred strictures.

The *result* is radiation sclerosis of the bowel.

■ **Radiation Bone Necrosis**

— *Early phase:* These lesions usually occur within three years of irradiation and may be masked by inflammatory reaction (radiation ostitis and/or radiation osteomyelitis). The necrotic bone is sequestered. Histologic examination reveals adhesions within its lamellar structure, and the osteolytic lacunae are empty (► C).

The *result* is radiation ostitis leading to radiation bone necrosis.

— *Late phase:* The medullary cavity appears scarred and fibrotic with interspersed areas of telangiectasia. The trabeculae show no signs of osteoblastic or osteoclastic activity.

The *result* is radiation osteosclerosis leading to radiation osteosarcoma (p. 358).

> **Note:** *Osteomyelitis* refers to inflammation of the bone including the medulla.

■ **Radiation-Induced Leukocyte Disease** The sensitivity of the hematopoietic and lymphopoietic cell systems to radiation depends on (a) the size of the specific proliferation compartment (p. 308) and (b) the dwell time of the affected cells in the differentiation compartment (p. 308). This time is significantly longer for erythrocytes than for leukocytes.

The *result* is radiation agranulocytosis within 2–3 weeks, later followed by radiation anemia.

> **Note:** The sequence of radiation-induced bloodcell lesions is:
> 1. Lymphopenia.
> 2. Thrombocytopenia.
> 3. Neutropenia.
> 4. Anemia.

> **Note:** Tissue structures that act as biologic radiation dosimeters (i.e., structures particularly sensitive to radiation) include the skin and mucous membranes.

> **Note:** Blood vessels are indicators of late sequelae of radiation (radiation-induced vascular disease).

Radiation Therapy

Radiation injuries to tumors are identical to those in normal tissue. Most obvious are the changes in the cell nucleus (p. 8). Such injury manifests itself primarily in abnormal mitotic figures, often in the form of triads shaped like a Mercedes star (► D), bizarre enlargements of the nucleus (giant cells; ► A1), and a chaotic nucleus (nuclear polymorphism).

Clinical complications include fibrosis of the irradiation tissue. *Example:* In peritubular testicular post-radiation fibrosis (► E), the testicular tubules are sclerosed and surrounded by collagen fibers (► E1). They contain only Sertoli cells (► E2) without any elements of spermatogenesis.

☺ **Prominent "patients":**
Atomic bomb victims: The Japanese cities of Hiroshima and Nagasaki were bombed during World War II in 1945. All that remained of one person was his watch (► F).
Victims of nuclear testing: US military personnel were knowingly exposed to radiation during above-ground testing of nuclear weapons in 1952 in Nevada.
Victims of nuclear waste accidents: Rescue workers were knowingly exposed to radiation following the large-scale nuclear accident at the reactor complex in Chernobyl in the Soviet Union in 1986.

The previous sections have shown that chemical and physical agents can produce tissue injuries accompanied by severe pain. The patient experiences the injury as "inflammation." The pathobiology of such injuries is the subject of the following chapters. First, we will discuss how the body detects foreign cells or autologous tissue distorted by injury (immune pathology), and then we will examine how it deals with such tissue (inflammation pathology).

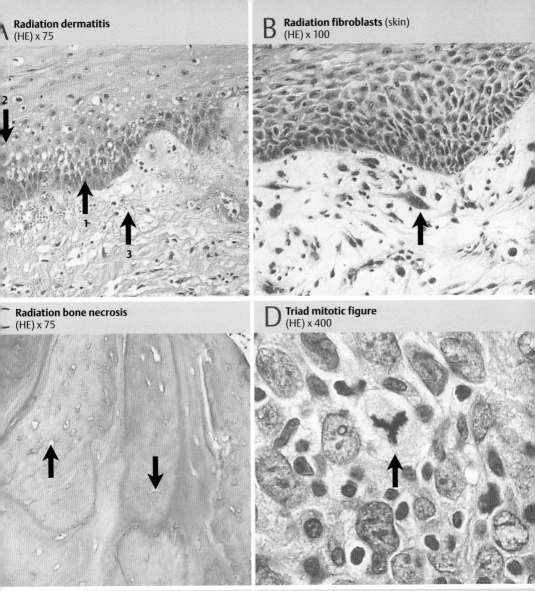

A Radiation dermatitis
(HE) x 75

B Radiation fibroblasts (skin)
(HE) x 100

C Radiation bone necrosis
(HE) x 75

D Triad mitotic figure
(HE) x 400

E Radiation fibrosis of the testis
(EvG) x 100

F Watch of atomic bomb victim

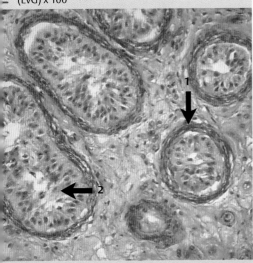

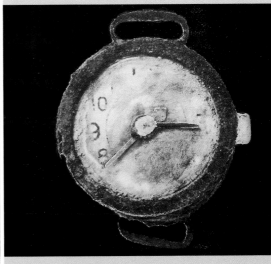

12 Self-Recognition and Self Defense
Immune Pathology

Summary

Myriads of microorganisms live on the gigantic surface structures of the human body. Because of this, the body must defend itself against its own skin and maintain its identity by means of nonspecific defense mechanisms (resistance) and specific defense mechanisms (immunity). Immunity is based on the body's ability to distinguish between autologous substances ("self") and exogenous substances ("non-self"). This is the task of the immune system. This system can be subdivided into two different families of cells, the B and T lymphocytes. The B cells are responsible for humoral immunity. Their effector mechanism consists of the antibodies they produce. These antibodies are supported by a system of complements activated in a cascade. Their effectiveness is attributable to the cytokines they generate and to killer cells among them. In light of this, it becomes apparent why defects in immunoglobulin synthesis, the complement system, and communication between leukocytes can lead to the following abnormal immune reactions:

▶ **Hypersensitivity reactions:** Here the organism responds to renewed contact with an antigen that it already knows and to which it is hypersensitive.

— *Type I hypersensitivity reactions* occur in patients who react to a certain antigen (or allergen) with abnormal production of IgE. IgE has a particular affinity for the mast cells and provokes the release of histamines.

— In *type II hypersensitivity reactions,* humoral antibodies against autologous antigens are created. When these antibodies bind to a target cell, macrophages interpret them as a signal to kill the cell.

— *Type III hypersensitivity reactions* lead to immune complex disease in which antigen–antibody complexes circulate in the body and cause vascular disease by deposits they form.

— *Type IV hypersensitivity reactions* are mediated by T lymphocytes that for a certain time have been "trained" on (a) pathogenic germs (infection allergy), (b) antigens that adhere to the skin (contact allergy), or (c) donor organ antigens (transplant allergy).

▶ **Autoimmune disorders:** In these disorders, the body violates the protection of its own identity and attacks itself. Accordingly, autoreactive antibodies or autoreactive lymphocytes that attack autologous substrates are crucial elements in the pathogenesis of these disorders.

▶ **Immunodeficiency disorders:** These disorders are attributable to a deficient immune response to various antigen stimuli. *Congenital B-cell defects* are clinically conspicuous because the reduced resistance to bacterial infection that they involve. In contrast, primary T-cell defects leave the patient unprotected against viruses and fungi. Patients with a combined B-cell and T-cell deficiency are poor candidates for survival. Among the *acquired immunodeficiency disorders,* gammopathy due to neoplastic proliferation of a plasma cell clone and AIDS due to infection with the human immunodeficiency virus (HIV) warrant special mention.

Antigen

Definition: A substance the body recognizes as "foreign" and that triggers a specific immune response (**anti**somato**gen**).

Complete antigen: A substance that induces an immune response and that can specifically react with the product of that response (the antibody).

Incomplete antigen (hapten): A low-molecular-weight substance (a short peptide or drug) that only acts as an antigen once it binds to macromolecules.

Antigen Neutralization

The body uses several strategies to render antigens harmless:

Humoral immunity: This involves the B lymphocytes, which create "antidotes" (antibodies) that circulate in body fluids.

Cell-mediated immunity: This involves the T lymphocytes that have learned to differentiate between autologous material ("self") and foreign material ("non-self").

This division of the immune system into B-cell and T-cell systems is made in the interest of clarity. From a biologic standpoint, it is an artificial distinction because the two component systems cooperate by means of a genetically determined control system (the HLA system) and special messenger substances (cytokines).

Immune Organs

Physiology: The human immune system consists of about 1×10^{12} lymphocytes and weighs about 1 kg. It is composed of tissues belonging to the lymphatic and reticuloendothelial systems. The lymphocytes circulate in the blood and also temporarily reside in the immune organs.

The immune organs include the following anatomic structures.

Central Immune Organs

■ Thymus

Until the end of the second month of embryonic development, the thymus is purely an epithelial organ. After that time, immature lymph cells migrate from hemopoietic embryonic tissue into the thymus. There they are cared for by nurse cells (interdigitating cells) and are programmed to distinguish between "self" and "non-self." They then enter the bloodstream as "fighting lymphocytes" (T lymphocytes) and settle in the peripheral lymphatic organs.

■ Bursa of Fabricius and Bone Marrow

The bursa of Fabricius occurs only in birds and is located near the cloaca. Bone marrow appears to have assumed the function of this organ in mammals and may therefore be regarded as its equivalent with respect to the ontogeny of the human immune system. Accordingly, the lymphocytes produced here are referred to as B lymphocytes.

Peripheral Immune Organs

■ Lymph Nodes

The follicular cortical region with primary and secondary follicles and the medullary region with the sinus of the node contain B lymphocytes. The paracortical region with its tertiary follicles supplied by venules harbors T lymphocytes.

■ Spleen

Branches of the trabecular artery, the periarterial lymph sheaths of the arteries of the splenic pulp belong to the T-cell system, whereas the splenic follicles and part of the red pulp belong to the B-cell system. The follicular arteries empty their blood directly into the splenic sinus (the fast compartment) or into the pulp strands (the slow compartment), from which it flows on through the trabecular vein.

■ MALT

Mucosa-associated lymphoid tissue includes the following structures:

— *Lymphatic pharyngeal ring* with the pharyngeal, lingual, and palatine tonsils;
— *Gut-associated lymphoid tissue (GALT),* including the Peyer's patches in the duodenum, the follicles of the appendix, the solitary follicles of the colon, and the immunocompetent cells of the intestinal mucosa;
— *Bronchi-associated lymphoid tissue (BALT),* including the lymphoid tissue in the peribronchial fascial sheath;
— *Exocrine glands* (salivary glands and pancreas);
— *Mammary glands.*

The MALT is characteristically located in the walls of hollow organs containing bacteria (gastrointestinal and respiratory tracts) and is in contact with pathogenic germs and other antigen material. Antigens from the intestinal tract are treated as follows:

The follicle-associated intestinal epithelium contains membranous cells (M cells), which pass antigens from the intestinal lumen to intraepithelial lymphocytes. The absorbed antigen is received by macrophages and dendritic cells and treated in such a manner that T cells and/or B cells in the adjacent lymph follicle are activated. They then enter the peripheral blood through the lymph system and search for these antigens. However, their homing receptors enable them to find their way back to the endothelium of their home vessels in the intestinal mucosa and in the other mucosa-associated lymphatic tissues. When they come into contact with an antigen, one of the substances they produce is IgA-type immunoglobulin (see below). This substance enters secretions such as milk, and is passed on to the infant. The infant then ingests the specific IgA antibodies against the disease with which the mother's immune system has already contended.

■ SALT

(**S**kin-**a**ssociated **l**ymphoid **t**issue).

 Note: *Lymphocytes* originate in either the **t**hymus (**T** lymphocytes) or the **b**one marrow (**B** lymphocytes).

Apart from this anatomic classification of the immune system, there is also a functional classification system based on the characteristics of the B lymphocytes (B cells) and T lymphocytes. This functional classification system is the subject of the next section.

Cell-Mediated Immunity

Definition: Immune reactions mediated by T lymphocytes within 24–48 hours of the antigen contact.

Note: *Cell-mediated immunity* is a delayed immune response.

T Lymphocytes

Physiology: The T lymphocytes stem from the pluripotent cells of the hemopoietic system. They migrate to the thymus, where they settle in the cortex.

There they are programmed to distinguish autologous antigens from exogenous antigens, which are presented to them in combination with a membrane antigen (human leukocyte antigen or HLA) that they themselves possess (this is the major histocompatibility complex or MHC restriction). This triggers two processes in the T cells.

— *Negative selection:* This process triggers apoptosis in those T-cell precursors that react against autologous antigen peptides in combination with autologous HLA.
— *Positive selection:* This process sends survival signals in the form of certain interleukins (IL) to those T-cell precursors that recognize autologous peptides in combination with autologous HLA molecules. The process triggers apoptosis in the other cells.
Result: Tolerance of autologous antigens.

Crucial to both selection processes is the configuration of the T-cell receptor resulting from rearrangement of the genomes that encode its α/β or γ/δ chains. These processes lead to mature T cells that express CD4 or CD8 molecules[1] according to their specific differentiation.

Initial Immune Response

A foreign antigen penetrating the body (► A1) is intercepted by antigen-presenting cells of the T-cell zone in the lymph nodes (interdigitating cells; ► A2) and by the Langerhans cells of the skin (► B1). It is then processed and presented to the T cells with the aid of HLA (► A2, B2). The foreign antigen then binds to the lymphocyte with the appropriate receptor (► A3), emitting a mitosis signal for a specific family of leukocytes (clone selection). This triggers their transformation to immunoblasts (► A4), resulting in proliferation of antigen-specific T-cell subpopulations (► A5).

■ Effector Mechanisms

▥ T Helper Cells

Synonyms: CD4+ T cells, T$_H$ cells

These cells receive T-cell receptors from α/β chains and express CD3 and CD4. The HLA class II structures present only the immunogenic peptide fragment of the foreign antigen digested by the antigen-presenting cells to the T cells (► B2). However, only the T$_H$ cells respond to this because their surfaces contain CD4 antigen that can bind to the class II molecules with CD3 as a co-ligand (► B3). This transmits a signal (► B4), causing the T$_H$ cells to release IL (► B5). These cells are classified according to their function.

— *T$_{H1}$ cells* defend against viruses and bacteria. They activate natural killer cells[2], resulting in release of interferon-γ and IL-2. This activates the T$_{H1}$ cells, which in turn activate macrophages and cytotoxic T cells. T$_{H1}$ cells are inhibited by IL-4.
— *T$_{H2}$ cells* defend against worms and other parasites. These invaders release IL-4, which (a) activates B cells, leading to production of IgG and IgE and (b) enlists the aid of eosinophilic mast cells. T$_{H2}$ cells are inhibited by interferon-γ.

▥ TCR γ/δ Cells

These lymphocytes contain T-cell receptors (TCR) of γ/δ chains and express neither CD4 nor CD8, which results in an HLA-independent reaction.

These cells occur in mucosa-associated lymphoid tissue (MALT).

▥ Cytotoxic T Lymphocytes

Synonym: CD8+ T cells.

These cells contain T-cell receptors of α/β chains and express CD3 and CD8.

Once a foreign antigen has been bound by an HLA class I molecule in a body cell, it is recognized by cytotoxic T cells because they have CD8 surface molecules that interact with HLA class I structures. In both the T cells that carry CD4 and those that carry CD8, the crucial activation signal is mediated via the CD3 surface molecule associated with the T-cell receptor after contact between HLA and foreign antigen. The cytotoxic T lymphocytes use membrane-perforating molecules (perforins or Fas-Ligand) to initiate the programmed destruction of adjacent cells (apoptosis; p. 128).

▥ Mediator Substances

The efficiency of the T-cell system depends heavily on cell-to-cell communication. This is controlled by two mechanisms: *interleukins,* signal substances created by lymphocytes and macrophages (► A6, B5), and *adhesion molecules,* such as the immunoglobulin superfamily, integrins, selectins, and cadherins.

■ Secondary Immune Response

The initial wave of proliferation also produces lymphocytes with high longevity, which as stationary stem cells have formed antigen-specific receptors on their surfaces. These are the memory cells (► A7), and they are responsible for the secondary immune response.

Note: Lymphokines are interleukins.

---

[1] CD = cluster of differentiation by which monoclonal antibodies are defined.
[2] Natural killer cells trigger apoptosis via perforin in cells without MHC.

A T-cell reaction

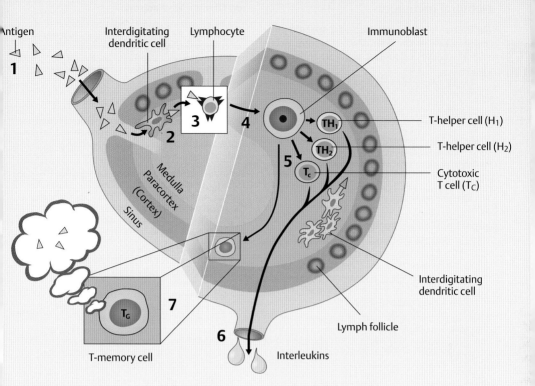

Antigen
1

Interdigitating dendritic cell

Lymphocyte

Immunoblast

3

4

2

TH$_1$ — T-helper cell (H$_1$)

TH$_2$ — T-helper cell (H$_2$)

5

T$_c$ — Cytotoxic T cell (T$_C$)

Medulla
Paracortex
(Cortex)
Sinus

Interdigitating dendritic cell

T$_G$

7

6

Lymph follicle

T-memory cell

Interleukins

B Mechanism of antigen presentation

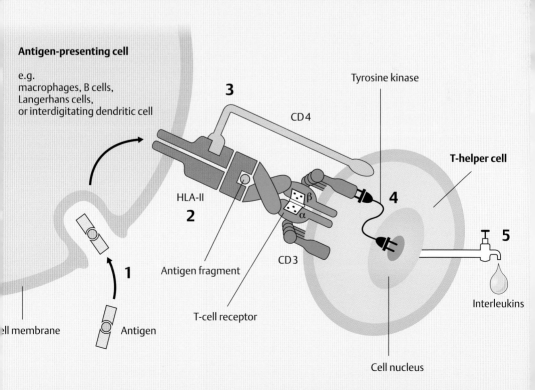

Antigen-presenting cell

e.g.
macrophages, B cells,
Langerhans cells,
or interdigitating dendritic cell

3

Tyrosine kinase

CD 4

T-helper cell

HLA-II

β
α

4

2

CD 3

Antigen fragment

5

Interleukins

T-cell receptor

1

Cell membrane   Antigen

Cell nucleus

Humoral Immunity

Definition: Immune reactions, by specific antibodies aided by the complement system, occur within minutes of contact with an antigen.

Note: *Humoral immunity* is an immediate immune response.

B Lymphocytes

Physiology: The B lymphocytes have large quantities of surface immunoglobulins. After contact with antigens (polysaccharides, drugs, pathogen toxins, or cell antigens), they transform themselves into antibody-secreting plasma cells via a series of intermediate proliferation and maturation phases.

Initial Immune Response

When an antigen enters the body, it is either transported to a lymph node or via the bloodstream to the spleen, where there are many B lymphocytes. They all can have the appropriate antibodies for a certain antigen as receptors on their surface, and after contact they can synthesize the appropriate antibodies.

B cells are excellent synthesizers of anti-protein antibodies. However, they are usually only able to do so after having enlisted the aid of T-helper cells. The intensity of the immune response hinges on how the antigens are presented. This role is assumed by antigen-presenting macrophages such as the marginal macrophages and follicular dendritic cells (► A, B1). They engulf the antigen (► A1), break it down by proteolysis (► A2), and present it to the T-helper cells (► A3, B2). B lymphocytes can do the same thing. In this manner, B cells and T cells cooperate (► B3). The B cells are stimulated both by the contact with the antigen and by the T-cell lymphokines (► A5), and they are either transformed into immunoblasts or form germinal centers (► B4).

— B immunoblasts pass through several intermediate stages to become plasma cells (► A6, B6). They lose their membrane-bound antibodies in the process, although they can synthesize humoral antibodies (► A7, B7).

— The centroblasts of the germinal centers create centrocytes that produce B immunoblasts (► B5) and B memory cells (B2 lymphocytes; ► B8). The B2 memory cells initiate a rapid immune response upon renewed contact with the antigen (a "anamnestic" response).

■ Effector Mechanisms

The B-cell system ensures humoral immunity using antibodies as its defensive weapons. Together with the complement system (described below), these antibodies destroy cells. Depending on the antigen, the B-cell system may be aided by macrophages and/or mast cells.

▓ Antibodies

Definition: Macromolecular serum proteins from the group of the γ-globulins (immunoglobulins) that specifically bond to matching antigen bonding sites (antigenic determinants or epitopes).

Structure of antibodies: Antibodies are composed of two identical light chains and two identical heavy chains. Human immunoglobulins are classified according to the respective heavy chain as IgG, IgA, IgM, IgD, and IgE. The heavy chains are identified with Greek letters: γ, α, μ, δ and ε.

Characteristics of antibodies:

— **IgM:** These are the first specific antibodies in the humoral immune reaction and the main antibodies in the primary response.

— **IgG:** These normally have the highest serum concentration of all immunoglobulins. They play an important role as neutralizing antibodies in defense against bacterial infections. In humoral immune reactions, they replace the IgM antibodies that arrive at the scene first. They are the main antibodies in the secondary response and can pass through the placental barrier.

— **IgA:** This is the main immunoglobulin in bodily secretions. In bacterial invasions, the classic role of IgA antibodies is to activate the complement system, triggering bacteriolysis and creating a protective immune layer for the mucous membranes.

— **IgD:** These antibodies often occur together with IgM on the surface of B lymphocytes. They regulate the interaction between B cells and T cells.

— **IgE:** These are formed primarily in the MALT (p. 157) of the respiratory and gastrointestinal tracts and can attach to mast cells (cytotropic antibodies). They also attach to the Langerhans cells that present antigens.

Formation of antibodies: Initial contact with an antigen induces the B cells to form IgM, which they later carry on their surface as an antigen receptor. Later, T-cell cytokines influence the B cells. When the antibody pattern is copied, the code for the type γ chain is replicated in place of the code for the heavy type μ chain. This results in formation of IgG antibodies. Following this isotype switch, the antibodies are then released into the serum with bonding specificity for the original antigen.

A Cooperation between macrophages and lymphocytes

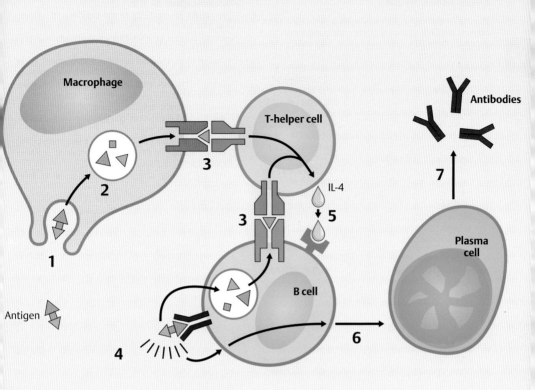

Macrophage

T-helper cell

Antibodies

3

2

IL-4

3

5

7

1

Plasma cell

Antigen

B cell

4

6

B B-cell reaction

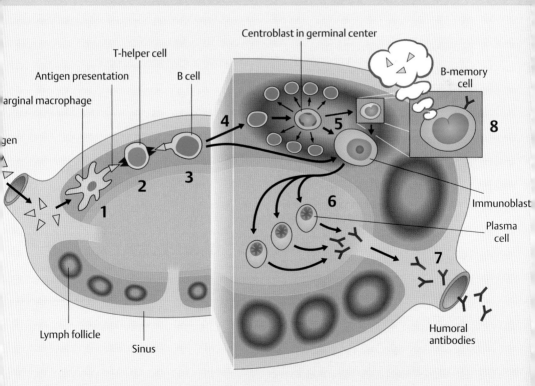

Centroblast in germinal center

T-helper cell

B-memory cell

Antigen presentation

B cell

Marginal macrophage

4

gen

5

8

2

3

Immunoblast

1

6

Plasma cell

7

Lymph follicle

Humoral antibodies

Sinus

Antigen–antibody reaction:

The antigen–antibody reaction leads to formation of an antigen–antibody complex or immune complex. Its fate depends on its size and solubility. The solubility of an immune complex is determined by the nature of components involved and by their relative quantities.

— With an *overabundance of antigen,* the bonding sites of the few antibodies are occupied by isolated antigens, and no immune complex will form (▶ A1).
— With an *overabundance of antibodies,* all determinants on the antigen are occupied by individual antibodies. This means that a cross-linked immune complex mesh will not form, and the immune complex remains small (▶ A2).
— Where the quantities of *antigens and antibodies* are nearly in equilibrium, a large immune complex will form. This will not remain in solution, but will precipitate out (▶ A3). A cross-linked immune complex or agglutination (▶ A4) will form even in reactions with cell-bound antibodies, such as blood-group antibodies.

Fate of an immune complex aggregation:
— *Large, precipitating immune complexes* are rapidly attacked by macrophages. Large quantities will produce an Arthus reaction (p. 174).
— *Large, soluble immune complexes* penetrate vessel walls, successively leading to deposits on the basement membrane and to tissue damage from ongoing formation of immune complex.
— *Small soluble immune complexes* are excreted. However, these complexes may also remain in the blood for an extended period of time without any consequences.

Subsequent reactions to immune complex:
— *Neutralization of antigen.*
— *Elimination.*
— *Opsonization:* The antibody deposits (IgG with complement action, IgM without it) on the surface of the pathogenic bacteria mark the antigens for macrophages, which phagocytize them.
— *Antibody-dependent cell-mediated cytotoxicity:* Killer cells (neither B cells nor T cells) with receptors for IgG antibodies cause the destruction of target cells occupied by specific antibodies without complement action.
— *Activation of complement system*

▨ Complement System

This effector system in the antigen–antibody conflict consists of nine plasma glycoproteins, C1–C9. Its components are activated in a cascade of reactions triggered in one of two ways.
— The *classic activation path* (▶ B) involves specific activation with involvement of humoral antibodies. The cascade begins with the recognition of an antibody bonded to an antigen by a C1 component (detection unit; ▶ C). This is followed by activation of C2 and C4 (activation unit), and then by dissociation of C3 and C5 into inflammation-controlling fragments. This leads to formation of a membrane-attack complex (MAC) (membrane destruction unit; ▶ D).
— The *alternate activation path* involves unspecific direct activation of the complement activation unit with dissociation of C3 and C5 into inflammation-controlling fragments. This activation is triggered by lipopolysaccharides such as endotoxins without involvement of the humoral antibodies.

Complement effects (▶ B):
— *Increased permeability* of the capillary structures: Activation of C2 creates a fragment that acts as a kinin (C-kinin, p. 202). This increases vascular permeability.
— *Anaphylactic reaction* (p. 166): The fragments C3a and C5a (anaphylatoxins) react with the receptors on the surface of mast cells and basophils, releasing histamine (p. 202). This is accompanied by contraction of smooth muscle, release of lysosomal enzymes, and formation of cytotoxic oxygen compounds.
— *Immune adherence:* C3b (and to a lesser extent C4b) on the surface of a target cell of immune complex causes inflammation cells to bond.
— *Opsonization* occurs primarily as a result of fragment C3b.
— *Chemotaxis:* Fragment C5a attracts neutrophils and macrophages into the inflamed region (p. 200).
— *Cytolysis* occurs as the membrane-attack complex penetrates the cell membrane, creating pores (▶ D). This leads to perforation of the cell membrane and disintegration of the cell.

▨ Immune Helper Cells

— *Macrophages* are antigen presenters and inflammation cells (p. 200). They phagocytize bacteria, cellular debris, foreign bodies, and immune complexes, and have receptors for IgG and C3b. They are attracted into the inflamed region by command substances (lymphokines) emitted by activated T lymphocytes. One factor attracts them by chemotaxis, whereas another keeps them migrating further; one encourages them to go to work, and another makes them cytotoxic.
— *Mast cells* are located near vascular structures, the skin, and the respiratory and gastrointestinal tracts. These cells have receptors for IgG, IgE, and C5a. Contact with cellular IgE leads to generation of inflammation mediators (p. 202).

Secondary Immune Response

When an antigen re-enters the body, the initial response is for circulating antibodies to intercept the antigens, forming an immune complex. These antibodies are bonded to Fc and complement receptors of the dendritic cells in the B areas of the lymph nodes and spleen. There they stimulate and trigger proliferation of B memory cells. These cells either transform themselves into immunoblasts, or they form germinal centers. Immunoblasts form plasma cells that produce IgG. Germinal centers create new memory cells.

The B cells and T cells do not form a uniform anatomic tissue group. The fact that they form an orchestrated functional unit is due to their special communication system. This consists of the immune-regulating antigens discussed in the next section.

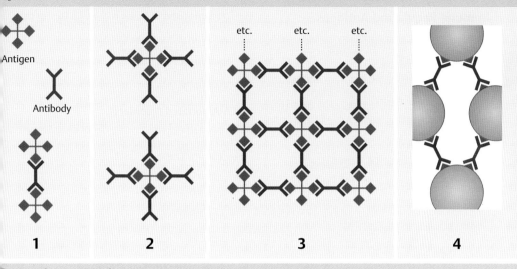

A Pattern of antigen-antibody reaction

Antigen

Antibody

etc.   etc.   etc.

1   **2**   **3**   **4**

B Complement cascade

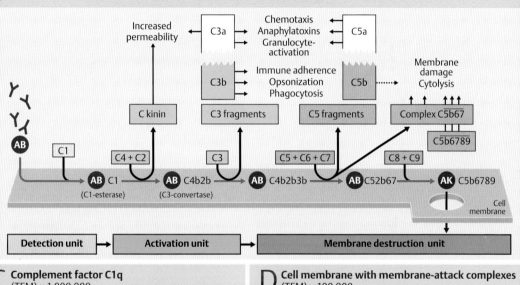

Increased
permeability

Chemotaxis
Anaphylatoxins
Granulocyte-
activation

C3a   C5a

Membrane
damage
Cytolysis

C3b → Immune adherence
Opsonization
Phagocytosis

C5b

C kinin   C3 fragments   C5 fragments   Complex C5b67

C5b6789

AB   C1   C4 + C2   C3   C5 + C6 + C7   C8 + C9

AB C1 → AB C4b2b → AB C4b2b3b → AB C52b67 → AK C5b6789
(C1-esterase)   (C3-convertase)

Cell
membrane

| Detection unit | → | Activation unit | → | Membrane destruction unit |

C Complement factor C1q
(TEM) x 1 000 000

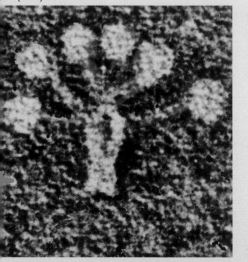

D Cell membrane with membrane-attack complexes
(TEM) x 100 000

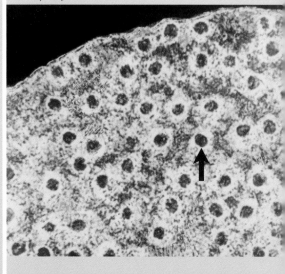

12

Immune Pathology

Immune-Regulating Antigens

Synonyms: major histocompatibility complex (MHC), human leukocyte antigen (HLA), transplantation antigen.

General definition: Cellular surface antigen that enables the T lymphocytes to identify foreign cells among the body's own cells and in so doing to distinguish between "self" and "non-self."

Classification of the HLA Genes

Class I: These occur in all nucleated cells and include the gene sites HLA-A, HLA-B, and HLA-C, L, H, and CD1-molecules and endogenous peptides present. They trigger the production of complement-binding antibodies in a foreign organism and stimulate cytotoxic T cells, initiating processes such as the destruction of donor cells.

Class II: These include the gene sites HLA-DP, HLA-DQ, and HLA-DR. They do not occur in all cells but are found primarily in B cells, macrophages, Langerhans cells of the skin, and interdigitating and dendritic reticulum cells. They present exogenous peptides, ingested and processed by antigen-presenting cells to CD4-helper cells.

Class III: These include the closely grouped gene loci for complement factors C2, C4, and factor B as well as the gene loci for cytokines TNF-α and TNF-β.

Function of the HLA Antigens

The macrophages track down antigen-bearing invaders in the body, process their antigens, and present them on their cell surface to the T helper cells. Yet they also pass their information on to other T cells and B cells. In order to mount an effective immune response, the T cell must recognize an identical immunologic complex of antigen and HLA class II molecule on the macrophages or on the B cells (this is the MHC restriction). The T cells only recognize a foreign antigen when they also find the body's own HLA (i.e., "self" characteristics) on the respective cell. In this manner, the B cells and T cells also use the HLA system as a private communication system to perform these tasks:
— *Antiviral protection* (▶ A): A body cell infected by a virus presents a viral antigen on its surface with the aid of an HLA I molecule. The antigen is recognized by the TCR in connection with the CD8 surface molecule of a cytotoxic T cell. This causes it to trigger apoptosis in the altered "self" cell by means of T-cell activated CASPASE (▶ A: penetrating arrow symbol).
— *Antibacterial protection* (▶ B): A foreign antigen (such as a bacterium) entering the body is phagocytized by macrophages. The macrophages then process the foreign antigen and present it to the TCR of a T helper cell with the aid of an HLA class II molecule (HLA II). The T cell recognizes the processed foreign antigen with its TCR in conjunction with the CD4 surface molecule. This causes it to secrete signal substances (lymphokines) for B cells (▶ B: droplet symbol), which activates the B cells and stimulates antibody production.

— *Protection against foreign cells* (▶ C): Foreign cells (such as transplant tissue) enter the body. With the aid of its TCR and the CD8 surface molecule, the cytotoxic T cell recognizes the other cell as foreign because of its incompatible HLA class I molecule (HLA I). The T cell then initiates apoptosis in the foreign cell (▶ C: penetrating arrow symbol).

HLA-Associated Disorders

General pathogenesis: A number of disorders are associated with certain types of HLA antigen expression. These include:

Inflammations with HLA-B27:
Occurrence: seronegative joint inflammations (arthritides) such as
— *Ankylosing spondylitis* in the form of ossification of the intervertebral spaces resulting in a stiff, immobile spine (primarily in the sacroiliac joint) and
— *Enteropathic arthritis* (primarily secondary to bowel inflammation).

Pathogenesis: Presumably the pathogen antigen and HLA type are cross-reactive.

Metabolic disease with HLA-A3:
Occurrence: hemochromatosis (p. 72).

Pathogenesis: unknown.

Autoimmune diseases with HLA-DR loci:
Occurrence (p. 180): Goodpasture syndrome, Sjögren syndrome, and autoimmune endocrinopathies.

Pathogenesis: Several mechanisms are possible.
— Immortalization of activated T cells.
— Imbalance between the activity of T helper cells and T suppressor cells may lead to inadequate stimulation of B cells.
— Pathogen antigen and HLA antigen type may be cross-reactive.
— There may be inadequate HLA class II expression.
— Release of self-antigen by tissue destruction.

> **Note:** *Lymphokines (interleukins)* are signal substances from leukocytes (lymphocytes, macrophages, and neutrophils) for leukocytes.

> **Note:** *Histocompatibility antigens* largely determine whether transplanted tissue is compatible.

The next section will examine diseases in which minor deviations in the immune response produce an excessive bodily hypersensitivity reaction. These diseases are pathogenic immune reactions. In contrast to the physiologic mechanisms described in the previous section, these aberrant reactions produce disease.

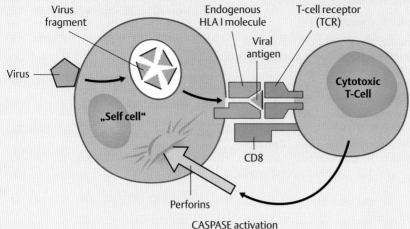

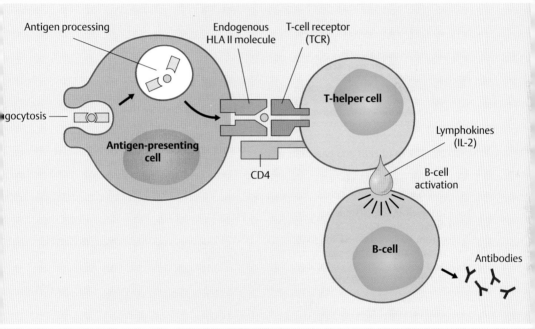

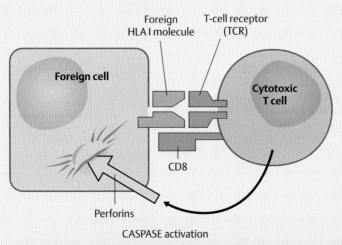

Pathogenic Immune Reactions

Hypersensitivity Reactions

General definition: Excessive pathogenic reaction of a sensitized body to renewed contact with the sensitizing antigen.

Type I Hypersensitivity Reactions

Synonyms: anaphylactic reaction, IgE allergy, IgE-mediated hypersensitivity reaction.

Definition: Induced by antigens, this chain reaction terminates in the IgE-induced release of inflammation-mediating substances from mast cells and/or basophils.

These substances include:

— *Histamine,* leading to increased vascular permeability, bronchial constriction, and secretion of mucus;
— *Prostaglandins* – primarily PGD_2, PGE_2, $PGF_{2\alpha}$ (p. 202), and thromboxane – leading to increased vascular permeability and bronchial dilation;
— *Leukotrienes* LTC_4, LTD_4, and LTE_4, leading to gradual bronchial constriction (p. 202);
— *LTB_4, a substance that attracts leukocytes,* for neutrophils, eosinophils, and macrophages;
— *Platelet-activating factor,* leading to platelet aggregation and increased vascular permeability;
— *Substances that activate kinin system,* leading to stimulation of "pain" nerves and increased vascular permeability.

Pathogenesis: The mast cells and basophils possess receptors for IgE and the anaphylatoxins from the complement cascade (C3a and C5a), which can also activate these cells.

Anyone can develop a type I hypersensitivity reaction. However, only about 15% of the population suffer from such reactions. The pathogenic antigens, usually allergens, are macromolecular (proteins and polysaccharides) or of low molecular weight (haptens) and occur in these substances:

— Plant pollen (grasses, trees, and flowers);
— Some foods;
— Some drugs (penicillin);
— Diagnostic agents (radiographic contrast media);
— Insect toxins (melittin);
— Mite feces in mattresses, animal fur, and head hair;
— Parasite antigens.

Initial antigen contact: After being phagocytized by an antigen-presenting cell, these antigens (► A1) are presented to a TH_2 cell (► A2). This stimulates the TH_2 cells, which secrete cytokines such as IL-4 (► A3). This causes, by T-B cell cooperation, plasma cells to express IgM-type antibodies on their surface upon initial contact with the triggering antigen. T cells incorrectly regulate cytokine production (IL-4) by a mechanism that is not understood. This induces B cells to effect an isotype switch and produce IgE with the same antigen specificity instead of IgM (► A4).

This isotype switch is brought about when B cells replace the type μ heavy chains with type ε chains when replicating the design of the antibody. This portion of the immunoglobulin also contains the Fc section to which the Fc receptors of the respective effector cell bond. Therefore, the IgE acquires a particular affinity for mast cells and basophils (and to a lesser extent thrombocytes and eosinophils). The result is a cytotropic IgE antibody.

Finally, the plasma cells secrete IgE, causing IgE antibodies to bond to the membrane of mast cells and basophils (► A5). Because allergens are rapidly broken down, no significant antigen–antibody reaction occurs.

Second antigen contact: In this case, overabundant IgE antibodies are formed that occupy the membrane surface of the mast cells and basophils so densely that the specific antogen (allergen), which bonds to the Fab-part of the IgE antibody, cross-links itself with its neighboring IgE molecule (IgE-"bridging"). This IgE bridging is the trigger for the release of inflammatory mediator substances out of the mast cells' basophilic granula, which causes the allergic reaction. This occurs in the following phases:

— **Immediate phase:** It involves the action of histamine, causing a reaction within minutes of contact with the allergen.
— **Late phase:** It involves the action of prostaglandin leukotrienes, causing a reaction within 5 hours of allergen contact at the earliest.

Note: The *function of a type I hypersensitivity reaction* is to flush out the antigen by exudation, cough it out bonded to mucus, and reduce the quantities inhaled by constricting the bronchi.

Note: There is an exception in which *IgE causes an immediate reaction:* IgE bonds to the Langerhans cells of the skin (p. 177). This means that inhaled allergens may also trigger eczematous late reactions in addition to the immediate reaction.

Initial antigen contact

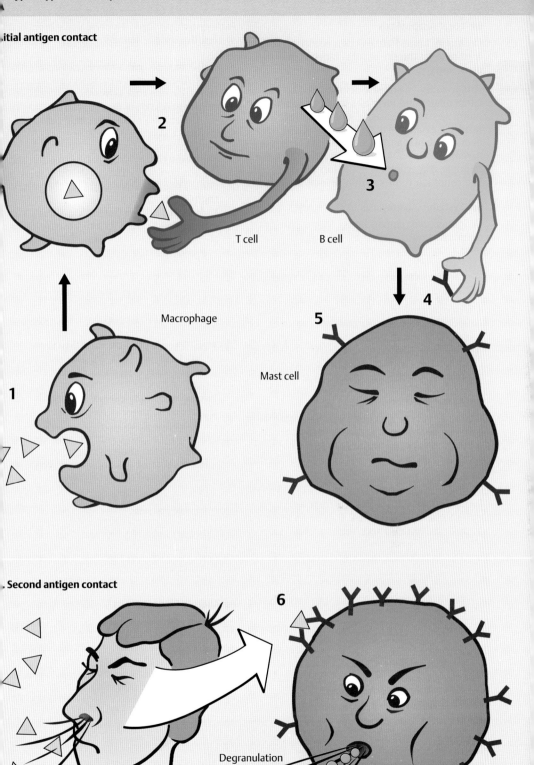

2

3

1

T cell

B cell

Macrophage

5

Mast cell

4

Second antigen contact

6

Degranulation

7

■ Local Anaphylaxis

Definition: Immediate reaction occurring within minutes at the site of subcutaneous injection of an antigen.

Pathogenesis: The release of inflammation mediators dilates and increases the permeability of minor vessels (capillaries and arterioles). This results in exudation of blood serum with subsequent erythema and tissue swelling (serous inflammation; p. 204). This generally results in multiple skin eruptions in the form of urticaria. The condition remits within several hours.

■ Systemic Anaphylaxis

Definition and pathogenesis: Immediate systemic reaction triggered by the following factors:
— local reinjection of an antigen;
— contact with large quantities of an antigen;
— intravenous administration of an antigen.

Affected organs in humans include the *lung,* where the resulting bronchial constriction causes difficulty in breathing, and the *peripheral cardiovascular system,* where the resulting disturbance in regulation of the microcirculation causes anaphylactic shock.

■ Atopic Reaction

Definition: Local reaction to environmental antigens occurring in patients with a genetic predisposition even in the absence of unusual exposure.

Pathogenesis: Only 10 % of the population suffers from atopic reaction; 50 % of them have a family history with a linkage to several gene loci such as 5931 (IL3, IL4, IL5) and 6p (HLA complex). Crucial factors include impaired T-cell function with preferential activation of the TH$_2$ cells. This leads to excessive and prolonged IgE production, in turn leading abnormal eosinophil activity that causes normal environmental substances to act as pathogens (p. 166).

Occurrence:
— Skin eczema (atopic dermatitis; ► A);
— Allergic rhinosinusitis;
— Bronchial asthma.

Disorders Associated with Type I Hypersensitivity Reaction

■ Bronchial Asthma (► C–E)

Definition: Disease of the respiratory system with hyperreactivity, characterized by recurrent transient dyspnea due to inflammatory bronchial obstruction.

Pathogenetic principle: Hyperreactive bronchial system due to the following trigger mechanisms:
— **Exogenous allergic asthma** (extrinsic asthma): Allergen contact triggers an anaphylactic reaction that activates mast cells, resulting in release of mediators (p. 202) with
  — Generation of spasmogenic substances and
  — Chemotactic factors (p. 200).
  This results in (a) bronchial obstruction and (b) eosinophilic infiltrate, leading to secondary release of mediators and the asthma triad (see below).
— **Endogenous asthma** (intrinsic asthma): The asthma triad occurs in the absence of an allergenic cause, without IgE-mediated bronchial obstruction.

Morphology: Asthma triad:

— **Hypertrophic bronchial musculature** (► E1) is present as a bronchial spasm sign (► D).
— **Excessive mucus production** leads to mucus plugs in the form of Curschmann spirals (► E2). These produce valve-like bronchial obstructions (► C, D, E). The pulmonary alveoli become distended, causing emphysema.
— **Mucous membrane edema:** Eosinophilic infiltrate in the mucous membrane (► B, C, E3) leads to generation of inflammation mediators (p. 202), successively causing swelling of the mucous membranes, and crystallization of eosinophilic enzymes, as diamond-shaped Charcot-Leyden crystals (► E4).

☺ **Prominent patients**:
Arnold Schönberg (1874–1951), musician and composer who introduced 12-tone, "atonal"-composition.
Marc Chagall (1887–1962), Russian-born French painter of surrealistic religious themes.
Mark A. Spitz, American swimmer and winner of seven gold medals at the 1972 Olympics.

■ Allergic Rhinosinusitis

Definition and pathogenesis: A local (atopic) anaphylactic reaction causes inflammation of the nasal and sinus mucosa with watery nasal discharge (p. 204), lymphocytic and eosinophilic infiltrate (► B), and hypertrophy of the mucus glands, producing the clinical picture of hay fever.

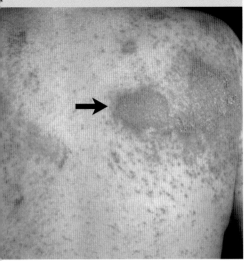

Atopic dermatitis (exposure test)

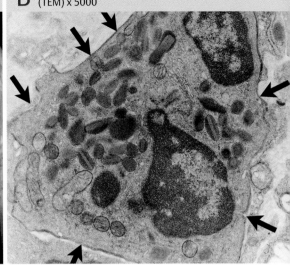

B **Eosinophilic granulocyte**
(TEM) x 5000

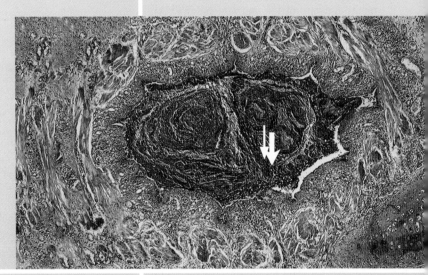

Bronchial asthma
(AS) x 50

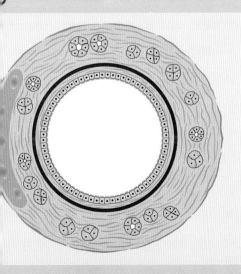

D **Normal bronchus**

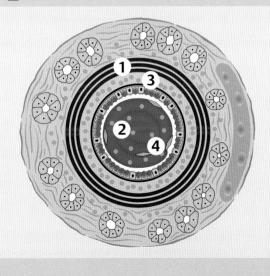

E **Bronchus in bronchial asthma**

12

Immune Pathology

Type II Hypersensitivity Reactions

Synonym: cytotoxic reaction, antibody-mediated cytotoxic hypersensitivity reaction, IgG-mediated and IgM-mediated hypersensitivity reaction.

Definition: Immune reactions triggered by humoral antibodies that are directed against tissue- or cellular-bounded antigens.

Pathogenesis: The following antigens may be responsible for triggering these immune reactions:
- Transplantation antigens;
- Blood group antigens;
- Tumor-associated antigens;
- Endogenous antigens (self antigens or autoantigens);
- Antibodies against complexes of drugs bonded to cell membranes.

The underlying mechanism in this type hypersensitivity reaction involves generation of a humoral antibody of IgE and IgM-type (▶ A1) whose specificity is directed against the antigen on the surface of cells (▶ A2) or other tissue components. To the extent that these humoral antibodies have bonded with the corresponding antigens, they cause cytotoxic cell injury with involvement of (a) the *complement cascade* (▶ A3) or (b) *macrophages.* In the first case the target cell is killed by the activated complement system's membrane-attack complex. In the latter case, the Fc portions of antibodies bonded to a foreign cell or foreign material (▶ A4) contact Fc receptors on macrophages (▶ A5).

Result: The cell is killed by apoptosis.

Examples:
- *Rhesus incompatibility:* Rh-positive erythrocytes that pass from the fetus through the placental barrier or enter the Rh-negative mother's bloodstream by transfusion cause the mother to produce Rhesus antibodies against Rh antigen. During a second pregnancy or blood transfusion, a cross-linked antigen–antibody complex forms (p. 162) with agglutination of the fetal erythrocytes, resulting in the dissolution of the erythrocytes (hemolysis).
- *Transfusion accidents* involving ABO incompatibilities result in agglutination of erythrocytes (▶ C, D).
- *Idiopathic thrombocytopenic purpura* may occur due to thrombocytic antibodies.
- *Goodpasture syndrome (p. 182).*

Type III Hypersensitivity Reactions

Synonym: immune complex reaction.

Review: Collagen necrosis (p. 46).

General definition: Immune reactions in which antigen–antibody complexes circulate in the blood and other bodily fluids where they are deposited in and/or around blood vessels, triggering an inflammatory reaction.

General pathogenesis: The following antigens may be responsible for triggering these immune reactions:

Not-self antigens include persistent infections from viruses (hepatitis B), bacteria (streptococci and staphylococci), fungi (Aspergillus), protozoans (malaria), and foreign protein (serum).

Self antigens include components of DNA, RNA, cytoplasm, and tissue.

Contact with one of these antigens triggers an antigen–antibody reaction that results in formation of a large soluble immune complex (▶ B1) of the IgG or IgM type. This exceeds the clearance capacity of the macrophage system, which is unable to eliminate the immune complex. The immune complex circulates in the blood, penetrating vessel walls in the kidneys, joints, and heart and producing deposits of immune complex (▶ B2) that may be demonstrated by fluorescence microscopy. These deposits activate the complement cascade until the anaphylatoxin C3a and C5a are formed (p. 162), triggering immune-complex vasculitis with secondary tissue damage that follows this pattern:
- *Leukocytoclasis:*[1] Deposits of immune complex in or around the blood vessel wall leads to neutrophil chemotaxis (▶ B3) and in turn to neutrophil apoptosis; the neutrophils disintegrate into fragments (▶ B4; hence the name leukocytoclasis), leading to:
- *Fibrinoid necrosis of the vessel wall.* Neutrophil proteases are released, immunecomplexes bind to thrombocytes, activating the coagulation cascade and producing microthrombi (▶ B5). This results in damage to the vessel wall and to:
- *Serous tissue inflammation.* The abnormal permeability due to the anaphylatoxins (▶ B6) leads to an exudative inflammatory reaction (p. 196) and subsequently to tissue damage.

---

[1] Leukocytoclasis: from leukocyte + *klasia* (Greek) = breaking.

A Cytotoxic reaction

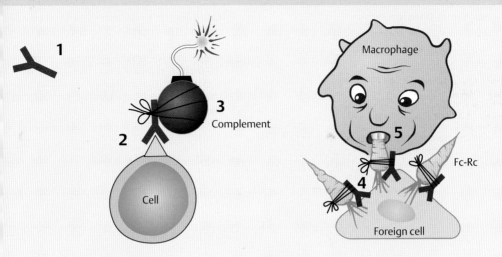

1
2 Cell
3 Complement
Macrophage
5
4
Fc-Rc
Foreign cell

B Pathogenesis of immune complex diseases

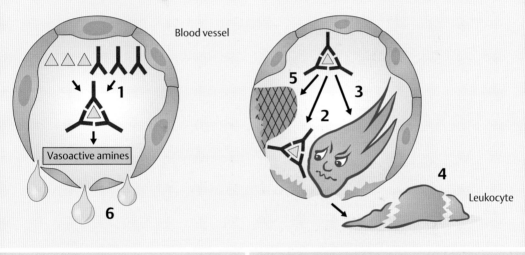

Blood vessel
1
Vasoactive amines
6
5
2
3
4
Leukocyte

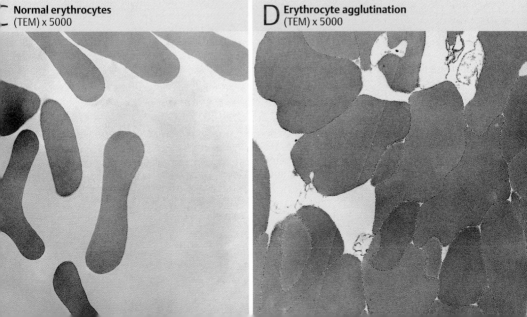

C Normal erythrocytes
(TEM) x 5000

D Erythrocyte agglutination
(TEM) x 5000

◼ Serum Disease

Synonym: systemic immune complex disease.

Definition: Immune reaction due to incompatibility of foreign serum.

Etiologic factors include:
— Foreign serum;
— Foreign globulins and other foreign proteins;
— Haptens like penicillin.

Pathogenesis: Repeated administration of foreign antigens leads to generation of soluble circulating immune complex. This in turn leads to deposits of immune complex and/or penetration of immune complex through the vessel wall, producing tissue damage (primarily in the kidneys, joints, and heart).

✚ **Clinical presentation:** Urticaria, joint pain, proteinuria, and hematuria occur within 3 days of administration of foreign protein.

Disorders Associated with Serum Disease

◼ Immune Complex Vasculitis

Pathogenesis: The extent of vascular damage caused by the immune complex essentially depends on how efficiently the immune complex and resulting damage are eliminated.

▦ **Urticaria** affects capillaries. Here immune complex is cleared rapidly, resulting in formation of itching wheals without persisting endothelial damage.

▦ **Leukocytoclastic vasculitis** affects venules (► A1). Immune complex is cleared slowly, resulting in endothelial damage successively leading to neutrophil chemotaxis (p. 200), extravascular leukocytoclasis (► A2) with precipitation of fibrin, and cutaneous purpura bleeding (p. 398) with a central area of necrosis.

▦ **Polyarteritis nodosa** affects medium-sized arteries of the internal organs. Failure to eliminate immune complex leads to fibrinoid necrosis of the vessel walls, in turn resulting in stenosing vascular repair (p. 58).

▦ **Lupus vasculitis (p. 180)** affects small and medium-sized arteries.
— *Early phase:* It is characterized by permanent presence of antigen without clearance of the immune complex. This produces sectors of fibrinoid necrosis of the vascular wall accompanied by a lymphocytic infiltrate (► B).

— *Late phase:* It is characterized by slow reparative mechanisms. The endothelial damage leads to activation of thrombocytes, which in turn results in release of platelet-derived growth factor. This causes proliferation of the medial myocytes, producing a concentric pattern of intimal and medial fibrosis ("onion-skin" arteriopathy). This leads to vascular stenosis (p. 180) without any significant infiltrate.

◼ Immune Complex Nephritis

Human pathogenetic prototype: Glomerulus inflammation secondary to a *Streptococcus* infection (p. 254; poststreptococcal glomerulonephritis).

Classic animal model: It involves *serum nephritis* with the following pathogenetic chain reaction:

Initial contact with antigen: Intravenous injection of bovine albumin as a foreign serum (overabundance of bovine antigens) in rabbits causes the rabbit to produce antibodies against the bovine albumin.

Second contact with antigen: Intravenous injection of these antibodies into cattle causes the cow to produce an overabundance of antibodies. This results in formation of a soluble circulating antigen–antibody complex. The immune complex passes through the glomerular basement membrane of the kidney, creating immune complex deposits on the outside of the basement membrane that form subepithelial humps. A peripheral granular pattern of deposits is visible under fluorescence microscopy (► C). Immune complexes activate the complement system, causing capillary damage with increased permeability. This in turn allows the escape of protein and erythrocytes, leading to hematuria and proteinuria.

Morphology of poststreptococcal glomerulonephritis:
— *Early phase:* It is characterized by swollen glomeruli with endothelial damage. Some of the capillary lumina are completely obstructed by granulocytes, monocytes, and microthrombi (► D). Subepithelial humps are present.
— *Late phase:* It is characterized by reactive proliferation of endothelial and mesangial cells.

The macroscopic features of the disorder include hyperemic swelling of the kidneys with punctate surface hemorrhages resembling fleabites (► F).

✚ **Clinical presentation:** *Poststreptococcal glomerulonephritis* occurs in adolescents, twice as often in boys than in girls. Symptoms include hematuria, proteinuria, hypertension, and edema. The disorder resolves completely in 80% of all cases.

A **Leukocytoclastic vasculitis**
(HE) x 75

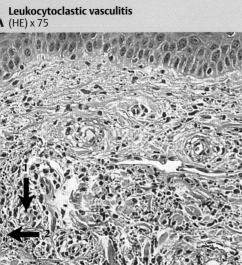

B **Lupus vasculitis**
(HE) x 50

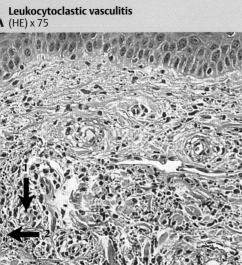

Immune complex nephritis
(IgG; IF) x 50

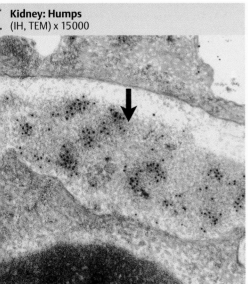

D **Immune complex nephritis**
(PAS) x 75

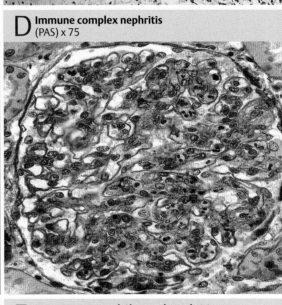

Kidney: Humps
(IH, TEM) x 15000

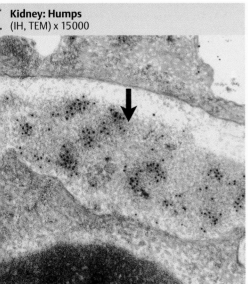

F **Poststreptococcal Glomerulonephritis**

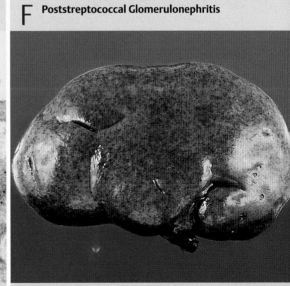

■ Local Immune Complex Disease

Pathogenesis:

Classic animal model: It involves the *Arthus reaction* with the following pathogenetic chain reaction:

Initial contact with antigen: Intravenous injection causes generation of circulating antibodies against the antigen.

Second contact with antigen: Antigens are injected subcutaneously 2 weeks after the initial injection. A few hours later, this leads to local precipitation of the immune complex, activating the complement cascade. This cause immune complex vasculitis, leading to tissue damage at the site of the injection.

Histologic findings vary. Mild forms are characterized by an acute serous inflammatory reaction (p. 204) with edematous tissue swelling. Severe forms involve hemorrhagic inflammation (p. 216) with granulocyte infiltration of the minor vessels, leading to rupture bleeding (hemorrhage; p. 398). The minor vessels become occluded with blood clots (thrombosis; p. 402), leading to necrosis.

Disorders Associated with Local Immune Complex Disease

■ Extrinsic Allergic Alveolitis

Synonym: hypersensitivity pneumonia.

Definition: Pulmonary disease due to inhalation of organic allergens.

Pathogenesis: Inhalation of actinomycetes or dusts containing Aspergillus or avian protein (p. 256, 272) leads to an abnormal chain reaction 24 hours later. IgG antibodies against foreign protein (precipitins) are created. The resulting immune complex results in lymphocyte and plasmacyte infiltration of the bronchioli that spreads to the alveoli. This causes fever, coughing, and shortness of breath. These symptoms are often accompanied by a type IV hypersensitivity reaction involving formation of epithelioid cellular granulomas[1] (► A; p. 176, 230).

In chronic exposure to allergens, the allergen phagocytizing macrophages secrete growth factors and cytokines, leading to proliferation of fibroblasts in the alveolar wall (p. 40), which in turn causes fibrosis of the lung (► B; p. 40).

✚ **Clinical presentation:** Risk groups include farmers (farmer's lung), cheese washers (cheese washer's lung), and bird breeders (pigeon breeder's or bird handler's lung; ► B).

Type IV Hypersensitivity Reaction

Synonym: cell-mediated hypersensitivity reaction, delayed hypersensitivity reaction.

Definition: Delayed hypersensitivity reaction mediated by specifically sensitized T lymphocytes (CD4 – TH1).

Pathogenetic principle: Contact with an antigen initiates the following chain reaction (► C).

Initial contact with antigen (► C1): Macrophages present the antigen to the T cells (► C2). This sensitizes naïve CD4-T cells and creates T memory cells (► C3).

Second contact with antigen: The antigen now encounters T memory cells from the initial contact (► C4). This triggers the transformation of lymphoblasts, which mature and proliferate (► C5). T memory cells become CD4–TH1-T lymphocytes (delayed immunity effector cells), resulting in the release of these macrophage-controlled cytokines:

— MAF (macrophage-activating factor), allowing these cells to kill germs (► C6);
— MCF (macrophage-chemotactic factor);
— MIF (migration-inhibitory factor), keeping macrophages in the vicinity of the inflammation (► C7);
— MFF (macrophage fusion factor), transforming macrophages into multinucleated giant cells (► C8).

In addition to this, cytotoxic CD8-T cells (killer cells) also appear in the inflammation area. The T cells and/or macrophages kill off target cells by the following mechanisms:

— ***Apoptosis*** (p. 128) after sensitized cytotoxic T cells "open fire" with membrane-perforating proteins (perforins)
— ***Proteolysis*** following phagocytosis (p. 26) by T-cell-activated macrophages.

Four forms of type-IV hypersensitivity reaction may be distinguished according to the time at which the cells involved in the hypersensitivity reaction appear. These include:
— Cutaneous basophilic hypersensitivity reaction;
— Contact allergy;
— Tuberculin reaction;
— Granulomatous hypersensitivity reaction.

---

[1] Granuloma (Latin), 'small corn': a nodular arrangement of inflammation cells.

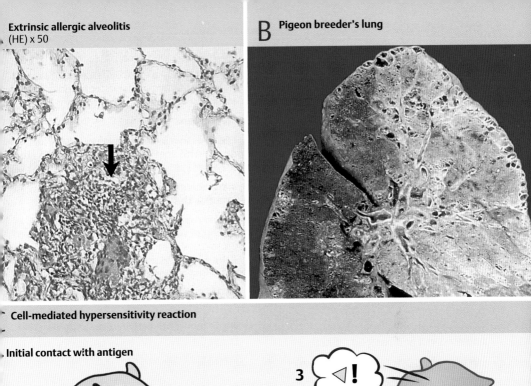

Extrinsic allergic alveolitis
(HE) x 50

B **Pigeon breeder's lung**

Cell-mediated hypersensitivity reaction

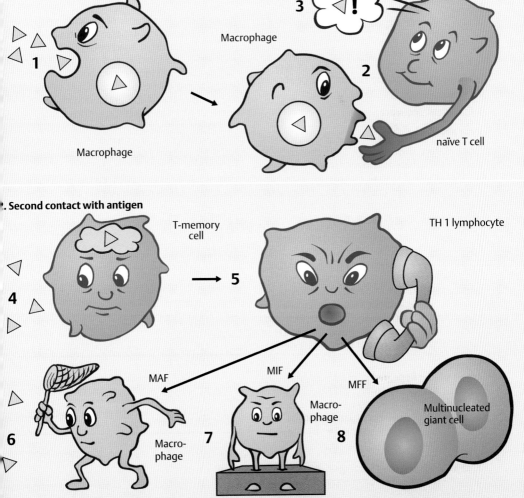

Initial contact with antigen

Macrophage

1

3 ◁!

2

Macrophage

naïve T cell

Second contact with antigen

T-memory cell

TH 1 lymphocyte

4

5

MAF

MIF

MFF

6

Macro-phage

7

Macro-phage

8

Multinucleated giant cell

12

Immune Pathology

■ Cutaneous Basophilic Hypersensitivity Reaction

Synonym: Jones-Mote reaction.

Definition: Cutaneous manifestation of the type IV hypersensitivity reaction involving the sequelae of activation of mast-cell basophils.

Pathogenesis:

Classic animal model: It involves a *Jones-Mote reaction* with the following pathogenetic chain reaction:

Initial contact with antigen: Subcutaneous injection of low-antigen foreign protein such as ovalbumin in Freund's adjuvant in guinea pigs.

Second contact with antigen (1 week later): Repeated subcutaneous injection of foreign protein leads to chemotaxis and activation of basophils and mast cells by T_D cells 24 hours after the injection. This produces an inflammatory reaction at the injection site with erythema and mast-cell and basophil infiltrate.

✚ **Clinical significance:** This reaction occurs in skin injuries from parasites such as ticks or insects and contact with their allergens.

■ Contact Allergy

Definition: Epidermal manifestation of type IV hypersensitivity reaction at the site of antigen contact.

Pathogenetic sequence:

Acute phase:

Initial contact with antigen: Skin contact with substances that act as antigens (usually haptens like nickel in jewelry; ► C) bond to body proteins, forming an immunogen (i.e., an antigen). The Langerhans cells in the skin present the antigen to the T cells (► A, B).

Second contact with antigen (2–3 days later): Influx of sensitized CD4-TH1 cells with homing receptors for cutaneous capillary endothelia and skin macrophages from cytokines. This results in an intercellular epidermal edema, resulting in cytotoxic spongiosis of the epithelium and blistering of the skin. This reaction produces a lymphocyte skin infiltrate (► D) at the site of the antigen contact (contact dermatitis; ► C).

Chronic phase: Repeated contact with the antigen leads to reactive "protective" thickening of the epidermis with excessive cornification of nucleated epidermal cells (parakeratosis). This leads to erythema and scaling (► E) or seborrheic eczema.

✚ **Clinical significance:** This occurs in allergy to jewelry metals, occupational disorders, and reaction to toxic plant substances.

■ Tuberculin Reaction

Definition: Cutaneous manifestation of a type IV hypersensitivity reaction after postinfection injection of antigen.

Pathogenesis:

Classic animal model: It involves a *tuberculin reaction* with the following pathogenetic chain reaction:

Initial contact with antigen: Guinea pigs are infected with tuberculin bacilli (p. 264).

Second contact with antigen: Intracutaneous injection of tuberculin as an antigen (tuberculoprotein). Within 2–3 days this produces an inflammatory reaction at the application site with erythema and nodular swelling.

✚ **Clinical significance:** tuberculin test.

■ Granulomatous Hypersensitivity Reaction

Definition: Type IV hypersensitivity reaction with nodular groupings of inflammatory cells where presence of the antigen persists (p. 226).

Pathogenesis: Persistence of the antigen leads to antigen–antibody complexes or nonimmunogenic substances in macrophages, leading to permanent stimulation and causing TH1 cells to release cytokines (see above). Within 2 weeks at the earliest, macrophages migrate to and congregate at the antigen site. The clustered macrophages are transformed into densely layered cytokine-producing epithelioid cells without any phagocytic tendencies. Some of these cells fuse into multinucleated giant cells, forming an inflammatory cell mass or granuloma with epithelioid cells at the center and lymphocytes on the periphery (p. 226).

✚ **Clinical significance:** This reaction is the formal pathogenetic principle in these infections:
- mycobacteriosis (leprosy or tuberculosis);
- spirochetosis (syphilis);
- brucellosis (Bang disease);
- yersiniosis (pseudotuberculosis);
- mycotic, parasitic, and some viral infections.

Transplantation of exogenous organs and tissues represents what may be regarded in a certain sense as an iatrogenic form of hypersensitivity reaction. In these cases, drugs are used to force the body to tolerate the foreign antigens. This type of hypersensitivity reaction is discussed in the next section.

Langerhans cells of the skin
(S-100; IH) x 100

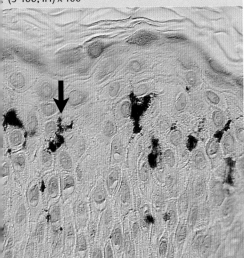

Contact eczema

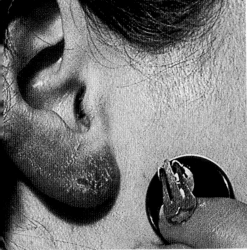

Contact dermatitis
(HE) x 50

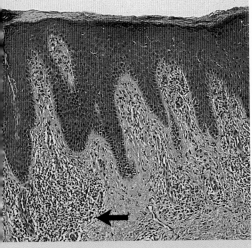

B **Langerhans cells of the skin**
(TEM) x 500

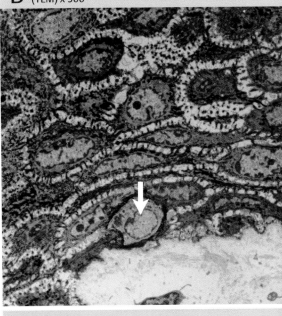

E **Seborrheic eczema**

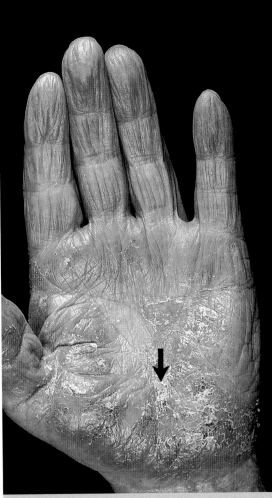

12

Immune Pathology

Transplantation Pathology

Definition: Transplantation is the transfer of organs and tissues to a different site within the same individual or from a donor to a recipient.

Autograft: The transplant consists of the individual's own tissue (such as a skin graft).

Isograft: The transplant consists of tissue transferred between genetically identical individuals (a graft from an identical twin).

Allograft: The transplant consists of tissue transferred between genetically dissimilar individuals of the same species (such as a human heart transplant).

Xenograft: The transplant consists of tissue transferred between different species (such as a porcine heart valve implanted in a human heart).

■ Transplant Allergy

Several rejection reactions may occur depending on the compatibility of donor and recipient HLA.

▦ Hyperacute Rejection

Pathogenesis: Patients who have already formed circulating antibodies against the organ transplant prior to transplantation experience a type II hypersensitivity reaction. Arteritis and arteriolitis with thrombosis occur within a period of minutes to hours after vascular communication has been established between the transplant and the recipient. This eliminates the vascular supply to the transplant, producing ischemic necrosis and creating a mottled yellow and red pattern in the organ tissue.

▦ Acute Rejection

Pathogenetic mechanisms:
— *Cellular immune reaction:* Persistence of donor HLA sensitizes cytotoxic CD8-T cells. This produces a type IV hypersensitivity reaction with an interstitial lymphocyte infiltrate, leading to lymphocytic endothelial damage and eventually to obliteration of vascular structures.
— *Humoral immune reaction:* Immune suppression induced; persistence of donor HLA results in formation of anti-HLA antibodies. This in turn leads to stenosing inflammation of the arterial intima (acute transplant vascular disease) and subsequently to thrombosis (p. 404) and infarction (► A; p. 412).

▦ Chronic Rejection

Pathogenesis: Formation of a complex of transplant antigens and host antibodies leads to permanent lymphocytic intimal damage in the transplant (► B). This results in obliterative arterial disease with a concentric or "onion-skin" pattern of intimal fibrosis (chronic transplant vascular disease). This condition leads to ischemic organ damage.

■ Graft-Versus-Host Disease

Definition: Cytotoxic immune reactions of implanted or infused immunocompetent T cells against the immunocompromised body of the host.

Pathogenesis: The primary cause of this disease is a cell-mediated immune reaction against the host with significant activation of macrophages. The donor cells sensitized against the host antigen become cytotoxic effector cells and destroy the host cells by triggering apoptosis (p. 128) in these cells, effectively causing autoimmune disease.

Result: Destruction of individual cells in host tissue in the vicinity of the lymphocytes (satellite necrosis).

Graft-versus-host (GVH) disease occurs primarily in these types of tissue:
— *Large bowel:* Lymphocytic apoptotic enterocyte destruction occurs primarily in the crypts (► C), leading to ulceration of the mucosa (► D) and diarrhea.
— *Epidermis:* Lymphocytic apoptotic damage to the epidermis produces dermatitis (► E), resulting in separation of the epithelium and ulceration (► F).
— *Liver:* Lymphocytic epithelial damage to the bile ducts causes bile duct destruction, successively leading to cholangiolitic hepatitis and cholestatic jaundice.

☺ **Prominent "patients":** In the People's Republic of China, organs are often removed from executed prisoners for use as transplants.

The next section examines diseases that result from the creation of antibodies against the body's own antigens. Formation of an immune complex in such cases causes systemic autoimmune disease. If the antibodies are directed against cell receptors for a specific organ, the lesion will be confined to that organ.

Transplant rejection (kidney)

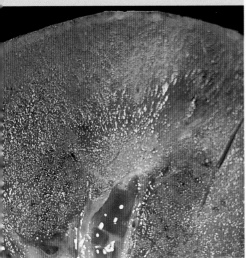

B **Transplant vasculitis**
(EvG) x 75

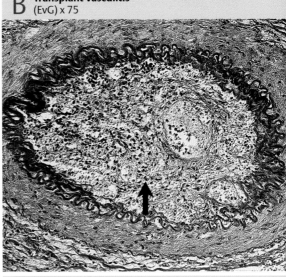

Graft-versus-host disease: colon
(HE) x 100

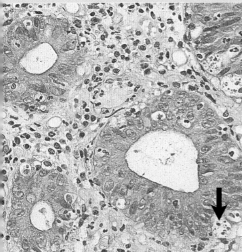

D **Graft-versus-host disease:** colon

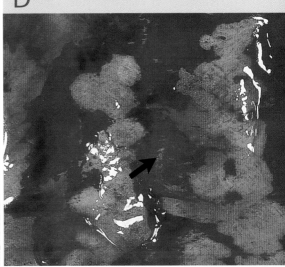

Graft-versus-host disease: skin (early)

F **Graft-versus-host disease:** skin (late)

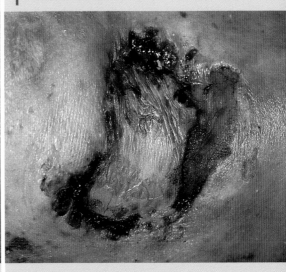

Autoimmune Disorders

General definition: Clinical syndromes that occur in the absence of exogenous influences and are maintained throughout the patient's life occur by humoral or cell-mediated immune reactions. These reactions are directed at specific endogenous substrates.

General pathogenesis: A normal body does not react against its own tissues. However, several mechanisms can compromise this autoimmune tolerance, causing endogenous tissue to act as a pathogen. These include:
— *No central immune tolerance*
— *Interruption of clonal Anergy* of autoreactive T cells
— *Immortalization of activated T cells*
— *Loss of activity of T-suppressor cells* with inhibition of proliferation of B-cell clones for endogenous substrates;
— *Formation of anti-antibodies* (anti-idiotypes);
— *Formation of cross-reactive antibodies* with specificity against pathogenic and endogenous HLA (molecular mimicry and antigen mimicry);
— *Release of autoantigens* such as mitochondrial components (AMA) and myosin (ASMA) from tissue destruction;
— *Inadequate HLA expression*, causing autoreactive T-helper cells to recognize potential autoantigens on cells that normally do not express HLA class-II antigens.

In terms of formal pathogenesis, autoimmune diseases are based on type II or III hypersensitivity reactions triggered by these mechanisms:
— *Complement-binding antibodies* directed against endogenous cells (primarily blood cells) and tissue components (primarily basement membranes) or
— *Non-complement-binding antibodies* directed against endogenous cell receptors (autoreactive antibodies). In the latter case, the antibodies created can act either as a stimulating cell signal or as a blocking signal.

Systemic Autoimmune Disorders

These include the following disease entities:
— Systemic lupus erythematosus;
— Progressive systemic sclerosis;
— Dermatomyositis;
— Goodpasture syndrome;
— Wegener granulomatosis;
— Rheumatoid arthritis;
— Sjögren syndrome.

■ Systemic Lupus Erythematosus

Textbook example of systemic autoimmune disease.

Definition: Systemic disorder characterized by cell damage induced by immune complex in which the presence of antinuclear antibodies (► A; p. 10) plays a crucial role. The disorder is rare.

Causal pathogenesis: For unknown reasons, antinuclear antibodies (= ANA) are primarily directed against double-stranded DNA (anti-dsDNA), nuclear ribonucleic protein, histone, and extractable nuclear proteins (= ENA) as non-histone proteins.

Formal pathogenesis: For unknown reasons, autoreactive antibodies are created, resulting in the formation of circulating immune complex. This successively leads to complement activation (p. 162), necrotizing immune complex vasculitis (lupus arteritis), and, in the terminal stage, "onion-skin" arteriopathy (► F; p. 172).

✚ Clinical presentation and morphology:
The disorder is more common in women than men, reaching its peak between the ages of 20 and 50.
– *Butterfly erythema:* Skin inflammation on the cheek side of the nose and over the zygoma (► C). Histologic findings include bands of immune complex deposits between the epidermis and the dermis, resulting in focal lymphocytic infiltrate (► D1) with fibrinoid collagen necrosis (p. 46). This leads to degeneration of the epidermal basal cells. Hyperkeratosis occurs in the funnels of the hair follicles (► D2).
– *Immune complex vasculitis* (lupus arteritis; p. 172).
– *Libman-Sacks endocarditis:* Rough wart-like deposits of fibrin on the margins of the mitral and tricuspid valves (► E) increase the risk of embolism.
– *Immune complex nephritis* of the focal segmental type[1] is present, with usually extensive subendothelial deposits of immune complex (lupus nephritis). This leads successively to renal insufficiency and uremia.
– Lupus arthritis.

❗ Note: In the *lupus erythematosus phenomenon,* the nuclei of damaged cells react with antinuclear antibodies and are transformed into homogeneous corpuscles (► B1) that can be stained with hematoxylin (hematoxylin bodies). Nuclei of this sort are phagocytized by neutrophilic granulocytes and macrophages, a process that can often only be demonstrated *in vitro* (► B2).

---

[1] Focal segmental glomerulonephritis: focal (not involving all glomeruli) and segmental (involving only portions of the glomerulus).

Antinuclear antibody
(immunofluorescence) x 100

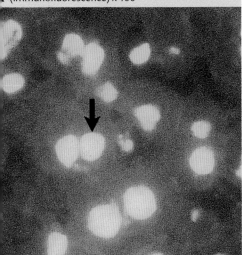

B **Lupus erythematosus phenomenon**
x 200

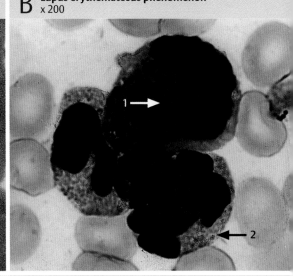

Butterfly erythema

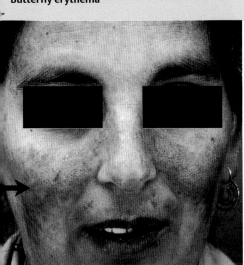

D **Dermatitis in lupus erythematosus**
(HE) x 50

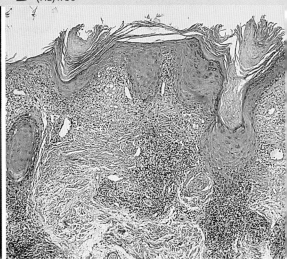

Lupus endocarditis

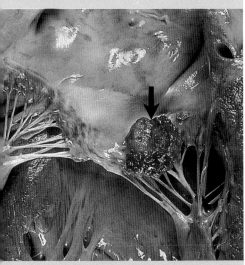

F **'Onion-skin' arteriopathy**
(PAS) x 50

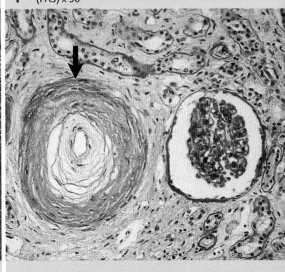

■ Progressive systemic sclerosis

Definition: Systemic immunologic disorder that begins with progressive sclerosis of the dermal connective tissue and spreads to the vascular connective tissue of internal organs.

Causal pathogenesis: The cause of the disorder in not known. The increased occurrence of several factors suggests the presence of an autoimmune process. These include:

— T lymphocytes against collagen;
— Antinuclear antibodies (p. 10) against topoisomerase I (anti-Scl-70 antibodies).
— Antinuclear antibodies against centromeres;

Formal pathogenesis: The disorder is characterized by two mechanisms:
— Formation of immune complex and, presumably induced by it,
— Excessive formation of abnormal collagen and microfibrils (p. 48).

Formation of immune complex leads to "onion-skin" arteriopathy in minor vessels in the wake of prior fibrinoid necrosis (see also lupus vasculitis, p. 172). This results in obstructive vascular fibrosis. Sequelae include:
— **Raynaud's phenomenon** with tricolor phenomenon (p. 148), leading to sclerosis of the skin and "rat bite" acral necrosis extending as far as the bones.
— **Fibrosis and infarction** of internal organs (esophagus, lungs, and kidneys).

✚ **Clinical presentation and morphology:** The disorder is more common in women than in men, reaching its peak between the ages of 30 and 50.
– *Skin:* Sclerosis of the skin of the fingers from collagen fibers with atrophy of the epidermal ridges (► B, C), leading to sclerodactyly (fingers appear "wooden"), a purse-string pattern of skin folds around the mouth, and a mask-like face (► A).
– *Gastrointestinal tract:* Elastosis and fibrosis of the walls of the bowel with collagen fibers leads to difficulties in swallowing and digestion, causing dysphagia and malabsorption (p. 82).
– *Respiratory tract:* Pulmonary elastosis and fibrosis leads to cor pulmonale (p. 390).
– *Kidney:* Chronic glomerulonephritis is usually present, leading to kidney failure.

✚ **Clinical variant:** CREST syndrome is characterized by calcinosis (finger, knee, and elbow), Raynaud's phenomenon, esophageal motility disorders, sclerodactyly, and telangiectasia.

☺ **Prominent patient** (► A): Paul Klee (1879–1940), Swiss painter.

■ Dermatomyositis

Synonym: polymyositis (with its sole manifestation in skeletal musculature).

Definition: Inflammatory autoimmune myopathy, usually with skin involvement.

Causal pathogenesis: The cause of the disorder in not known. The increased occurrence of several factors suggests the presence of an autoimmune process. These include:
— Anti-myoglobulin antibodies in patient serum;
— Antinuclear antibodies (ANA-type Jo-1) in patient serum;
— T lymphocytes sensitized against skeletal musculature in tissue.

✚ **Clinical presentation and morphology:** The disorder is more common in women than in men, reaching its peak between the ages of 30 and 50.
– *Skeletal musculature:* Acute edematous muscle swelling occurs, causing a painful sensation of heaviness in the limbs. Chronic symptoms include fibrous atrophic musculature, leading to painful fatigue.
Histologic findings include muscle necrosis, phagocytosis of muscle cell fragments, regenerative changes with large nuclei close to the sarcolemma (► D1), CD8-cytotoxic lymphocytes and histiocytes (► D2). Inflammatory infiltrate is present in the intramuscular connective tissue. Focal calcifications may occur.
– *Skin* (usually the dorsum of the nose and eyelids are affected): pinkish erythema and swelling produce an expressionless face.
Histologic findings include CD8-cytotoxic lymphocytic inflammatory infiltrate around the dermal blood vessels progressing to fibrosis with partial calcification.

■ Goodpasture's Syndrome

Definition: Autoimmune disorder with hematuria and pulmonary bleeding.

Pathogenesis: Expression of the Goodpasture antigen (NC1 of the α3 IV chain of collagen type IV of the basal membrane) occurs for unknown reasons. This triggers creation of anti-basal membrane antibodies, leading formation of an immune complex, deposits of which accumulate along the pulmonary alveolar and glomerular basal membranes (► E).

✚ **Clinical presentation and morphology:**
The disorder occurs primarily in young men.
– *Kidney:* Immune complex deposits produce a linear pattern of immunofluorescence (► F) and cause the glomerular loops to rupture. This in turn produces hematuria and reactive crescentic proliferation of the glomerular capsular epithelium (► G). The glomerulus scleroses, causing rapidly progressing kidney failure and uremia.
– *Lung:* Immune complex causes alveolar rupture, leading to alveolar hemorrhaging, which appears in chest radiographs as miliary foci in the lung around the hilum.

A Progressive systemic sclerosis

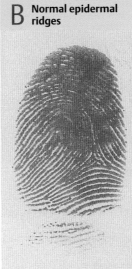

B Normal epidermal ridges

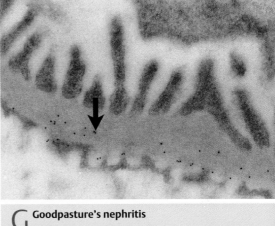

C Atrophic epidermal ridges

D Dermatomyositis
x 150

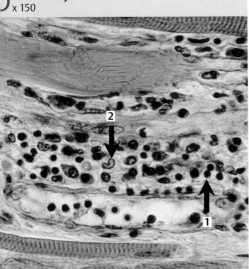

1

2

E Anti-basal membrane antibodies
(IH;TEM) x 10000

F Anti-basal membrane antibodies
(IH) x 75

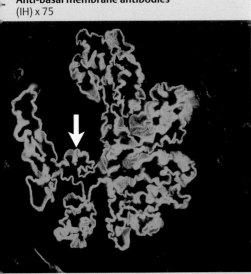

G Goodpasture's nephritis

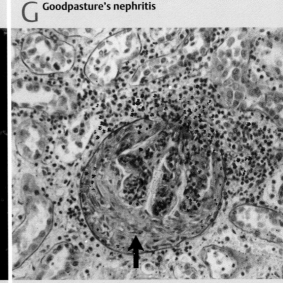

12

Immune Pathology

■ Wegener's Granulomatosis

Definition: Systemic autoimmune inflammation characterized by anti-cytoplasmic antibodies, granulomatous inflammation, and necrotizing vasculitis that usually begins in the upper respiratory tract.

Pathogenesis: For unknown reasons, autoimmune antibodies (c-ANCA p-ANCA[1]) (► A) activate granulocytes by a mechanism that is not understood. This produces granulomatous inflammation with cell-mediated vasculitis (► B) by an unknown mechanism, usually perivascular granulomas of the tuberculous type (p. 232), and infiltrate-containing lymphocytes, plasmacytes, and granulocytes. Sequelae of the vasculitis include infarction-like necrotic areas in and around granulomas in which the structure of the tissue remains intact.

✚ **Clinical presentation and morphology:**
Interstitial stage: Focal inflammation is present with local and regional rhinitis and sinusitis (diagnosis is made by mucosal biopsy). This leads to necrosis of the nasal cartilage, producing a swayback nose. Later this spreads intracanalicularly and leads to laryngotracheal bronchitis, often with necrotic foci in the lungs (where proliferation of T helper cells in the lungs occurs).

Systemic stage: Necrotizing granulomatous inflammation spreads primarily to these organs:
- In the lungs, it manifests itself as alveolar bleeding.
- In the kidneys, it produces immune complex glomerulonephritis with fibrinoid necrosis of the glomerular loops (► D1), successively leading to bleeding on the kidney surface (► C) and hematuria. This later produces adhesions of the glomerular loops (► D2) and reactive crescentic proliferation of the glomerular capsular epithelium.
- In blood vessels, it manifests itself as generalized vasculitis.

■ Rheumatoid Arthritis

Definition: One of the collagen diseases, this systemic inflammatory autoimmune disorder primarily attacks the synovial membrane of the minor joints in successive episodes, leading to joint stiffening.

Pathogenetic chain reaction: In patients with a genetic predisposition (HLA-DRB1 0401, 0404 and 0101, it is presumed that an initial viral infection somehow stimulates autoreactive Th1 cells. This generates autoantigens (see below), successively causing lymphocytic synovitis and proliferation of lymphocytes mit formation of lymphocytic follicles in the synovial membrane. This causes B cells to form autoreactive antibodies (rheumatism factors), including anti-idiotypes (primarily IgM against IgG as well as IgG anti-IgG and IgA

anti-IgA), antinuclear antibodies, and anti-collagen type II antibodies.

These antibodies cross-link to form deposits on collagen fibers (fibrinoid necrosis), leading to formation of rheumatoid granulomas (p. 234). This activates the complement system (p. 162), which perpetuates the inflammation.

✚ **Clinical presentation:** The disorder manifests itself primarily in the small joints and in mechanically exposed areas of the subcutis like the elbow, where rheumatoid nodules appear. Visceral involvement is rare but may include necrotizing vasculitis, interstitial pulmonary fibrosis (p. 40), serositis, myositis, and uveitis.

■ Sjögren's Syndrome

Definition: Systemic autoimmune disorder with symmetrical involvement of the salivary and lacrimal glands and desiccation of the conjunctiva and oropharynx.
- **Primary form** involves an isolated keratoconjunctivitis sicca syndrome;
- **Secondary form** involves a keratoconjunctivitis sicca syndrome in conjunction with other autoimmune disorders such as rheumatoid arthritis or systemic lupus erythematosus.

Pathogenesis: The cause of the disorder is not known. Patients with a genetic predisposition (primarily HLA-DR3) form autoreactive antibodies mainly against splicosomal proteins such as Ro/SS-A and La/SS-B as well as against the excretory epithelia of the salivary and lacrimal glands.

Morphologic findings include destructive inflammation with lymphocytes and plasmacytes (► E1) in the form of a lymphoepithelial lesion, primarily around the excretory ducts (► F) with progressive glandular atrophy. This leads to regenerative proliferation of uninvolved acinar duct cells resembling myoepithelium (► E2).

✚ **Clinical presentation:** Keratoconjunctivitis sicca and dacryoadenitis sicca, often progressing to a MALT lymphoma.

❗ **Note:** *Sjögren's syndrome is diagnosed* by a lip biopsy with >50 lymphocytic, plasmacytic, and histiocytic cells in the vicinity of the salivary gland.

❗ **Note:** The manifestation pattern of autoimmune disorders includes:
- Circulating immune complexes, leading to systemic autoimmune disorders (with vasculitis);
- Antibodies against tissue epitopes, tending to lead to autoimmune disorders that primarily affect certain organs;
- antibodies against cell regions, leading to autoimmune disorders of a specific organ.

---

[1] c-ANCA: antineutrophil cytoplasmic autoantibody against neutral lysosomal granulocyte serin protease-3 (PR3); p-ANCA against myeloperoxidase in granulocytes.

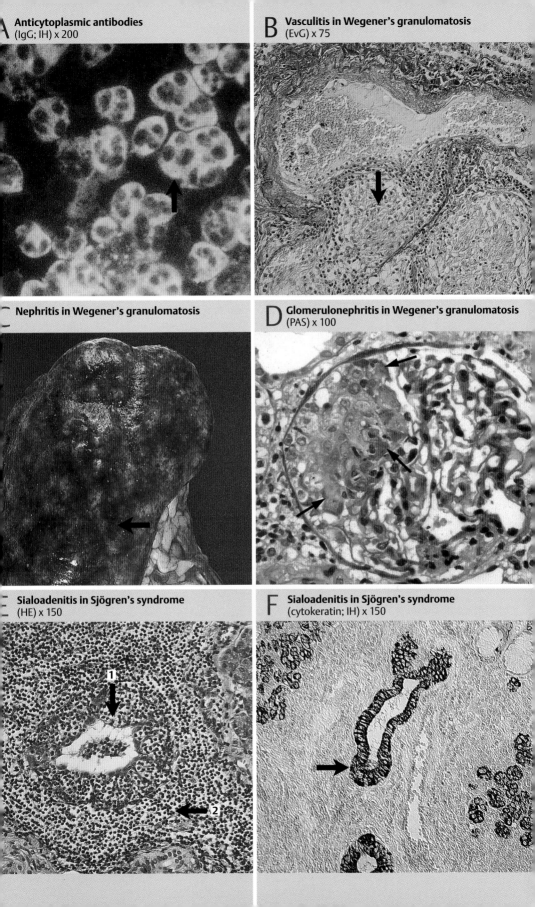

A Anticytoplasmic antibodies
(IgG; IH) x 200

B Vasculitis in Wegener's granulomatosis
(EvG) x 75

C Nephritis in Wegener's granulomatosis

D Glomerulonephritis in Wegener's granulomatosis
(PAS) x 100

E Sialoadenitis in Sjögren's syndrome
(HE) x 150

F Sialoadenitis in Sjögren's syndrome
(cytokeratin; IH) x 150

Autoimmune Disorders Organ specific

■ Hashimoto Thyroiditis

Synonym: lymphocytic thyroiditis.

Definition: autoimmune inflammation of the thyroid.

Etiologic factors include exogenous factors such as viruses and endogenous factors such as HLA-DR5 predominance.

Pathogenesis: Autoreactive antibodies are formed.

✚ Clinical presentation and morphology:
- *Antibodies against thyroglobulin* (► A);
- *Antibodies against peroxidase and the cell nucleus* (► C) of the thyroid cells lead to lymphocytic infiltrate with formation of germinal centers (► B). This causes destruction of the thyroid follicles (► B), later leading to oncocytic transformation of the remaining thyroid cells. The result is a pale brown enlarged thyroid with a rubbery consistency.
- *Antibodies against TSH receptors* cause permanent stimulation of the thyroid. This successively leads to increased hormone production, thyroid enlargement (goiter), and occasionally to transient thyroid hyperactivity.
- *Antibodies against iodine transporter* lead to hypothyroidism. The *late stage* of this disorder is characterized by fibrotic replacement of the destroyed inflamed parenchyma, leading to thyroid atrophy and hypothyroidism.

■ Autoimmune Adrenalitis

Definition: Autoimmune inflammation of the adrenal gland with clinical symptoms of insufficiency.

Pathogenesis: For unknown reasons, autoreactive antibodies against the adrenal gland are formed.

✚ Clinical presentation and morphology: Lymphocytic inflammation produces scarring and fibrous atrophy, leading to hypocorticism in the form of Addison's disease (p. 24, 112).

■ Type I Diabetes Mellitus

Definition: Autoimmune insulitis with development of insulin-dependent diabetes mellitus (p. 78).

Etiologic factors include exogenous factors such as viruses, environmental agents, endogenous factors such as HLA-DR4 and/or HLA-DR3 genetic predisposition.

Pathogenesis: The autoimmune response includes
- *Autoreactive antibodies* (against tyrosine phosphatase = islet cell cytoplasm, glutamic acid decarboxylase and insulin) and
- *Autoreactive CD8-cytotoxic lymphocytes* against insulin-forming islet cells, leading to lymphocytic insulitis.

■ Myasthenia Gravis

Definition: Autoimmune disorder of voluntary muscles involving abnormal muscular weakness.

Pathogenesis: Thymus hyperplasia and/or neoplasia lead to formation of autoreactive antibodies for reasons that are not clear.

✚ Clinical presentation and morphology:
- *Antibodies against acetylcholine* receptors block the transmission of impulses from nerve to muscle. This results in abnormal muscular weakness and fatigue following repeated activation and protracted contraction. This results in reduced facial expression, drooping of the eyelids, impaired vision, speech deficiencies, and difficulties in swallowing.
- *Complement activation* leads to destruction of the postsynaptic membrane. This results in few lymphocytic infiltrates along the muscle fibers.

■ Autoimmune Gastritis

Synonym: type A gastritis.

Definition: Autoimmune inflammation of the gastric mucosa progressing to pernicious anemia.

Pathogenesis: For unknown reasons, autoreactive antibodies are formed.

✚ Clinical presentation and morphology:
- *Antibodies against the parietal cells of the stomach* causes lymphocytic and plasmacytic destruction of the stomach glands (► E). In the *early stage*, inflammation of the superficial gastric mucosa is present as "superficial gastritis" (► D1), leading to destruction of the peptic cells and parietal cells. In the *late phase*, these cells are replaced by mucoid glandular epithelia (atrophic gastritis).
- *Antibodies against intrinsic factor*[1] lead to megaloblastic anemia.

■ Multiple Sclerosis

Synonym: disseminated encephalomyelitis.

Definition: Episodically progressing brain disease with disseminated focal demyelination in all sections of the white matter.

Etiologic factors include exogenous factors such as viruses (although which specific ones is not known) and endogenous factors such as HLA-A3, B7, DW2, and DR2 genetic predisposition.

Pathogenesis of this disorder is not clear.

✚ Clinical presentation and morphology:
Early stage: Lymphocytic and plasmacytic perivascular infiltrates primarily in the white matter lead to disintegration of the myelin and phagocytosis by fatty granular cells. This produces multiple, sharply demarcated foci of demyelination that spare the axons. Primary sites include:
- The lateral ventricular walls and the subcortical region along the border between cortex and medulla;
- The deep medulla of the cerebellum (producing ataxia, dysarthria, and spastic paralysis), spinal cord, and brain stem;
- the optic nerve (leading to impaired vision).
Later symptoms include proliferation of astroglia, leading to formation of fibrous glial tissue at the focus of demyelination or glial sclerosis (hence the name "multiple sclerosis").

---

[1] Intrinsic factor: a protein that controls absorption of vitamin B_{12}.

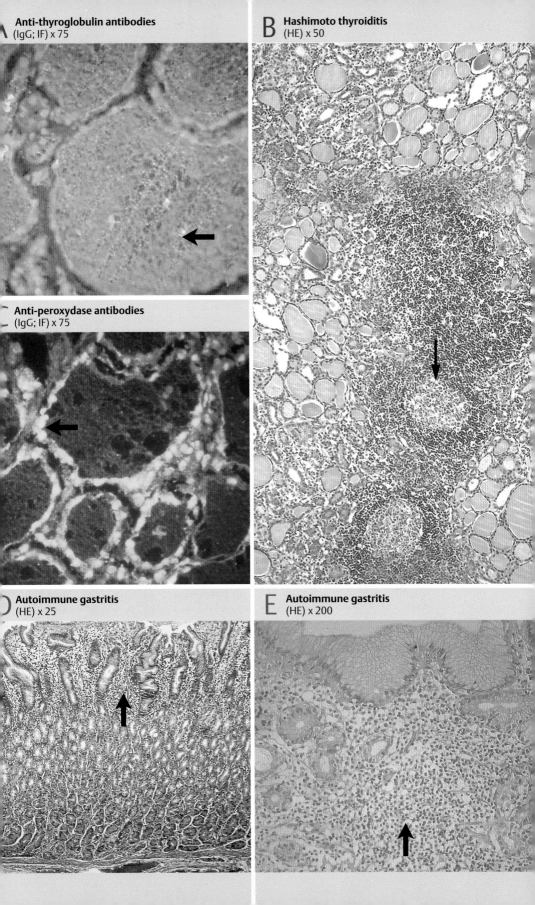

A Anti-thyroglobulin antibodies
(IgG; IF) x 75

Anti-peroxydase antibodies
(IgG; IF) x 75

B Hashimoto thyroiditis
(HE) x 50

D Autoimmune gastritis
(HE) x 25

E Autoimmune gastritis
(HE) x 200

Immunodeficiency Disorders

Synonym: immunodeficiency syndromes.

General definition: These are clinical syndromes due to an absent or insufficient immune response to various antigen stimuli.

Usually rare, these disorders serve to illustrate the function of that part of the immune system affected by the underlying defect and its effect on the organism. In this respect they may be regarded as pathogenetic models.

Primary Immunodeficiency Disorders

■ X-Linked Agammaglobulinemia

Textbook example of a hereditary B-cell defect.

Definition: General absence of immunoglobulin in young boys (Bruton agammaglobulinemia) due to defective B-cell maturation.

Pathogenesis: A genetic defect of a tyrokinase involved in signal transduction of B-cell maturation results in the absence of mature B cells, plasma cells, and and under-developed MALT system. As a result, serum levels of all immunoglobulins are drastically reduced.

Morphologic consequences of this B-cell maturation defect include a lack of secondary follicles with reaction centers in the secondary immune organs. The T-cell system remains morphologically and functionally intact.

✚ **Clinical presentation:** The disorder exhibits an X-linked inheritance pattern, with recurrent infections of the respiratory tract, otitis (middle ear infections), pyodermia (purulent skin inflammations), lambliasis, and sepsis (p. 222).

■ Transient Hypogammaglobulinemia

Definition and pathogenesis: When the level of the mother's antibodies in the infant's blood decreases, the infant can exhibit delayed intrinsic antibody creation for reasons that remain unclear. This results in transient hypogammaglobulinemia.

✚ **Clinical presentation:** The disorder manifests itself at the age of 3 months in the form of persistent otitis, bronchitis, and pneumonia (lung inflammation).

■ Heavy-Chain Defect

Definition and pathogenesis: The disorder is caused by various deletions of the heavy-chain genes on chromosome 14. Depending on the location of the genetic defect, there will be a corresponding absence of specific immunoglobulin isotypes or subtypes.

✚ **Clinical presentation:** The disorder exhibits an autosomal recessive inheritance pattern. Only a few patients suffer repeated infections.

■ κ Chain Defect

Definition and pathogenesis: The disorder is caused by single-point mutations of the κ chain gene on chromosome 2. Only immunoglobulins with λ chains are found in the blood.

■ IgG Subclass Defect

Definition: A group of immunodeficiency syndromes with reduced serum levels of IgG2, IgG3, and IgG4 (individually or together) in the presence of normal overall serum IgG levels.

Pathogenesis: The disorder lacks a uniform causal mechanism. It may be due to homozygous deletion of genes that encode the constant region of the various γ chains, or to defective regulation of B-cell differentiation.

✚ **Clinical presentation:** Patients present with recurrent infections of the respiratory tract and occasionally with IgA deficiency as well.

■ Hyper IgM Syndrome

Definition and pathogenesis: This group of diseases involves an isotype switch defect (p. 160) with the B cells. This leads to elevated serum levels of IgM and reduced serum levels of IgG, IgA, and IgE.

✚ **Clinical presentation:** The disorder occurs sporadically and exhibits an X-linked or autosomal inheritance pattern. Symptoms resemble those of hypogammaglobulinemia.

■ Isolated IgA Deficiency

Definition and pathogenesis: This is the most common primary immunodeficiency syndrome. Patients develop atopy, nontropical sprue (celiac disease, p. 82), and autoimmune diseases.

■ Common Variable Immunodeficiency

Synonym: CVID.

Definition: Heterogeneous group of syndromes with hereditary or acquired antibody deficiency associated with panhypogammaglobulinemia.

Pathogenesis: The following underlying defects are involved association with distinct HLA genes;
— Defective B-cell maturation in immunoglobulin-secreting plasma cells;
— Increased effect of T suppressor cells;
— Deficient effect of T-helper cells on B cells (cognate T- B-cell interation).

Morphologic characteristics:
— **Lymphadenopathy** with nonmalignant proliferation of lymphocytes and severe follicular hyperplasia.
— **Intestinal mucosa:** polypous, nodular lymphatic hyperplasia.
— **Splenomegaly.**
— **Plasma-cell deficiency** (hardly any immunoglobulin is formed) in bone marrow, lymph nodes, and GALT[1].

✚ **Clinical presentation:** These disorders are equally common in women and men, reaching their peak between the ages of 20 and 30. All forms of CVID have several characteristics in common:
– *Immunoglobulin deficiency* with low levels of IgG, IgA, and often IgM as well;
– *Sinopulmonary infections* leading to chronic obstructive lung disease;
– *Gastrointestinal disorders* (50% of all patients) such as diarrhea and malabsorption (p. 82);
– *Giardiasis:* intestinal infestation with the protozoan *Giardia lamblia* (p. 274) is common due to the IgA defect of the GALT;
– *Autoimmune diseases* are common (p. 180), including rheumatoid arthritis, pernicious anemia, autoimmune anemia, autoimmune thrombocytopenia, and neutropenia;
– *Increased risk of tumor.*

Primary Immunodeficiency Syndromes: T-Cell Defects

■ DiGeorge Syndrome

Textbook example of a congenital T-cell defect.

Definition: A malformation in the pharyngeal pouch region in particular, with defective T-cell maturation resulting from thymus aplasia (p. 300).

Pathogenesis: The products of the HOX 1.5 gene control the migration and differentiation processes of certain tissues that evolve from the neural crest, such as the third and fourth pharyngeal pouches (p. 296). Deletion of this gene leads to a condition in which the thymus is aplastic or hypoplastic. This results in an absence of mature T cells in the regions of the peripheral lymph organs controlled by the thymus.

✚ **Clinical presentation:** The disorder is characterized by neonatal tetany (persistent muscle cramps). Patients are susceptible to viral and mycotic infections and exhibit facial deformities, including
– Hypertelorism (widely spaced eyes),
– Micrognathia (narrow, fish-like jaw),
– Deep-seated ears, and often cardiovascular deformities (primarily of the aortic arch and ventricular septum).

■ Nezelof Syndrome

Definition: Combined immunodeficiency syndrome due to a genetic developmental anomaly of the thymus, characterized by absence of further deformities.

Pathogenesis: Failure of the thymus to differentiate into cortex and medulla leads to an absence of T cells. This results in a lymphocyte deficiency in the regions of the peripheral lymph organs controlled by the thymus and lack of interaction between T cells and B cells.

✚ **Clinical presentation:** The disorder exhibits a recessive or X-linked recessive inheritance pattern. Serum immunoglobulin concentrations are nearly normal. However, antibodies against vaccines fail to form, making patients susceptible to infection (primarily with *Candida albicans;* p. 270).

■ Chronic Myocutaneous Candidiasis

Definition and pathogenesis: Isolated defect in cell-mediated immunity against fungi of the genus Candida. Humoral immunity remains intact.

✚ **Clinical presentation:** patients present with Candida infection (p. 270) of the skin and mucous membranes, primarily in the respiratory and gastrointestinal tracts.

❗ **Note:** *Clinical presentation of B-cell defects* primarily involves recurrent bronchopulmonary infections.

❗ **Note:** *Clinical presentation of T-cell defects* primarily involves recurrent mycotic infections.

Primary Immunodeficiency Syndromes: B-Cell and T-Cell Defects

■ Severe combined immunodeficiency (= SCID)

Definition: Genetic heterogeneous syndrome characterized by the absence of humoral an cell-mediated immunity

Pathogenetic basis: It consists of mutated:
— Enzymes of lymphatic cells;
— Cytokine receptors in precursor T cell;
— Recombinase followed by deficient rearrangements of T-cell and B-cell receptors;
— Kinase of signal transduction in T cell;
— Transcription factors for MHC molecules.

The two most frequent of these rare disorders are:
— *Chromosomally-inherited form* (50 % of all SCID cases): More common in boys, it is based on a mutation in the α-chain of those cytokine receptors that control the differentiation and proliferation of T cells, intervening consequentially in the early phase of T-cell and the late phase of B-cell development. THe result is the drastically reduced number of T cell cooperation. B-cell and T-cell zones are absent in the peripheral lymphatic organs (► A, C).
— *Autosomally-recessive inherited forms:* Most common of these is adenosine deaminase deficiency (ADA deficiency), causing, during purine metabolism, the accumulation of deoxyadenosine and deoxy-ATP (dATP) in precursor T cells, which leads to T-cell destruction.

✚ **Clinical presentation:** Most children with SCID have a serious shortage of T cells in the peripheral blood. Consequently, all T-cell function tests yield negative or pathologic results. These children die within one to two years due to recurrent infections by viruses such as CMV, bacteria such as Pseudomonas, fungi such as candida, and protozoans such as Pneumocystis carinii. Treatment: semi-allogenic stem cells from the parents.

■ Ataxia Telangiectasia

Synonym: Louis-Bar syndrome.

Textbook example of a precancerous condition involving a DNA repair defect.

Definition and pathogenesis: The disorder involves a hereditary DNA repair mechanism deficiency with progressive cerebellar atrophy, thymus dysplasia with lymphopenia (primarily involving CD4 lymphocytes), IgA deficiency and oculocutaneous telangiectasia (primarily of the conjunctiva).

✚ **Clinical presentation:** The disorder exhibits an autosomal recessive inheritance pattern. Patients suffer from frequent bronchopulmonary infections and ataxia (► B).
- *Children* frequently develop hematologic neoplasms such as malignant lymphomas (p. 364) and myelomonocytic leukemia.
- *Adults* frequently develop solid tumors (primarily breast carcinoma).

■ Wiskott-Aldrich Syndrome

Definition: Rare X-chromosomal recessive (inherited) immunodeficiency with thrombocytopenia, eczema, and recurrent infections.

Pathogenesis: This disorder is the result of mutation on Xp11.23 of the "Wiskott-Aldrich" gene, whose product is involved in the signal transduction of hematopoietic cells. The resulting pathogenetic mechanism is unclear. In the course of the disease, peripheral blood and the lymph node's paracortical zones are deprived of T Cells. T-Cell dependent immunity is rendered ineffective and fails to form antibodies against polysaccharide-rich antigens.

✚ **Clinical presentation:** Serum: normal IgG level, low IgM level, raised IgA and IgE levels. Typical symptoms: eczema, thrombocytopenia, recurrent infections. Early death; high risk for malignant lymphomas.

Secondary Immunodeficiency Syndromes

General definition: Acquired antibody deficiency that manifests itself only in adolescence or later.

Etiologic factors:

Humoral immunodeficiencies are caused by:
— *Deficient protein intake* in starvation, dietary deficiencies, and tumor cachexia;
— *Protein loss* due to
    — Exudative gastroenteropathy (disorder of variable etiology involving massive intestinal protein loss) or
    — Nephrotic syndrome (disorder of variable etiology involving massive renal protein loss):
— *Gammopathy,* involving tumor synthesis of defective immunoglobulins.

Cellular immunodeficiencies may be caused by
— *Impaired T-cell proliferation* in corticosteroid-induced immunosuppression, from cytostatic agents, or with T-cell tumors, or they may be caused by
— *Impaired T-cell function* due to viruses or chronic infection.

The result is diminished resistance against bacterial, viral, and mycotic infections and against opportunistic microorganisms such as *Pneumocystis carinii* (p. 278).

■ Monoclonal Gammopathy

Definition: Disorders with increased formation of immunoglobulins of one class, one type, and one specificity resulting from neoplastic proliferation of a single plasmacell clone.

Benign monoclonal gammopathy involves expansion of a morphologically normal plasmacell clone. This produces a slight elevation in the level of serum monoclonal immunoglobulins (<3 g), with at most minimal Bence Jones proteinuria.

Plasmocytoma is the most common generalized bone tumor. It usually develops in bone marrow (p. 364).

Waldenström macroglobulinemia is a group of neoplastic B-cell disorders, most commonly a neoplastic lymphocytoid or plasmacytoid immunocyte (p. 364), with monoclonal proliferation of IgM (► D, E).

Heavy-chain disorders involve neoplastic B-cell disorders that form heavy chains (γ, α, and μ chain types) that are not bonded to light chains.

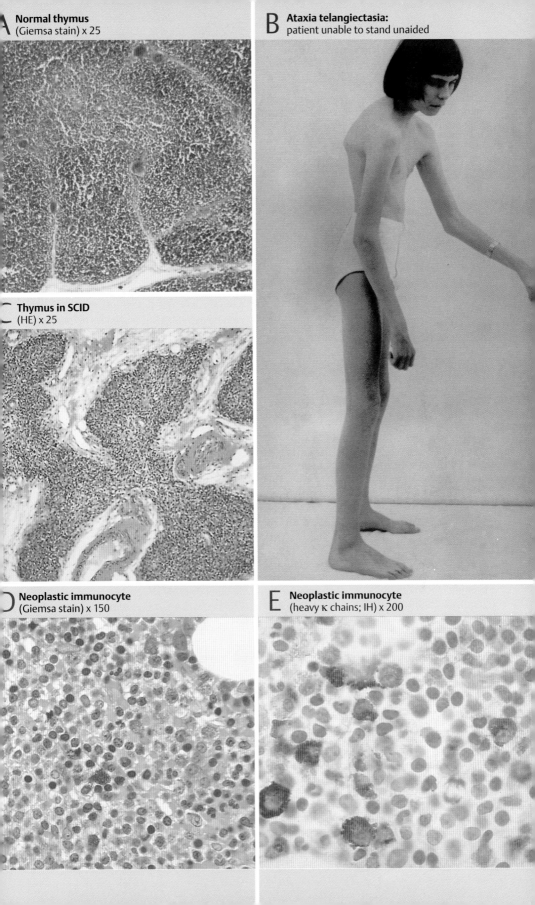

A **Normal thymus**
(Giemsa stain) x 25

B **Ataxia telangiectasia:**
patient unable to stand unaided

C **Thymus in SCID**
(HE) x 25

D **Neoplastic immunocyte**
(Giemsa stain) x 150

E **Neoplastic immunocyte**
(heavy κ chains; IH) x 200

Acquired Immunodeficiency Syndrome (AIDS)

Textbook example of an acquired T-cell defect.

Definition: Common secondary immunodeficiency syndrome resulting from viral infection, characterized by defective cellular immunity.

Pathogenesis (p. 244).

Sequelae of AIDS

— HIV lymphadenopathy
— Kaposi's sarcoma
— HIV-associated pneumopathy
— HIV encephalitis

HIV Lymphadenopathy

This progresses in three stages (► A):

1: Irregular follicular hyperplasia: Initially, B cells receive excessive continuous stimulation in the lymph nodes. This leads to gigantic follicular hypertrophy. In time, the mantle zones around the follicle atrophy, resulting in follicles consisting of bare germinal centers and resembling tulips. This leads to enlargement of the lymph nodes (HIV lymphadenopathy).

✚ **Clinical presentation:** Generalized lymphadenopathy stage.

2: Progressive follicular destruction: In time, the structure of the grossly enlarged follicle breaks apart, causing viruses in the lymph nodes to stimulate production of vasoformative factor. This leads to proliferation of venules and to destruction of the giant follicle.

✚ **Clinical presentation:** AIDS-related complex (ARC) stage.

3: Follicular atrophy: The cortical B-cell zone and paracortical T-cell zone disappear (► B). The resulting shrunken follicles are replaced by lymphocyte infiltrate rich in plasma cells and proliferating venules due to stimulation of vasoformative factor (► B1). This leads to lymph nodes that are free of follicles and high atrophic. This complete immune defect makes the body vulnerable to opportunistic infections. Non-Hodgkin lymphomas of the B-cell type also occur, primarily in the gastrointestinal tract.

Kaposi's Sarcoma

This malignant tumor (occurring in 25% of all cases) is the result of HIV infection and simultaneous infection with human herpes virus type 8 (HHV-8). Kaposi's sarcoma is a sarcomatous tumor, initially infiltrated with lymphocytes and later consisting of spindle cells, that expresses CD34. It arises from proliferating vascular endothelial tissue and forms irregular vascular spaces (► C). The tumor occurs at multiple foci, initially in the skin, later in the lymph nodes and intestinal tract as well. Stromal bleeding gives the skin foci a brownish appearance (► D).

HIV-Associated Pneumopathy

One or more of the following lung lesions often occurs in AIDS patients:

— Diffuse alveolar damage syndrome;
— Chronic interstitial pneumonia;
— Pneumonia with opportunistic pathogens (primarily Pneumocystis carinii; p. 278);
— Hyperplasia of the bronchi-associated lymphoid tissue.

HIV Encephalitis

This is recognizable by the diffuse lymphocytic infiltrates in the leptomeningeal and medullary substance with multiple nodules of cells (► F1) consisting of microglia and macroglia, and of lymphocytes and histiocytes. Typical findings include individual macrophages or macrophage groups (some multinucleated) with expression of viral p21 protein (► F2), especially in the cerebral medulla. Where these findings are accompanied by medullary lesions in the cerebrum, the condition is referred to as HIV encephalopathy.

❗ **Note:** *AIDS-related complexes* include episodic fever, diarrhea without evidence of a pathogen, weight loss, anemia, leukopenia, thrombopenia, and helper cell deficiency.

❗ **Note:** Opportunistic pathogens associated with AIDS include:
– *Toxoplasma gondii* (toxoplasmosis);
– *Cryptosporidium* (cryptosporidiosis);
– *Pneumocystis carinii* (pneumonia);
– *Candida albicans* (respiratory and digestive tract);
– *Cryptococcus* (cryptococcosis);
– *Mycobacterium tuberculosis*;
– *Mycobacterium avium-intracellulare*;
– *Herpes simplex*;
– *Cytomegalovirus*;
– *Papovavirus* (warts and oral hairy leukoplakia);
– *hepatitis viruses* (HBV and HBC).

❗ **Note:** *HIV encephalitis* is macrophage encephalitis.

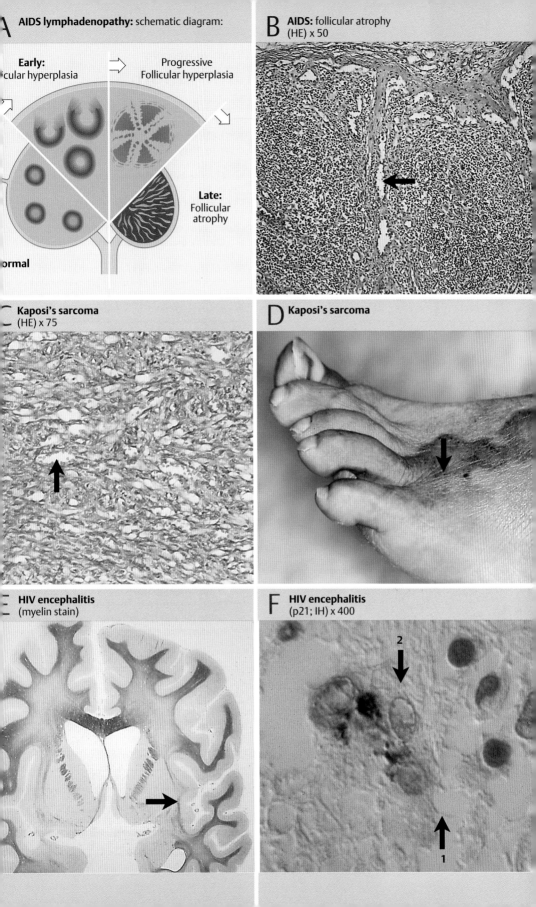

A AIDS lymphadenopathy: schematic diagram:

Early: follicular hyperplasia → Progressive Follicular hyperplasia

Late: Follicular atrophy

Normal

B AIDS: follicular atrophy (HE) x 50

C Kaposi's sarcoma (HE) x 75

D Kaposi's sarcoma

E HIV encephalitis (myelin stain)

F HIV encephalitis (p21; IH) x 400

Pathology of Inflammation

Summary

An inflammation is a defensive process in which the organism's immune system is involved. Without this process, it would succumb to foreign organisms. There are several basic forms of inflammation:

▶ **Acute exudative inflammatory reaction**: The biologic purpose of such a reaction is to locally increase vascular permeability. This allows sufficient fluid to escape, reducing the concentration of the noxious agent at the inflammation site (exudation). The slowed circulation also hinders the spread of the noxious agent in tissue. Leukocytes attracted to the inflamed area are responsible for specifically eliminating the noxious agent. Acute forms of inflammation are classified according to the dominant component in their exudate. An acute inflammation that

fails to heal either progresses to chronic inflammation or it complicates the course of the primary disorder by triggering secondary immunologic disorders.

▶ **Chronic inflammations** that form granulation tissue are characterized by formation of a capillary-rich mesenchyma in the form of granulation tissue. The chances of defective healing depend on the potential for this tissue's being absorbed.

▶ **Chronic granulomatous inflammations** are associated with nodular deposits of inflammatory cells (granulomas). These form when contaminants that are not immediately destroyed are surrounded by groups of macrophages. These "squads" receive their orders to attack from surrounding lymphocytes.

Definition of Inflammation

Inflammation is a defensive process that a living body initiates against local tissue damage. It takes the form of a complex reaction of blood vessels, certain plasma components and blood cells, and cellular and structural components of connective tissue. Terms ending in the suffix **"–it is"** denote inflammation.

Etiology of Inflammation

An inflammation may be triggered by several mechanisms. These include:

— Noxious physical agents (p. 146);
— Noxious chemical agents (p. 140);
— Accumulated products of metabolism;
— Immunologic tissue injury;
— Tissue injury from infection;
— Tissue necrosis.

Spread of Inflammation

■ **Local inflammation:** This inflammation is limited to a circumscribed area of tissue in the vicinity of its port of entry. The spread of a local inflammation is passively controlled by organ capsules and fascial septa. The following forms of dissemination are differentiated:

— *Hematogenous* dissemination occurs through blood vessels.
— *Lymphatic* dissemination occurs through lymph system.
— *Neurogenic* dissemination occurs via the flow of axoplasm in the nerves.
— *Ductal* dissemination occurs through ductal or canalicular systems in organs, leading to ascending inflammation.
— *Direct contagion* may also occur.

■ **Metastatic inflammation:** An inflammatory reaction often spreads from the local focus of inflammation. This results in transmission of the inflammatory pathogens into other organs and tissues (metastasis), where the pathogen can trigger a metastatic inflammation (septicopyemia; p. 222).

■ **Generalized infection:** In this case, the pathogen spreads diffusely throughout the entire body.

Symptoms of Inflammation

Inflammation produces local clinical and morphologic changes (▶ A). These include:

— *Tumor,* inflammatory tissue swelling;
— *Rubor,* inflammatory hyperemic erythema;
— *Calor,* inflammatory heat in the tissue;
— *Dolor,* pain in the inflamed area;
— *Functio laesa,* functional impairment of the inflamed organ or tissue.

Note: Terms ending in the suffix "–it is" denote inflammation.

Note: The inflammatory tumorescence is always tender upon palpation, in contrast to a neoplastic tumor.

The five cardinal symptoms of inflammation (▶ A) are attributable to the reaction of the vascular mesenchyma and blood cells. Together, they constitute the acute exudative inflammatory reaction described in the next section.

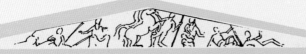

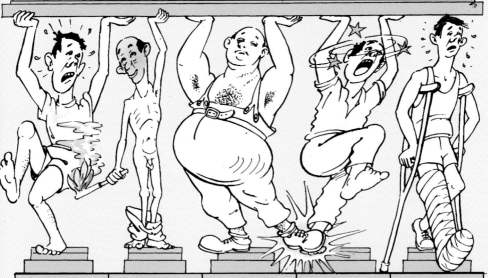

Calor	Rubor	Tumor	Dolor	Functio laesa
Local hypothermia, fever	Hyperemia (redness)	Tissue swelling (inflammatory tumor)	Burning pain	Functional impairment

Exudative Inflammatory Reaction

Definition: Response pattern of acute inflammation, characterized by exudation of blood components and emigration of blood cells.

Biologic purpose: This is the result of the interplay of four factors:

— *Increased perfusion* due to hyperemia achieves rapid removal of the noxious agent from the site.
— *Exudation* of blood serum achieves rapid dilution of the noxious agent.
— *Elimination of pathogens* by phagocytosis achieves rapid destruction of the noxious agent.
— *Sequestration* by a "strike force" of inflammatory cells achieves rapid containment of the noxious agent.

The acute exudative inflammatory reaction consists of these formal pathogenetic elements:

— Changes in microcirculation;
— Changes in permeability;
— Leukocyte transmigration.

Changes in Microcirculation

Physiology: The microvasculature lies between the terminal arterioles and postcapillary venules. It comprises the capillary network and an anastomosing vessel between the respective arteriole and venule. Blood flow through the microvasculature is adapted to specific needs. Normally, the main bloodstream is fed through the capillary system after the precapillary sphincters are closed. The capillaries only receive blood intermittently. Additionally, the arterioles and venules constantly alternate between vasoconstriction and vasodilatation. These "throttle" mechanisms regulate blood flow and filtration pressure, which directly affects the transudation of soluble substances into the surrounding tissue.

Many humoral factors and chemical substances are involved in this regulation process (p. 202). The interplay of these factors and substances causes a typical pattern of changes in the capillary structures that occurs in three phases.

First phase of changes in microcirculation: This involves transient arteriolar vasoconstriction (▶ A) lasting from a few seconds to a few minutes. This phase is not detectable in every inflammatory reaction.

Scenario: The noxious agent *enters* the tissue. The "faucet" is turned off by means of arteriolar vasoconstriction, preventing further spread of the noxious agent.
Result: Brief paling of the inflamed area.

Second phase of changes in microcirculation: This begins a few minutes after the first phase. Inflammation mediators lead to vasodilatation of the arterioles, capillaries, and postcapillary venules. This causes exudation of blood serum that leads to inflammatory tissue swelling (▶ B) with stimulation of the nociceptive nerves (pain nerves).

Scenario: The noxious agent *is in* the tissue. All "faucets" are turned on by means of vasodilatation of the arterioles, capillaries, and venules to thoroughly flush out the noxious agent.
Result: Erythema, swelling, and pain in the inflamed area.

Third phase of changes in microcirculation: This begins several hours after the onset of inflammation and lasts for a period of several hours. It is brought about by vasodilatation of the capillaries and arterioles and is accompanied by vasoconstriction of the venules. This slows the circulation, elevates filtration pressure, and increases vascular permeability in the inflamed area (▶ C).

The pathogenetic chain reaction to the slowed circulation in the microvasculature involves several events:

— *Sealing of vascular structures:* Laminar aggregations of erythrocytes change into what appear under light microscopy to be homogeneous cylindrical vascular castings ("red sludge"). This causes endothelial damage, making the endothelium "wettable". This causes thrombocytes to aggregate, leading to thrombosis. This seals off the leaking vascular structures in the inflamed area.
— *Leukocyte extravasation:* Leukocytes migrate out of the microvasculature and into the inflamed area.

Scenario: The noxious agent *remains in* the tissue. All "faucets" are turned and sealed off by means of vasoconstriction of the venules and formation of microthrombi.
Result: The area damaged by the noxious agent is sealed off, paving the way for the "strike force" of leukocytes.

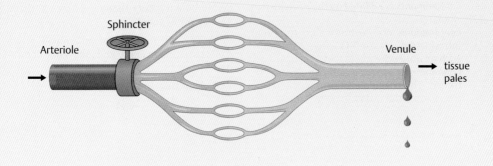

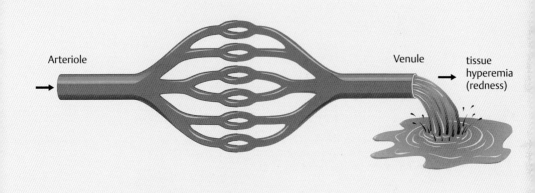

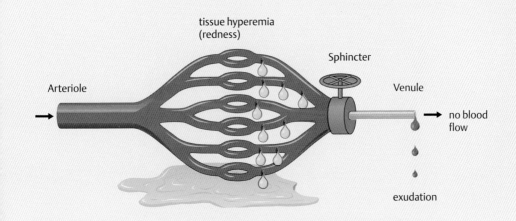

Increased Permeability

The biologic purpose of exudation is the result of the interplay of a trio of factors:

— **Contaminants are diluted** by the protein-rich exudate.
— **Contaminants are neutralized** by the rapid introduction of counteractive substances such as antibodies.
— **Contaminants are fixed** and damage is controlled. The coagulated fibrin in the tissue demarcates the inflammatory damage and fixes the pathogens.

> **Note:** Exudate is composed of water, fibrinogen and other coagulating proteins, immunoglobulins, complement factors and cleavage products, and macroglobulins and microglobulins.

Pathogenetic principle: The increased vascular permeability in the inflammatory process primarily affects the postcapillary venules. It primarily involves extravasation of substances between the endothelial cells (p. 424). Two mechanisms regulate this extravasation:

— **Endothelial cell contraction:** The cytoskeleton of the endothelial cells of the postcapillary venules contains actin. These cells can contract under the influence of most inflammation mediators, opening pores in the walls of the capillaries (▶ A1).
  Result: Regulated, moderate fluid exudation.
— **Endothelial necrosis:** The noxious agent that triggers inflammation damages the endothelium and causes endothelial swelling (▶ A2). This later leads to irreversible endothelial damage in the form of endothelial necrosis (▶ A3), with formation of holes in the capillary.
  Result: Unregulated, excessive fluid exudation.

A hemodynamic factor (p. 424) is present in addition to these cellular factors. It consists of a local increase in intravascular pressure, leading to extravasation of blood serum in the form of an inflammatory exudate.

These changes in permeability permit the exudation of blood serum and/or plasma components into tissue.

Result: Inflammatory tissue swelling or inflammatory tumescence.

Depending on the type of inflammation, the changes in permeability will follow one of three patterns:

Immediate Transient Type

Occurrence: slight exposure to ultraviolet light (sunlight erythema) and type I hypersensitivity.

This permeability pattern persists only briefly, lasting a maximum of 1 hour (▶ B1), and occurs in the postcapillary venules. It is primarily regulated by cell-derived inflammation mediators (▶ C). Like histamine (p. 202), these mediators are already present in active form in mobile connective-tissue cells such as mast cells (p. 200) and basophilic granulocytes. They take effect immediately upon being released.

Result: Endothelial contraction (▶ A1).

Delayed Persistent Type

Occurrence: sunburn and type IV hypersensitivity.

This permeability pattern is delayed several hours in its onset, persists for of hours (▶ B2), occurs primarily in the capillaries and venules, and is regulated by plasma-derived mediators (p. 202) what follows is the activation of a complement system and if arachidonate cascade, generating eicosanoids (▶ C).

Result: Contraction and subsequent endothelial damage (▶ A2).

Immediate Persistent Type

Occurrence: trauma (lacerating crush injuries), burns (p. 146), and chemical injuries.

This permeability pattern occurs without any mediation from inflammation mediators (▶ C) within minutes following massive tissue injury (▶ B3). It occurs in the endothelial cells of the microvasculature (capillaries and venules) and lasts for several days.

Result: Endothelial and vascular necrosis (▶ A3) with serum leakage. This leakage is later sealed by intravascular blood coagulation and endothelial proliferation.

Endothelial damage leading to vascular permeability

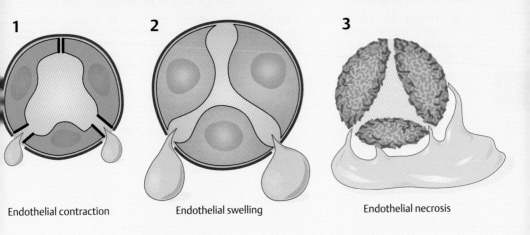

1 Endothelial contraction **2** Endothelial swelling **3** Endothelial necrosis

Types of changes in permeability

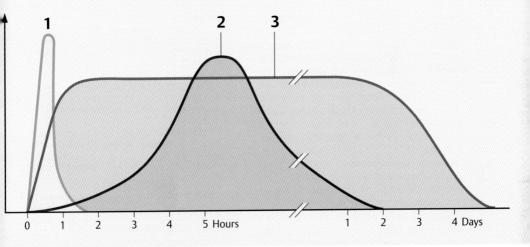

Mediators of permeability changes

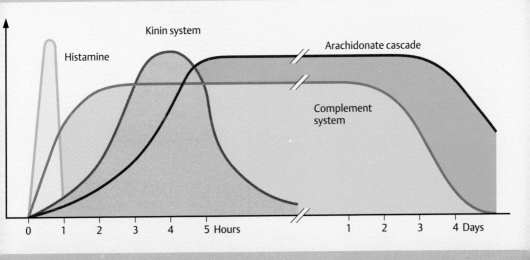

Leukocyte Transmigration

Biologic purpose: The leucocytes traveling into the inflamed regions, exiting the blood via the vascular wall, must construct a temporary and efficient "defensive system".

Pathogenetic principle: Under the influence of particular signal substances, the circulating leucocytes are "arrested" at the inflammatory site and then "lured" into the damaged area. This process takes the following steps:

— *Leukocyte margination:* The inactive sperical granulocytes normally travel in the axial current of a vessel. In the second phase of microcirculation changes, a few minutes after inflammation onset, mediators such as histamine, PAF, TNF-α, IL-1, and C5a induce the expression of "semi-stick" adhesion molecules (first P-selectin, later E-, L-selectin) on the endothelial surface, and trigger their "initial adhesion" onto the endothelium. The increased perfusion in this phase, however, tears them loose, causing them to roll along the endothelial surface like stones along a river bed (► A, B).

— *Leukocyte adhesion:* Thirty minutes later, the granulocytes are activated and assume the shape of fried eggs (► C, D). The same cytokines TNF-α and IL-1 stimulate the endothelia to express "sticky" adhesion molecules such as ICAM-1 (**i**ntercellular **a**dhesion **mo**lecule) on their surface. They cause the granulocytes to firmly adhere to the endothelial surface ("stable adhesion").

— *Leukocyte transmigration:* The granulocytes are attracted along a concentration gradient into the inflamed region by endo- and/or exogenous factors. To the former belong distinct bacterial products (N-formyl peptide). To the latter belong complement factors (C5a), eicosanoids (leucotrienes) and cytokines (chemokines). By binding on endothelial ICAM-1 and PECAM-1 (**p**latelet **e**ndothelial **c**ell **a**dhesion **mo**lecules), the granulocytes trigger focal contraction of endothelial (► E). They create gaps in their surface through which the granulocytes slip like amebas and, dissolving the subendothelial basement membrane, they migrate (► F) toward the source of chemoattractant factors. Once there, they are prevented from escaping by migration-inhibiting factors.

Biologic Role of Inflammatory Cells

Endothelial cells, which may be thought of as "border guards", are proinflammatory cells that generate selectins, which cause adhesion of lymphocytes and granulocytes, and a factor VIII activator, which activates the complement and kinin cascade (p. 202) that increases permeability. "

Thrombocytes may be thought of as "dike builders," leading to platelet thrombi; they are proinflammatory cells that generate inflammation mediators (see below) and platelet-derived growth factor (PDGF), which stimulates fibroblasts, smooth muscle cells, and endothelial cells.

Neutrophils, which may be thought of as "micro-macrophages", generate several substances:
— Lysozyme, an unspecific germicide;
— Tissue catabolizing enzymes for "waste removal";
— NO synthase, which in turn produces nitrous oxide and peroxy nitrile, a bactericide;
— The NADPH oxidase system, which uses myeloperoxidase to produce oxygen metabolites, in turn producing HOCl, a bactericide (p. 26);

Macrophages have a long life span and can proliferate in the inflamed region. They may be thought of as large "devouting cells" and antigen presenters for T lymphocytes. They generate several substances:
— Tissue catabolizing enzymes for "waste removal";
— The NADPH oxidase system, which uses myeloperoxidase to produce oxygen metabolites, in turn producing HOCl, a bactericide (p. 26);
— NO synthase, which in turn produces nitrous oxide and peroxy nitrile, a bactericide;
— Macrophage-derived growth factor (MDGF) for fibroblasts;
— Chemotactic factors, which attract neutrophils;
— Activating cytokines for lymphocytes and granulocytes;
— Arachidonate derivatives (see below), which cause inflammation.

Eosinophils may be thought of as the mast cells' "foremen" and parasite killers; they accumulate in bacteria-infested mucous membranes. Via their receptors, they react to IgG, IgA, complement factors, and PAF (see below). They generate cytotoxic and antimicrobial oxygen metabolites. The contents of their granulae destroy parasites.

Mast cells and basophils may be thought of as "water cannons." They have granulae containing heparin, histamine (which increases permeability), substances that attract eosinophils and neutrophils, and substances that cause platelet aggregation.

Lymphocytes and plasma cells maintain the cellular and humoral immune system in the inflamed area (p. 158, 160).

Leukocyte margination

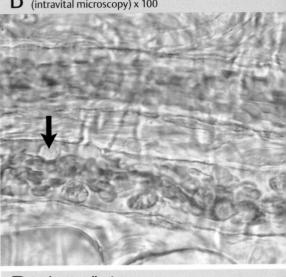

B Leukocyte margination
(intravital microscopy) x 100

Leukocyte adhesion

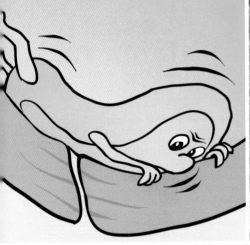

D Leukocyte adhesion
(HE) x 100

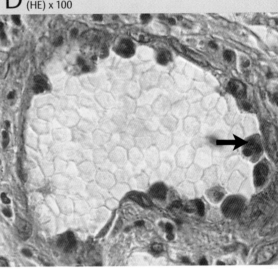

Leukocyte transmigration

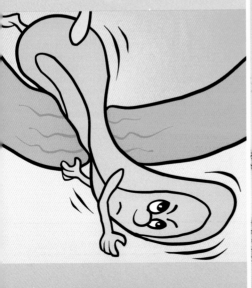

F Leukocyte transmigration
(TEM) x 5000

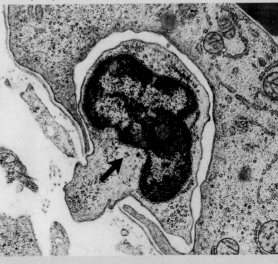

Inflammation Mediators

General definition: Chemical substances that trigger certain processes in an inflammatory reaction.

In an uncomplicated inflammation, these substances mutually activate each other so that individual steps in an inflammation combine to form a coordinated defensive reaction (▶ A). They may be derived from dead tissue (as are kinins) or be formed by living tissue. The following classes of mediators are differentiated according to their origin:
— necrosis-derived mediators (see kinins);
— cell-derived mediators;
— plasma-derived mediators.

■ Cell-Derived Mediators

Definition: These are either mediators stored in certain cells that release them in activated form, or mediators synthesized *ad hoc* by cells.

Histamine is stored in the granulae of mast cells and basophils. It plays a key role in allergic forms of inflammation. Histamine may be released by
— *Antigen–antibody complexes,* and requires prior sensitization of the cells by membrane-bound IgM molecules, or by
— *Direct cell injury* (also in the process of complement activation). Its effects include:
   – Contraction of smooth musculature (blood vessels, bowel, and bronchioles);
   – Dilation of arterioles, and later venules as well;
   – Immediate transient increase in vascular permeability;
   – Pruritus (itching);
   – Eosinophil chemotaxis.

Serotonin comes from the enterochromaffin cells of the small bowel and from thrombocytes. Its effects are similar to those of histamine and lead to increased vascular permeability.

Neutrophilic proteases destroy proteins and cell membranes and are responsible for proteolytic activation of the complement, coagulation, and kinin cascade (see below).

Interleukins (known as IL or lymphokines) control several functions of inflammatory cells:
— Destruction of target cells;
— Proliferation of inflammatory cells;
— Modulation of inflammation (IL-1 and TNF-α).

Interleukin-1 (IL-1) from macrophages activates the arachidonate cascade, forms platelet activating factor (PAF), and activates the kinin system.

Tumor necrosis factor (TNF-α) from macrophages activates granulocytes. This triggers generation of cytotoxic antimicrobial O_2 and N_2 compounds and generation of prostaglandins and leukotrienes.

Chemokines: These, formed by macrophages, lymphocytes, and endothelial cells, represent a "superfamily" of smaller proteins of similar structure. They can chemotactically attract and chemokinetically activate various types of leucocytes. The chemokines trigger the cell's answer by binding onto certain receptors on the target cells (CXC-R and CC-R) as mediated by the G-proteins. Certain viruses such as HIV use chemokine receptors as co-receptors.

Arachidonic acid derivatives: Every cell injury activates phospholipase A_2, resulting in the formation of 20-carbon polyunsaturated fatty acids such as arachidonic acid. This acid is metabolized in two ways.
— Lipoxygenase breaks it to down into *leukotrienes* (LT).
— Cyclooxygenase breaks it down into *prostaglandins* (found in almost all cells) in a process that can be inhibited by nonsteroidal antiinflammatory agents. Prostacyclins are formed in the capillary endothelia and vascular walls, and thromboxane is formed in thrombocytes.

Effects of prostaglandins include:
— Generalized vasodilatation;
— Sensitization of pain receptors;
— Increase in body temperature (fever).

Effects of leukotrienes include:
— Chemotaxis and chemokinesis for neutrophilic and eosinophilic granulocytes;
— Vasoconstriction;
— Bronchoconstriction.

Platelet activating factor (PAF): A phospholipid catalyzed by phospholipase A_2 that is formed by thrombocytes, granulocytes, macrophages, and endothelial cells. Its effects include:
— Increasing vascular permeability;
— Platelet aggregation;
— Bronchoconstriction.

■ Plasma-Derived Mediators

Definition: Some of these mediators are synthesized as inactive precursors. Before they go into action in the inflammation process, they must be activated by enzymes or combined to form active complexes.

Kinin system (activated by necrosis): The cascade-like kinin system is based on a series of plasma proteins formed in the liver as inactive preliminary stages in the form of high milecular kininogen (= HMWK). Prekallikrein is converted into the active specific protease kallikrein (serine protease) under the influence of avtivated clotting factor XII. The kallikrein in turn converts the HMWK-kininogens proteolytically into vasoactive peptide bradykinin. Bradykinin and the other kinins are short-lived because they are quickly inactivated by kinases. Effects of the kinin system include:
— vasodilatation, causing a drop in blood pressure;
— bronchoconstriction and bowel spasms;
— increased permeability;
— activation of pain receptors.

Complement system (p. 162):

C-reactive protein (CRP): Hepatocytes form this substance as an unspecific response by the body to inflammatory processes, necrosis, and cancer (acute phase reaction). CRP is related in its molecular structure to serum amyloid P component. Its effects include:
— activation of the complement system;
— opsonization to facilitate phagocytosis;
— activation of killer lymphocytes;
— formation of thromboxane, causing platelet aggregation.

> **Note:** Side effects of nonsteroidal antiinflammatory agents include peptic ulcer and analgesic nephropathy (from overuse).

The next section examines acute inflammatory reactions according to the specific mechanisms they involve.

A Activation cascades of the various inflammation mediators
(mediator activation is terminated by a control loop mechanism)

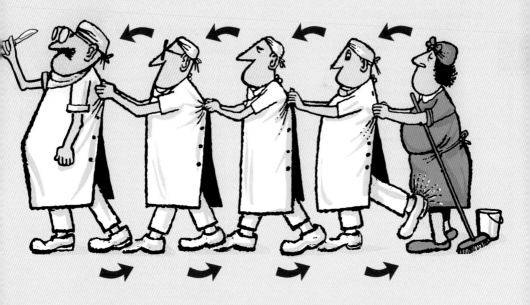

B Pathogenetic types of inflammtory mediators

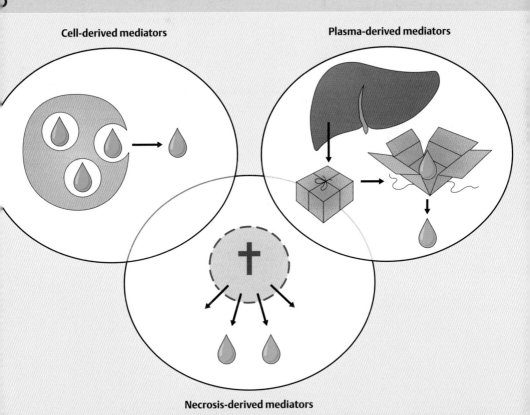

Cell-derived mediators

Plasma-derived mediators

Necrosis-derived mediators

Acute Exudative Inflammations

General definition: Acute inflammations whose principal histologic findings include exudation of blood serum and extravasation of blood cells into the inflamed area.

Acute inflammations may be classified as follows according to the principal components of the exudate:
— serous inflammation;
— seromucous inflammation;
— fibrinous inflammation;
— fibrinous suppurative or fibrinous purulent inflammation;
— suppurative or purulent inflammation;
— hemorrhagic inflammation.

Serous Inflammation

Definition: Acute inflammation with exudate of fibrin-free serum (▶ A).

Biologic purpose: Immediate dilution of the noxious agent at the site of inflammation.

Etiologic factors include:
— hypersensitivity reactions;
— bacterial and viral tissue injury;
— physical and chemical tissue injury.

Morphology (according to tissue):
— *Serosa:* Erythema (hyperemia) and inflammatory swelling from effusion with large numbers of displaced serosal covering cells and few macrophages in the exudate.
— *Skin:* Erythema and swelling that varies according to epidermal involvement.
  — Wheals (urticaria) form where there is isolated exudation without epidermal damage. Here the exudate takes the form of an effusion.
  — Vesicles form where the exudation occurs from dermal capillaries with epidermal injury. This causes separation of the epidermis. Here the exudate is the contents of the vesicle.
— *Mucous membrane:* Erythema and swelling lead to mucosal edema with risk of stenosis.
— *Parenchyma:* Erythema and swelling are present with sparse leukocytic infiltrate. This expands the organ capsule, which is tender to palpation due to its sensory innervation. Here the exudate takes the form of an edema.

Examples:
— *Initial transitory stage* preceding other forms of inflammation, collateral inflammation surrounding a focal inflammation of another type.
— *Inflammation of serous membranes* such as the pleura, pericardium, peritoneum, and joints.
— *Organ inflammation* such as serous hepatitis, nephritis (acute interstitial nephritis), myocarditis, encephalitis. Serous alveolitis (exudative pulmonary alveolitis) leads to toxic pulmonary edema with exudation into the interstitium of the alveolar wall, causing expansion of the alveolar wall (▶ C, D) and impairing diffusion (p. 40).

— *Vesicular skin infections.*
— *Serous mucosal inflammations* can lead to acute glottal and laryngeal edema (▶ B) with risk of asphyxia.

Seromucous Inflammation

Definition: Acute inflammation occurring exclusively on the mucous membranes of the respiratory and gastrointestinal tracts and producing a watery exudate of serum and mucus (▶ E).

Etiologic factors include:
— Hypersensitivity reactions;
— Bacterial and viral tissue injury;
— Physical and chemical tissue injury.

Morphology: The mucosa and submucosa appear reddened and swollen, with a slight degree of lymphocytic infiltration. Part of the surface epithelium may die, and epithelial tissue may be sloughed off. As a result, the mucous exudate may contain epithelial cells.

Examples:
— Acute rhinitis (common cold);
— Acute catarrhal bronchitis;
— Enteritis.

Associated Disorder

▬ Acute Rhinitis

Synonym: common cold.

Definition: Viral serous catarrhal inflammation of the nasal mucosa.

Pathogenesis and morphology: The disorder is caused by droplet infection by rhinoviruses (p. 240). The viruses penetrate the epithelium of the upper respiratory tract, triggering inflammation with hyperemia of the mucous membrane and serous exudation. This leads to obstruction of the nasal passage, creating optimum conditions for proliferation of the virus. The cytopathic effect of the viruses (lytic infection) leads to epithelial necrosis, which in turn releases viruses. Inflammatory irritation of the mucous glands and goblet cell hyperplasia (▶ F) cause the hypersecretion of mucus typical of a "runny nose", sign of serous catarrhal inflammation. This triggers the sneezing reflex. Sneezing both releases pathogen and exudate and completes the cycle of droplet infection by which the virus spreads.

> **Note:** Complications of a cold include bacterial superinfection progressing to purulent catarrhal inflammation (with yellowish-green mucus) due to an epithelial defect.

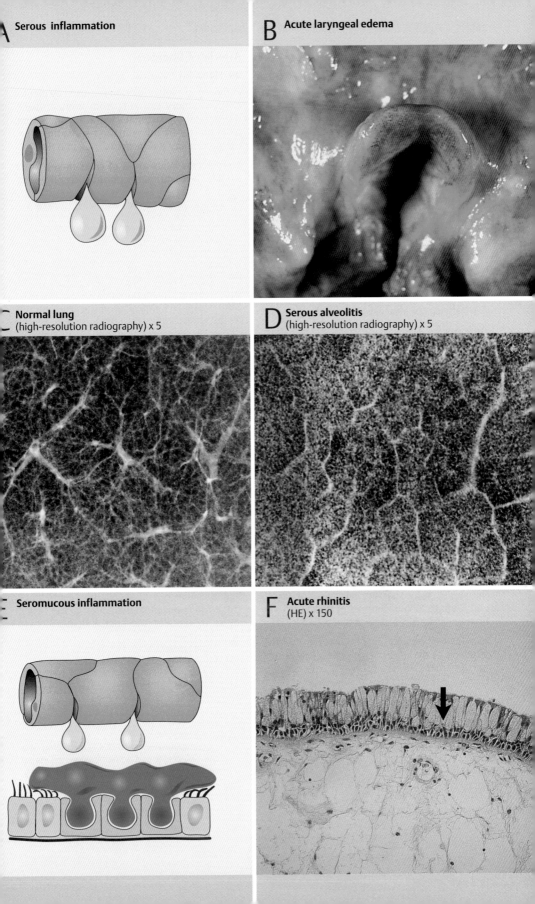

A Serous inflammation

B Acute laryngeal edema

C Normal lung
(high-resolution radiography) x 5

D Serous alveolitis
(high-resolution radiography) x 5

E Seromucous inflammation

F Acute rhinitis
(HE) x 150

Fibrinous Inflammation

Definition: Acute inflammation with exudation of fibrinogen-containing serum that polymerizes to fibrin outside the blood vessels (▶ A, B). Here the exudate takes the form of serum-containing fibrinogen.

Biologic purpose: Immediate temporary barrier against additional effects of inflammation.

Etiologic factors include:
- Infectious toxic tissue injury;
- Tissue injury from physical trauma;
- Chemical and toxic tissue injury;
- Excretion of toxic metabolites (uremic toxins);
- Ischemic tissue injury.

Fibrinous Parenchymal Inflammation

Definition: Acute inflammation with exudation of fibrin on the inner surfaces of the pulmonary parenchyma (pulmonary alveoli).

Pathogenesis: This usually occurs as a transitory stage following infectious toxic injury (lobar pneumonia) or radiation injury (radiation pneumonitis) of the pulmonary microvasculature with diffuse exudation of fibrin on the surface of the alveoli (croupous inflammation).

Examples include
- *Lobar pneumonia* in the gray hepatization stage (p. 210) and
- *Radiation pneumonitis.*

Fibrinous Serosal Inflammation

Definition: Acute fibrinous inflammations of the serous membranes may occur as a reaction of the serosa to other underlying disorders (serositis) or in the presence of tissue injury occurring in the serosa (such as infarction).

Macroscopically, the serosa will only appear dull where slight amounts of fibrin are present (as in the pleura; ▶ E); massive exudation of serum will produce villous deposits of fibrin (as in fibrinous pericarditis or "hairy heart"; ▶ C, D).

Microscopic findings include widespread destruction of the mesothelial cells at the site of the fibrin deposits. The submesothelial connective tissue is covered by a felt-like layer of fibrin of varying thickness, which with time becomes homogenized (▶ F). Later the fibrin deposits are absorbed by histiocytes and transformed into scar tissue, creating adhesions between the layers of the serosa.

Associated Disorders

▬ Fibrinous Pleuritis

Pathogenesis: Inflammation is caused by pleural capillary injury resulting from uremic toxins, direct viral or bacterial pleural inflammation, or indirectly by inflammation spreading from the pulmonary parenchyma (pneumonia).

Morphology: Wide areas of cross-linked fibrin exudate (▶ E), primarily on the visceral pleura.

✚ **Clinical presentation:** *Auscultatory findings* include sounds of pleural friction resembling creaking leather. Respiratory excursion is painful. *Late sequelae* include pleural adhesions, leading to impairment of pulmonary expansion and dyspnea.

▬ Fibrinous Pericarditis

Pathogenesis: Inflammation is caused by pericardial capillary injury resulting from uremic toxins, direct viral or bacterial pleural inflammation, or iatrogenic alteration (heart surgery).

Morphology: Wide areas of cross-linked fibrin exudate (▶ C, D), primarily on the epicardium later lead to adhesions between the pericardium and epicardium that interfere with ventricular contraction.

✚ **Clinical presentation:** *Auscultatory findings* include sounds of pericardial friction resembling creaking leather. Patients report chest pain, and the heart is enlarged.

▬ Fibrinous Peritonitis

Pathogenesis: Inflammation is caused by peritoneal capillary injury resulting from uremic toxins, direct (iatrogenic) or bacterial peritoneal inflammation.

Morphology: Wide areas of cross-linked fibrin exudate, primarily on the visceral peritoneum, lead to adhesions between the bowel loops. These can result in strangulation of the bowel, impairing motility (mechanical ileus).

✚ **Clinical presentation:** *Percutaneous findings* include pain upon palpation. Spontaneous abdomen pain can be partially alleviated when the patient assumes a lateral fetal position.

⚠ **Note:** *Membrane – Pseudomembrane:*
- Membrane: It is an existing physiologic sheet of tissue;
- Pseudomembrane: It is a skin-like covering of a tissue defect (see pseudomembranous inflammation, p. 208).

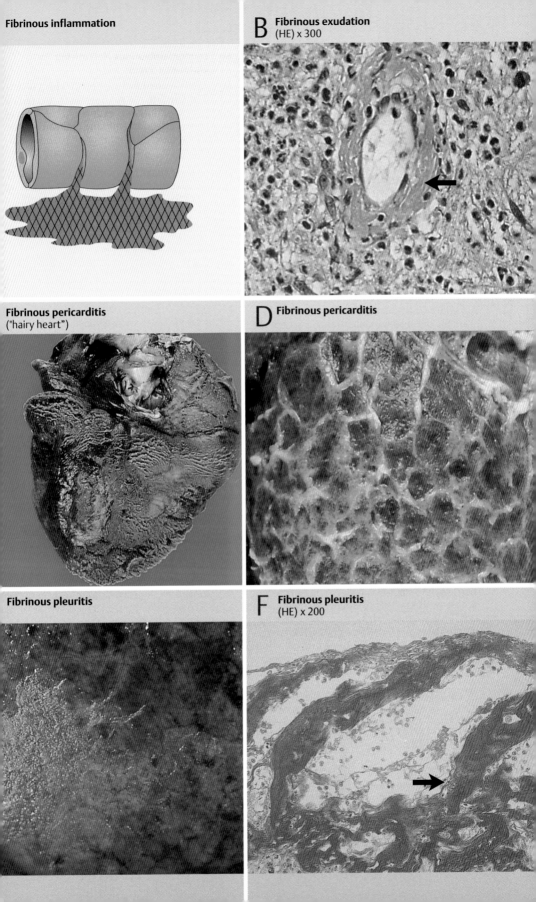

Fibrinous inflammation

B Fibrinous exudation
(HE) x 300

Fibrinous pericarditis
("hairy heart")

D Fibrinous pericarditis

Fibrinous pleuritis

F Fibrinous pleuritis
(HE) x 200

Fibrinous Mucosal Inflammation

General pathogenesis: In fibrinous inflammations in the mucosa, the fibrinous exudation process is usually preceded by superficial necrosis.

Several forms are differentiated based on the relation of fibrin exudation and necrosis.

■ Pseudomembranous Croupous Form (Influenza Type)

Definition: Acute inflammation in which a wide area of fibrinous exudate forms an easily removable pseudomembrane covering the necrosis, which is limited to the mucosal epithelium (► A, B1).

Pathogenetic chain reaction: The inflammatory necrosis only involves part of the mucosa; islands of epithelium remain unaffected (► B2). The submucosal vascular structures become abnormally permeable while the structure of the submucosa remains largely intact. This leads to exudation of fibrin on the surface of the mucosa and formation of a pseudomembrane (► B1) as protection against infection.

Examples:
— Influenzal tracheobronchitis (► B)
— Amebic dysentery (p. 276)
— Ischemic pseudomembranous colitis.

Associated Disorder

▒ Influenzal Tracheobronchitis

Definition: Febrile inflammation of the trachea and bronchi caused by viral infection and producing a fibrinous pseudomembrane.

Pathogenesis and morphology: Infection with type A influenza virus (p. 242) causes viral epithelial injury with an intact mucosa. Initially there is only hyperemia and serous (lymphocytic and plasmacytic) inflammation of the mucosa. This is followed by a wide area of fibrinous exudate on the basement membrane of the largely de-epithelialized mucosa. This leads to formation of a grayish-white diphtheroid pseudomembrane that can be easily removed without bleeding (► C).

✚ **Clinical presentation:** Croup is an inflammatory stenosis of the larynx with shortness of breath, a whistling sound during inspiration (stridor) and a barking cough. Complications include bacterial superinfection.

❗ **Note:** There are several forms of croup:
- *Genuine croup* is croup in laryngeal diphtheria.
- *Pseudocroup* involves croup syndrome in
  - *Infections* (influenza, measles, and Staphylococcus or Haemophilus influenza) or
  - *Allergies*, which lead to spasmodic croup.

■ Pseudomembranous Necrotizing Form (Diphtheria Type)

Definition: Acute inflammation in which necrosis extending into the submucosa is covered by a wide area of fibrinous exudate in the form of an adhesive pseudomembrane that can only be forcibly removed (diphtheric pseudomembrane).

Pathogenetic chain reaction: The inflammatory necrosis extends to the submucosa, causing erosion of the submucosal vessels and resulting in the escape of fibrinous exudate over a wide area. The exudate spreads over the surface of the mucosa, forming a diphtheric pseudomembrane with root-like adhesions in vascular branches of the submucosal tissue (► D). This causes bleeding when the pseudomembrane is forcibly removed.

Examples:
— Diphtheric laryngotracheitis (diphtheria, p. 256)
— Antibiotic enterocolitis

Associated Disorders

▒ Diphtheric Laryngotracheitis

Pathogenesis: Infection with corynebacteria (p. 256) causes tracheal diphtheria.

✚ **Clinical presentation:** Croup (genuine croup) is present with neuritis of the cranial nerves. This leads to aphonia (loss of voice) and development of a pseudomembrane. Risk of asphyxiation is present, and emergency tracheotomy may be indicated.

☺ **Prominent patient:** Medical Professor M. Wilms, who first described the Wilms tumor, died in 1918 of diphtheria contracted while performing an emergency tracheotomy on a French prisoner of war. The patient survived.

▒ Antibiotic associated Enterocolitis

Definition: Infectious toxic inflammation of the large bowel (and often the small bowel as well) during antibiotic therapy.

Pathogenesis and morphology: Antibiotic therapy suppresses normal intestinal organisms, creating a selective advantage for organisms such as Clostridium difficile. Clostridia release enterotoxin that destroys the epithelium of the crypts, causing neutrophils to accumulate therein. This results in crypt abscesses. Necrosis then spreads to the intestinal mucosa, resulting in fibrin permeation and demarcation by leukocytes. The eroded mucosa is then covered by a whitish pseudomembrane (► E) of fibrin and detritus.

✚ **Clinical presentation:** Patients present with bloody diarrhea.

Diphtheroid pseudomembrane

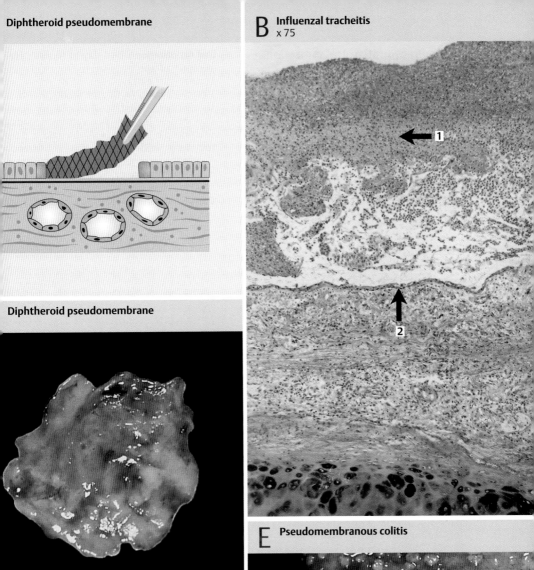

B **Influenzal tracheitis**
x 75

Diphtheroid pseudomembrane

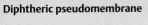

Diphtheric pseudomembrane

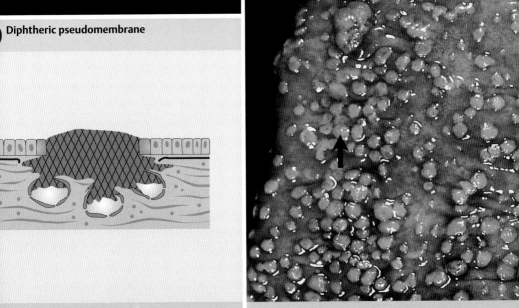

E **Pseudomembranous colitis**

Fibrinous Suppurative Inflammation

Definition: Acute inflammation with copious fibrin exudate and neutrophilic leukotaxis.

Associated Disorder

■ **Lobar Pneumonia**

Text book exampel of a disease exhibiting every phases of an exudative inflammatory reaction.

Definition: An inflammation with sudden onset that rapidly involves an entire pulmonary lobe (rarely several lobes). Left untreated, it progresses through several stages.

Etiologic factors include:
— *Streptococcus pneumoniae* type I (90 % of all cases);
— *Klebsiella* (5 % of all cases).

Predisposing factors include: .
— protein-rich pulmonary edema (heart failure);
— compromised immune system (alcoholics and neonates).

Pathogenesis: Lobar pneumonia develops in several stages:
— **"Surprise" phase:**
   The pathogens encounter a patient with insufficient immune protection and release toxins. This causes changes in vascular permeability with generalized vasodilatation in the microvasculature. These changes cause hyperemia with a serous exudative inflammatory reaction in the alveoli, producing optimum growth conditions for the pathogens. The ensuing damage to the alveolar epithelium prevents production of surfactant, which causes the interalveolar pores of Kohn to open. The inflammation is thus able to spread rapidly throughout an entire pulmonary lobe.
— **"Combat" phase:**
   The increasing effect of the toxin damages the microvasculature, causing fibrinous inflammation. The fibrinous exudate fixes the pathogens.
— **"Conquering" phase:**
   In the interim, the immune system has learned to produce specific antibodies against pneumococci. This means that pathogens can be marked for phagocytosis by macrophages (opsonization; p. 26). The macrophages release chemokinetic substances that attract neutrophils, resulting in a suppurative inflammation in which the pathogens are destroyed and the exudate is dissolved.

Morphology of lobar pneumonia:
— **Initial congestion** (first to second day of illness): Hyperemic alveolar vessels produce a protein-rich exudate that is released into the alveolar lumen and contains hardly any neutrophils (serous inflammation).
   Macroscopic findings include a dark red, fluid-filled soft lung.

— **Red hepatization** (third day of illness): Hyperemia of the alveolar microvasculature occurs with extravasation of blood serum into the alveoli (► B) and production of a serofibrinous exudate. Auscultatory findings include high-pitched rattling sounds.
   Macroscopic findings (► A) include a dark red lung with a liver-like consistency (hence the term "hepatization"). Percussion is without resonance. Auscultatory findings include sounds resembling rubbing leather.
— **Gray hepatization** (fourth to fifth day of illness): Massive fibrinous exudation into the alveolar lumen is present, and macrophages and neutrophils are found in the inflamed area. The alveoli are lined with fibrinous lattices (► D1), and fibrin passes through open pores of Kohn into the adjacent alveoli.
   Macroscopic findings include a gray nodular appearance of the cut surface of the lung, which has the consistency of liver (► C).
— **Yellow hepatization** (seventh day of illness): A massive suppurative inflammatory reaction is present with large numbers of neutrophils (see below; ► F). The exudate is dissolved by proteolysis, with resulting destruction of cells and tissue. Detritus forms and microcirculation returns to near normal.
   Macroscopic findings include a dirty yellow appearance of the cut surface of the lung, which still has a firm consistency (► E).
— **Resolution** (between the seventh and ninth days of illness): This involves massive fibrinolytic dissolution of the exudate by macrophages and neutrophils. The alveoli are cleared, and the patient either coughs up the dissolved exudate in the form of rust brown sputum or it is absorbed through the lymph system. The alveoli expand again. Auscultatory findings include the crackling sounds of expanding alveoli.

✚ **Complications:**
– *Chronic pneumonia:* The exudate cannot be dissolved and is organized by granulation tissue, producing a flesh-like cut surface (organizing pneumonia).
– *Pulmonary abscess:* The exudation process is superseded by necrosis, resulting in tissue liquefaction.
– *Pleural empyema* may occur following erosion of an abscess.

☺ **Prominent patient:** Franz Liszt (1811–1886), Hungarian composer, conductor and pianist.

❗ **Note:** Lobar pneumonia is simultaneous inflammation of one lobe; bronchopneumonia involves inflammatory foci of varying stages in one or more lobes.

Red hepatization (lung)

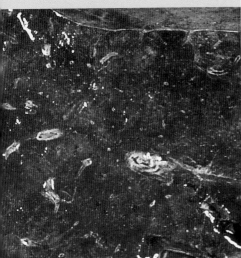

B **Red hepatization**
(HE) x 75

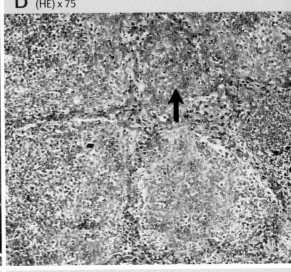

Gray hepatization (lung)

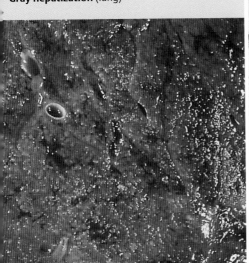

D **Gray hepatization**
x 150

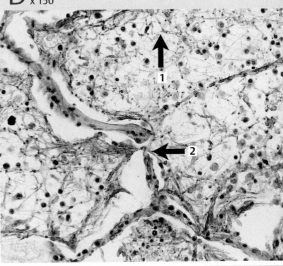

Yellow hepatization (lung)

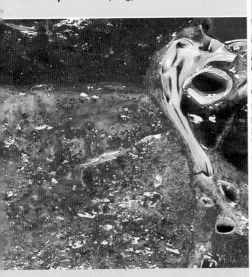

F **Yellow hepatization**
x 150

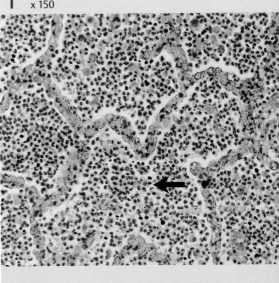

Suppurative Inflammation

Synonym: purulent inflammation.

General definition: Inflammation with exudate consisting primarily of neutrophils and cellular debris (detritus).

Biologic purpose: Damaged tissue is dissolved along with the pathogen. This clears the way for repair.

Etiologic factors usually include pyogenic pathogens such as
— *Staphylococci* (p. 254), which produce thick yellowish pus that leads to abscess-forming inflammation, and
— *Streptococci* (p. 254), which produce yellowish fluid fibrin-free pus that usually leads to suppurative inflammation.

The *general morphology* of a suppurative inflammation typically involves several layers:
— A *necrotic zone* is a central focus of proteolytic liquefaction with lipid-rich detritus producing yellowish pus.
— A *pus zone* contains large numbers of neutrophils and surrounds the central necrotic area.
— A *hyperemic zone* with perifocal edema of serous exudate is also present.

Mucopurulent Inflammation

Definition: Acute inflammation of a mucous membrane with exudate of mucus, granulocytes, and cellular detritus (▶ A).

Examples (usually secondary to viral infection) include purulent catarrhal rhinitis (p. 204) and purulent catarrhal tracheobronchitis (▶ B).

Empyema

Definition: Suppurative inflammation in a body cavity.

Pathogenesis: An empyema usually occurs where a suppurative inflammation of an organ breaks through into an adjacent cavity.

Examples:
— Pericardial, peritoneal, and pleural empyema (▶ C);
— Gallbladder and appendiceal empyema;
— Middle ear and nasal sinus empyema;
— Pyosalpinx (pus in the uterine tube);
— Pyocephalus (pus in the cranial vault);
— Hypopyon (pus in the anterior chamber of the eye).

Phlegmon

Definition: Diffuse suppurative inflammation without tissue liquefaction that spreads primarily in loose fibrous connective tissue.

Pathogenetic chain reaction: Infection (usually by streptococci) results in the release of hyaluronidase and fibrinolysin by the pathogens. This destroys the germ barrier of fibrin exudate, hyaluronates, and proteoglycans, allowing the inflammation to spread rapidly with negligible pus formation. The exudate primarily consists of granulocytes and proteolytic serum components.

Examples:
— Erysipelas, inflammation in the connective tissue of the skin usually caused by β-hemolytic streptococci (rarely anthrax bacilli) involving a map-like pattern of erythema and swelling (▶ D);
— Muscular phlegmon;
— Phlegmon of the floor of the mouth;
— Mediastinal phlegmon;
— Phlegmon of the walls of hollow organs (such as phlegmon in cholecystitis, appendicitis).

Abscess-Forming Inflammation

Definition: An abscess is an accumulation of pus from tissue destruction.

Pathogenetic chain reaction: Direct infection (primarily by *Staphylococcus aureus*) triggers an inflammatory reaction accompanied by focal circulatory disruption that produces necrosis. Staphylococci emit substances that attract granulocytes (chemokines), resulting in granulocytic and proteolytic dissolving of tissue (▶ E) into bacteria-containing pus. Later the granulocytes and histiocytes sequester the site, forming an abscess membrane (p. 226). This creates a cavity that remains after the abscess drains.

Examples:
— *Pulmonary abscesses* occur after pulmonary infarction or lobar pneumonia; sepsis (p. 222) produces hematogenous abscesses.
— *Cerebral abscesses* occur following open cranial and cerebral trauma. Such abscesses may also spread from a suppurative facial or cranial inflammation; sepsis produces hematogenous abscesses.
— *Kidney abscesses* may spread from purulent pyelonephritis (▶ E); sepsis produces hematogenous abscesses.
— *Liver abscesses* may spread from a suppurative inflammation in the region drained by the portal vein, such as amebic dysentery (p. 276). It may also spread from suppurative cholangitis; sepsis produces hematogenous abscesses.
— *Septicopyemic abscesses* occur focally in the subpleural lung, as medullary strip lesions in the kidney, as punctate subendocardial lesions in the heart, and as punctate subcapsular lesions in the liver.
— *Perityphlitic abscess* may occur in suppurative appendicitis.
— *Furuncles* are abscess-forming inflammations of the hair follicle usually following staphylococcal infection.

Note: Pus consists of phagocytizing neutrophils with cellular debris (detritus).

Mucopurulent inflammation

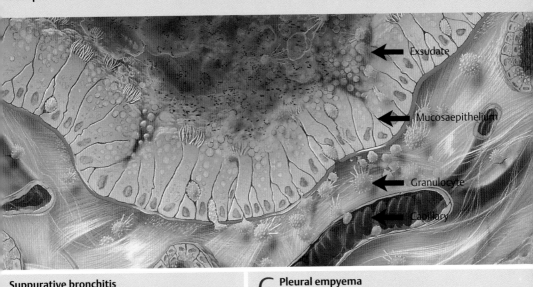

Exsudate

Mucosaepithelium

Granulocyte

Capillary

Suppurative bronchitis

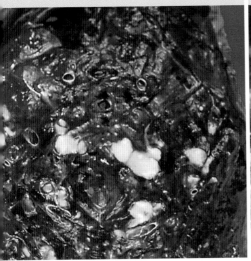

C Pleural empyema

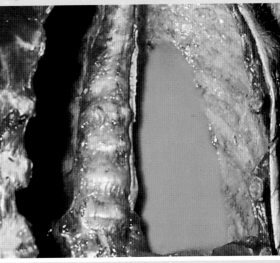

D Erysipelas of the neck

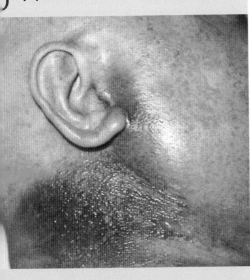

E Soft tissue abscess

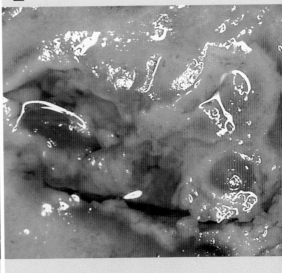

Associated Disorders

■ Appendicitis

Model disorder is which all the forms of suppurative inflammation occur sequentially as phases of the disease.

Definition: Isolated inflammation of the cecal vermiform appendix.

Pathogenetic chain reaction: Impaired motility and stool passage (due to coproliths, oxyuriasis, scarring, or hypertrophy of mucosa-associated lymphoid tissue or MALT) leads to injury of the wall of the bowel and colonization with intestinal flora (*Escherichia coli* and enterococci; p. 260).

Morphology: The inflammation progresses in several stages:

— *Erosive appendicitis* occurs within 6 hours and involves mucosal erosion in the crypts with wedge-shaped area of fibrinous suppurative inflammation (► A).
— *Phlegmon* occurs within 12 hours with transmural inflammation (► B).
— *Phlegmon with ulceration* occurs within 24 hours. The mucosal erosions enlarge into ulcers, leading to an ulcerous, necrotizing, suppurative inflammation of the bowel wall with increased risk of perforation. Where the bowel is obstructed, accumulation of pus leads to appendiceal empyema.
— *Abscess formation* occurs within 48 hours. Microabscesses form in the wall of the appendix. Fibrinous suppurative serositis leads to focal adhesions between the bowel loops interspersed with pockets of accumulated pus (empyema).
— *Gangrenous appendicitis* occurs within 72 hours. Tissue liquefaction leads to infestation with putrefactive bacteria (see below). This leads to perforation and peritonitis.

■ Acute Pyogenic Pyelonephritis

Definition: Acute abscess-forming inflammation of the renal interstitium, tubules, and, occasionally, the renal pelvis caused by bacterial infection.

Etiologic factors include pathogenic *E. coli,* primarily in the presence of a pre-existing metabolic condition such as diabetes mellitus, gout, or cortisone treatment.

Pathogenetic forms:

— *Ascending infection* involves impaired outflow of urine with ascending bacterial colonization through the lower urinary tract (acute recurrence is common). Coalescent clusters of focal inflammation the size of a pinhead are present with hemorrhagic halos. The cut surface exhibits radial strip-like focal abscesses (► C) in the medulla.

Histologic findings include abscess-forming strips of inflammation with destructive liquefaction of the interstitium and tubules (► D1), leading to masses of neutrophils within the lumen that form cylindrical castings (► D2). These leucocyte cylinders are present in urinary sediment.

— *Hematogenous infection* involves septicopyemic spread of bacteria (p. 222). The bacteria are intercepted in (a) the first capillary filter, the glomeruli, causing embolic suppurative focal glomerulitis and (b) the second capillary filter, the vasa recta, causing embolic suppurative medullary nephritis.

✚ **Complications:** The condition may recur and become chronic.
Chronic bacterial pyelonephritis:
Definition and pathogenesis: Bacteria and/or their components trigger inflammation of the renal interstitium with progressive, episodic parenchymal destruction.
Morphology: Large, flat, pale red vascularized scars lead to shrinkage of the kidney. *Histologic findings* include sclerotic glomeruli with thickened Tamm-Horsfall mucoprotein in distended tubules. This leads to histologic findings similar to colloid-filled follicles in a pseudogoiter.

■ Acute Pyogenic Meningitis

Synonym: purulent meningitis.

Definition: Suppurative inflammation of the central nervous system with focal manifestation in the meninges. This can spread to the substance of the brain, causing meningoencephalitis.

Pathogenetic forms:

— *Hematogenous bacterial form:* Infection with *Neisseria meningitidis* (p. 256) triggers suppurative inflammation in the subarachnoid space primarily through the convexities, producing a hood-like pattern of metastatic meningitis (► E). The inflammation spreads to adjacent brain tissue, resulting in metastatic focal encephalitis (see septicopyemic metastasis, p. 222).
— *Transmitted bacterial form:* Ear or nasal infections can produce a suppurative inflammation in the subarachnoid space of the base of the brain (► F).
— *Direct bacterial form:* this may occur secondary to penetrating craniocerebral trauma (p. 316).

❗ **Note:** Acute inflammatory reaction in physiologically avascular tissue (such as heart valves or cornea) involves proteolytic lesion of the extracellular matrix, precipitation of fibrin on the inflamed surface, and reactive capillary formation.

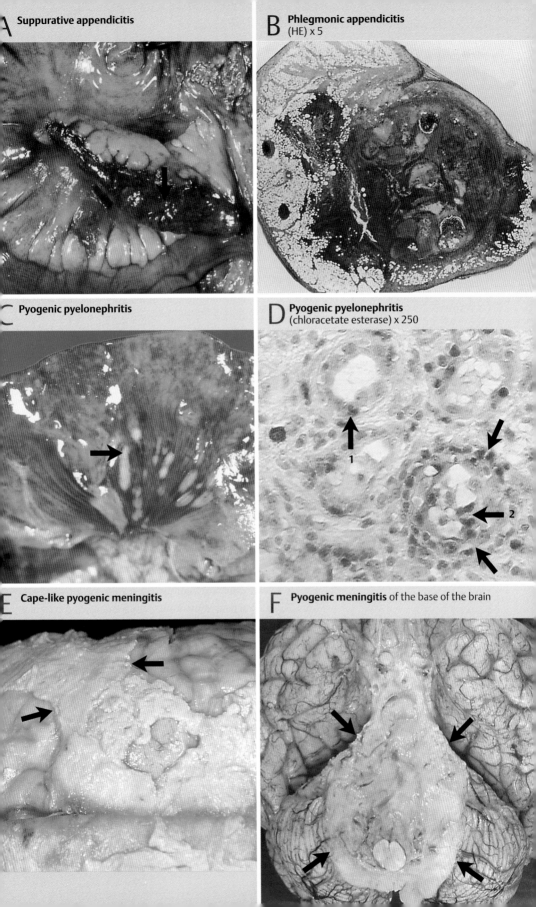

A Suppurative appendicitis

B Phlegmonic appendicitis
(HE) × 5

C Pyogenic pyelonephritis

D Pyogenic pyelonephritis
(chloracetate esterase) × 250

E Cape-like pyogenic meningitis

F Pyogenic meningitis of the base of the brain

Hemorrhagic Inflammation

Definition: Acute inflammation involving microvascular injury with massive microvascular bleeding, producing an exudate with a high erythrocyte content (▶ A).

Biologic purpose: Exudative inflammation despite severe vascular injury.

Morphology: The inflamed area is usually necrotic and filled with blood.

Etiologic factors include:
— bacterial exotoxins and endotoxins;
— viral cytopathic effect on endothelium;
— proteolytic tissue destruction;
— cytotoxic injury in hypersensitivity type III.

Associated Disorders

■ Scarlet Fever

Pathogenesis: β-hemolytic group A streptococci (p. 254) create erythrogenic toxins that damage capillary walls and cause hemolysis, producing patchy erythema of the skin (exanthema).

✚ **Clinical presentation:** This exanthematous disorder occurs in children.

■ Waterhouse-Friderichsen Syndrome

Pathogenesis: Sepsis with Neisseria meningitidis (p. 256) in children immediately inundates the blood with endotoxin that is toxic to endothelium. The resulting blood poisoning causes toxic microvascular injury.

✚ **Clinical sequelae:**
– *Petechial cutaneous hemorrhage.*
– *Disseminated intravascular coagulation* (p. 400) leads to profuse bleeding into tissue and diffuse cutaneous hemorrhage in the form of suggillations or ecchymoses (p. 398).
– *Bilateral hemorrhagic adrenal necrosis* (▶ B) leads to acute hypocorticism (Addison's crisis) with electrolyte imbalance and spontaneous hypoglycemia (p. 112).
– *Circulatory shock* (septic and endocrine; p. 392).
– *Symptoms* include vomiting, high fever, and meningism.

■ Plague

Textbook example of a highly infectious disease.

Pathogenesis: Infection with Yersinia pestis produces exotoxin leading to painful hemorrhagic lymphadenitis (bubonic plaque) in which mere traces of the lymph node structure remain, (▶ C) and hemorrhagic pneumonia (pneumonic plague).

■ Influenzal Pneumonia

Pathogenesis: Infection with influenza virus (p. 242) creates capillary defects, leading to hemorrhagic pneumonia with bleeding into the alveoli (▶ D).

■ Disorders Associated with Enterohemorrhagic E. Coli

Pathogenesis: Overuse of antibiotics in commercial pig raising leads to selection of resistant strains of *E. coli* (p. 260) that produce a toxin with neurotoxic, enterotoxic, and cytotoxic effects. This results in endothelial injury and microangiopathy.

✚ **Clinical sequelae:** *Hemorrhagic enterocolitis* occurs due to intestinal microangiopathy and enterocyte necrosis. *Hemolytic-uremic syndrome* occurs due to glomerular microangiopathy. The glomerular loops become congested with erythrocyte fragments, hemolysis, and microthrombi, leading to kidney failure.

■ Hemorrhagic Viral Urocystitis

Pathogenesis: Infection with BK viruses (especially in immunosuppressed patients; p. 250) causes diffuse mucosal bleeding (▶ E).

■ Anthrax

Pathogenesis: Infection with Bacillus anthracis (p. 258) produces exotoxins that are toxic to endothelia. This causes hemorrhagic inflammatory necrosis in the skin, bowel, and lungs.

■ Viral Hemorrhagic Fever

Pathogenesis: Infection with an arenavirus or togavirus spread by mosquitoes or ticks (p. 242).

■ Acute Pancreatitis

Etiology is unclear. Contributing factors include:
— alcohol abuse (p. 144);
— defective secretion (hypersecretion or accumulated secretions);
— biliary disorders.

Pathogenetic chain reaction: Focal cell necrosis occurring for unknown reasons leads to release and activation of autocatalytic proteases. This activates the kinin, complement, and coagulation systems (p. 202), whose interaction produces a serous inflammation (pancreatic edema). This leads to lipolytic necrosis in the intrapancreatic and peripancreatic fatty tissue (▶ F2; p. 132).

✚ **Clinical presentation:** Symptoms include painful acute abdomen and massively elevated serum amylase and lipase levels.

✚ **Complications** may occur if the inflammation fails to subside. These include
– *Proteolysis,* partial digestion of the walls of blood vessels in and around the pancreas with bleeding and thrombosis leading to tissue necrosis and hemorrhagic pancreatitis (▶ F1). This in turn leads to
– *Disseminated intravascular coagulation* (p. 400), which can progress to *circulatory shock* (p. 392).

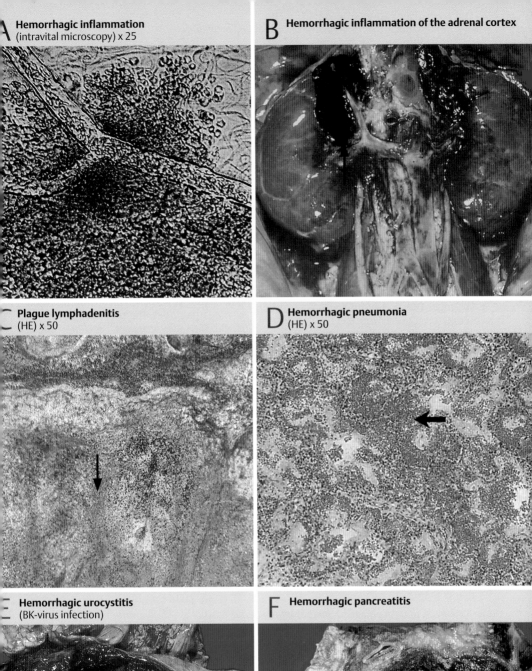

A Hemorrhagic inflammation
(intravital microscopy) x 25

B Hemorrhagic inflammation of the adrenal cortex

C Plague lymphadenitis
(HE) x 50

D Hemorrhagic pneumonia
(HE) x 50

E Hemorrhagic urocystitis
(BK-virus infection)

F Hemorrhagic pancreatitis

Special Forms of Acute Inflammation

Necrotizing Inflammation

Definition: Acute inflammation in which tissue necrosis predominates.

Several types are differentiated according to demarcation of the inflammation or infestation with putrefactive bacteria. These include:
— Ulcerous necrotizing type;
— Diffuse necrotizing type;
— Nonreactive necrotizing type;
— Gangrenous type.

Ulcerous Necrotizing Inflammation

Definition: Acute inflammation with focal necrosis extending into the submucosa or deeper and covered with fibrinous exudate (scab).

Pathogenesis: The ulcerous tissue defect may be caused by several mechanisms:
— Sloughing off of focal mucosal necroses in the gastrointestinal region;
— Sloughing off of diphtheroid pseudomembrane in the gastrointestinal region (prototype is typhoid fever; p. 260);
— Sloughing off of damaged oropharyngeal mucosa by vesicular separation, leaving a greasy grayish-white ulcer (aphtha).

Associated Disorders

■ Acute Necrotizing Ulcerous Gingivitis

Synonym: Vincent angina.

Definition: Destructive Ulcerous inflammation of the gingiva and tonsils caused by endogenous anaerobic bacteria.

Etiologic factors include a weakened immune system, leading to mixed infection with Borrelia vincenti and fusiform bacteria of the physiologic oral flora (► A2).

Morphology: A foul-smelling, crater-shaped ulcer (► A1) with a fibrin scab is present, containing fusiform bacteria (► A2). Tonsillar ulcers are usually unilateral.

■ Peptic Gastroduodenal Ulcer

Definition: Gastroduodenal inflammation caused by stomach acid and/or Helicobacter pylori (p. 262) that produces an ulcerous mucosal defect.

Etiologic factors include an imbalance between the aggressive and defensive factors in the mucosa.
— *Aggressive factors* include hydrochloric acid, pepsin, bile, duodenal reflux, salicylates, ischemia, and Helicobacter pylori.
— *Defensive factors* include the mucosal barrier due to regeneration, bicarbonates, and E prostaglandins (p. 202).

Pathogenesis: The locally uninhibited action of pepsin results in partial digestion of the gastro-duodenal mucosa, producing erosive inflammation. This progresses to ulcerous inflammation extending into the submucosa (► C1), producing one or often several round ulcers with a soft mucosal margin with a step off due to retraction of the muscularis mucosa and granulation tissue (p. 224, 312) on its floor. Later, the lesion progresses to a chromic ulcer with a hard, undermined margin (► C2).

Primary sites of ulcers include the lesser curvature and peripyloric antrum of the stomach and the duodenal bulb.

☺ **Prominent patients:**
Henri Matisse (1869–1954), French painter.
Pol Pot (1925–1998), Cambodian dictator.

■ Ulcerous Colitis

Definition: Ulcerative, idiopathic inflammatory bowel disease primarily involving the mucosa of the large bowel. The course of the disorder is chronic and recurrent, and the affected area spreads from distal to proximal.

Etiologic factors: genetic: mutation of intestinal main-genes (MUC-3A); *nutritional factors:* lots of refined sugar and saturated fats; *cigarette smoking; immunologic* tolerance impairment.

Ensuing pathogenetic reaction: The epithelium of the colon is destroyed at the base of the crypts. Initially lymphocytic and plasmocytic infiltrate is present in the crypts, later eosinophilic and granulocytic infiltrate (► F). These crypt abscesses cause epithelial necrosis that leads to ulceration (► D1, E1). Simultaneous epithelial regeneration and wound healing lead to reactive mucosal hyperplasia (► D2, E2) and proliferation of granulation tissue (p. 119). This results in inflammatory pseudo-polyps. Later, the chronic disorder results in fibrosis of the wall of the bowel.

✚ **Clinical presentation:** The disorder is more common in women than men. Symptoms include bloody, mucous diarrhea. Patients are at increased risk of colorectal carcinoma (p. 380). The diagnosis is made by rectosigmoidoscopy with biopsy.

Diffuse Necrotizing Inflammation

Definition: Acute inflammation with rapidly spreading necrosis and an ineffective or absent leukocyte reaction.

Associated Disorder

■ Necrotizing Fasciitis

Definition: Rare disease entity caused by various bacteria (gram positive cocci) with fulminant necrosis in the extremities.

Morphology: Soft tissue necrosis destroying the structure of the tissue and progressing to complete sclerosis (► B).

A Vincent angina
(PAS) x 600

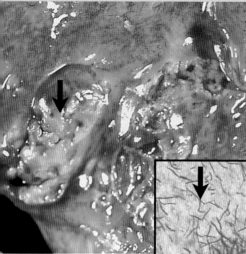

B Necrotizing fasciitis in the shoulder

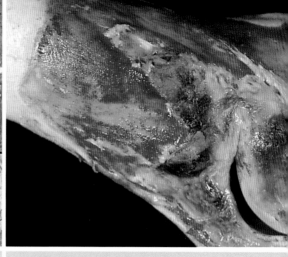

C Stomach ulcer

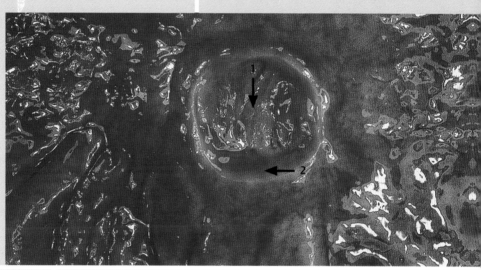

D Ulcerous colitis
(axial view)

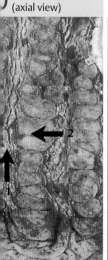

E Ulcerous colitis
(cross section)

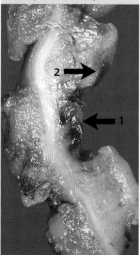

F Ulcerous colitis
(HE) x 200

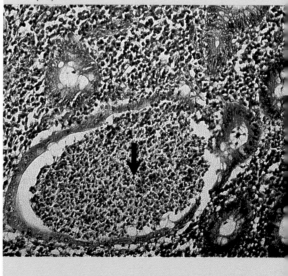

Areactive Necrotizing Inflammation

Definition: Acute necrotizing inflammatory reaction without appreciable accompanying leukocytic fibrinous reaction.

Etiologic factors include:
— Inflammatory cell deficiency (as in agranulocytosis);
— Cytotoxic bacterial toxins;
— Complement-activating antigen-antibody complexes (as in necrotizing vasculitis);
— T-cell-mediated hypersensitivity reaction (such as caseous necrosis in tuberculous granulomas).

Pathogenesis: The lack of an exudative inflammatory reaction leads to necrosis without leukocyte transmigration and fibrin exudation, i.e., nonreactive inflammation.

Gangrenous Inflammation

Definition: Putrid disintegration of a necrotizing inflammation due to infestation with anaerobic putrefactive bacteria.

Etiologic factors include:
— Generally weakened immune system;
— Diabetes mellitus;
— Local circulatory disruption;
— Inflammatory, ischemic, tumorous necrosis.

Pathogenesis: Patients with a predisposition suffer infection with spore-forming and non-spore-forming anaerobes. This results in putrid gangrenous tissue destruction with formation of amine, mercaptan, or gas in the tissue that leads to liquefactive necrosis (p. 132).

Examples:
— *Gangrenous inflammation* of the genitals (Fournier gangrene; ► A)
— *Gangrenous muscular inflammation.* The inflammation in the illustration (► B) is limited to one muscle compartment (► B1). The rest of the musculature is intact (► B2).

> **Note:** Gangrene may occur as ischemic dry gangrene or putrefactive wet gangrene (► A, B).

Lymphocytic Inflammation

Definition: Inflammation with an infiltrate of lymphocytes and (seldom) plasmocytes (round-cell inflammation).

Biologic "purpose": cellular inflammatory "specialists" create an inflammatory reaction.

Acute forms: These involve a lymphocytic round-cell infiltrate with numerous apoptotic cells (indicative of an autoimmune process, viral infection, allergic hypersensitivity reaction) without collagen fiber proliferation in the inflamed area.

Chronic forms: These involve a lympho-plasmocytic, round-cell infiltrate with proliferation and widening of collagen fibers (sclerosis; p. 40) in the inflamed area.

Examples include chronic inflammation of the uterine tube (salpingitis) in which there are large quantities of lymphocytes in an edematous stroma (► C, D).

> **Note:**
> – *Granulocytic (or leukocytic) inflammation* leads to tissue destruction with reparative scarring and a structural defect.
> – *Lympho-plasmocytic inflammation* is not associated with tissue liquefaction. In chronic disease, it leads to fibrosis (sclerosis) without a structural defect.

Fetal Inflammation

Embryo and fetus: Macrophage precursor cells appear in the yolk sac mesenchyma after the fourth week of gestation and in the bone marrow after the fifteenth week of gestation. Neutrophilic granulocytes are only released into circulating blood with the beginning of hemopoiesis in the bone marrow. As a result, the fetus can combat pathogens only by means of phagocytosis by macrophages. However, the macrophages are not yet able to present antigens to trigger antibody formation.

The fetus has a cellular defensive mechanism. After the sixth week of gestation, the earliest T-cell precursors appear in the yolk sac and the liver. However, they still must be "trained" in the thymus. The earliest B-cell precursors appear in the liver after the seventh week of gestation, in the spleen after the eleventh to fifteenth week, and in the bone marrow after the 30th week. At this stage, they can already react with antigens although they can only form IgM immunoglobulins. After the 28th week, IgG from the mother reaches the fetus (IgA and IgM cannot pass through the placental barrier). This means that the fetus cannot yet mount an immune defense; pathogens such as herpes virus, cytomegalovirus, toxoplasmas, listerias, and treponemes can survive and proliferate, causing fetal disease (p. 306).

Neonates: The humoral immune system develops only after birth.

Pathogenesis and morphology:
— *Viral infection* has a cytopathic effect and produces necrosis, which in turn leads to calcification (see toxoplasmosis, p. 306).
— *Bacterial infection* can induce two patterns of reaction:
  — *Histiocytic granuloma* (p. 228), a nodular aggregation of immature macrophages surrounding the pathogen, or
  — *Dystopic extramedullary hemopoietic foci* (► E in the kidney, F in the liver). In the latter case, immature blood cells are sent to the inflamed area. Blood cells proliferate at the site, leading to hemopoiesis.

> **Note:** Extramedullary hemopoietic foci can produce a particular manifestation of inflammation in fetuses and neonates.

The further course of inflammatory reaction is discussed in the next section.

Gangrenous genital inflammation

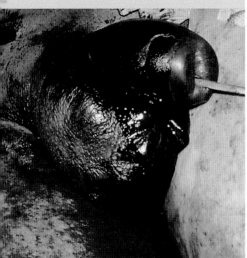

Gangrenous muscular inflammation

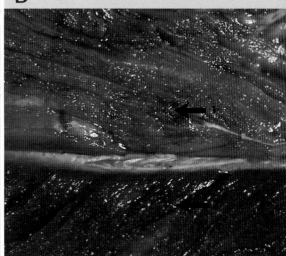

Chronic salpingitis
(Giemsa stain) x 75

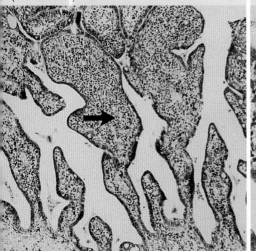

Chronic salpingitis
(Giemsa stain) x 200

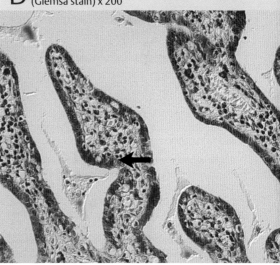

Fetal inflammation of the liver
(HE) x 75

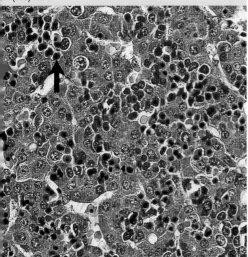

Fetal inflammation of the liver
(HE) x 150

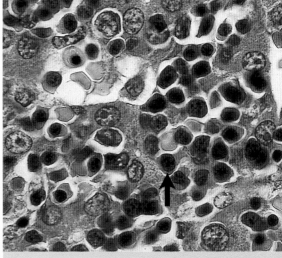

Courses of Acute Inflammation

■ Dissolution of the exudate:

In the absence of complications or defects in the immune system, the inflammatory exudate is eliminated by macrophages. The dissolved components of the inflammatory exudate are transported via the lymph vessels to the regional lymph nodes, resulting in regional lymphadenitis.

■ Regeneration: Once the exudate has been

dissolved, the tissue may either regenerate completely, or replacement tissue may form to fill the defect (p. 309).

■ Secondary postinfectious disorders: Circu-

lating antigen-antibody complexes formed during the course of inflammation may trigger a type III hypersensitivity reaction (p. 170), leading to a secondary disorder.

■ Chronic inflammation: An acute inflamma-

tion that fails to heal may become chronic.

■ Hematogenous Dissemination

Definition: Dissemination of pathogens from the point of entry to other parts of the body via the circulatory system. This may be accompanied by septicopyemic foci (see below) or by generalized tissue damage without suppurative inflammatory reaction (sepsis).

Pathogenesis: whether a pathogen leads to hematogenous dissemination and general malaise depends on several factors:
— *Virulence of the pathogen,* i.e., the aggressiveness of the pathogen and its tendency to proliferate.
— *Pathogenic toxins:* Gram-positive bacteria (such as diphtheria bacteria) form exotoxins with massive antigen characteristics. These are neutralized by specific antibodies. Gram-negative bacteria (such as salmonellas) form endotoxins with slight antigen effect. When these endotoxins (► A1) bond to the cell membrane (► A2), they trigger generalized reactions such as fever, skin rashes, and circulatory shock (p. 394).
— *Resistance,* i.e., the body's unspecific ability to resist an infection, determines the further course of contact with a pathogen.

▥ Bacteremia

Definition: The brief, asymptomatic presence of bacteria in the bloodstream ($<10^5$ pathogens per ml of blood).

▥ Fungemia

Definition: Presence of fungi in the bloodstream due to a weakened immune system. This invariably leads to clinical symptoms in the form of fungal sepsis.

▥ Sepsis

Definition: Clinical evidence (prior to antibacterial therapy) of pathogenic bacteria or fungi in the peripheral circulatory system ($>10^5$ pathogens per ml of blood) in the presence of corresponding systemic symptoms (fever).

Pathogenesis include release of endotoxins into the blood, referred to as endotoxemia or blood poisoning.

Morphology: Morphologic evidence of sepsis will only be present after morphologic correlates in the form of septic shock have occurred (p. 394).

> **Note:** The term sepsis does not apply to viruses, rickettsial organisms, or cell-bound parasitic bacteria where the pathogens survive within the blood cells without causing symptoms of sepsis.

▥ Septicopyemia

Definition: Pathoanatomic condition in which bacteria or fungi spread from a focus of origin to a metastatic site (► D2), where they cause a reactive suppurative inflammation in various organs (► B, C, D1).

Morphology: Septicopyemic foci are detectable primarily in organs with exchange functions, such as:
— *Kidneys,* in the medullary cone (► B);
— *Lungs,* in the subpleural tissue (► C);
— *Heart,* in the subendocardial myocardium (► D1).

> ☺ **Prominent patient:** Gustav Mahler (1860–1911), Austrian composer, suffered from streptococcal sepsis.

> **Note:** Hyperacute tubercular sepsis (p. 232) is a special form of septicopyemia associated with small focal areas of nonreactive necrosis surrounding bacterial foci occurring primarily in the liver (► E1), lung, and spleen.

> **Note:** The primary systemic effects of acute inflammatory reaction include:
> - *Presence of acute phase proteins*: IL-6 from lymphocytes leads to generation of C-reactive protein, complement factor C3, serum amyloid A, fibrinogen, and protease inhibitor.
> - **Fever**: Endotoxin leads to release of IL-1 and TNF-α from macrophages, leading to release of hypothalamic PGI_2 that stimulates the vasomotor center, producing fever and tachycardia.
> - *Blood leukocytosis.*

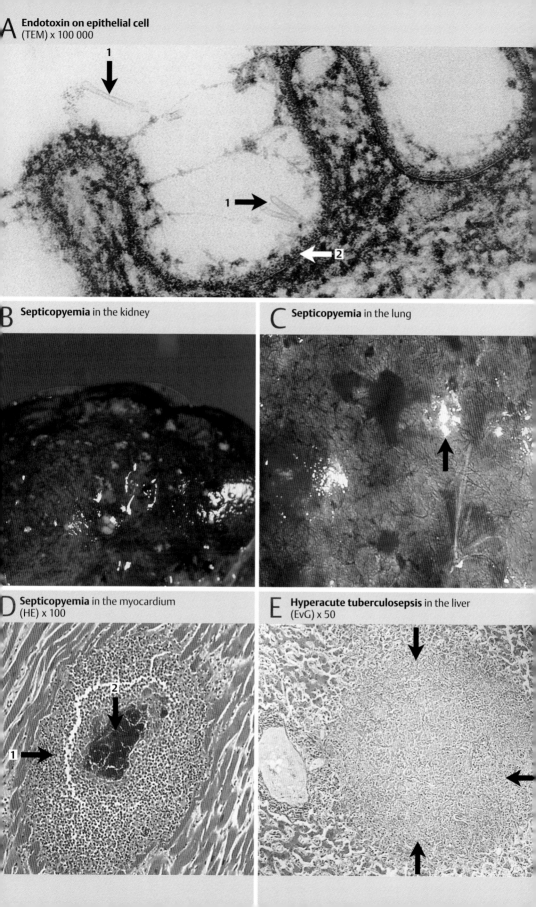

A **Endotoxin on epithelial cell**
(TEM) x 100 000

B **Septicopyemia** in the kidney

C **Septicopyemia** in the lung

D **Septicopyemia** in the myocardium
(HE) x 100

E **Hyperacute tuberculosepsis** in the liver
(EvG) x 50

Chronic Inflammation

Biologic purpose: Where the immediate reaction of acute inflammation fails to achieve the desired effect, the body resorts to what resembles "commando tactics." The inflammatory noxious agent is surrounded by specialized attack cells in the form of macrophages, lymphocytes, and plasma cells. Using their specialized weapons (proteases, cytotoxicity, and antibodies) they gradually wear down and destroy the noxious agent.

This longer-term inflammation process may be identified by distinctive histologic findings that occur in these chronic forms of inflammation:
— Chronic nonsuppurative inflammation;
— Chronic suppurative inflammation;
— Granulomatous inflammation.

Chronic Nonsuppurative Inflammation

Definition: Chronic inflammation without suppurative tissue liquefaction.

Pathogenetic factors include (a) an immune inflammatory reaction with cytotoxic lymphocytes and/or antigen-antibody reaction and (b) noxious environmental agents and certain pathogens.

Associated Disorder

■ **Chronic Bronchitis**

WHO definition: Disease of the respiratory tract with persistent or recurrent cough and expectoration on most days of at least three consecutive months during at least two successive years.

Etiologic factors:
— Endogenous factors (predisposition) include allergy, atopy, cystic fibrosis, IgA deficiency, and congenital or acquired kinociliary dysplasia in the nasotracheal and bronchial mucosa.
— Exogenous factors include primarily cigarette smoking but also airborne industrial pollutants, fog, viruses, and bacteria.

Pathogenetic chain reaction: In "smoker's bronchitis" (▶ A, B), cigarette smoke inhibits the activity of the kinocilia on the ciliated respiratory epithelium (▶ A1). This interferes with ciliary clearance of mucus (▶ A2), causing inhaled toxins to remain on the nasotracheal and bronchial mucosa. This leads to chronic injury to the ciliated epithelium and replacement of the ciliated epithelia with mucus-secreting goblet cells (▶ B1) in the form of goblet-cell metaplasia (p. 318) and reactive hypertrophy of the mucus glands in the bronchial wall (▶ B2), leading to increased mucus production. The cough reflex zone only begins in the bronchi, meaning that the contaminated mucus remains on the bronchial mucosa. The resulting blockage of ciliary mucus clearance successively leads to chronic inflammation with infiltration of lymphocytes and plasma cells (▶ B3), chronic coughing, hypertrophy of the musculature of the bronchial wall (▶ B), and a hernia-like widening of the excretory ducts of the bronchial glands.

✚ **Complications** include *chronic mucopurulent bronchitis.* The chronic catarrhal inflammation provides optimum conditions for the growth of opportunistic pathogens such as Haemophilus influenzae. This results in bacterial infestation and neutrophil chemotaxis. Neutrophils migrate into the inflamed area, leading to chronic mucopurulent bronchitis (see below) with a putrid greenish-yellow expectorate.

☺ **Prominent patients:**
Giacomo Puccini (1858–1924), Italian composer.
Henri Matisse (1869–1954), French painter.

Chronic Suppurative Inflammation

This may occur as a chronic mucopurulent inflammation or a chronic granulomatous inflammation (a special form of suppurative inflammation).

Chronic Mucopurulent Inflammation

Pathogenesis: Infestation of the mucosal hollow organs with pyogenic pathogens leads to a suppurative inflammatory reaction. Chronic recurrent mucosal injury leads to replacement of the epithelium with squamous epithelium (▶ C1) and to mucosal fibrosis (▶ C2). Persistent inflammation leads to atrophy of the mucosa with progression to chronic atrophic inflammation.

Examples include chronic mucopurulent bronchitis and chronic mucopurulent rhinosinusitis.

✚ **Complications:**
– In *chronic atrophic rhinitis,* infestation of the thickened nasal secretion with putrefactive bacteria (*Klebsiella pneumoniae ozaenae*) can lead to a sweet smell of decay.
– In *chronic atrophic bronchitis* (▶ C), bronchial wall atrophy can progress to the point of bronchial wall collapse.

❗ **Note:** An *active chronic inflammation* is a chronic inflammation with progressive tissue destruction with or without simultaneous presence of a neutrophilic infiltrate.

A Normal bronchus

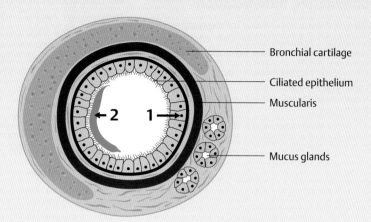

Bronchial cartilage

Ciliated epithelium

Muscularis

Mucus glands

2   1

B Chronic hypertrophic bronchitis

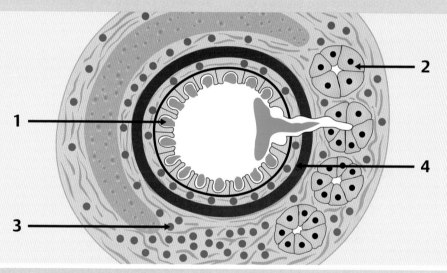

1

2

3

4

C Chronic atrophic bronchitis

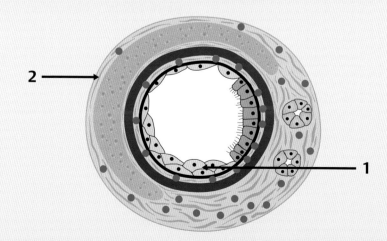

2

1

Granulating Inflammations

General definition: Chronic inflammations characterized by formation of new capillary-rich, absorptive mesenchyma (granulation tissue).

General histologic findings: The following three-layer structure of the inflammatory granulation tissue is common to all chronic granulating inflammations:

- *Resorption zone* (▶ A1, B1): This innermost zone borders directly on the necrotic material and primarily consists of phagocytic histiocytes. These cells store the poorly soluble fat in lysosomal vacuoles and are known as "foam cells" because of the foamy vacuolar appearance of their cytoplasm.
- *Granulation zone* (▶ A2, B2): This zone consists of granulation tissue rich in capillaries and fibroblasts. The tissue has a resorptive and reparative function; branching capillaries have the superficial appearance of granules (hence the term granulation tissue).
- *Mature connective tissue zone* (▶ A3): This oldest and outermost layer of tissue consists of granulation tissue that has matured to highly fibrous connective tissue, giving it a high degree of mechanical strength.

> **Note:** *Granulating inflammation occurs* as a secondary reaction to large tissue defects. In a certain sense it corresponds to wound healing.

> **Note:** *Granulation tissue has several functions:*
> - *Demarcation* of healthy tissue from necrotic tissue.
> - *Resorption* of necrotic tissue by organizing it.
> - *Repair* of tissue defects.

There are several morphologic variants of granulating inflammations, including:
- Demarcation of necrosis;
- Chronic abscess;
- Chronic fistula;
- Chronic ulcer.

■ Demarcation of Necrosis

Pathogenesis: Necrosis, bleeding into tissue (hematoma), and macroscopic areas of fibrinous exudation are sequestered from vital tissue by a "hemorrhagic halo" of capillary-rich granulation tissue, which absorbs the necrosis or exudate (▶ C; myocardial necrosis in a heart attack).

> **Note:** Necrosis is a tissue "wound." In terms of formal pathogenesis, a granulating inflammation corresponds to wound healing.

■ Chronic Abscess

Pathogenesis: In the absence of spontaneous or iatrogenic emptying, the abscess forms an abscess membrane (▶ D; chronic liver abscess) of granulation tissue around the necrotic area. Phagocytic histiocytes engorged with the lipid membranes of necrotic cells appears as foam cells and give the abscess membrane a yellowish color.

■ Chronic Fistula

Definition and pathogenesis: Abnormal communication between the necrotic focus of inflammation and an outer or inner surface of the body. Especially in the case of abscess-forming inflammations, the contents of the abscess can spontaneously empty outside the body through a cutaneous fistula or into a hollow organ through an internal fistula. The wall of the fistula consists of granulation tissue. The fistula canal may be partially lined with ingrowing surface epithelium.

■ Chronic Ulcer

Pathogenesis: This refers to an epithelial or tissue defect on an outer or inner surface of the body that fails to heal or whose healing is delayed (▶ E) and which is demarcated by granulation tissue with the three typical layers. The resorption zone includes the area of fibrinoid connective-tissue necrosis on the floor of the ulcer.

> **Note:**
> - *Tumerous ulcer* margin is hardened, raised, and medullar;
> - *Inflammatory ulcer* margin is soft, reddened, and raised.

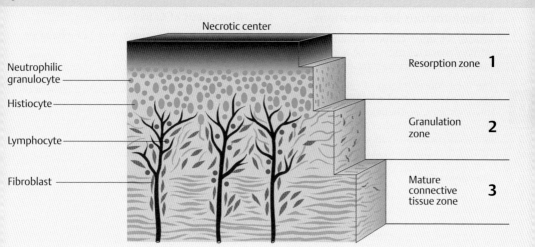

A The three layers of granulation tissue

Necrotic center

Neutrophilic granulocyte

Histiocyte

Lymphocyte

Fibroblast

Resorption zone **1**

Granulation zone **2**

Mature connective tissue zone **3**

B Granulation tissue
(HE) x 50

1

2

C Demarcation of necrosis in a myocardial infarction

D Chronic liver abscess

E Chronic ulcer (lateral malleolus)

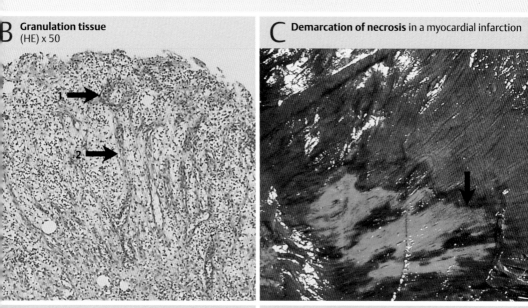

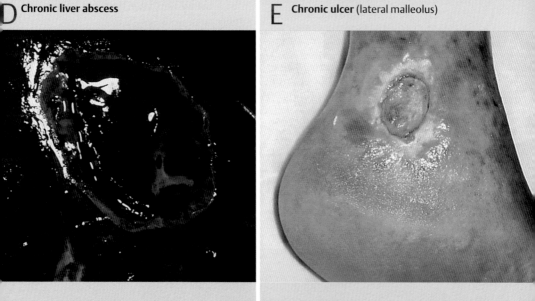

Granulomatous Inflammations

General definition: Chronic inflammation whose primary characteristic is large nodule of inflammatory cells, often measuring several millimeters.

The focal concentration of cells of the macrophage system involved in forming the granuloma (macrophages, epithelioid cells, and multinucleated giant cells) varies among individual inflammations. As a result, a granuloma may be sharply demarcated or diffuse and ill-defined.

Granuloma Cells

Macrophages transform themselves under the influence of cytokines or T lymphocytes to specialized cells for phagocytosis and antigen presentation. However, where they are forced to phagocytize persistent antigens, they transform themselves into epithelioid cells.

Epithelioid cells have lost important membrane receptors for phagocytosis. However, their cytoplasm has entirely adapted to the secretion of proteases and cytokines. To improve the efficiency of their enzymes, they form a dense epithelial wall of cells (hence their name) with ill-defined margins between individual cells. This isolates the focus of the inflammation and forms a microbicidal microenvironment. Histologic findings in these cells include a large nucleus resembling the sole of a shoe and containing loosely-packed chromatin.

Multinucleated giant cells are created by macrophages and epithelioid cells that fuse to form a syncytium. Older giant cells provide a bed for incoming macrophages. These giant cells fuse with macrophages that recently entered the inflamed area.

Two types of giants cells occurring in granulomas may be distinguished according to their morphogenesis.
— *Unorganized giant cells* have nuclei that are irregularly distributed throughout the cytoplasm. Foreign-body giant cells are a prime example of this type.
— *Organized giant cells* exhibit a ring-like or wreath-like configuration of nuclei in the periphery of the cell, depending on the orientation of the imaging plane. Langerhans giant cells are prime examples of this type of giant cell.

Cell sequesters are occasionally observed in the cytoplasm. These include asteroid or star-shaped bodies of cytoskeletal components and conchoidal or Schaumann bodies (clam-shaped calcified cytoplasmic components).

> **Note:** *The multinucleated giant cells* of fused macrophages do not migrate or phagocytize as readily as their mononuclear precursors. However, they produce large quantities of cytotoxic and microbicidal O_2 and N_2 compounds.

Histogenesis of Granulomas

The cellular composition of a granuloma depends on these factors:

— The state of the body's immune system;
— The antigenic character of the irritant;
— The relative quantities of antigen and antibodies in the immune reaction;
— The efficiency of neutrophils;
— The reactivity of the T cells.

The following types of granulomas may occur depending on the toxicity of the irritant.

■ Epithelioid granulomas

Definition: Sharply demarcated nodules consisting largely of densely grouped, specialized macrophages (epithelioid cells).

Pathogenesis and morphology: Some of these granulomas are caused by relatively toxic substances such as mycobacterial components (tuberculin). Only a few macrophages in the granuloma contain the irritant.

Epithelioid granulomas include:
— Sarcoidal granulomas and
— Tubercular granulomas.

Depending on the specific etiology, epithelioid granulomas are transformed by leukocytic infiltrates and/or necrosis.
— *Caseous granulomas* occur in the presence of cell-mediated immunity against components of inflammatory pathogens (such as tuberculosis). These granulomas become largely necrotic due to the production of cytokine by T lymphocytes and the release of proteases by macrophages.
— *Abscess-forming granulomas* occur in the presence of infection with certain pathogens in which neutrophils are also attracted into the granuloma.

This results in an abscess-forming histiocytic inflammatory reaction in the center of the granuloma.

■ Histiocytic Granulomas

Definition: Ill-defined nodular accumulations of primarily phagocytic histiocytes (foreign-body granuloma).

Pathogenesis and morphology: These granulomas primarily consist of histiocytes and are caused by minimally toxic foreign substances such as urate or substances not recognized as endogenous such as collagen covered by immune complex. Nearly all the histiocytes in them (macrophages) are covered with irritant or are involved in phagocytizing it.

Histiocytic granulomas include:
— Rheumatic granuloma;
— Rheumatoid granuloma;
— Foreign-body granuloma.

Morphology of Granulomas

Granulomatous inflammations may be classified according to etiologic aspects. They may also be classified according to their most conspicuous characteristic, the morphology of the granuloma.

Formal pathogenetic classification of granulomatous inflammatory reactions (according to Müller-Hermelink).

Type of granulomatous inflammation	Granuloma histology
Epithelioid granulomas	
Small focal epithelioid cell reactions	
— Infectious	Small, ill-defined small epithelioid granulomas
— Tumor-associated	
Granulomatous epithelioid cell reactions	
— Infectious epithelioid cell reaction	Large circumscribed epithelioid
— Tuberculoid foreign-body granulomas	granulomas with or without necrosis
— Tumor-associated granulomas	
— Hypersensitivity granulomas	
Mixed-cell granulomas	Histiocytic epithelioid granulomas with or without granulocytes
Histiocytic granulomas	
— Rheumatic granulomas	Histiocytic granulomas with or
— Rheumatoid granulomas	without granulocytes
— Foreign-body granulomas	
— Hyperergic histiocytosis	

Note: A granulomatous inflammation is not the same as a granulating inflammation.

Note: *Granuloma ↔ granulation tissue:* A granulomatous inflammation is granulation tissue specific to or typical of inflammation present in a more or less clearly defined nodular form.

Note: *Granuloma ↔ inflammation specificity:* The granuloma is a sign but not proof of a specific inflammatory etiology.

Note: Causes of granulomatous lymphadenitis include:
- Infections (primarily tuberculosis, syphilis, toxoplasmosis, and fungal diseases);
- Sarcoidosis and Crohn disease;
- Reaction to foreign bodies;
- Reaction to tumor material.

Note:
- Langerhans cells are antigen-presenting cells in the epidermis;
- Langhans giant cells are organized multinucleated giant cells.

The following section examines those granulomas that exhibit distinctive histologic findings and are characteristic identifiers of certain diseases.

Sarcoid Granulomas

Definition: Small granulomas of epithelioid cells (noncaseating epithelioid granulomas) without central necrosis (caseation) and with an outer layer of collagen fibers and a tendency toward centripetal fibrosis.

Pathogenetic chain reaction: An unidentified primary immune system dysfunction leads to antigen contact. This leads to proliferation of T helper cells, in turn leading to production of cytokines that attract macrophages. The macrophages are attracted to the site by chemokine and held there by a migration-inhibiting factor. A fusion factor induces them to form giant cells. Platelet-derived growth factor induces local fibrosis. An activation factor induces the transformation of macrophages into epithelioid cells, leading to formation of a granuloma (► A).

Histology of granuloma: These granulomas consist of a focal accumulation of epithelioid cells (► C1, F) with unorganized and organized Langhans giant cells (► C2), often with conchoidal and asteroid bodies (► C3) and a peripheral wall of lymphocytes. The sarcoid granulomas are usually covered with an outer layer of collagen fibers. This results in granulomas that tend to fibrose toward their centers and exhibit hyalinization; they do not exhibit central necrosis.

Examples:
— *Sarcoidosis.*
— *Crohn's disease.*
— *Berylliosis* following injury involving fluorescent lamps containing beryllium.
— *Primary biliary cirrhosis:* Progressive autoimmune destruction of the bile ducts involving release of bile into the hepatic parenchyma, followed by cirrhotic repair of the hepatic parenchyma (p. 22).
— *Extrinsic allergic alveolitis.*

Associated Disorders

Sarcoidosis

Definition: More or less generalized mycobacterial disorder associated with a granulomatous inflammatory reaction, primarily in the lung and lymph nodes but also in other organs.

Pathogenesis: See above.

Morphologic stages:
— **Initial stage:** lymphocytic alveolitis.
— **Granulomatous inflammatory stage:** Noncaseating epithelioid granulomas come together primarily in the bronchial mucosa, pulmonary parenchyma, and lymph nodes, giving a fleshy appearance to the affected lymph nodes (► E), hence the name sarcoidosis (from the French *sarx*, flesh).
— **Scarring stage:** Centripetal fibrosis and scarring of the granulomas leads to interstitial pulmonary fibrosis with perifocal emphysema. This in turn leads to restrictive respiratory insufficiency.

Crohn's Disease

Definition: Chronic granulomatous gastrointestinal inflammation (granulomatous enterocolitis) primarily affecting the terminal ileus (terminal ileitis) and with segmental involvement (regional ileitis). An example of an idiopathic inflammatory bowel disease.

Pathogenetic factors:
— *genetic:* familial aggregation with mutation of the NOD-gene, a intracellular receptor for bacterial products → activation of "NFκB";
— *infection:* atypical mycobacteria, latent measle viruses;
— *nutritional factors:* lots of refined sugar and saturated fats;
— *cigarette smoking;*
— *immunologic* tolerance impairment.

Morphology: The disorder is characterized by discontinuous inflammation with a lymphocytic infiltrate. Initially an aphthoid mucosal lesion is present, leading to ulcer formation. Large quantities of granulation tissue lie between the individual ulcers. This gives the surface of the mucosa a cobblestone appearance (► B). A wedge-shaped projection of the inflammation (fissural inflammation, ► D) causes perforation, creating fistulas into adjacent bowel loops and forming abscesses between the bowel loops. These abscesses produce adhesions, leading to an inflammatory "conglomerate tumor." Epithelioid granulomas develop in 40% of all cases. Later, reparative fibrosis creates a rigid bowel wall with stenosis. This leads to a typical radiographic "garden hose" phenomenon.

☺ **Prominent patient:**
Dwight D. Eisenhower (1890–1969), 34th President of the United States and WWII Supreme Commander of Allied Forces.

Note: *Crohn's disease* is characterized by *"skip lesions"* in which affected bowel segments are interspersed with normal segments (which can give rise to false negative diagnostic findings) and, where the disorder persists, by *precancerous conditions.*

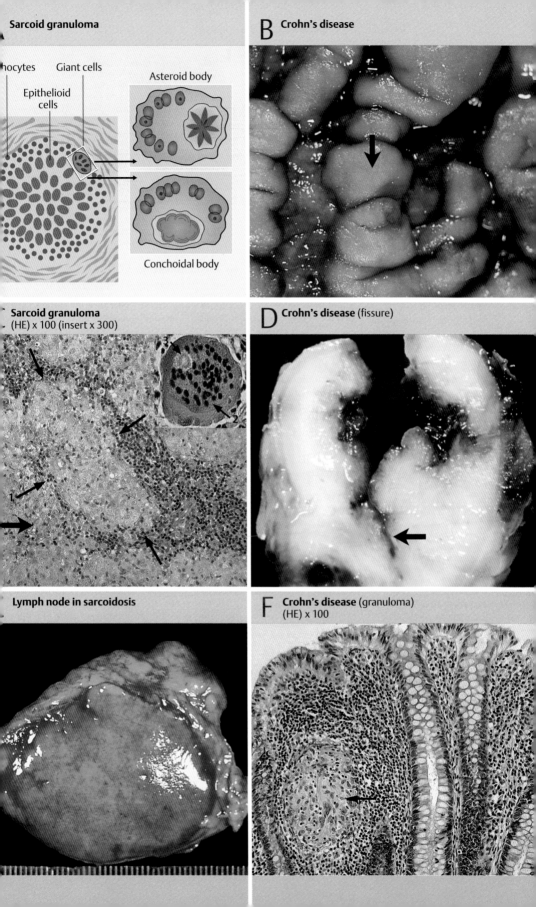

Sarcoid granuloma

hocytes   Giant cells

Epithelioid cells

Asteroid body

Conchoidal body

B **Crohn's disease**

Sarcoid granuloma
(HE) x 100 (insert x 300)

D **Crohn's disease** (fissure)

Lymph node in sarcoidosis

F **Crohn's disease** (granuloma)
(HE) x 100

■ **Tuberculous Granuloma**

Definition: Large circumscribed granulomas consisting of epithelioid cells with central caseous necrosis and an outer layer of lymphocytic cells.

Pathogenetic chain reaction: The disorder is caused by pathogens, some of which survive phagocytosis within the cell. As a result, pathogens may be released or "spit out" after phagocytosis. Macrophages communicate with T lymphocytes, resulting in production of cytokines (chemotactic agents, migration-inhibiting factors, and activating factors). This results in accumulation of epithelioid cells, which form nodules (epithelioid tubercles). Eventually the B cells come into contact with the pathogenic antigen, and humoral antibodies against the antigen are produced. This activates the complement system, inducing macrophages to phagocytosis. This leads to coagulation necrosis within the granulomas, which by this time are macroscopically discernible (► A, C). This progresses to caseation (p. 130) and later to calcification (p. 136).

Histology of granuloma: These granulomas exhibit central caseous necrosis (► B) containing neutralized pathogens and debris from macrophages surrounded by a solid wall (► D1) of bactericidal macrophages (epithelioid cells), some of which have fused to form organized multinucleated Langhans giant cells (► D2). The periphery of the granuloma consists of a wall of lymphocytes (► D3).

Examples:
— Tuberculosis (p. 264)
— Leprosy (p. 264)
— Syphilis (p. 262)

☺ **Prominent patients** with pulmonary tuberculosis:
Carl Maria von Weber (1786–1826), composer.
Frederic Chopin (1810–1849), Polish composer.
Ernst Ludwig Kirchner (1880–1938), German painter.
Franz Kafka (1883–1924), Czech-born German-speaking author.

❗ **Note:**
– The *granuloma in tuberculosis* is referred to as a *tubercle*. It lacks a central blood vessel and has peripheral lymphocytes.
– The *granuloma in syphilis* is referred to as a *gumma*. It contains central blood vessels and peripheral plasma cells.

❗ **Note:** Areactive granulomas in hyperacute tuberculous sepsis (p. 223) represent a *special form of tuberculous granuloma*. In this clinical syndrome, the immunocompromised body is overwhelmed by the pathogen, leading to hematogenous dissemination of the pathogen. Organs such as the lungs, liver, spleen, and lymph nodes are covered with focal necroses measuring 1–2 mm.
– The *center of the necrosis* includes massive quantities of acid-resistant rods;
– the *periphery of the necrosis* usually lacks any cellular immune reaction (hardly any giant cells and epithelioid cells are present).

❗ **Note:** Calcified tuberculous focal necroses can also contain infectious tuberculosis organisms.

■ **Pseudotuberculous Granuloma**

Synonym: Reticocytically abessing granuloma.

Definition: Often ill-defined granulomas consisting of macrophages and epithelioid cells with central necrosis with granulocytes.

Pathogenetic chain reaction: Some bacteria and fungi contain chitin polysaccharides in their capsule, enabling them to survive phagocytosis. The result is that pathogens are transported to the regional lymph nodes, where they are intercepted by sinus histiocytes. This may result in formation of characteristic inclusion bodies, which in turn successively leads to nodular proliferation of histiocytes and a histiocytic granuloma (► E). The histiocytes attempt to neutralize the pathogen with toxic O_2 and N_2 metabolites and lysosomal proteases, causing the histiocytes to release chemotactic agents and migration-inhibiting factors. This attracts neutrophils into the center of the granuloma and holds them there. The freshly-created histiocytic nodules become infiltrated by granulocytes and are necrotized by them (► F1). Later cell-mediated immunity comes into play, and the histiocytes are transformed into epithelioid cells that seal the granuloma off from the surrounding tissue like a palisade (► F2). Almost no giant cells are formed.

In many cases, the abscess formed partially empties through fistulas to the outside, causing scarring.

Histology granuloma: These granulomas are more or less well-circumscribed. The center contains abscess-forming necrosis with neutrophils (► F1). This is surrounded by a wall of histiocytes, some of which have been transformed into epithelioid cells (► F2).

Examples:
— Yersinia pseudotuberculosis (p. 260)
— Brucellosis
— Listeriosis (p. 256)
— Histoplasmosis (p. 272)
— Cryptococcosis (p. 270)
— Typhoid fever (p. 260)

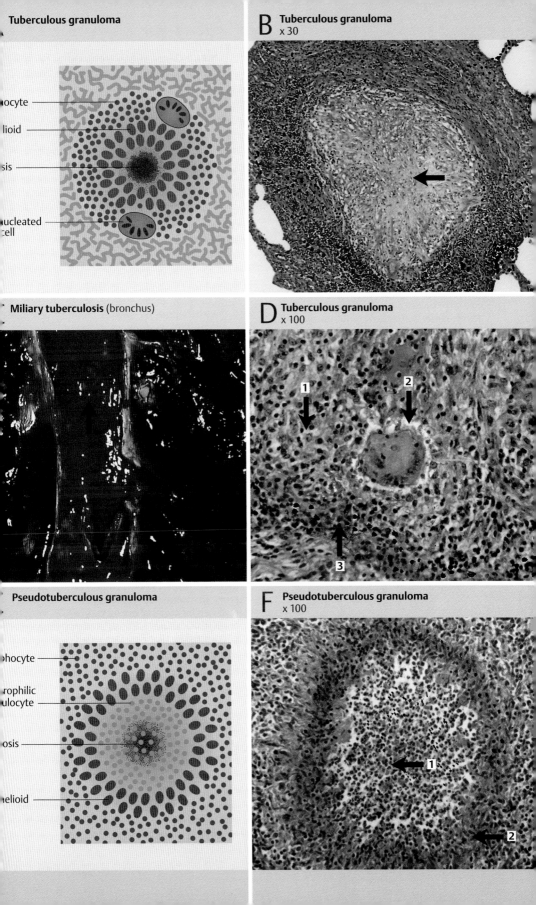

Tuberculous granuloma

ocyte

lioid

sis

ucleated
cell

B Tuberculous granuloma
x 30

Miliary tuberculosis (bronchus)

D Tuberculous granuloma
x 100

1

2

3

Pseudotuberculous granuloma

hocyte

rophilic
ulocyte

osis

helioid

F Pseudotuberculous granuloma
x 100

1

2

■ **Rheumatic Granuloma**

Synonym: Aschoff's lesion.

Definition: Histiocytic granuloma around a core of fibrinoid collagen necrosis, occurring primarily in the myocardium and only with rheumatic fever (acute articular rheumatism).

Pathogenetic chain reaction:

Phase 1 is characterized by pharyngeal infection with β-hemolytic streptococci (group A) leading to formation of antibodies that are directed against streptococcal antigens and against endogenous tissue antigens as a result of an autoimmune cross-reaction. M protein cross-reacts with cardial myosin and sarcolemma's; hyaluronate cross-reacts with connective tissue proteoglycans.

Phase 2, two weeks after the infection, involves postinfectious secondary disease in the form of acute febrile polyarthritis of the major joints (rheumatic fever), endomyocarditis, uveitis (inflammation of the vascular tunic of the eye), or acute glomerulonephritis. Rarely, the brain may be involved in the form of Sydenham chorea (rapid, purposeless contractions of individual muscle groups with grimacing).

Histology granuloma (► A, B): The granuloma occurs in the myocardial interstitium primarily adjacent to minor arteries (► B).
- **Exudative phase:** It is characterized by serofibrinous exudate, with deposits of immune precipitate on collagen fibers that lead to fibrinoid necrosis.
- **Granulomatous phase:** The fibrinoid necrosis is demarcated by specialized histiocytes and a sparse lymphocytic infiltrate (► B) with isolated granulocytes and, rarely, inflammatory giant cells (Aschoff cells).
  The *specialized histiocytes* or Anitchkov cells resemble epithelioid cells. Their elongated oval nuclei exhibit a flattened bottle-brush-like chromatin structure. The morphology changes according to the orientation of the imaging plane. Their cross section resembles a caterpillar; their longitudinal section resembles an owl's eye.
- **Scarring phase:** It is characterized by tissue repair with a spindle-shaped pattern of perivascular scarring (finely nodular fibrosis). Recurrence of the inflammation leads to recurrence of the granuloma.

Note: *Rheumatic fever* is said to "lick the knee but bite the heart."

Note: *The clinical course of rheumatic fever* involves a childhood infection with complications in adulthood (cardiac defect).

Note: Ischemia → myocardial scarring far from vascular structures; rheumatic fever → scarring close to vascular structures.

Note: Rheumatic fever in *children* proceeds from the myocardium to the endocardium to the joints; in *adults,* it proceeds from the joints to the endocardium to the myocardium.

■ **Rheumatoid Granuloma**

Definition: Histiocytic granuloma around a core of fibrinoid collagen necrosis, often occurring at multiple locations in the subcutaneous tissue and in articular nodules in rheumatoid arthritis (hence the term nodose rheumatism).

Pathogenesis: Endogenous antigens and autoreactive antibodies formed in the same tissue trigger an autoimmune inflammation.
- **Exudative inflammatory phase:** It begins with neutrophil and macrophage chemotaxis. The resulting activation of leukocytes and synoviocytes leads to proteolytic cartilage destruction in the small joints. Synovial macrophages phagocytize the immune complex, and macrophages migrating to the site surround collagen fibers enveloped with immune complex to form a rheumatoid granuloma.
- **Proliferative inflammatory phase:** It is characterized by transformation of the synovial cells into a highly proliferative mesenchyma or pannus. This pannus (► E1) grows into the joint space, irreparably destroying the articular cartilage (► E2). This causes stiffening of the joint (ankylosis) and deformity (► F). The inflammatory process in the subcutaneous tissue leads to the formation of rheumatoid nodules at exposed sites.

Histology granuloma (► C): The granulomas measure several centimeters. The center contains fibrinoid collagen necrosis (► D1) surrounded by a wall of histiocytes (► D2). Peripherally, the lesion is encapsulated with new connective tissue that contains small quantities of lymphocytes.

☺ **Prominent patient:** Auguste Renoir (1841-1919), French Impressionist painter.

Note: *Rheumatoid arthritis* is primary chronic arthritis of the small joints, especially the fingers.

Note: *Rheumatoid granulomas* are larger than rheumatic granulomas.

Note: In the interest of uniform *terminology,* some authors refer to both rheumatoid granulomas and rheumatic granulomas as "rheumatic granulomas."

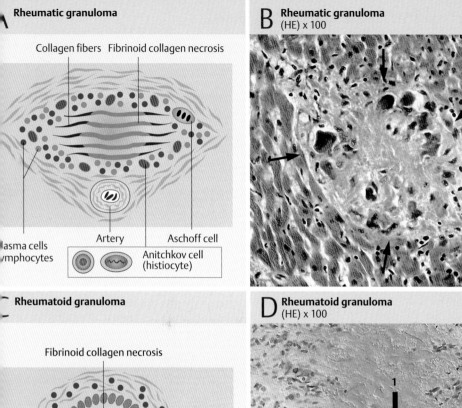

A Rheumatic granuloma

Collagen fibers   Fibrinoid collagen necrosis

asma cells
mphocytes

Artery   Aschoff cell

Anitchkov cell
(histiocyte)

B Rheumatic granuloma
(HE) x 100

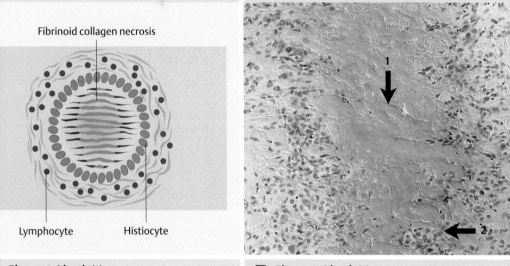

C Rheumatoid granuloma

Fibrinoid collagen necrosis

Lymphocyte   Histiocyte

D Rheumatoid granuloma
(HE) x 100

1

2

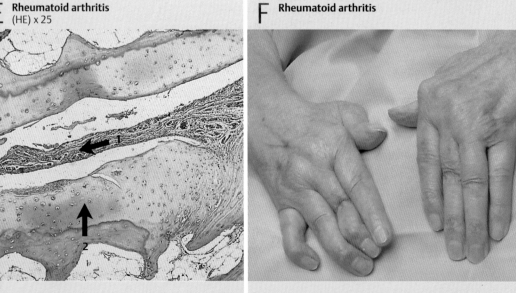

E Rheumatoid arthritis
(HE) x 25

1

2

F Rheumatoid arthritis

■ Foreign-Body Granuloma

Definition: Histiocytic granuloma surrounding material that the body can break down only with difficulty or not at all and that has lodged in or been released into tissue.

Substances eliciting foreign-body reactions may be crystalline or metallic, or they may be polymerized substances.

Pathogenetic chain reaction: Foreign material enters tissue and lodges there. This induces macrophages to accumulate, which attempt to phagocytize the foreign body. However, they are unable to engulf the material and break it down. The activated macrophages trigger the release of proteases and mediators. This leads to a) tissue destruction and b) fibrosis.

— **Tissue destruction** is one result. The release of proteases leads to partial digestion of the foreign body. This triggers an inflammatory reaction with progressive destruction of the foreign body (and usually of the surrounding tissue as well).

— **Fibrosis** is another result. Generation of cytokines (IL-1) and growth factors (platelet-derived growth factor) activate fibroblasts, leading to demarcation of the foreign body and/or reparative perifocal fibrosis. This often leads to progressive organ fibrosis.

Where the foreign bodies are larger than the macrophages, the macrophages fuse to form multinucleated foreign-body giant cells (unorganized giant cells). These cells adhere to the foreign body individually or in clusters like leeches.

Histology granuloma (▶ A): The foreign body is often detectable in the center of the granuloma under polarized light. It is surrounded by giant cells and macrophages that have been attracted to the site. These in turn are enveloped in a lymphocytic infiltrate together with penetrating capillaries and fibroblasts that form a fibrous capsule around the foreign body.

✚ **Clinical presentation and morphologic findings:**

Crystalline foreign bodies:
— *Glass fibers:* Skin injury leads to a cutaneous granuloma.
— *Silicate dust:* Inhalation triggers phagocytosis by alveolar macrophages (coniophages are dust-eating alveolar macrophages), producing perivascular accumulations of coniophages. These bloated cells die, and the released dust material is consumed by incoming phagocytes (p. 30). This re-

sults in release of proteases and generation of platelet-derived growth factor, leading to formation of granulomas (silicate granulomas) with progressive hyalinizing fibrosis. This progresses to inflammation of the pulmonary parenchyma with perifocal scarring and to pulmonary silicosis (p. 40).
— *Urates* (p. 102): Deposits in joint capsules and cartilage lead to gouty tophi and gouty arthritis.
— *Cholesterol* released in bile, in the form of cholesterol deposits (p. 90), from the remains of lipophages, and from membranes of necrotic cells, can produce a cholesterol granuloma.
— *Metals* may enter tissue in penetrating trauma or iatrogenically in the form of metal implants. This leads to phagocytosis (▶ C). Some of the metal is transported away in venules, and some remains in the tissue. Depending on the type of metal, an inflammatory reaction with vasculitis occurs (▶ D) in which the body attempts to bring the metal to its inner or outer surface (this occurs in implant loosening). Inert metals such as titanium are tolerated by tissue, and surrounding tissue will produce little or no inflammation.

Noncrystalline foreign bodies:
— *Starch* (impurities in heroin or glove powder) produces tuberculous granulomas that may be confused with tuberculosis.
— *Wood splinters* enter the body in penetrating trauma (▶ B1) and produce a mixed-cell granuloma with neutrophils.
— *Suture material* is absorbed by multinucleated giant cells (▶ F) in a suture granuloma.
— *Horn* (keratin) from broken epidermal cysts leads to resorptive inflammation.
— *Epithelial mucus:* Trauma and inflammation lead to a lesion of the excretory ducts and a mucus granuloma.
— *Oil droplets:* Trauma and inflammation lead to a fatty tissue lesion in which oil is phagocytized by macrophages (lipophage), transforming them into foam cells. The histiocytes fuse into multinucleated giant cells with foamy cytoplasm (Touton giant cells; p. 91), producing a granuloma of fat-filled histiocytes (lipophage granuloma).
— *Silicone:* The breast implant material can produce mixed-cell granulomas with a resorptive giant-cell inflammation surrounding rectangular silicone particles (▶ F). This results in inflammation of the tissue beneath the implant with painful and cosmetically unfavorable perifocal scarring in breast tissue.

This concludes the discussion of the morphologic fundamentals required to understand the inflammatory reactions caused by specific pathogens discussed in Chapters 12–16. These chapters represent what may be referred to as the applied pathology of inflammation.

A **Foreign-body granuloma**

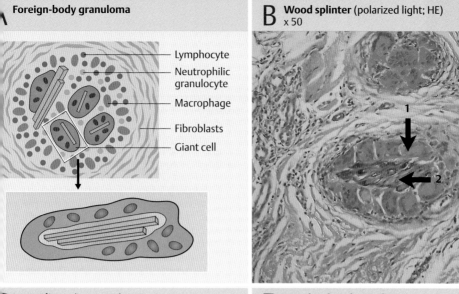

- Lymphocyte
- Neutrophilic granulocyte
- Macrophage
- Fibroblasts
- Giant cell

B **Wood splinter** (polarized light; HE) x 50

1
2

C **Iron splinter** (iron stain) x 70

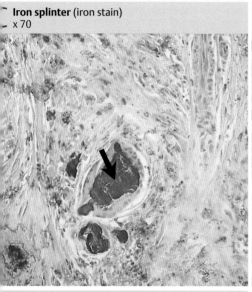

D **Metal-induced vasculitis** (HE) x 100

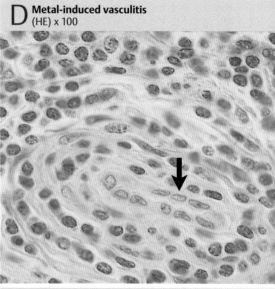

E **Suture granuloma** (polarized light) (HE) x 150

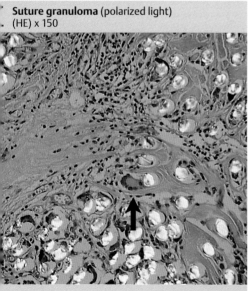

F **Silicon granuloma** (HE) x 50

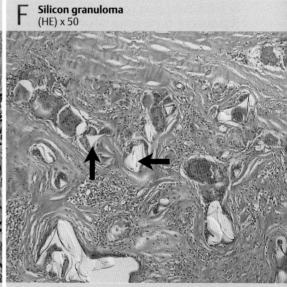

Viral Infection

Summary

A virus can infect a cell in several ways.

- *Latent infection* (▶ A1, B1) does not involve formation of new viruses or morphologic changes in the cell.
- *Noncytocidal infection* (▶ A2) involves virus reproduction without disturbing normal cell function.
- *Lytic infection* (▶ B2) leads to cell death following virus reproduction.
- *Transforming infection* (▶ A3, B3) results in uncontrolled cell growth.

A virus initially replicates in the tissue at the point of entry and in the local lymph nodes. This is followed by primary viremia and a central focus of virus proliferation. This progresses to secondary viremia with infection of the final target organ.

Dissemination of the virus occurs partially within the cytoplasm. Some viruses express a fusion factor on their surfaces, causing infected cells to fuse with uninfected cells to form large virus replication factories. Some viral infections involve only one organ system (referred to as organotropism). Normally, virus proliferation ceases in the acute stage of the disorder unless the immune defense becomes ineffective or deranged (in autoimmune disorders).

Several lines of defense are involved in combating invading viruses. These include a) the T-cell system in cooperation with the macrophages, b) virus-neutralizing antibodies and c-antibody dependent, cell-mediated cytotoxicity. When a virus infects a cell, it forces the host cell to express viral membrane antigens, effectively leaving "footprints" on the surface of the cell. T cells can detect these viral membrane antigens. Macrophages join the defensive effort within about two days. They phagocytize affected cells and present viral fragments to the T-helper cells so they can recognize them. Once the helper cells have "discovered" the viral antigen, they induce the development of cytotoxic T cells. These cells use their membrane-piercing toxins (perforins) to destroy all the cells corrupted by viral antigen they can detect.

In the time span between absorption of the virus and replication of the new viruses, no virus particles capable of replication are detectable in the body. The virus can be eliminated from the body if the infected cells are destroyed during this eclipse phase. The outcome of a viral infection is essentially determined by whether the T lymphocytes or the viruses win the race of cellular destruction.

Uncoated Single-Stranded RNA Viruses

Picornaviridae

■ Poliomyelitis Virus

Pathogen that causes poliomyelitis.

Pathogenesis: Droplet and smear infection occurs through direct contact with affected persons. Flu-like symptoms are initially present, after which the fever remits. This is then followed by either
- *aseptic meningitis* or
- *acute anterior poliomyelitis:*

Viral infection of the motor nerve endings leads to retrograde transport of the virus through the nerves to the ganglion cells of the anterior horns of the spinal cord (▶ C1). There, they cause necrosis of the ganglion cells and a reactive perivascular inflammatory infiltrate that initially contains granulocytes and later lymphocytes and plasma cells. This later triggers reactive proliferation of glial cells (▶ D1). The glial cells phagocytize the remains of the ganglion cells in a process known as neuronophagy (▶ D2). This is later followed by reparative gliosis of the anterior horn.

✚ **Clinical result:** Patients exhibit flaccid paralysis (usually in the extremities). Respiratory paralysis can be fatal.

☺ **Prominent patient:** Franklin D. Roosevelt (1882–1945), US President.

❗ **Note:** *Viral encephalitis* is classified as follows:
Polioencephalitis is encephalitis of the gray matter.
Leukoencephalitis is encephalitis of the white matter.
- *Perivenous encephalitis* (postinfectious encephalitis or postvaccinal encephalitis) involves formation of autoreactive antibodies, leading to disseminated perivascular lymphocytic infiltrates (primarily around the veins). This damages the surrounding myelin and axons, producing small perivascular foci of demyelination.
- *Hemorrhagic encephalitis* (as an anaphylactic reaction secondary to influenza infection or penicillin allergy) damages the microvasculature, leading to disseminated diapedesis (p. 398). Bleeding occurs in the form of minor massive hemorrhages, annular hemorrhages, focal bleeding, and in a fleabite pattern (cerebral purpura). This leads to disseminated tissue necrosis and eventually to fatal cerebral edema.

Panencephalitis is encephalitis of the gray and white matter.

A RNA virus infection

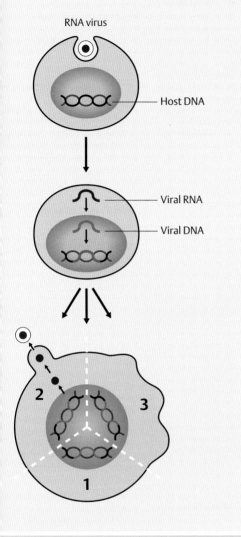

RNA virus

Host DNA

Viral RNA

Viral DNA

2

3

1

B DNA virus infection

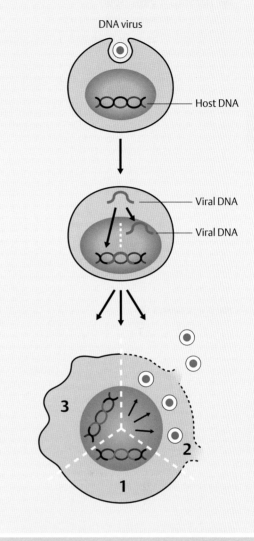

DNA virus

Host DNA

Viral DNA

Viral DNA

3

2

1

Poliomyelitis
(HE) x 50

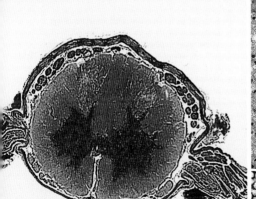

D Poliomyelitis
(HE) x 200 (insert: TEM, x 100000)

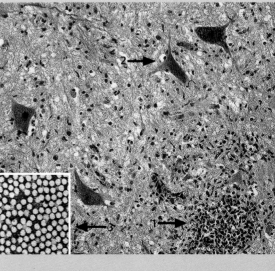

■ Hepatitis A Virus (HAV)

Pathogen that causes viral hepatitis A.

Pathogenesis: The virus is spread by fecal-oral contamination. It initially multiples in the bowel, causing brief viremia. The virus is hepatotropic, i.e., it attacks only the liver. Viruses are excreted in the stool via bile.

Morphology: Acute hepatitis with apoptosis of single cells (= Councilman bodies, single-cell-necrosis; p. 128, 132) surrounded by lymphocytes and Kupffer cells leads to hyperbilirubinemia (p. 108). Later the histiocytes (Kupffer cells) clear away the apoptotic cells, leading to storage of ceroid in histiocytes (p. 28) and liver-cell regeneration.

Pathogen indication: apoptotic Councilman bodies (▶ A).

✚ **Clinical presentation:** The disorder resembles hepatitis B (p. 248) but is more benign. Its clinical course is never chronic.

■ Rhinoviruses

Pathogen that causes viral rhinitis (coryza).

Pathogenesis: The virus spreads from one person to the next by droplet infection, primarily in the winter months. The virus adheres to the ICAM-1 molecule (adhesion molecule), penetrates the cell, and causes cell injury. This results in serous catarrhal rhinitis (p. 204).

✚ **Clinical presentation:** Symptoms include rhinitis with a watery mucous secretion (coryza). Immunity is specific to the virus and lasts only briefly. This and the broad range of rhinoviruses (over 100 serotypes) are responsible for recurrent colds in the same patient.

Uncoated Double-Stranded RNA Viruses

Reoviridae

■ Rotavirus

Pathogen that causes diarrhea in infants (▶ B).

Pathogenesis: The virus enters the mouth by droplet infection. It multiplies in the villi of the small bowel, causing serous enteritis.

✚ **Clinical result:** Infants suffer massive diarrhea. Massive fluid loss leads to life-threatening dehydration with persistent skin folds (desiccation).

Coated Single-Strand RNA Viruses

Togaviridae

Also referred to as arboviruses (**ar**thropod-**bo**rne viruses).

■ Alpha virus

Pathogen is transmitted by insect bites and leads to (mostly) asymptomatic or benign infections, fever, exanthema, and arthralgias.

■ Rubivirus

Pathogen that causes rubella ("German" measles; ▶ C).

Pathogenesis: Virus enters through the nasopharynx, multiplying in local lymphatic tissues. Viremia occurs, spreading the virus throughout the body. Immunity is lifelong. Rubella viruses are embryotrophic (they have an affinity for embryonic tissue). Clinical syndrome depends on the patient's age.

✚ **Clinical presentation and morphology:**
Rubella: Infection during childhood or adolescence presents as a harmless infectious disease with exanthema progressing inferiorly, and lymphadenitis of the throat. The disease creates permanent immunity. Postinfectious encephalitis is a rare sequela.
Rubella placentitis: Initial infection occurring during the first trimester of pregnancy results in passage of the virus through the placental barrier, where it causes nonreactive villous necrosis of the placenta (nonreactive due to the fetal immune system's immaturity); can lead to spontaneous abortion.
Congenital rubella syndome: Deformity syndrome resulting from initial infection during weeks 0-8 of pregnancy, characterized by a quartet of symptoms:
– *Rubella cataract* due to necrosis of the epithelium of the lens in the lenticular nucleus (▶ D,F).
– *Ventricular septum defects* (▶ E) due to virus-induced proliferation inhibition in the embryonic heart.
– *Rubella hepatitis* (less frequent) may be anicteric in its clinical course, or may involve cholestasis or cholangiolitis, leading to bile duct destruction an atresia.

Flaviviridae

Pathogens are transmitted by insect bites (dengue or breakbone fever, Russian spring-summer encephalitis virus ("RSSE"), yellow fever) or by feces (hepatitis C,G).

✚ **Clinical presentation and morphology:**
– *Dengue:* Febrile arthritis and myositis.
– *Meningoencephalitis of early summer:* Risk groups include forestry workers and hikers. Ticks are the vectors of this often lethal disease.
– *Yellow fever:* Mosquitoes act as vectors; infection produces necrotizing hepatitis with fine-droplet fatty degeneration an apoptotic liver cell necrosis in the central portions of the lobes without significant cellular inflammatory reaction. Severe cases also show planobular necrosis (necrosis of the entire hepatic lobe) and hemorrhagic fever like that caused by arenaviruses (p. 242).

Hepatitis A (Councilman body)
(HE) x 300

B **Rotaviruses**
(TEM) x 200000

Rubella viruses
(TEM) x 100000

D **Rubella cataract** (early)

Rubella: Ventricular septum defect

F **Rubella cataract** (late)

Orthomyxoviridae

■ Influenza Virus

Pathogen that causes type A, B, and C viral influenza (► A).

Pathogenesis: Droplet infection (► B) leads to adhesion of the virus (► A) to the ciliated epithelium by means of two surface proteins it uses as "spikes." These include neuraminidase, which exposes sugar, and hemagglutinin (viral lectin), which leads to adhesion of the virus to the exposed sugars (glycophorin A).

The virus then migrates into the cytoplasm when the viral fusion peptide is released by lysosomal proteolysis. This results in the formation of giant cells from infected host cells.

Pathogen indication: hemorrhagic necrotizing inflammation.

✚ **Clinical presentation:** Because of the genetic instability of the virus, its pathogenicity and antigenicity vary from one epidemic to the next, meaning that there is effectively no immunity against it.

Aggressive strains cause hemorrhagic and usually pseudomembranous tracheobronchitis, leading to postviral superinfection with staphylococci and/or Hemophilus influenzae. Rarely, death may result from hemorrhagic leukoencephalitis.

Paramyxoviridae

■ Parainfluenza Virus

Pathogen that causes flu and croup syndrome.

✚ **Clinical presentation and morphology:** These viruses (types I-IV a and b) are genetically stable. They multiply in the respiratory ciliated epithelia, damaging it and causing flu-like disorders and croup syndrome, primarily in children (p. 208).

■ Mumps Virus

Pathogen that causes epidemic parotidis (mumps).

Pathogenesis: Droplet infection leads to adhesion of the virus to the ciliated respiratory epithelium. The virus multiplies with cytolysis, leading to viremia. The virus is organotrophic.

✚ **Clinical presentation and morphology:** This highly contagious virus causes a febrile inflammation with painful, serous, and later fibrous, parotidis with cytolysis. This produces an infiltrate with granulocytes, lymphocytes, and histiocytes and parotid swelling. Chewing elicits pain, and patients have a set facial expression.

✚ **Complications:** Orchitis (► C) occurs in 40% of all cases and oophoritis in 5%. Rare complications include pancreatitis, perivenous meningoencephalitis, and leukoencephalitis.

■ Respiratory Syncytial Virus (RSV)

Pathogen of the pneumovirus group.

✚ **Clinical presentation and morphology:** This infection commonly occurs in infants, who develop peribronchiolitis with epithelial necrosis. This results in formation of syncytial giant cells and intraluminal pseudopapillary epithelial regenerative tissue that obstructs the distal bronchioles and causes the lung to collapse (resorption atelectasis). The peribronchial inflammation then progresses to peribronchial pneumonia.

■ Measles Virus

Pathogen that causes measles (highly contagious ► D).

Pathogenesis: The viral envelope does not contain any neuraminidase. However it does contain H antigen, which causes hemagglutination, and F antigen, which leads to cell fusion and formation of giant cells.

Spread by droplet infection, the virus uses its F antigen to penetrate the ciliated respiratory epithelium, inducing infected cells to fuse with uninfected cells to form giant cells. The virus replicates within these giant cells, causing primary viremia and infecting primarily the T cells in lymphatic organs. This then leads to secondary viremia.

Pathogen indication: Warthin-Finkeldey cells with multiple clustered nuclei (► E).

✚ **Clinical presentation and morphology:** The exanthema stage follows a 10-day incubation period.
- *Measles enanthema (Koplik spots)* begins in the oral mucos later progressing to
- *Measles exanthema* (flat and macular) with mottled erythema covering the face and body.

✚ **Complications:**
Measles croup can occur in infants (p. 208).
Measles giant-cell pneumonia (► F) is an often fatal interstitial pneumonia occurring prior to outbreak of the exanthema stage. It occurs primarily in children whose immune resistance is weakened.
Acute perivenous measles encephalitis is rare but fatal in infants and adults.
Subacute sclerosing panencephalitis (Dawson encephalitis) is a rare complication, occurring primarily in children and young adults. It is triggered by hypermutated defective measles virus (slow virus) and leads to perivenous lymphocytic infiltration with destruction of neurons and myelin. This causes secondary sclerosis of the white matter, which leads to dementia and death within six months to a year.

Arenaviridae

Pathogen: Spherical to pleomorphic RNA viruses with a granular sand-like internal structure. Small rodents act as vectors.

✚ **Clinical presentation and morphology:**
Meningitis: The LCM virus (in Europe and North America) produces lymphocytic choriomeningitis (inflammation of the meninges and choroid plexus).
Viral hemorrhagic fever: The Lassa virus in Africa, Junin virus in Argentina, and Machupo virus in Bolivia lead to inflammation of primarily the lung and liver that progresses to multiple organ failure.

Influenza viruses
(TEM) x 200000

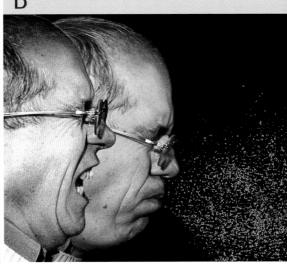

B **Droplet infection**

Mumps orchitis

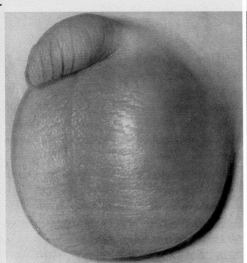

D Measles virus
(TEM) x 200000

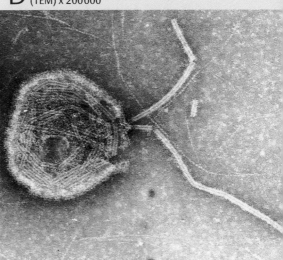

Warthin-Finkeldey cells (measles)
(PAS) x 200

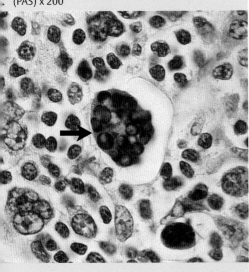

F Measles giant cell pneumonia
(HE) x 100

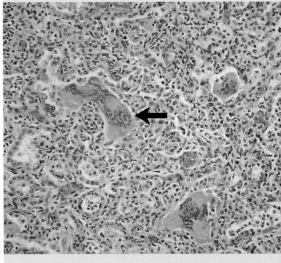

Rhabdoviridae

Pathogen: Bullet-shaped single-stranded RNA viruses.

■ Rabies Virus

Pathogen that causes rabies (► A).

The virus causes disease in humans and other mammals.

Textbook example of an infectious disease with a very high mortality rate.

Pathogenesis: The virus is spread by a bite or by contamination with the saliva of a rabid domesticated or wild animal. The virus initially multiplies in the tissue at the point of entry, for example in muscle cells. From there it migrates via the nerve fibers into the central nervous system. The virus replicates in the ganglion cells (acetylcholine receptors are virus receptors). These newly formed viruses spread back via autonomous nerves to peripheral organs (primarily the salivary glands, leading to excretion of virus in saliva).

Morphology of rabies encephalitis: Signs of hyperemia are present with minor bleeding, infiltrate containing lymphocytes and histiocytes, and occasionally destruction of neurons. In at least 75% of all cases, the nonnecrotic ganglion cells (primarily in the cornu ammonis, hippocampus, and brain stem) and the Purkinje cells (in the cerebellar cortex) contain inclusion bodies of replicating viruses.

Pathogen indication: Negri bodies, inclusion bodies within the cytoplasm of the ganglion cells, especially in the cornu Ammonis.

✚ **Clinical presentation:** The clinical syndrome is characterized by encephalitis, which is almost invariably fatal for humans and animals once it has broken out. The disorder passes through three stages following an incubation period of 1–2 months.
– *Prodromal stage* involves burning sensation in the bite wound, nausea, and vomiting.
– *Excitation stage* involves spasms in the pharyngeal muscles that may be easily precipitated by the sight of water (hydrophobia). Affected humans and animals are irritable with fits of uncontrolled anger.
– *Paralytic stage* ends with fatal respiratory paralysis.

Retroviridae

Definition: Viruses that employ the enzyme reverse transcriptase during their replication cycle, reversing the normal transcription process and encoding DNA from their RNA.

■ Oncornaviruses

Acronym: **onco**genic **RNA** viruses.

Pathogen: RNA viruses with characteristics that induce tumor and leukemia. These include the human T-cell lymphotropic viruses (HTLV), which cause disease in humans.

— *HTLV-1* causes acute T-cell lymphoma leukemia in southwestern Japan, the Caribbean, and in many sub-Saharan African populations.
— *HTLV-2* has been isolated in some cases of chronic T-cell lymphoma or leukemia.

Pathogenesis: Refer to the chapter on tumors (p. 334).

■ Human Immunodeficiency Virus (HIV)

Pathogen that causes AIDS, a pandemic sexually transmitted disease (p. 192; ► C, D).

The pathogen is genetically unstable.
— *HIV-1* causes the most cases in the Western industrialized countries;
— *HIV-2* is endemic in Africa and parts of Asia.

Transmission mechanisms include:
— *Blood and blood components,* such as transfusions, unsterile syringes among intravenous drug users, clotting factors (in hemophiliacs; p. 192);
— *Semen* (especially in anal intercourse);
— *Mother-to-infant transmission* by intrauterine or perinatal infection, or postnatal infection by breast feeding.

Pathogenesis: The CD4 antigen on certain cells such as T cells, macrophages, Langerhans cells, and follicular reticulum cells provides the main receptor for the gp120 glycoprotein on the HIV viruses. This antigen enables the virus to invade the cell. Infected CD4 cells express gp120 on their surfaces, spreading the infection from cell to cell and causing cells to fuse together into viral giant cells (p. 10), primarily in the brain. The virus initially remains latent; patients are clinically normal but are virus carriers. After an incubation period of 7–8 years, cytokines or activating proteins of other viruses (perhaps herpes viruses) are expressed for reasons still unknown. This activates the HIV virus, leading to a

Pathogenetic chain reaction: HIV replication causes progressive destruction of the T_4 helper cells and leads to numeric atrophy of the lymphatic tissue (► B; Appendix) by an apoptotic mechanism not yet understood. The immune system is therefore no longer able to mount a T-cell-mediated response to certain soluble antigens. This effectively disables the body's defenses against intracellular parasitic and opportunistic pathogens (p. 192), leading to fatal infection.

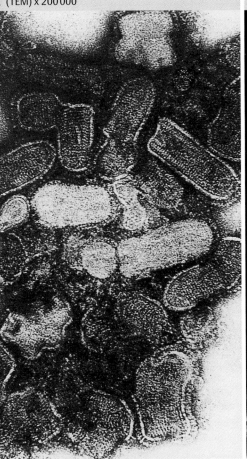

Rabies virus
(TEM) x 200 000

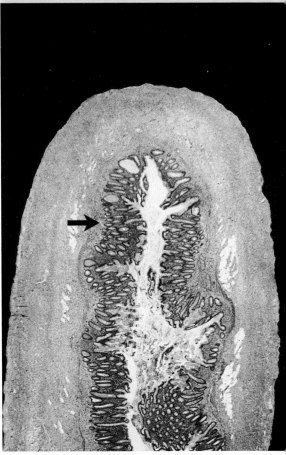

B **AIDS appendicitis**
x 25

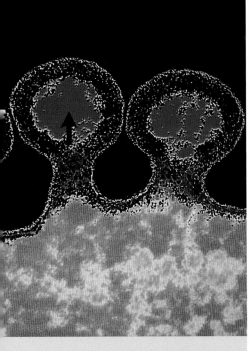

HIV- budding
idealized color-distorted image, (TEM) x 50 000

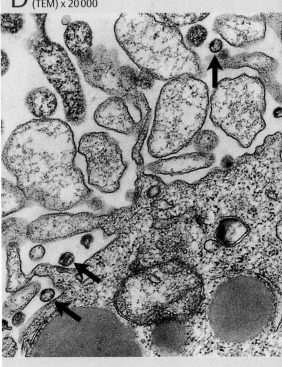

D **HIV-budding**
(TEM) x 20 000

Coated Double-Stranded RNA Viruses

Poxviridae

■ Variola Virus

Pathogen that causes smallpox. This virus multiplies in the cytoplasm of the host cells, causing a vesicular and later pustular skin inflammation.

According to the World Health Organization, the virus has been fully eradicated since 1977. Before that time, it triggered epidemics of usually fatal disease.

■ Molluscum Contagiosum Virus

Pathogen causing contagious viral warts.

Morphology: The central depression (► A) of the infectious skin tumors contains infected cells with eosinophilic cytoplasmic inclusion bodies of viral material. The infectious lesions can discharge these infected cells with cellular detritus (hence the name of the disorder).

Pathogen indication: Eosinophilic cytoplasmic inclusion bodies in tumor-cell detritus (► A2).

✚ **Clinical presentation:** The disorder occurs in children and AIDS patients, exhibiting pinhead-sized nodular lesions with central depressions. The disease resolves spontaneously.

Herpesviridae

■ Herpes Simplex Virus (HSV)

Pathogens causing vesicular skin and mucosal inflammations and, rarely, encephalitis. There, the virus multiplies by budding (► B) a few days before the typical rashes appear. The virus rapidly spreads via sensory and autonomous neurons to the cells of regional ganglia, which the virus uses as a temporary replication site (replication may include cytolysis). From the ganglia, the virus spreads to the ganglion cells of other regions of neural supply. Within a short time a persistent latent infection without further replication of the virus becomes established. Several factors may reactivate the virus.

These include:
— Ultraviolet radiation;
— Febrile infectious factors;
— Menstruation;
— Emotional irritation;
— Immunosuppression.

These factors reactivate replication of the virus, resulting in transport of the virus to the surface of the body and causing recurrence of the rash.

Morphology: Occasionally infected cells will fuse into multinucleated giant cells (► C1). The cytopathic effect of the virus disrupts the contact between the cells, causing formation of epidermal vesicles containing infected cells with replicating viruses (► C2, D).

Pathogen identification: Herpes infected cells have homogeneous cytoplasm resembling ground-glass with homogeneous nucleic inclusion bodies (Cowdry bodies). Immunohistochemical findings include antibodies against HSV-1 and HSV-2.

✚ **Clinical presentation and morphology of HSV-1:** *Herpetic gingivostomatitis:* Vesicular aphthoid inflammation of the oral mucosa and gums (► D). *Herpetic esophagitis:* Vesicular inflammation of the esophageal mucosa (► E), later progressing to aphthoid ulcerous inflammation (► F). *Herpetic keratoconjunctivitis:* Necrotizing inflammation of the cornea and conjunctiva of the eye. *Herpetic encephalitis:* Acute cerebral inflammation with bilateral necroses, primarily in the temporal regions. The disorder is usually fatal.

✚ **Clinical presentation and morphology of HSV-2:** *Vulvovaginitis* and *herpetic balanitis:* This disorder primarily occurs in AIDS patients. It is a sexually transmitted vesicular inflammation of the genitals. Sequelae may include recurrent genital herpes and, rarely, generalized herpes.

■ Varicella Zoster Virus

Pathogen causing chicken pox and herpes zoster (shingles).

The varicella zoster virus is also known as α-herpes virus. The varicella virus is identical to the zoster virus. This is the contagious volatile virus best known for causing chicken pox.

✚ **Clinical presentation and morphology:** (► G): *Chicken pox:* The initial infection occurs in the mucosa of the upper respiratory tract. From there, the disease spreads by hematogenous dissemination. Symptoms include:
– *Enanthema* (spotty erythema) in the ears, nasopharynx, and conjunctiva;
– *Exanthema* with pox-like vesicles (hence the name chickenpox) on the face, trunk, and extremities (but not on the hands or feet);
– *Lymphadenopathy* (generalized and cervical, and nuchal).

The primary mucosal lesions are presumably the point of origin for neural transport of the viruses to the spinal ganglia. This produces a latent infection of the ganglion cells and, rarely, postinfectious encephalitis. Decades later, the virus may be reactivated by radiation, immunosuppression, or malignant lymphoma, and produce herpes zoster.

Herpes zoster: This necrotizing skin inflammation (► G) covers a belt of skin corresponding to the area supplied by the respective nerve root. It is painful and associated with ganglionitis.

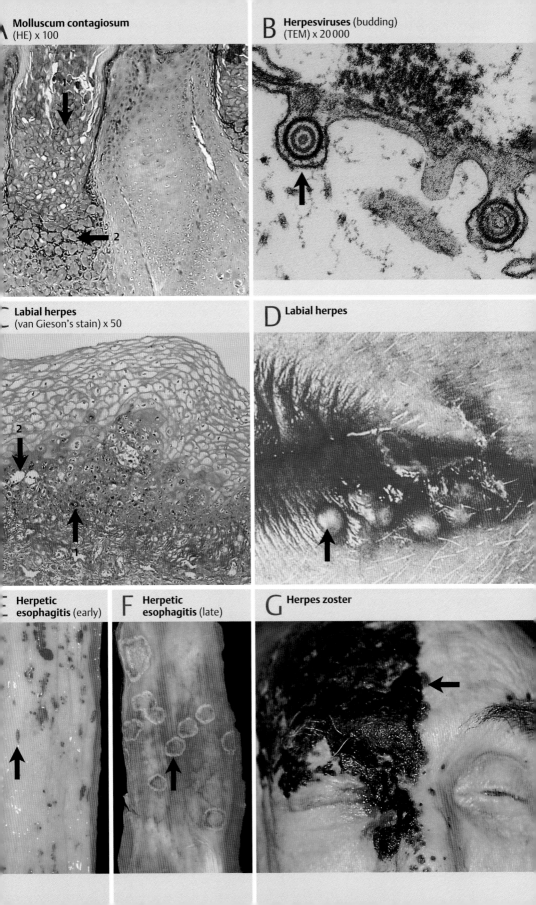

A Molluscum contagiosum (HE) x 100

B Herpesviruses (budding) (TEM) x 20 000

C Labial herpes (van Gieson's stain) x 50

D Labial herpes

E Herpetic esophagitis (early)

F Herpetic esophagitis (late)

G Herpes zoster

■ **Cytomegalovirus** (CMV)

Pathogen is a β-herpes virus (▶ A).

Pathogenesis: Cytomegalovirus is present in saliva, urine (used to confirm diagnosis), semen, and breast milk. Infection occurs by contact with secretions or through the placenta. The cytopathic effect of the virus leads to creation of infected giant cells.

Pathogen identification: includes mononuclear cytomegalic giant cells with large intranuclear viral inclusion bodies ("owl's eye cells"; ▶ B). Immunohistochemical findings include anti-CMV antibodies (p. 10).

✚ **Clinical presentation and course:** This depends on the relative degree of immunocompetence:
– *Intrauterine infection* as a primary infection in an immunocompromised mother leads to fetal death or generalized infection in the newborn with encephalitis and hepatitis.
– *Initial infection in immunocompetent patients* (children and adults) usually begins unnoticed with the virus remaining latent. Decreased immunocompetence leads to activation of the virus and usually harmless viremia. This usually results in CMV infection of isolated organs (primarily the salivary glands). Viruses are contained in the saliva and may spread by droplet infection in places such as day care centers. Transfusion of CMV-contaminated blood produces mononucleosis-like lymphadenitis (see below).
– *Initial infection in immunocompetent patients* or reactivation of the virus leads to generalized inflammation, leading to ulcerous gastrointestinal inflammation with bleeding, chorioretinitis (causing blindness), and death.

■ **Epstein-Barr Virus** (EBV)

Pathogen (γ-herpes virus) causes infectious mononucleosis, Burkitt lymphoma, and, occasionally, nasopharyngeal carcinoma (▶ C).

EBV are also involved in the development of peripheral T-cell lymphomas of the nasopharynx, subtypes of Hodgkin lymphomas, and primary cerebral B-cell lymphomas.

Pathogenesis of infectious mononucleosis: The main point of entry is the oropharynx (hence the synonym "kissing disease"). The target cells are B cells (keratinocytes).

Infection causes B cells to express the viral apoptosis blocker LMP-1. This transforms them into cells that theoretically are permanently proliferative. As a result, large quantities of virus-specific T cells appear in the blood (blood lymphocytosis). Special T cells stop this B-cell proliferation, and cytotoxic T cells disable the apoptosis inhibition, causing B-cell destruction.

Pathogen identification: includes immunohistochemical findings of viral LMP-1 (late membrane protein).

✚ **Clinical presentation and morphology:**
Infectious mononucleosis is a generalized febrile disorder associated with the formation of heterophil agglutinin (Paul-Bunnel test) and several lesions including:
– *Blood lymphocytosis* with mobilization of monocytic T cells leading to infectious mononucleosis;
– *Lymphadenitis of the throat* with widening of the paracortical zone due to proliferation of T cells, T immunoblasts (▶ D), and lymphatic plasma cells;
– *Splenomegaly* with inflammatory swelling.
Concomitant viral hepatitis may occur.

Coated Single-Stranded DNA Viruses

Hepadnaviridae

■ **Hepatitis B Virus** (HBV)

Pathogen that causes hepatitis B (serum hepatitis).

The pathogen occurs in blood and glandular secretions and is transmitted through wounds, blood transfusions, and contact between mucous membranes, i.e., via sexual contact.

Pathogenesis: After infection, the virus enters cells of the hepatic parenchyma and multiplies therein, producing what are referred to as "ground-glass" hepatocytes (p. 14). Viral proliferation causes cytolysis. The infection may be overcome by antibodies that neutralize the HBV and/or by a cytotoxic immune reaction, in which infected cells and hunted down and destroyed.

Morphology: HBc antibodies appear with the onset of the disease. Apoptosis occurs in individual hepatocytes in the center of the lobe, usually mediated by lymphocytes (p. 128, 132). These cells appear as eosinophilic Councilman bodies. In severe courses of the disease, lytic necrosis of groups of liver cells occurs (▶ F). The dead infected cells are phagocytized by Kupffer cells and broken down to ceroid pigment (p. 28). Lymphocytic infiltrate is present in the portal regions.

Pathogen indication: includes Councilman bodies and ground-glass hepatocytes (p. 14). Immunohistochemical findings include anti-HBV antibodies (▶ E).

✚ **Clinical presentation and course:** Where there is *complete elimination of the virus,* the clinical course is uncomplicated. Following fever, nausea, loss of appetite, joint pain, and often jaundice, the liver regenerates.
Where the *virus is not eliminated,* the disorder becomes chronic, usually lasting over 6 months. It then progresses to two main forms of chronic hepatitis.
– *Inactive form:* It is characterized by inflammation only in the portal region; its prognosis for healing is usually good. In the
– *Active form:* The inflammation spreads from the portal region to the hepatic lobes, leading to liver cirrhosis (p. 42) and hepatocellular carcinoma (p. 328, 332).

☺ **Prominent patient:** Wolfgang Borchert (1921–1947), postwar German author.

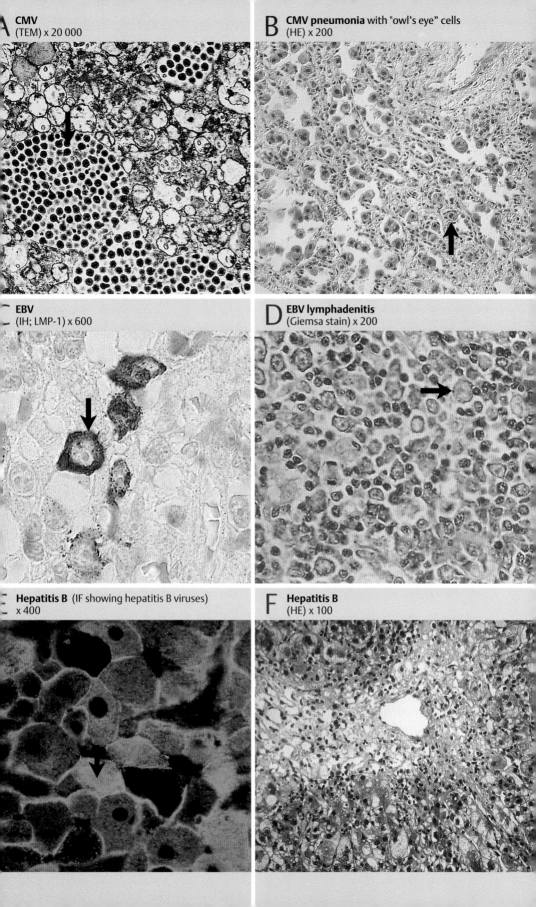

A CMV
(TEM) x 20 000

B CMV pneumonia with "owl's eye" cells
(HE) x 200

C EBV
(IH; LMP-1) x 600

D EBV lymphadenitis
(Giemsa stain) x 200

E Hepatitis B (IF showing hepatitis B viruses)
x 400

F Hepatitis B
(HE) x 100

Uncoated Double-Stranded DNA Viruses

Adenoviridae

Pathogenesis: A lytic infection transforms infected cells into a homogeneous mass with dense smudged nucleus ("smudge cells"), leading to necrotizing inflammation (p. 218).

Pathogen indication: includes "smudge cells" (► B) with a large homogeneous basophilic cell nucleus (and crystalline accumulation of virus) and type A Cowdry inclusions, eosinophilic viral nuclear inclusions (► A1) surrounded by a ring (► A2) and a halo of chromatin.

✚ **Clinical presentation:** Viruses produce the following disorders in infants and children that are invariably associated with lymphadenitis:
- Infections of the upper respiratory tract;
- Pharyngoconjunctival fever;
- Hemorrhagic urocystitis;
- Gastroenteritis;
- Epidemic keratoconjunctivitis in young adults (such as military recruits).

Papovaviridae

Pathogens that cause papillomas in the upper respiratory tract, skin warts, and anal or genital condylomas. Papillomaviruses also have a carcinogenic effect (p. 332, 370).

✚ **Clinical presentation and morphology:**
Common warts (verruca vulgaris; ► C): HPV type 2 and type 4 enter skin keratocytes through direct contact (such as walking barefoot around a public swimming pool). This results in virus-induced keratocyte proliferation. The locally proliferating epidermis forms epithelial folds with the subepidermal stromal layers that are passively involved (papilloma, p. 370) and becomes cornified, exhibiting parakeratosis. At the same time, viruses replicate in large quantities in the superficial epithelial cells. This leads to formation of inclusion bodies (► D).

Pathogen indication: nuclear inclusion bodies (homogenous masses of viruses in crystalline beds) and basophilic cytoplasmic inclusion bodies consisting of oversized nonviral keratohyalin granules (► D).

✚ **Condyloma acuminatum** is also known as venereal wart. These occur in dense groups of projecting warts (► E) in the anogenital region and may be spread by sexual contact.

Pathogen indication: includes koilocytes, squamous cells with a perinuclear vacuole (► F) and heterochromic nucleus.

✚ **Flat condyloma** is a flat, circumscribed whitish thickening of the epithelium of the uterine cervix, or other site, with enlargement, heterochromia (p. 8), and koilocytosis of the cell nuclei (► F). Depending on the type of virus involved (type 16, 18, 31, or 33), the lesion should be evaluated as a precancerous condition.

Miopapovaviridae

Pathogen that causes multiple tumors in laboratory animals (young hamsters).

Pathogenesis: The initial infection is latent despite the high degree of contamination in humans (with serum antibodies). The disease is initially asymptotic but reduced resistance leads to reactivation of the virus with symptomatic outbreak of the disorder (virus is detectable in urine).

✚ **Clinical presentation and morphology:**
- *JC virus type:* It causes opportunistic infection in immunocompromised patients (AIDS or tumor patients; p. 354). The virus multiplies in oligodendrocytes, producing viral inclusion bodies. This leads to oligodendrocyte necrosis and focal demyelination in the white matter. This progressive multifocal leukoencephalopathy causes death within a period of months.
- *BK virus type:* It infects the epithelium of the urogenital. This infection is initially latent in most cases. Immunosuppression (especially in transplant recipients) reactivates the virus, which leads to hemorrhagic urocystitis.

Uncoated Single-Stranded DNA Viruses

Parvoviridae

▬ Parvovirus B19

Pathogen that causes a) erythema infectiosum in children and b) hemolytic anemia primarily in fetuses.

Pathogenesis: The disorder spreads by droplet infection. The virus attacks erythroblasts and replicates, causing a lytic infection that destroys erythroblasts in bone marrow. Specific antibodies are formed within a week; these allow regeneration of the erythroblasts so that erythroblast destruction remains a transient feature of the disorder.

Pathogen indication: includes abnormally large proerythroblasts in bone marrow, especially toward the end of the phase of erythroblast destruction.

✚ **Complications:**
- *Severe anemic crises* may occur in cases with reduced erythrocyte longevity (e.g. spherocytosis) and compensatory increased erythropoiesis.
- *Hemolytic anemia* can occur in fetuses, ranging from generalized edemas to fetal hydrops (abnormal accumulation of serous fluid in fetal tissues; p. 424).

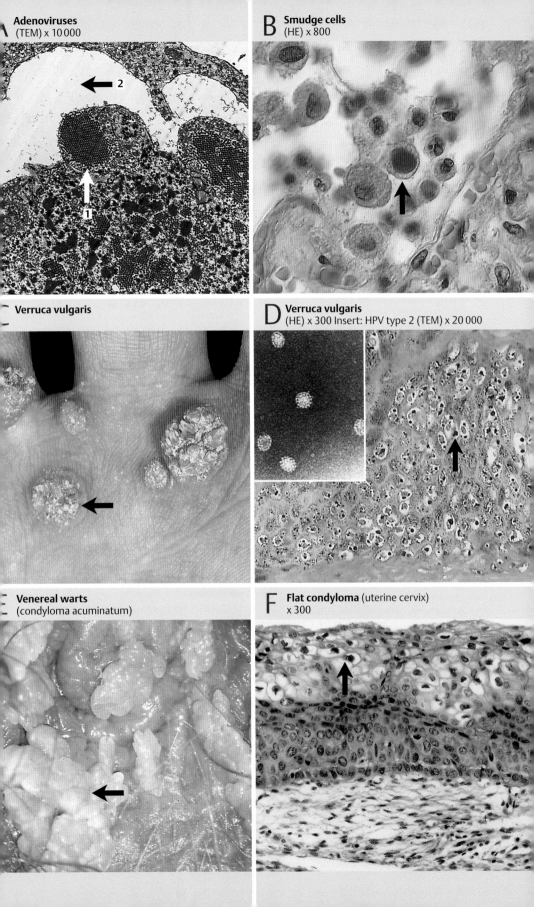

A Adenoviruses (TEM) x 10 000

B Smudge cells (HE) x 800

Verruca vulgaris

D Verruca vulgaris (HE) x 300 Insert: HPV type 2 (TEM) x 20 000

E Venereal warts (condyloma acuminatum)

F Flat condyloma (uterine cervix) x 300

Prion Diseases

Synonym: spongiform encephalopathy.

Definition: Generic term for spongiform encephalopathies with the following characteristics:
— **transmissible** by prions;[1]
— **typical lesions** involving spongiform tissue damage without inflammatory and/or immune reaction;
— **clinical course** involving an incubation period of months to a few years (5–10 years) and ending in death (formerly referred to as slow virus infection).

Routes of infection:
— **Hematogenous infection** is thought to occur during treatment with somatotropic hormones from human pituitary glands.
— **Infection from inhaling** contaminated feed meal is thought to occur.
— **Infection from corneal transplants** taken from prion-infected donor cadavers is thought to occur, with the prion traveling through the recipient's optic nerve to the brain.
— **Peroral infection** has been thought to occur via the following pathogenetic chain reaction. British sheep infected with scrapie (see below) were slaughtered and processed into feed meal without sufficient thermal processing. This animal- protein meal was then fed to cattle, effectively turning these natural herbivores into carnivores. The cattle then developed "mad cow disease" or bovine spongiform encephalopathy (BSE).
The increased incidence of prion diseases among British beef eaters shows that the disease can be transmitted to humans.

Pathogenesis: Prion protein is an infectious glycoprotein, PrP^{Sc}. Its physiologic counterpart is the protein PrP^C in the cell membrane, which has homologies to an acetylcholine receptor. Physiologic PrP^C is involved in cell adhesion and restricts the function of synapses. PrP^{Sc} is resistant to protease, which cause it to accumulate in lysosomes. Association with heparan-containing proteoglycans produces amyloid fibers, which in turn combine to form amyloid plaques (p. 48).

Morphology: Brain atrophy occurs with ventricular expansion (► B, C). Spongy dystrophic tissue is present in the gray matter (especially in the cerebral cortex and basal ganglia). This spongiform dystrophy (► D) leads to regional destruction of nerve cells (► A). The Purkinje cells become rarified, astroglia proliferation occurs (► A4), and Kuru plaques of PrP^{Sc} amyloid

develop in the subcortical cerebral medulla, especially in the cerebrum and cerebellum (► A1, A2).

Pathogen indication: includes Kuru plaques and a spongiform lesion in the brain's gray matter.

Disorders Associated with Prions

■ Creutzfeldt-Jakob Disease

Definition: Acquired human prion disease with encephalopathy that leads to dementia at an early age.

✚ Clinical presentation:
Without exposure to BSE, disease onset is after the age of 70 and its clinical course lasts several months.
With exposure to BSE, onset of the disease is after the age of 20 and its clinical course lasts several years.
- *Early symptoms* include neurologic deficits (gait and speech abnormalities) that progress to spastic paralysis and myoclonus.
- *Late symptoms* include dementia, progressing to decerebrate rigidity and eventually death.

■ Gerstmann's Hereditary Senile Ataxia

Definition: Inherited form of human prion disease with encephalopathy leading to early dementia.

✚ Clinical presentation: Patients present with cerebellar ataxia that progresses to dementia and eventually death.

■ Kuru

Definition: Epidemic human prion disease occurring among the indigenous population of New Guinea as a result of the ritual consumption of human brains.

✚ Clinical presentation: Dementia begins in adolescence and progresses to death.

■ Scrapie

Definition: Epidemic prion disease among sheep and goats.

✚ Clinical presentation: Affected animals exhibit pruritus, causing them to rub off their wool. Gait abnormalities are present, progressing to ataxia and eventually death.

■ Bovine Spongiform Encephalopathy

Synonyms: BSE, mad cow disease.

Definition: Epidemic prion disease occurring among cattle fed with meal containing animal protein.

✚ Clinical presentation: Affected animals exhibit pruritus and gait abnormalities, progressing to ataxia and eventually death.

---

1 Prion = **pr**otein**a**ceous **i**nfectious **a**ge**nt**

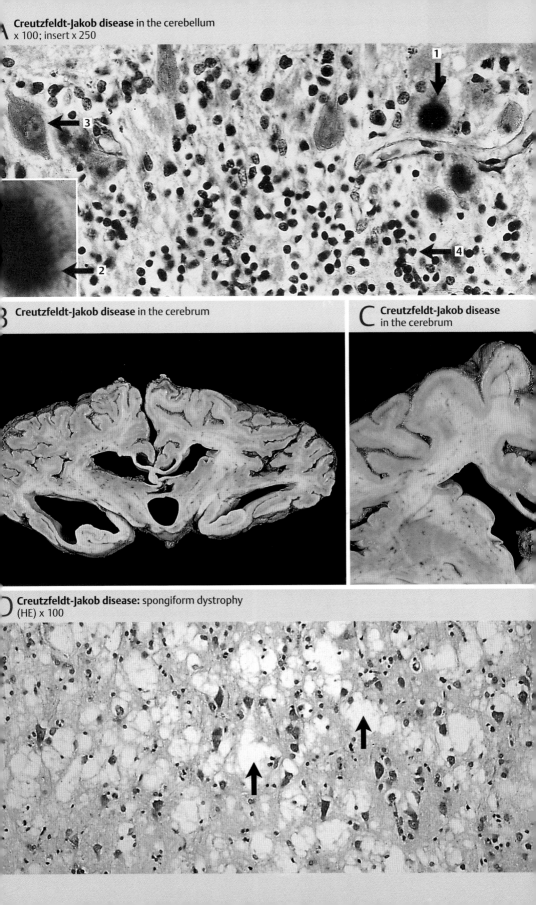

A **Creutzfeldt-Jakob disease** in the cerebellum
x 100; insert x 250

B **Creutzfeldt-Jakob disease** in the cerebrum

C **Creutzfeldt-Jakob disease** in the cerebrum

D **Creutzfeldt-Jakob disease:** spongiform dystrophy
(HE) x 100

15 Attack From an Ecological Niche
Bacterial Infection

Summary

To survive in the body, bacteria must first be able to adhere to the cell membrane. Then they must deceive the body's immune mechanisms (virus "virulence") or use toxins to neutralize them so that the bacteria can thrive in this new environment (referred to as colonization). Depending on their specific survival strategy, the bacteria will produce certain inflammatory tissue reactions:

- Invasive bacteria enter the blood stream and can cause sepsis.
- Noninvasive bacteria destroy tissue with their toxins and exotoxins.
- Intracellular bacteria (phagocyte parasites) trigger granulomatous inflammations.

Gram-Positive Cocci

Staphylococci

■ Staphylococcus epidermidis

Pathogen that causes suppurative inflammations and can produce sepsis.

Occurrence: This coagulase-negative pathogen occurs in normal skin flora. It adheres to such structures as plastic catheters, producing sepsis. Its specific capsular characteristics allow it to avoid phagocytosis.

■ Staphylococcus aureus

Pathogen that causes suppurative abscess-forming inflammations (creating a creamy pus) that result in intoxication.

Occurrence: This clustered, coagulase-negative pathogen occurs in skin and mucosal flora (▶ A).

Pathogenesis: Staphylococci form several types of lytic enzymes and toxins that they use to cause tissue liquefaction, which forms abscesses.

- **Coagulase** causes intravascular fibrin thrombi.
- **Staphylokinase** dissolves fibrin.
- **α-Hemolysin** destroys granulocytes and histiocytes.
- **Enterotoxin** produce food poisoning.
- **Toxic shock syndrome toxin** is a powerful antigen.
- **Exfoliative toxins** (causing dermal necrosis) produce epidermal vesicles, leading to necrotizing epidermolysis over the entire body (▶ D) and exfoliative dermatitis or staphylococcal scalded skin syndrome.

➕ **Clinical presentation:** Invasive infections produce abscess-forming inflammation (▶ E). Intoxications produce clinical syndromes at locations remote from the point of entry of the pathogen.

Streptococci

Pathogens that cause suppurative inflammations, leading to secondary immune disorders.

Occurrence: Most of these ubiquitous catalase-negative pathogens are found in the oral flora.

Classification of streptococci:

- **α-Hemolysis:** The membrane of the erythrocyte remains largely intact; the pathogen forms colonies on blood agar, producing a green envelope in which hemoglobin is reduced to a compound resembling biliverdin.
- **β-Hemolysis:** The erythrocyte is destroyed and hemoglobin broken down; the pathogen forms colonies on blood agar, producing a large yellow envelope of hemolysis.
- **γ-Hemolysis:** No hemolysis occurs.

■ Streptococcus pyogenes

Pathogen that causes suppurative inflammations (producing runny greenish pus), leading to secondary immune disorders.

Occurrence: The concatenating pathogen (▶ B) is ubiquitous; it belongs to antigen group A and causes β-hemolysis.

Pathogenesis: The capsular substances, toxins, and enzymes of this bacterium are important pathogenetic substances.

- **M protein** is a capsular substance and the main virulence factor. It inhibits phagocytosis and the alternate pathway of complement activation.
- **Capsular hyaluronate** is a secondary virulence factor inhibiting phagocytosis of the pathogen.
- **Lipoteichoic acid** is the adhesion molecule for the pathogen, enabling it to adhere to fibronectin.
- **Streptolysin O and S** are cytotoxins affecting erythrocytes (in which they cause β-hemolysis), macrophages, and granulocytes.
- **Hyaluronidase** promotes dissemination of the pathogen and so doing promotes acute cellulitis (▶ F, focal myositis).
- **DNAase** causes liquefaction of cell nuclei.
- **Streptokinase** or fibrinolysin dissolves the fibrin exudate (resulting in fibrin-free pus), leading to disseminated intravascular coagulation (p. 402).
- **Pyrogenic streptococcal exotoxins A and C**, produced by β-hemolytic group A streptococci, lead to scarlet fever exanthema and enanthema (p. 216).

➕ **Clinical presentation:** Invasive infections include impetigo (purulent skin infections are characterized by formation of crusty lesions; ▶ D), erysipelas, focal inflammation, otitis media, tonsillitis, generalized infectious disease (scarlet fever), and sepsis. Secondary diseases include acute glomerulonephritis (p. 172) and acute rheumatic fever (p. 234).

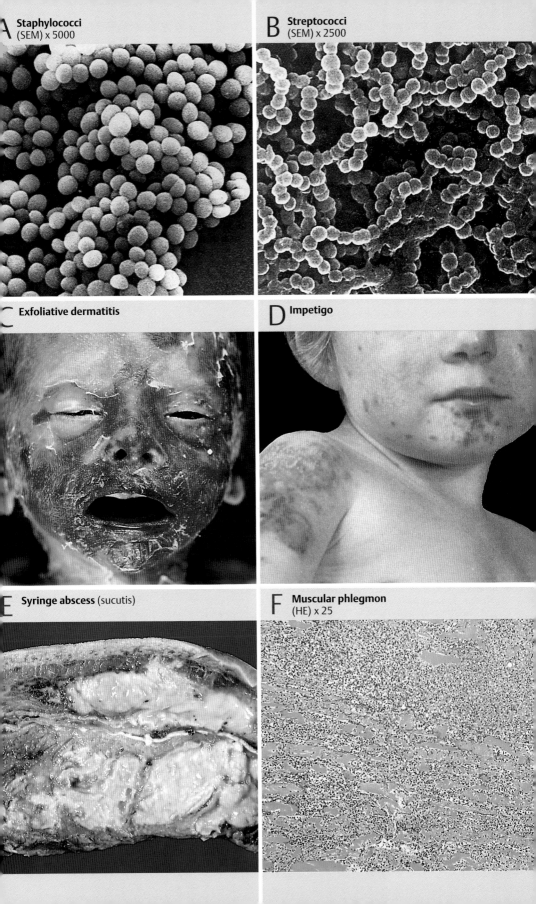

A **Staphylococci** (SEM) x 5000

B **Streptococci** (SEM) x 2500

C **Exfoliative dermatitis**

D **Impetigo**

E **Syringe abscess** (sucutis)

F **Muscular phlegmon** (HE) x 25

Gram-Negative Cocci

Neisseriaceae

■ Neisseria gonorrhoeae

Pathogen that causes gonorrhea; also known as gonococcus.

Pathogenesis: The pathogen is absorbed through phagocytosis by histiocytes and granulocytes (p. 26). It then proliferates in phagocytic vacuoles. The pathogens produce IgA protease, which destroys antibodies in the mucosal secretions. This results in specific colonization of the urogenital tract, peritoneal cavity, rectal mucosa, pharyngeal mucosa, and conjunctiva.

Pathogen identification: is obtained with a pus smear. Gram-negative diplococci are visible in neutrophils (► A).

✚ **Clinical presentation and morphology**:
– *In men*, onset of the disease involves urethritis and purulent discharge, leading to prostatitis and epididymitis.
– *In women*, onset of the disease involves cervicitis and purulent discharge, leading to purulent salpingitis and peritonitis.
– *Perinatal infection* manifests itself in neonates as purulent conjunctivitis (gonococcal conjunctivitis), which can progress to blindness.

■ Neisseria meningitidis

Pathogen that causes meningitis and sepsis; also known as meningococcus or diplococcus.

Occurrence: The organisms are pathogens of the nasopharynx.

Pathogenesis: The pathogen is spread by droplet infection. Absence of antibodies leads to bacteremia, then sepsis (p. 222).

✚ **Clinical presentation:** In addition to harmless diseases of the respiratory tract, there are two fatal disorders. These are
– **Cerebrospinal meningitis** (p. 214) and
– **Waterhouse-Friderichsen syndrome.** The latter involves sepsis accompanied by severe hemorrhagic necrosis, primarily in the adrenal cortex (p. 222).

Gram-Positive Rods

■ Corynebacterium diphtheriae

Pathogen that causes diphtheria (► B).

Pathogenetic chain reaction: The pathogen's exotoxin causes irreversible blockage of cellular protein biosynthesis. This successively leads to cell death, tissue necrosis, and fibrinous pseudomembranous necrotizing inflammation in the upper respiratory tract (p. 208).

Pathogen identification: includes drumstick-like pathogens arranged in configurations resembling Chinese characters (► B).

✚ **Clinical presentation and morphology:** The disease begins as nasal diphtheria and successively spreads to the pharynx, larynx, trachea, and bronchi, where there is risk of asphyxiation. Systemic manifestations can include toxic myocarditis and neuritis of the oculomotor, trigeminal, facial, and glossopharyngeal nerves.

■ Listeria monocytogenes

Pathogen that causes listeriosis and fetal disease.

Sources of infection include domestic animals, dairy products (certain cheeses), and bacterial carriers.

Pathogenesis: The pathogens are opportunistic organisms combatted by phagocytic monocytes (► D) without T-cell activation. *Listeria* contain a
– **Highly toxic endotoxin** that causes hemolysis and lipolysis. They also release a
– **Lipoid** when the bacteria die. This substance produces sepsis in a variety of organs, multiple abscesses, and granulomas.

Pathogen identification: presence of silvery rods in organ cells.

✚ **Clinical presentation and morphology**:
– **Listeriosis** is a generalized febrile infection resembling influenza. In immunocompromised patients, there is a risk of sepsis with meningoencephalitis.
– **Listerial placental inflammation.**
– **Septic infant granulomatosis** is a generalized inflammation in fetuses and neonates with miliary histiocytic and epithelioid granulomas (mixed-cell granulomas) occurring primarily in the skin, lung, and liver (► C).

■ Actinomyces israelii

Pathogen that causes cervicofacial actinomycosis. This anaerobic bacterium has murein typically found in walls of bacteria.

Occurrence: normal oral mucosal flora.

Pathogenesis: The pathogen usually invades through minor injuries of the oral mucosa. It colonizes tissues with a low redox potential (due to hypoxia or accompanying bacteria), producing a chronic granulating fistula-forming inflammation with absorptive fatty degenerative histiocytes.

Pathogen identification: includes the following findings: sulfurous yellow granules the size of rice grains in the pus (histologically, these are a conglomerate of small *Actinomyces* colonies). The pathogen forms the histologic structure of a fungus with branching filaments resembling mycelium surrounded by hyalin protein precipitates (Splendore-Hoeppli phenomenon; ► F2).

✚ **Clinical presentation and morphology:** The main location of lesions is at the angle of the mandible. The pathogen spreads along tissue planes (Skin!), creating fistulas (p. 226) with tunnel-like passages; outward drainage (► E). No lymphadenitis in contributing lymph nodes.

A **Gonococci**
(Gram stain) x 800

B **Corynebacterium diphtheriae**
(Neisser stain) x 800

C **Listeria granuloma** in the liver
(HE) x 100

D **Listeria** in the liver
(silver stain) x 400

E **Actinomycosis of the neck**

F **Actinomyces**
(PAS) x 100

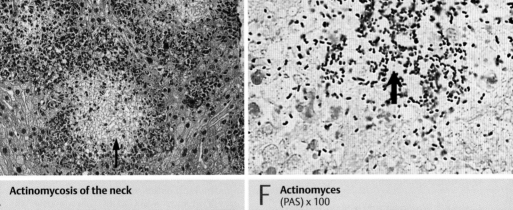

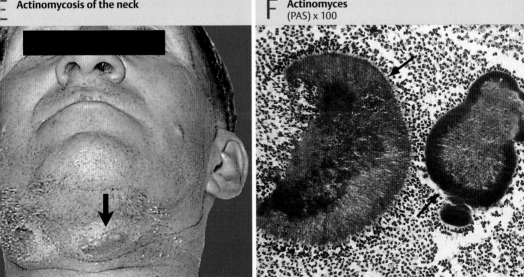

■ Bacillus anthracis

Pathogen that causes anthrax.

Occurrence: domestic animals in southern Europe and South America.

Pathogenesis: The infection can affect the skin, the respiratory tract, or the intestinal tract. The pathogenicity of this highly infectious aerobic organism is due to its

— *Polypeptide capsule,* which protects it against phagocytosis, and an
— *Exotoxin causing tissue necrosis,* which causes microvascular injury. This produces a serous hemorrhagic inflammatory reaction (p. 216).

✚ **Clinical presentation and morphology**: Infection spreads to humans from diseased domestic animals or from contamination from animal products. As a result, the disorder is regarded as an occupational disease of furriers, slaughterhouse workers, wool sorters, and second-hand clothing merchants (hence its popular name "wool sorter's disease").
– *Cutaneous anthrax* presents with painless black and red necrosis of the skin with blackish scabbing. Patients tend to develop erysipelas.
– *Pulmonary anthrax* results from inhalation of contaminated dust, producing hemorrhagic focal pneumonia.
– *Intestinal anthrax* presents with hemorrhagic enteritis and bloody diarrhea.

Clostridia

General pathogen in the form of anaerobic gram-positive rods.

Occurrence: These organisms survive in spores in soil and in a vegetative form in the human intestinal tract.

General pathogenesis: These pathogens cannot break down oxygen metabolites, which are toxic for them. The pathogenicity of this organism is due to the histotoxins, neurotoxins, or exotoxins it produces.

Clostridia – associated Disorders

■ Clostridial Gas Gangrene

Pathogens primarily include Clostridium perfringens, C. novyi, C. septicum, and *C. histolyticum.*

Pathogenesis: Pathogens enter the anaerobic environment of wounds with or without fecal or soil contamination. There they emit exozymes (collagenase, hyaluronidase), δ-toxin (cell membrane rupture), and θ-toxins (porous damage to neutrophils). This produces acutely painful myositis in the form of coagulation necrosis (► A1; p. 130) with dissolution of the myofilament (► B, C). This is accompanied by formation of gas from bacterial fermentation (histologic findings include gas vesicles; ► A2). Palpation findings include subcutaneous gas pockets. The disease is life threatening and often fatal.

■ Tetanus

Synonym: Lockjaw.

Pathogen: Clostridium tetani (► D).

Pathogenesis: Pathogens enter the anaerobic environment of wounds with fecal or soil contamination. There they generate a neurotoxin (tetanospasmin). Retrograde transport of the toxin occurs in the peripheral nerves, where it blocks the synapses of inhibiting interneurons and motor end-plates.

✚ **Clinical result:** Patients present with muscle spasms. Facial spasms produce a characteristic "grinning" expression known as risus sardonicus (► E). Spasms of the rectus abdominis produce a scaphoid posture.

■ Botulism

Pathogen: Clostridium botulinum.

Pathogenesis: Foods that have spoiled in an anaerobic environment (primarily old canned vegetables) result in proliferation of the pathogen, which produces a thermolabile neurotoxin (botulinum toxin). The toxin stops exocytosis of vesicles containing acetylcholine, blocking the motor end-plates and causing muscle paralysis.

❗ **Note:** Botulinum toxin is the strongest known lethal poison.

❗ **Note:** Botulism is an intoxication, not an infection.

■ Antibiotic associated Enterocolitis

Pathogens primarily include *Clostridium difficile* (► F).

Pathogenesis: Antibiotic therapy selects in favor of certain pathogens which produce toxins.
— *Toxin A* is an enterotoxin that disrupts the transport of water and electrolytes through the epithelium, resulting in loss of water.
— *Toxin B* is a cytotoxin that destroys the superficial intestinal mucosa beginning in the crypts. This leads to erosion and development of pityroid pseudomembranes of fibrin and cellular detritus (► G; p. 208).

Result: is infectious diarrhea.

❗ **Note:** Diarrhea is defined as abnormally frequent discharge of mostly fluid fecal material from the bowel.

❗ **Note:** The biologic purpose of diarrhea is to rapidly "flush the pathogen out of the bowel." When noninvasive pathogens are involved and sufficient liquid and electrolytes are replaced, most cases resolve spontaneously.

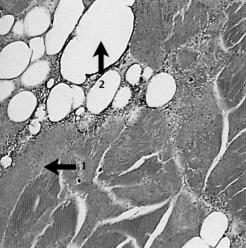

A **Clostridial gas gangrene** (skeletal muscle)
(HE) x 100

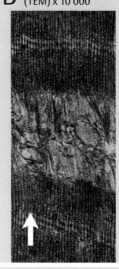

B **Normal muscle**
(TEM) x 10 000

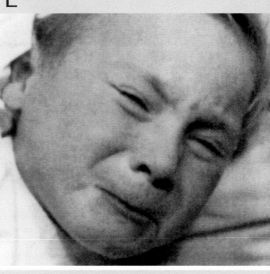

C **Muscle in clostridial gas gangrene** (TEM)

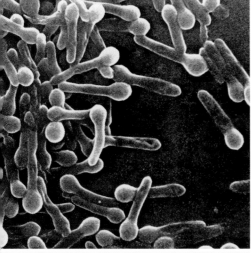

D **Clostridium tetani**
(SEM) x 40 000

E **Risus sardonicus** (tetanus)

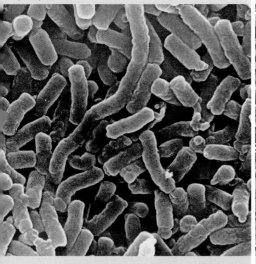

F **Clostridium difficile**
(SEM) x 40 000

G Antibiotic associated enteritis

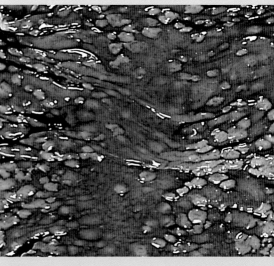

15

Gram-Negative Rod-shaped Bacteria

Enterobacteriaceae

Pathogens that cause most intestinal disorders and often nosocomial infections.

Occurrence: gastrointestinal tracts of humans and animals.

This group includes the following pathogens:
— *Escherichia coli* (► A), which causes diarrhea;
— *Salmonella typhi* (► B), which causes typhoid fever;
— *Salmonella paratyphi* (► B), which causes paratyphoid fever;
— *Shigella*, which cause bacterial dysentery;
— *Yersinia*, which cause enteritis and plague;
— *Klebsiella*, which cause pneumonia.

Pathogenetic factors:
— **Surface antigens** include surface lipopolysaccharide chains, flagellar (H-)antigen, capsular antigen, and fimbriae (hairlike adherent structures).
— **Endotoxin** is a part of the lipopolysaccharide complex integrated into the bacterium's outer membrane.
— **Virulence factors** include colonization factors such as adhesive fimbriae, enterotoxins that disrupt electrolyte transport, cytotoxins that damage the colonic enterocytes and the microvascular endothelium, neurotoxins that cause nerve injury, and invasive factors such as invasion of mucosal tissues.

✚ **Clinical forms** of Enterobacter disease:
– **Noninvasive enteritis** involves damage to the enterocytes from enterotoxins.
– **Invasive enteritis** involves penetration of the pathogens into the mucosa and submucosa.
– **Sepsis:** a systemic infection by bacteremia.
– **Hemorrhagic colitis** is caused by enterohemorrhagic *E. coli* or EHEC and involves cell injury from verotoxins.
– **Hemolytic-uremic syndrome** (p. 216) is a sequela to EHEC infection.

Disorders Associated with Enterobacteriaceae

■ **Typhoid Fever**

Definition: Infectious invasive enteritis (and, rarely, enterocolitis) caused by Salmonella typhi with systemic organ manifestations following hematogenous dissemination.

Occurrence: Humans act as reservoirs for the pathogen.

Pathogenetic chain reaction: Oral infection leads to penetration of the pathogen into intestinal enterocytes. It is then transported through the lymph system via Peyer's patches, regional lymph nodes, and the thoracic duct into the bloodstream, where it causes sepsis (p. 222). The pathogen multiplies in the blood and in the histiocytes of the wall of the bowel, leading to excretion of pathogens into the bowel via the bile. One week later, a massive B-cell reaction occurs in the mucosa-associated lymphoid tissue (MALT), resulting in increased titer of humoral antibodies (Widal reaction). Antibodies destroy the pathogen, releasing endotoxins

(p. 222). This endotoxemia causes a high fever and destruction of the intestinal MALT together with a pathogen-specific antigen-antibody reaction.

Morphologic stages:

Initial stage: It is characterized by medullary *swelling* of Peyer's patches (► C) and of the mesenteric lymph nodes by histiocytic granulomas that are usually ill-defined (► E; p. 228). These granulomas consist of large histiocytes (► E1) that phagocytize the remains of neutrophils ("Rindfleisch" cells; ► F) and of endogenous lymphocytes and plasma cells (► E2). Granuloma necrosis is rare.

Second stage: It involves *scabbing* of the superficial layer of the intestinal wall due to the destruction of mucosa-associated lymphoid tissue (MALT). This scabbing appears in the form of grayish yellow necrosis extending the muscularis.

Third stage: It is characterized by *ulceration* resulting from granulocytic demarcation of the necrotic areas. The necrotic tissue is sloughed off, producing longitudinal mucosal ulcerations (► D) that lead to bleeding.

Fourth stage: A layer of *scarring* granulation tissue covers the ulcers, which then become re-epithelialized.

✚ **Clinical presentation:** Patients present with a high fever, bradycardia, disorientation (*typhos* is Greek for fog), erythematous macular skin exanthema (roseola), leukopenia, diarrhea ("pea-soup" stools) with traces of blood (indicative of ulcers), and inflammatory splenomegaly.

✚ **Complications** in the absence of antibiotic therapy include:
– Intestinal perforation leading to fecal peritonitis;
– Splenomegaly leading to anemic infarction and rupture of the spleen;
– Necrotizing muscular inflammations in the myocardium and abdominal musculature (Zenker degeneration).

❗ **Note:** Differential diagnosis of ulcers of the small bowel should distinguish between **typhoid ulcers**, which develop along the longitudinal axis of the bowel, and transverse **tuberculosis ulcers.**

■ **Salmonella Enteritis**

Definition: Noninvasive salmonella enteritis (caused primarily by Salmonella enteritidis) in the form of food poisoning with diarrhea and vomiting.

Pathogenesis: Oral infection leads to irritation of the intestinal mucosa, causing diarrhea (with risk of desiccation). This flushes out the pathogens, allowing the disorder to resolve spontaneously.

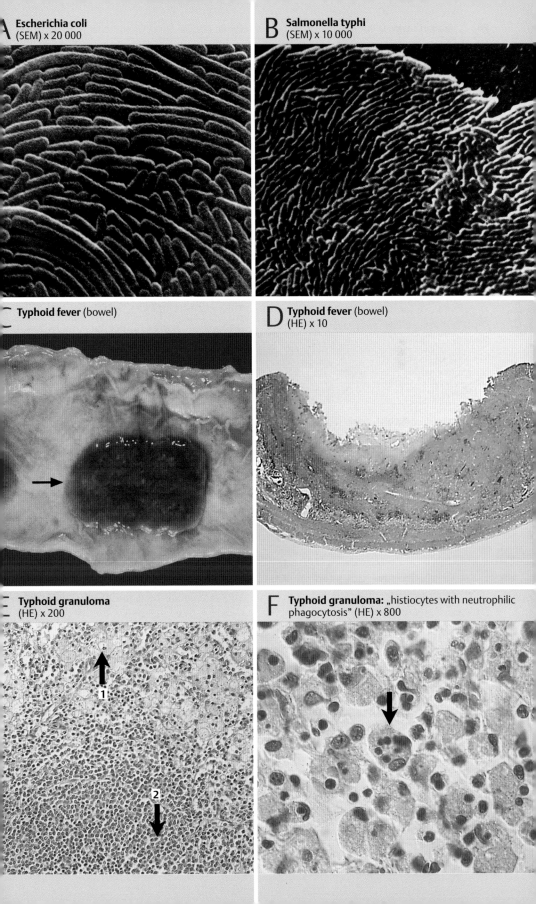

A Escherichia coli
(SEM) x 20 000

B Salmonella typhi
(SEM) x 10 000

C Typhoid fever (bowel)

D Typhoid fever (bowel)
(HE) x 10

E Typhoid granuloma
(HE) x 200

F Typhoid granuloma: „histiocytes with neutrophilic phagocytosis" (HE) x 800

Short-Curved Gram-Negative Rod-shaped Bacteria

■ Vibrio cholerae

Pathogen that causes cholera (► A).

Pathogenesis: The pathogen is transmitted in contaminated water and multiplies in the lumen of the bowel. There the B component of its enterotoxin (choleragen) allows it to adhere to a GM-1 monosialoganglioside molecule on the intestinal enterocytes. The A component of the cholera enterotoxin invades the cell where it activates adenylate cyclase, stimulating chronic production of cAMP. This in turn results in permanent protein kinase stimulation, successively leading to chronic opening of the ion channels and excessive passage of electrolytes and water from the enterocytes into the lumen of the bowel.

✚ **Clinical presentation:** Patients present with diarrhea and vomiting. Fecal discharge is cloudy and watery, contains massive quantities of pathogens, and reaches a volume of up to 20 l per day. Microscopic examination reveals groups of rods resembling schools of fish. Humans are the reservoir of the pathogen.

☺ **Prominent patient:** Peter Ilich Tchaikovsky (1840–1893), Russian composer.

■ Campylobacter jejuni coli

Pathogens that cause Campylobacter enteritis.

✚ **Clinical presentation and morphology:**
Slightly erosive granulocytic enteritis with bloody diarrhea.

■ Helicobacter pylori

Pathogen that causes active bacterial gastritis (► B) and is associated with intestinal MALT syndrome and gastric carcinoma.

Pathogenetic chain reaction:

— H. pylori bacilli adhere to sialic acid and the blood group O antigen of the parietal cells of the stomach.
— Their cytotoxic effects include high urease activity, which triggers local NH_4 production and increases pH. This damages the ion pump and successively leads to neutrophil chemotaxis and epithelial damage to pits of the gastric mucosa (► D). The resulting destruction of the mucosa leads to erosive gastritis and gastroduodenal ulcer (p. 218).

Pathogen identification: The presence of silvery rods in the pits of the gastric mucosa (► B). A urease test provides clinical evidence.

✚ **Clinical presentation:** The pathogen is prevalent in patients with blood group O, where it produces gastritis and gastric ulcer disease that may progress to MALT lymphoma and antral carcinoma.

Flexible Spiral Gram-Negative Bacteria

■ Borrelia burgdorferi

Pathogen that causes Lyme disease, which is spread by tick bites from the species *Ixodes domini* (► C).

✚ **Clinical presentation and morphology:**
– The *initial stage* (3–30 days) is characterized by a slowly spreading erythema with a pale center at the site of the bite (► E).
– The *second stage* (a period of weeks to months) involves leptomeningitis with lymphocytes and plasma cells, and pancarditis.
– The *third stage* (a period of months to years) involves polyarthritis and atrophic acrodermatitis (peripheral papery inflammatory skin atrophy).

■ Treponema pallidum

Pathogen that causes syphilis, a sexually transmitted disease (► F1).

Pathogenetic factors include humoral and cell-mediated immunity.

— ***Humoral immunity*** in the form of a plasma-cell infiltrate primarily around minor vessels leads to intimal inflammatory infiltration. This in turn causes obliterative endarteritis.
— ***Cell-mediated immunity*** in the form of granulomas with central caseous necrosis (p. 232): first, an immune response is mounted that cannot overcome the treponemes. Later, cell-mediated immunity continuously decreases.

Pathogen identification: includes anti-treponeme antibodies (► F1) and anti-lipoid antibodies.

✚ **Clinical course:**
Primary syphilis begins with a hard chancre, usually on the genitals (► F2), and a variety of cutaneous manifestations.
Secondary syphilis (4–8 weeks later) exhibits flat, oozing, infectious macerated lesions (condylomata lata) that develop in moist areas such as the axilla, vulva, and around the anus.
Tertiary syphilis occurs after several months or years of clinically asymptomatic disease (latent syphilis). Following this latent period, syphilitic granulomas (p. 232) develop in the skin, mucosa, and in nearly all organs. Particularly dangerous sequelae include syphilitic aortitis (p. 58) and *neurosyphilis*. *Fetal syphilis* is discussed on p. 306.

☺ **Prominent patients:**
Ignaz P. Semmelweis (1818–1865), Hungarian physician.
Friedrich Smetana (1824–1884), Czech composer.
Friedrich Nietzsche (1844–1900), German philosopher.
Paul Gauguin (1848–1903), French painter.
399 African-American syphilitics were subjects of a U.S. Dept. of Public Health-led study during which they were intentionally denied treatment (Tuskegee, Alabama, 1932–1972).

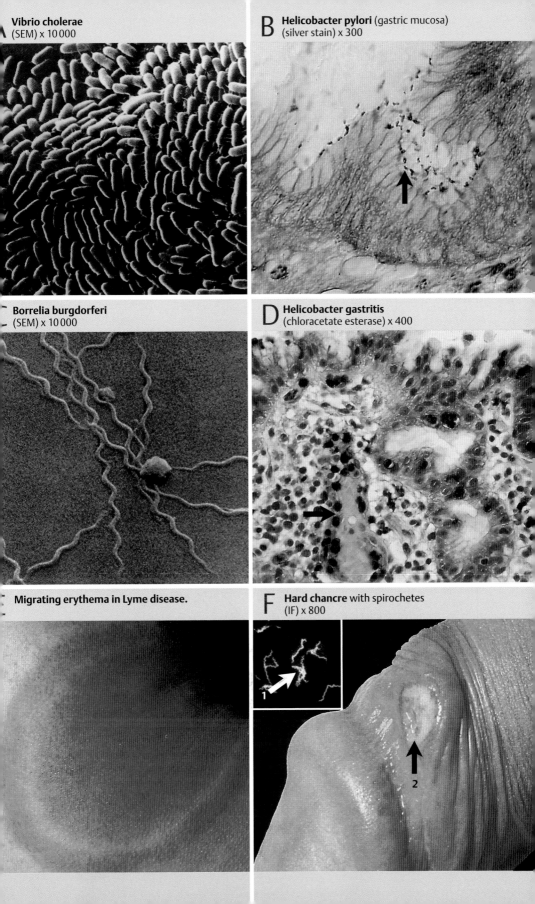

A **Vibrio cholerae** (SEM) x 10 000

B **Helicobacter pylori** (gastric mucosa) (silver stain) x 300

C **Borrelia burgdorferi** (SEM) x 10 000

D **Helicobacter gastritis** (chloracetate esterase) x 400

E **Migrating erythema in Lyme disease.**

F **Hard chancre** with spirochetes (IF) x 800

Mycobacteria (Acid-Resistant Rods)

■ Tuberculosis Bacteria

Pathogens that cause human tuberculosis (TB). These purely aerobic organisms (► A) are intracellular parasites. There are three types:

— *Mycobacterium tuberculosis,* the human type;
— *Mycobacterium bovis,* occurring in unpasteurized cow's milk;
— *Mycobacterium africanum,* native to Africa.

Pathogenesis: The disease usually spreads as a droplet infection by inhalation, rarely through oral infection by drinking contaminated milk. Several factors are decisive for the formal pathogenesis of tuberculosis.

— **Waxy coat:** It resists stomach acid, prevents desiccation, and resists lysosomal enzymes. This waxy coat allows tuberculosis pathogens to survive in macrophages.
— **Cord factor** (trehalose 6,6'-dimycolate) is a virulence factor that slows granulocyte chemotaxis and causes formation of granulomas.

This makes the tuberculosis inflammatory reaction a race between the proliferating tuberculosis pathogens and macrophage activation by T lymphocytes. This race defines the formal pathogenesis of tuberculosis, which may exhibit these forms:

— An **exudative caseous inflammatory reaction** with formation of multiple infectious foci or progressive tissue disintegration occurs in the absence of an immune defense or where this defense is weak. This results in unimpeded proliferation of the pathogen. The patient coughs up necrotic material, leaving behind cavernous tissue defects (► D).
— A **granulomatous inflammatory reaction** occurs where the immune defense keeps pace with the progress of the infection. The granulomas (p. 232) are the size of millet kernels and are therefore visible to the naked eye (► C).
— A **proliferative productive reaction** occurs when the damaged organ tissue is gradually repaired with scarring.

Pathogen identification: Red rods under Ziehl-Neelsen stain. Fluorescent yellow rods are visible under auramine rhodamine stain (► B).

➕ **Clinical course:**
Primary stage (primary tuberculosis)
- *Primary TB complex* begins with a *primary subpleural focus* (Ghon complex) in the central parenchyma of the lung. This leads to *lymphangitis* and caseous hilar *lymphadenitis.*

Secondary stage (hematogenous generalization)
- *Localized formation of hematogenous foci* in the presence of strong resistance leads to apical reinfection of the lung.
- *Disseminated formation of hematogenous foci* in the body in the presence of weak resistance leads to formation of granulomas the size of millet

kernels in a condition that manifests itself as miliary tuberculosis.
- *Pulmonary TB* involves granulomas that cover the lung (► C).
- *Urogenital TB* involves caseous inflammation of the renal parenchyma that finally progresses to caseous pyonephrosis.
- *Basal cerebral TB* produces cerebrospinal fluid with a spider-web pattern of fibrin coagulation and pleocytosis (overabundance of cells).
- *Landouzy sepsis,* which occurs with high virulence and weak resistance, leads to hyperacute sepsis (p. 223, 232).

Third stage (postprimary or organ TB)
Persistent infection leads to pulmonary TB manifestation. Infraclavicular or Assmann tuberculous infiltrate results from bronchogenic dissemination from a prominent TB focus. Cavernous pulmonary TB with inflammatory tissue necrosis causes patients to cough up the necrotic material. This creates cavernous tuberculous defects (► D) and leads to bronchogenic dissemination of the pathogen with clover-leaf foci (acinous nodular TB).

☺ **Prominent patients** (p. 232).

■ Mycobacterium leprae

Pathogen that causes leprosy. This organism is an intracellular parasite.

Pathogenesis: As in tuberculosis, cell-mediated immunity plays an important part in the creation of the typical tissue lesion of leprosy. Depending on the state of the patient's immune system, one of the following inflammatory reactions will occur.

Lepromatous reaction: An adequate T-lymphocyte response is lacking. Histologic findings include massive quantities of infiltrate composed of macrophages that contain parasitic pathogens in their foamy cytoplasm (Virchow cells).

Pathogen identification: Red rods under Ziehl-Neelsen stain (► F); PCR.

➕ **Clinical course:** The disorder is malignant and progresses throughout the life of the patient.
- The *skin* develops thickened nodules (erythema nodosum leprosum).
- *Peripheral nerves* exhibit cord-like thickening leading to sensory deficits and mutilation (mutilating acral necrosis).

— **Tuberculoid reaction:** The T-cell system remains intact, through functionally unable to fully eliminate the leprosy bacteria. Formation of caseous epithelioid granulomas is evidence of the immune system's attempt to eliminate the pathogen.

➕ **Clinical course:** The disorder remains benign and does not progress throughout the life of the patient.

Mycobacterium tuberculosis
(TEM) x 20 000

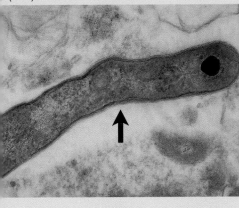

B Mycobacterium tuberculosis (auramine-rhodamine and fluorescence) x 1000

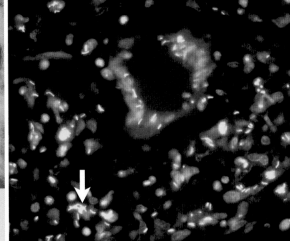

Miliary tuberculosis

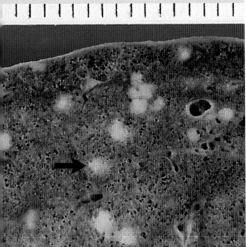

D Tuberculous cavernous defect

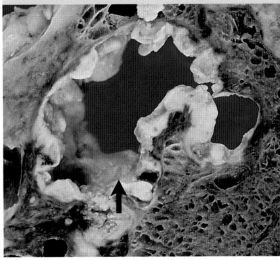

Cutaneous leprosy
Ziehl-Neelsen's stain x 200

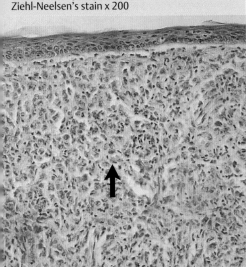

F Mycobacterium leprae in the skin
(Ziehl-Neelsen's stain) x 800

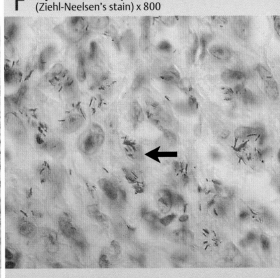

Obligatory Intracellular Bacteria

■ Rickettsia prowazekii

Pathogen that causes epidemic typhus. This organism is an obligatory intracellular parasite.

Pathogenesis: The pathogen is transmitted to humans via body lice. It causes rickettsemia, which allows the pathogens to invade the endothelial cells of the microvasculature. There they multiply, where their endotoxic cytotoxins cause lysis of the endothelial cells and release more bacteria into the bloodstream. These bacteria then infect other endothelial cells, producing generalized vasculitis. The resulting thrombosis progresses to obliterative vasculitis, palpable as "typhus nodules." Punctate necroses with petechial hemorrhages occur primarily in the skin (petechial exanthema), and in the brain and myocardium.

✚ **Clinical presentation and morphology:** *Epidemic typhus* is an infectious disease characterized by high fever with punctate erythematous lesions the size of a pinhead on the trunk and extremities. Hepatosplenomegaly is present, and circulatory shock may occur. Panencephalitis is a rare complication.

☺ **Prominent patients:**
Alexander the Great of Macedonia (356–323 BC) died of typhus.

■ Calymmatobacterium granulomatis

Pathogen that causes granuloma inguinale. The organism is a gram-negative intracellular coccobacillus.

Occurrence: The disorder occurs primarily in indigenous populations in the tropics.

Pathogenesis: The pathogen is transmitted primarily by sexual intercourse.

✚ **Clinical presentation and morphology:** *Granuloma inguinale* manifests itself:
– *initially* as painless reddened papules or subcutaneous nodules in the inguinal, genital, and perianal region.
– *Later* symptoms include skin ulcerations with excessive proliferation of granulation tissue in the absence of lymphadenitis.

Histologic findings in the ulcer include putrid granulation tissue with vacuolated histiocytes containing inclusion bodies (▶ A1) and pseudo-epitheliomatous epithelial regeneration along the margins (▶ A2).

Pathogen identification: Silver-staining bean-shaped pathogens (Donovan inclusion bodies; ▶ B) in histiocytes.

■ Chlamydia

Pathogens that differ from other bacteria in that they are very small, obligatory intracellular parasites with a unique reproductive cycle.

There are two forms of this pathogen:
– *elementary bodies:* infections form. After having attached themselves to certain cell receptors, they are phagocytized by the host cells, leading to reproduction and transformation into initial bodies in the phagosome (▶ C).
– *initial bodies:* these are found only in the host cells' phagosomes, and they change back into elementary bodies; the host cells eventually perish.

✚ **Clinical presentation and morphology** vary with the pathogen.
Trachoma is a chronic inflammation of the conjunctiva and cornea (keratoconjunctivitis) that occurs in Africa and eastern Asia. The *pathogen*, C. trachomatis serotype A, triggers the following pathogenetic chain reaction: Keratoconjunctivitis leads to deformative scarring of the eyelids and growth of granulation tissue (pannus) into the cornea, which leads to blindness. The disorder is common. Pathogen indication: inclusion bodies in cells in Giemsa-stain smears.
Inclusion conjunctivitis is caused by the pathogen C. trachomatis serotype A–C from genital secretions in unchlorinated swimming pools. This organism does not cause scarring or pannus.
Inclusion bodies are positive evidence of the pathogen.
Chlamydia genital inflammation is caused by the pathogen C. trachomatis serotype B, C, D, and E. In men, it produces non-gonococcal urethritis; in women, it produces urethritis, proctitis, and cervicitis with distinctive flame-red erythema of the surface of the cervix (▶ D).
Lymphogranuloma venereum is caused by the pathogen C. lymphogranulomatis. The infection is a sexually transmitted disease and begins as a genital ulcer. Later it progresses to lymphadenitis with pseudotuberculous granulomas. This produces chronic inflammation with rectal and genital scarring, which disrupts lymph drainage and produces anogenital elephantiasis.

Pathogen identification: The Frei intracutaneous test.

Bacteria Without a Cell Wall

■ Mycoplasma pneumoniae

Pathogen that causes atypical forms of pneumonia.

In contrast to other bacteria, mycoplasmas lack a rigid murein-containing cell wall (▶ E1). This gives it its distinctive coccal to filamentous shape and makes it resistant to antibiotics that inhibit murein synthesis.

Pathogenesis: The pathogen enters the respiratory tract by aerogenic transmission and adheres to the ciliated respiratory epithelium (▶ E2). This damages the ciliated structures, blocking mucociliary clearance. In turn, this leads to pulmonary inflammation with lymphocytic infiltrate in the interstitium of the pulmonary alveoli (▶ F).

✚ **Clinical presentation:** *Atypical pneumonia* is characterized by insidious onset without chills and usually without rattling sounds. Chest radiographs show a veil-like infiltrate of low density.

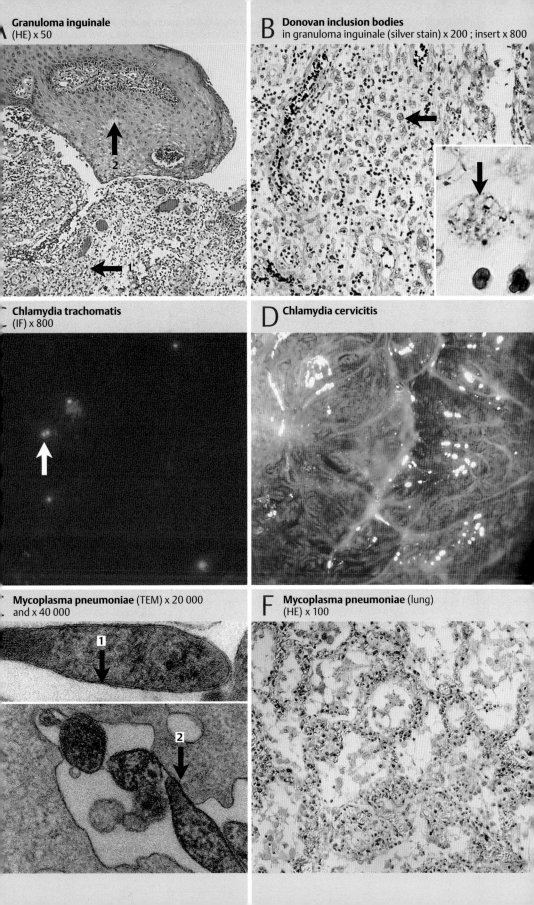

A **Granuloma inguinale**
(HE) x 50

B **Donovan inclusion bodies**
in granuloma inguinale (silver stain) x 200 ; insert x 800

Chlamydia trachomatis
(IF) x 800

D **Chlamydia cervicitis**

Mycoplasma pneumoniae (TEM) x 20 000
and x 40 000

F **Mycoplasma pneumoniae** (lung)
(HE) x 100

Summary

The hypha is the basic morphologic element of multicellular fungi in the vegetative phase. It is a multi-branched tubular structure subdivided by transverse septa. These structures form a network known as a mycelium. The unicellular hyphae are oval to round, but often adhere together in the form of hypha-like chains (pseudo-hyphae). Most of the fungi that cause disease in humans have only slight pathogenic potential and can only invade tissue in an immuno-compromised host or after destruction of competing bacterial flora. These are known as opportunistic pathogens. Tissue destruction by mycotic pathogens is partially attributable to toxic fungal products that cause disease by mechanisms that are not always well understood. It is also partially attributable to abnormal immune reactions. Antigens of the fungus capsule stimulate a population of B lymphocytes to form antibodies. This leads to precipitating and complement-binding antibodies, whose presence aids in diagnosing these disorders.

▶ The spores of saprophytic fungi such as Aspergillus, Candida, Coccidioides, and Penicillium cause allergic hypersensitivity reactions in predisposed patients and lead to mycotic allergies. A cell-mediated type IV hypersensitivity reaction also plays a decisive role in combating mycotic infections, as does uncompromised granulocyte function.

▶ Histologic findings of a "ruthlessly proliferative" mycelium that does not respect tissue septa, organ capsules, or vascular walls are common to all infectious diseases caused by mycelium-forming fungi (mycoses). The mycelium grows through these structures and typically exhibits a ring-like or spherical pattern of proliferation.

Skin Mycoses (Superficial Mycoses)

Pathogenesis: Forms of mycosis are differentiated according to the pathogen and depth of penetration in the tissue.

— **Superficial epidermal mycosis** is infestation of the horny layer of the epidermis with fungus organisms (not dermatophytes or fungi that produce deeper types of mycosis).

— **Cutaneous mycosis** refers to infestation of the entire epidermis and/or hair with fungal organisms (primarily dermatophytes, which cause dermatophytosis, and Candida, which causes candidosis).

Dermatophytoses

Pathogens (dermatophytes): They only infect tissue containing large amounts of keratin such as the epidermis (Epidermophyton floccosum), hair (Trichophyton rubrum), and nails (Trichophyton mentagrophytes).

Pathogenesis: Dermatophytoses are the only fungal infections that are spread by human-to-human or animal-to-human contact.

Pathogen identification: All dermatophytes are hyphomycetes and form septated hyphae in the skin lesions they create. These hyphae will be positive in a periodic acid-Schiff reaction (PAS).

✚ **Clinical presentation and morphology:**
Dermatomycoses (skin mycoses) are caused by variety of pathogens that produce morphologically similar cutaneous lesions (referred to as a tinea and further specified according to location). These tineas consist of round or oval erythematous rashes that are often concentric (▶ A).
Onychomycosis (nail mycosis) is an infection of the nails of the fingers or toes causing yellowish-white opacification and flaking of the nail (▶ B). The disorder begins as distal unguinal, proximal unguinal, or superficial onychomycosis and later progresses to dystrophic onychomycosis.
Deep trichophytosis is dermatophytosis with bacterial superinfection that results in a suppurative abscess-forming inflammation with mycelium at the depth of the hair follicles.

Subcutaneous and Mucosal Mycoses

General pathogenesis: Fungi grow beyond the epidermis and penetrate into deeper layers of subcutaneous connective tissue through skin wounds. This results in a focal chronic inflammatory reaction around the mycelium (▶ C2); granulomatous inflammatory reactions (▶ C1) may occur in patients with stronger immune systems.

Organ and Systemic Mycoses

General pathogenesis: Fungal penetration may occur by several mechanisms.

— **Aerogenic penetration** leads to fungal bronchitis (▶ D1) with invasion of the bronchial wall (▶ D2) progressing to invasion of surrounding pulmonary tissue.

— **Iatrogenic penetration** of fungi present in the oral flora can occur during endoscopic retrograde cholangiopancreatography (ERCP).

— **Hematogenous penetration** can occur in vascular invasion, which may successively lead to fungal vasculitis (▶ E), fungemia (fungal sepsis), and fungal colonization of organs such as the liver (▶ F).

⚠ **Note:** The general principle of mycosis due to mycelium-forming fungi involves these elements:
– *Relentless* invasion of tissue septa, organ capsules, and vessel walls;
– *Organ* invasion → spherical pattern;
– *Skin* invasion → circular pattern.

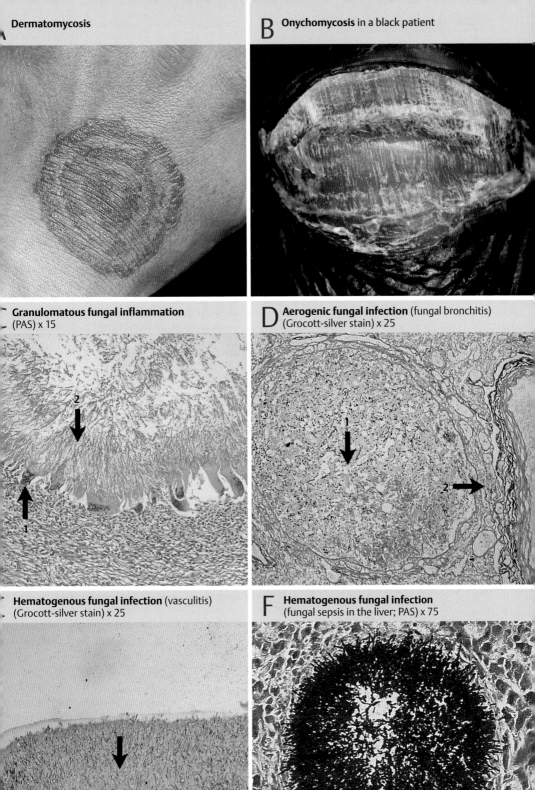

A Dermatomycosis

B Onychomycosis in a black patient

C Granulomatous fungal inflammation
(PAS) x 15

D Aerogenic fungal infection (fungal bronchitis)
(Grocott-silver stain) x 25

E Hematogenous fungal infection (vasculitis)
(Grocott-silver stain) x 25

F Hematogenous fungal infection
(fungal sepsis in the liver; PAS) x 75

Yeasts

Pathogen: Yeasts are monocellular fungi that reproduce by budding. They combine to form chains that resemble hyphae.

■ Candida albicans

Pathogen that causes Candida infections in humans.

Occurrence: The organism is a saprophyte normally found on the squamous epithelium of human oral and rectal mucosa.

Pathogenesis: This opportunistic fungus can become a pathogen. For example, Candida from the oropharyngeal mucosa may be swallowed and passed to the rectum, from which it can infest the vaginal mucosa. Other modes of infection are also possible; all require certain conditions such as:

— An immunocompromised host;
— Immunodeficiency disorders of the T-cell system;
— Therapy with corticosteroids and/or immunosuppressive agents that suppress lymphocytopoiesis;
— agranulocytosis (severe neutrophil deficiency);
— Antibiotic therapy that suppresses and disrupts the balance of oral and gastrointestinal flora;
— Endocrine disorders (primarily diabetes mellitus).

Virulence factors include:
— Formation of hyphae;
— Hyphae-forming pathogens adhere more readily to the target cells, and their surface proteases and lipases make them particularly invasive;
— Lectin-like adherence factors;
— Molecular mimicry; the pathogens bind thrombocytes with their fibrinogen ligands, creating a surface "camouflage" that renders them invisible to immune defenses.

Pathogen identification: include slightly basophilic organisms under hematoxylin and eosin stain and purplish red organisms in a periodic acid-Schiff reaction (► A). The fungus may be present in the form of an oval yeast (► A1), a pseudomycelium with pseudo-hyphae (► A2), and occasionally one with septate mycelia as well. The mycelium will be thinner than Aspergillus.

✚ **Clinical presentation and morphology:** Candida fungi cause several cutaneous, subcutaneous, and systemic mycoses.
Oral candidiasis (thrush) occurs in two forms.
– *Superficial candidiasis* is characterized by whitish-gray patches that are readily removed (► C). These lesions occur primarily on the mucosa of the cheeks, gums, and tongue. Histologic findings include fibrinous pseudomembranes with mycelium growing perpendicular to the surface (► B) and slight amounts of inflammatory infiltrate.
– *Deep candidiasis* involves hard grayish-white plaques (primarily on the back of the tongue and in the corners of the mouth). This chronic disorder is accompanied by foreign-body inflammation with giant cells (p. 236).

– *Candidal colpitis* involves vulvovaginitis. Among the possible modes of infection are descending infection from the gastrointestinal tract and contamination from prior anal intercourse.
Candidal balanoposthitis occurs in men; in homosexual males it may occur as result of anal intercourse.
Candidal dermatomycosis may occur in the nail bed in the form of onychomycosis, as intertrigo (inflammatory erosive dermatitis) between folds of skin, and as diaper dermatitis in the form of erosive erythema.
Candidal pneumonia occurs as mycotic tracheobronchitis with pseudomembranous deposits (► D). This leads to descending aspiration infection (rarely, in the presence of fungemia), progressing to mycotic pneumonia.
Candidal sepsis occurs with generalized fungemia.

Note: Candida infestation in a necrotic gastric biopsy suggests carcinoma.

Note: Diabetes mellitus should always be excluded where findings include Candida intertrigo.

■ Cryptococcus neoformans

Pathogen that causes cryptococcosis (torulosis). The organism is an encapsulated yeast.

Occurrence: The organism is present throughout the world in pigeon feces and contaminated soil.

Pathogenesis: The organism is an obligatory pathogen. Patents with T-cell defects are predisposed to infection. Virulence factors include the organism's polysaccharide capsule (which inhibits phagocytosis), its neutralization of opsonizing antibodies, and its activation of the complement system (p. 162) via the alternate path. Where the host's immune system is sufficiently strong, small histiocytic granulomas will form, which lead to necrotic calcification (p. 134).

Pathogen identification: includes small round fungi with a ragged mucoid capsule that appear to have an "empty" halo under hematoxylin and eosin stain and appear reddish under mucicarmine stain (► E).

✚ **Clinical presentation and morphology:** The disorder is more common in men than in women. Infection occurs by inhaling the pathogen; symptomatic cases exhibit three stages:
– The *initial stage* usually involves occult pulmonary cryptococcosis. Radiographs show a focal shadow in the inferior portions of the lung. This leads to hematogenous dissemination to other organs.
– The *second stage* is characterized by cerebral cryptococcosis in the form of meningoencephalitis with nonreactive cystic myxoid gelatinous focal necroses (► F).
– In the *third stage*, the disorder progresses to generalized disease.

Note: *Cryptococcal meningitis* is the most frequent manifestation of cryptococcosis.

Candida albicans
(PAS) x 400

B Candidal esophagitis
(Grocott-silver stain) x 100

Candidal esophagitis

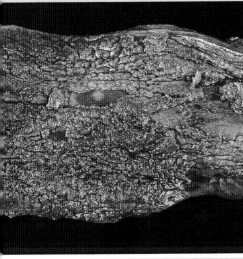

D Candidal tracheitis

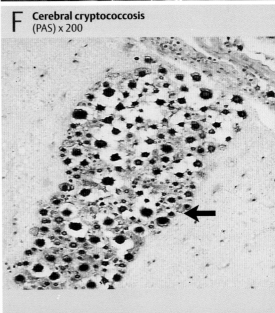

Cryptococcus neoformans
(HE) x 800

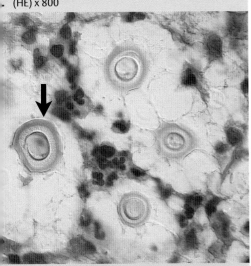

F Cerebral cryptococcosis
(PAS) x 200

Molds

Pathogens of lattice-forming hyphae (mycelia) that are usually divided by septa.

■ Aspergillus Fungi (▶ A)

Pathogens that cause aspergilloses.

Occurrence: These fungi are ubiquitous and produce several toxins: aflatoxin, which causes liver carcinoma (p. 328), elastase, and gliotoxin.

Pathogenesis: Predispositions include agranulocytosis and/or a T-cell defect. Infection is by inhalation. The fungal toxins destroy tissue and interfere with the alternate activation path of the complement system, disrupting the body's immune system.

Pathogen identification: includes a branching mycelium of septate hyphae that appears purplish-red under PAS and black under Grocott-silver stain. Where sufficient oxygen is present, the organism will form a head resembling the crown of a tree (▶ A).

✚ **Clinical presentation and morphology** depend on the state of the patient's immune system. Disorders include
allergic bronchopulmonary aspergillosis or extrinsic allergic alveolitis in the presence of hyperergia (caused by A. clavatus).
Aspergilloma (caused by A. fumigatus) occurs in patients with normal sensitivity. This involves infestation of necrotic material in a body cavity such as paranasal sinuses, ear canal, or the cavern of the lung (▶ B) without invasion of blood vessels. The result is a round focus, referred to as an aspergilloma.
Invasive necrotizing Aspergillus pneumonia occurs in insensitive patients, primarily in the presence of immunodeficiencies. The pathogen, A. fumigatus, invades the vessel wall (▶ C1), causing mycotic thrombotic vascular obstruction (▶ C2) and infarctoid necrosis. The result is what is known as a "target lesion" (▶ E). The inner layer consists of infarction necrosis with mycelium, the middle layer of fibrinous exudate, and the outer layer of hemorrhagic exudate.
Aspergillus sepsis involves multiple foci with infarctoid necrosis, primarily in the kidneys and central nervous system (▶ D).

■ Mucor (Zygomycetes)

Pathogen is a ubiquitous mold.

Pathogenesis: Predispositions include immune deficiencies and diabetic acidosis.

Pathogen identification: includes mycelium of thick, perpendicular aseptate hyphae.

✚ **Clinical presentation and morphology:** Infection occurs by inhalation of the pathogen, which then infests blood vessels. This causes paradox thrombosis (thrombus + hemorrhage) and tissue infarction and leads to rhinocerebral, pulmonary, or cutaneous manifestations (as opportunistic infections).

Dimorphic Fungi

Pathogens that grow as a parasitic yeast in the host and exogenously as a saprophytic mycelium.

■ Histoplasma capsulatum

Pathogen that causes histoplasmosis.

Occurrence: The pathogen occurs naturally in soil.

Pathogenesis: Infection is by inhalation. The pathogen is phagocytized by alveolar macrophages, where it multiplies by budding. This produces and inflammatory reaction that can involve pseudotuberculous granulomas progressing to calcifying necrosis.

Pathogen identification: The pathogen is invisible under hematoxylin and eosin stain but appears black under Grocott-silver stain. In tissue, it appears as a small ovoid corpuscle in histiocytes.

✚ **Clinical presentation and morphology:** Histoplasmosis manifests itself primarily in the lung in the form of bronchopneumonic miliary foci that heal with calcification. Splenomegaly is also present. The disseminated form infests all organ systems, primarily the bone marrow and adrenal gland.

■ Coccidioides immitis

Pathogen that causes coccidioidomycosis, a highly infectious disease.

Occurrence: The pathogen occurs in the southern United States and Central America.

Pathogenesis: Infection is by inhalation, which causes pneumonia. In about 5% of all cases, the patient develops a cavernous lung inflammation with pseudotuberculous granulomas progressing to calcifying necrosis.

Pathogen identification: In tissue, the fungus does form a mycelium, rather a spherical, double-walled configuration known as a sporangium or spherule with a number of spherical endospores (▶ F). The spherule capsule exhibits a Splendore-Hoeppli phenomenon.

✚ **Clinical presentation and morphology:**
Pulmonary coccidioidomycosis presents as a cold-like disorder with bronchopneumonic foci of caseous necrosis leading to formation of cavernous defects and miliary dissemination, leading to:
disseminated coccidioidomycosis with foci occurring primarily in the skin, bone, and brain.

■ Rhinosporidium seeberi

Pathogen that causes in rhinosporidiosis humans and animals. The taxonomic position of the organism is uncertain.

Occurrence: The organism is ubiquitous, occurring more frequently in India and Sri Lanka.

Pathogen identification: (▶ G) includes cystic structures under hematoxylin and eosin stain that represent mature spherule (sporangia with small round endospores).

✚ **Clinical presentation and morphology:** Infection occurs through the nose and mouth. The pathogen infests the oropharynx, forming polyploid granulation tissue that interferes with nasal breathing.

The next section will examine diseases that are caused by protozoans or worms. These organisms create injury merely by entering the body. In contrast to infectious diseases, their offspring (such as eggs) leave the host. For this reason, these disorders are referred to as infestations (i.e., invasive disorders).

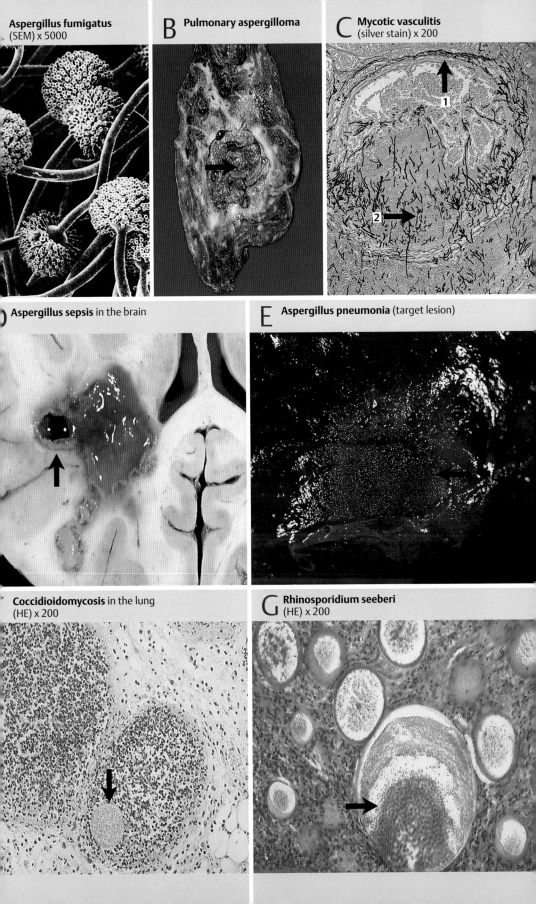

A Aspergillus fumigatus (SEM) x 5000

B Pulmonary aspergilloma

C Mycotic vasculitis (silver stain) x 200

D Aspergillus sepsis in the brain

E Aspergillus pneumonia (target lesion)

F Coccidioidomycosis in the lung (HE) x 200

G Rhinosporidium seeberi (HE) x 200

Protozoan Infection

Summary

Protozoans that cause disease in humans improve their opportunities for proliferation by changing hosts and by utilizing vectors in the form of blood-sucking insects. Other waterborne ameboid protozoans seek out their own hosts. These organisms exploit weak points in the human immune system to parasitize the body. There they often multiply until a new generation of offspring has been produced. The diseases they cause (protozoan infections) are the result of their energetic parasitism and, occasionally, of an excessive immune reaction.

Zoomastigophora

■ Trypanosoma cruzi

Pathogen that causes Chagas disease (South American trypanosomiasis).

Occurrence: South and Central American slums and in the southern United States.

Pathogenesis: Infection is spread by bites of insects of the genus Triatoma or by rat bites. When the insect sucks blood, the trypanosomes enter its intestine. There they change their form and multiply. When the insect next bites a human, it deposits feces containing trypanosomes on its victim's skin. Scratching the bite smears the pathogen into minor skin lesions. From there, the trypanosomes drill their way into the microvasculature. Parasitemia results, and the organisms colonize their target cells in the skeletal and cardiac muscle (primarily the myocardium) and in the smooth muscle (primarily the intestinal tract), leading to cellular parasitism.

Pathogen identification: includes pseudocysts in striated muscles with punctate amastigotes (► B1) surrounded by necrosis with resorptive inflammation (► B2).

✚ **Clinical presentation**: *Chagas disease* exhibits an *acute phase* characterized by inflammatory subcutaneous nodules (chagomas) with regional lymphadenitis or unilateral conjunctivitis at the point of entry. In the *chronic phase*, Chagas myocarditis occurs with apical cardiac aneurysm, in some cases accompanied by megaesophagus and megacolon.

■ Leishmania

Pathogen that causes leishmaniasis.

Pathogenesis: The pathogen is passed to humans by sand fleas. When the insect sucks blood, the Leishmania organisms enter its intestine. There they develop, multiply, and metamorphose into the flagellated promastigote form. When the insect bites, these organisms pass to the definitive host (a human or other vertebrate), where they are phagocytized by macrophages. In the phagocytic vacuoles, they metamorphose into unflagellated amastigotes. There they multiply within the cell until the macrophage bursts. This releases the pathogens and leads to infection of new macrophages.

Pathogen identification: includes the "period and comma" phenomenon (► C). The oval nucleus of the amastigote represents the "period" (► A1); the "comma" is formed by rod-shaped cinetoplast of the mitochondrial apparatus and helical mitochondrial DNA (► A2).

✚ **Clinical presentation and morphology:**
Visceral leishmaniasis (kala-azar) occurs in Central and South America, Africa, Asia, and in the Mediterranean region.
– A *primary focal lesion* develops in the form a granulomatous inflammation at the point of entry.
– In its *generalized form*, the disorder is characterized by hepatosplenomegaly, lymphadenia (pathogen identification is obtained by splenic or lymph-node aspiration), hyperplastic bone marrow, and pancytopenia. *Skin symptoms* include dry skin with hyperpigmentation and papules. Episodic fever is also present.

Cutaneous leishmaniasis occurs in tropical regions. It is a *purely cutaneous infection* characterized by a disintegrating ulcerated papule (► E).

■ Trichomonas vaginalis

Pathogen that causes trichomoniasis.

Pathogen identification: includes a pear-shaped organism with multiple flagella and an ovoid cell nucleus (► D).

✚ **Clinical presentation:** The disease is transmitted by sexual intercourse. Trichomoniasis manifests itself in women as vaginitis and less often as urethritis, leading to vaginal discharge (25% of all infections are asymptomatic). In men, infection is usually asymptomatic, rarely manifesting itself as urethritis.

■ Giardia lamblia

Pathogen is a pear-shaped organism with multiple flagella and two symmetrical nuclei (► F).

Occurrence: Small rodents and cats are reservoirs of the pathogen.

Pathogenesis: Predispositions include immunodeficiency such as common variable immunodeficiency (CVID) and AIDS. The pathogen enters through the mouth or rectum (homosexual practices have been implicated), from which it then colonizes the upper mucosa of the small bowel.

✚ **Clinical presentation:** This facultative pathogen usually produces asymptomatic infection, but can also result in intermittent diarrhea and occasional malabsorption.

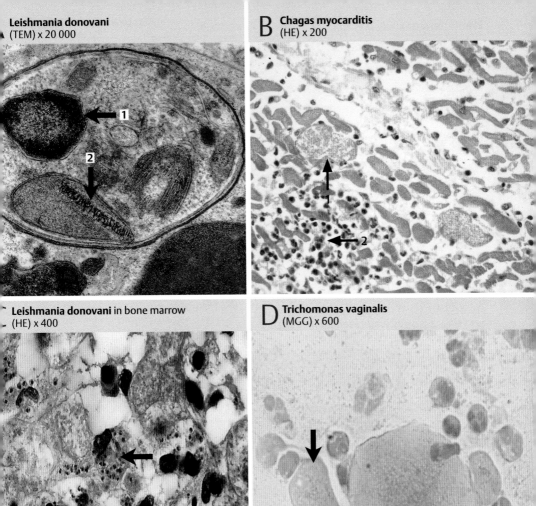

Leishmania donovani
(TEM) x 20 000

B Chagas myocarditis
(HE) x 200

Leishmania donovani in bone marrow
(HE) x 400

D Trichomonas vaginalis
(MGG) x 600

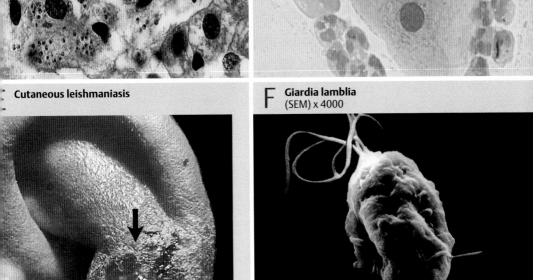

Cutaneous leishmaniasis

F Giardia lamblia
(SEM) x 4000

Lobosea

■ Entamoeba histolytica

Pathogen that causes amebic dysentery (► A1).

Occurrence: The organism occurs primarily in tropical and subtropical regions.

Pathogenesis: The pathogen is ingested in its mature cystic form, which is resistant to gastric acid. The amebas usually emerge from their cysts in the small bowel and pass to the large bowel. There they change into the smaller parasitic form that lives in the lumen of the bowel and infests either the mucosa or the contents thereof. The resulting change in the intestinal flora increases the virulence of the pathogen. The organism then changes into the larger form, which lyses tissue with its collagenases and pore-forming proteins (hence the name histolytica). The pathogen "crawls through" the bowel wall, producing ulcerous amebic colitis (► E) that results in a reactive inflammation of the surrounding tissue and omentum, leading to ameboma. Dissemination of the pathogen via the portal vein produces multiple encapsulated hepatic necroses (liver abscesses).

Pathogen identification: includes trophozoites in stool and tissue in the form of a round PAS-positive ameba with a round nucleus and cysts (in the stool only) with numerous small nuclei (► C).

✚ Clinical presentation:
Noninvasive intestinal amebiasis is asymptomatic.
Invasive intestinal amebiasis involves chronic recurrent diarrhea (dysentery) with soft, watery stools vaguely resembling raspberry jam because of the blood they include.
Hepatic amebiasis occurs secondary to hematogenous infection and results in an abscess-forming inflammation of the liver.

☺ Prominent patient:
Vincenzo Bellini (1801–1835), Italian opera composer, died of this disease.

Sporozoa

■ Toxoplasma gondii

Pathogen that causes toxoplasmosis (► B).

Occurrence: The organism is found in humans and domestic animals.

Pathogenesis: The pathogen produces a new generation of offspring and changes hosts. It exists in three forms:

— *Tachyzoite:* This is a crescent-shaped cell that can penetrate host cells. These cells multiply asexually and thrive only in the body of the host. They do not survive gastric acid.
— *Bradyzoite:* This is a smaller form of the parasite that occurs within intracellular cysts (► D). It is a form with a high longevity and does not damage tissue.

— *Oocyst:* This is a form that multiplies sexually in the bowel of cats (its specific host). It has a resistant capsule and is excreted with feces, where it forms spores that cause disease in humans.

Infection in humans occurs by ingestion. After penetrating the wall of the bowel, the pathogen is temporarily present in the blood and/or lymph. From there, the pathogens penetrate host cells primarily in the central nervous system and cardiac and skeletal muscle. There they multiply in the cytoplasm, causing the host cell to burst. This releases the pathogens, which then invade and damage neighboring cells, creating areas of focal tissue necrosis. This proliferation process lasts until the host dies. Where the host is able to mount an adequate immune response, the bloodstream will be cleared of free pathogens, and the organisms will be forced to live in cysts, where they multiply. However, once immunity is compromised, these cysts open and the struggle begins again.

Pathogen identification: includes tiny, crescent-shaped tachyzoites and intracellular cysts filled with kernel-like PAS-positive bradyzoites (► D).

✚ Clinical presentation and morphology:
Prenatal toxoplasmosis results in fetopathy.
– *Infection* prior to the *second trimester* leads to abortion.
– *Infection* after the *second trimester* leads to generalized fetal disease. One aspect of the disease is necrotizing encephalitis with calcifying foci of tissue liquefaction, which leads to cavernous defects known as "Swiss cheese brain" and ventricular widening. Another aspect is posterior uveitis with a triad of symptoms, including hydrocephalus, intracerebral calcifications, and posterior uveitis.
– *Infection shortly before birth* leads to generalized visceral toxoplasmosis.
Postnatal infection may be latent or symptomatic. The symptomatic form primarily manifests itself as lymphadenitis in the back of the neck with small focal epithelioid granulomas (► F).
Systemic toxoplasmosis occurs in immunocompromised patients and secondary to bone marrow transplants. It manifests itself as meningoencephalitis and nonreactive necrotic inflammations in internal organs (pneumonia, myocarditis, and hepatitis).

❢ Note: Risk groups include cat owners and diners who enjoy steak tartare.

❢ Note: A history of toxoplasmosis prior to pregnancy poses no risk to the fetus.

❢ Note: AIDS must be considered in patients presenting with toxoplasmic meningoencephalitis.

A **Entamoeba histolytica**
(diagram) x 1000

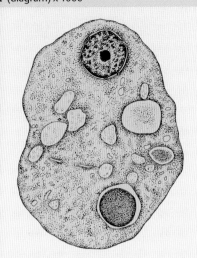

B **Toxoplasma gondii**
(diagram) x 1000

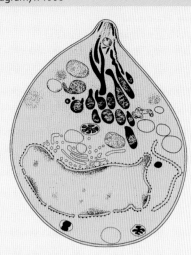

C **Entamoeba histolytica**
(PAS) x 600

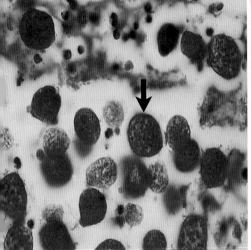

D **Toxoplasmic myocarditis**
(PAS) x 800

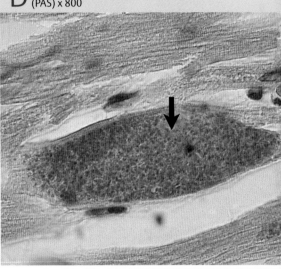

E **Amebic abscess** in the small bowel
(PAS) x 60

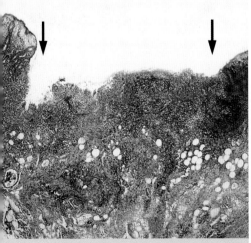

F **Toxoplasmic lymphadenitis**
(HE) x 200

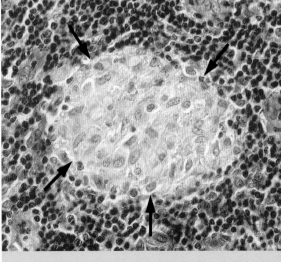

■ Plasmodia

Pathogens that causes malaria.

Occurrence: Tropical Africa, southern Asia, and Central and South America. Most deaths from malaria are due to infection with Plasmodium falciparum.

Pathogenesis: Malaria parasites are transmitted to humans in the saliva of the female *Anopheles* mosquito, which feeds on human blood. The malaria parasites employ a double strategy to evade the immune system. The organisms shed part of their capsule with its antigens, and they emit a "braking" factor for the T cells pursuing them.

Malaria parasites enter the parenchymal cells of the liver within 15 minutes of the mosquito bite. There they multiply and disguise themselves by altering their capsular antigens. One sporozoite produces up to 30 000 merozoites, which then enter the bloodstream as "unidentified newcomers." There they invade the erythrocytes (► A1, A2) within 10 minutes and digest their hemoglobin, leaving malaria pigment (p. 106). In their new hiding place, they can continue to multiply undisturbed. The erythrocytes alter their surface antigen structure after they are invaded. Normally, this causes the spleen to filter out these altered erythrocytes. However, the malaria parasites avoid this defense by triggering erythrocyte clumping. This causes aggregates of altered erythrocytes with their cargo of pathogens to lodge in the microvasculature of vital organs such as the brain, kidneys, heart, and lungs (► B), where they cause microinfarctions. Once sufficient merozoites have formed, the erythrocyte carrying them bursts. This releases pyrogenic substances that result in episodic bouts of fever. The resulting hemolysis leads to anemia.

Finally, the merozoites mature into female macrogametocytes and male microgametocytes. These sexually mature forms of the parasite again enter the female mosquito when it next bites an infected human. The organisms mate in the mosquito (insects lacking an efficient plasmoid defense mechanism), and the fertilized macrogametocytes (zygotes) encyst in the wall of the mosquito's stomach. There they transform themselves into oocysts in which sporozoites multiply by the thousands. When the cyst bursts, these sporozoites are released into the mosquito's lymph system, from which they pass into its salivary glands. There they are ready to complete the cycle of human infection with the next mosquito bite.

Pathogen identification: includes black malaria pigment (hematozoidin) in the macrophages of the reticuloendothelial system and plasmodia in the erythrocytes that are ring-shaped due to a central vacuole (► A1).

✚ **Clinical presentation:** Depending on the specific pathogen, patients present with episodic fever recurring at intervals of two or three days or with continuous fever. This is accompanied by hemolytic anemia.

☺ **Prominent patients:**
Emperor Heinrich VI (1165–1197) of the Holy Roman Empire contracted the disease while laying siege to Naples, forcing him to withdraw his troops.
Albrecht Dürer (1471–1528), German artist, contracted malaria during his travels in Italy.
John F. Kennedy (1917–1963), US President.

❗ **Note:** Malaria should be considered in patients presenting with fever and malaise who have recently traveled to tropical countries. In areas that abound with mosquitoes, the disease may be spread to other persons in the vicinity.

Mycoid Parasites

■ Pneumocystis carinii

Pathogen that causes Pneumocystis carinii pneumonia.

Due to its analogous ribosomal RNA sequences, the pathogen is most closely related to lower fungi such as Saccharomyces cerevisiae and to amebas.

Occurrence: The organism is ubiquitous and is found in the lungs of many mammals, including humans.

Pathogenesis: Pneumocystis carinii is an opportunistic parasite. Infection occurs by inhalation of P. carinii cysts, each of which releases eight small intracystic bodies that transform themselves into ameboid trophozoites. These trophozoites use their filopodia to attach themselves to the alveolar cells in the lung. Pairs of trophozoites fuse to form zygotes, which surround themselves with a thin cyst-like wall (pre-cyst). The pathogens multiply within this wall and form a genuine cyst (► C, D, E1, and F1). Reinfection occurs when the patient coughs up the cysts or they burst.

Pathogen identification: is obtained by lung biopsy. Findings include large cysts (usually within the alveoli), which under Grocott-silver stain are seen to contain small, black organisms (► D; bronchial lavage). The cyst contents will appear reddish and foamy in a periodic acid-Schiff reaction (► C).

✚ **Clinical presentation and morphology:** This is the commonest opportunistic infection encountered in AIDS patients. Every infection with P. carinii reduces immunity to a lower level.
Pneumocystis carinii pneumonia in AIDS patients is characterized by interstitial pneumonia with sparse lymphocytic inflammation in widened alveolar septa (► E2).
Pneumocystis carinii pneumonia in newborns is characterized by interstitial pneumonia with severe inflammation containing lymphocytes and plasma cells in widened alveolar septa (► F2).

A **Malaria falciparum** (Papanicolaou smear) x 500

B **Malaria falciparum** in a brain capillary (PAS) x 200

C **Pneumocystis carinii** (PAS) x 300

D **Pneumocystis carinii** in a bronchial lavage (Grocott-silver stain) x 400

E **Pneumocystis carinii pneumonia** in an AIDS patient (silver stain) x 100

F **Pneumocystis carinii pneumonia** in a newborn (HE) x 100

Summary

All parasitic worms causing disease in humans have one characteristic in common: They increase their range of efficacity and chances of survival by changing hosts. They reach sexual maturity in the host and multiply in the larval stage in an intermediate host independently of the adult generation by means of parthenogenesis. The parasites live off their host and only kill it in the long run if at all. Macrophages and eosinophilic granulocytes with their parasiticidal proteins play an important role in combating worm infestation (helminthic infection).

Trematodes

■ Schistosomes

Pathogen that causes bilharziosis.

Occurrence: tropical regions.

When schistosomes mate, the male envelopes the smaller thread-like female with its body, which resembles a pea pod.

Pathogenesis (host cycle): The eggs of the worm enter water in human feces. The single-cell miracidia that emerge from these eggs infest a certain species of freshwater snail as an intermediate host. There they form cysts and multiply as cercaria. The cysts then burst, releasing multinucleated cercaria into the water. Upon contact with humans, these organisms penetrate the skin and enter the human cardiovascular system, where they elicit an allergic reaction (p. 166). In the bloodstream, they transform themselves into schistosomula, which eventually enter the portal vein. They then mature into schistosomes and mate. The host's antibody-mediated cytotoxic immune response is ineffective against these organisms, and they often continue to produce eggs for years. The eggs migrate upstream through the circulatory system into the mucosa of the large bowel. There they trigger an immune response from the host and cause a granulomatous inflammatory reaction (p. 232) with eosinophilic infiltrate. The eggs then die in the tissue with regressive calcification, producing what may be referred to as egg granulomas. Where the normal migration path of the eggs is disturbed, such egg granulomas can occur in organs such as the liver, lungs, and urinary bladder.

Pathogen identification:
— **S. mansoni:** oval egg with a lateral spur (▶ A).
— **S. haematobium:** oval egg with a terminal spur (▶ B).
— **S. japonicum:** round egg without a spur (▶ C).

✛ Clinical presentation and morphology:
Urogenital bilharziosis is caused by *S. haematobium* (occurring in Africa). Eggs are deposited in the superior rectal vein. From there, they pass through anastomoses into the veins of the wall of urinary bladder. There they cause granulomatous urocystitis in the form of egg tubercles that are visible under endos-

copy (▶ D). This "sand grain" urocystitis leads to hydronephrosis that later progresses to carcinoma of bladder.
Hepatosplenic schistosomiasis is caused by *S. mansoni* or *S. japonicum* (occurring in China and Japan). Eggs are only deposited in the superior mesenteric and splenic veins. This causes granulomatous inflammation along venules of the portal vein with a pipestem pattern of fibrotic scarring, which leads to hepatosplenomegaly and portal venous hypertension (p. 392).
Intestinal schistosomiasis is primarily caused by *S. mansoni* (occurring in South America and Africa) and leads to submucosal granulomas.

Cestodes

■ Taenia saginata

Synonym: Beef tapeworm.

Pathogen that causes *Taenia saginata* infection (taeniasis saginata).

Occurrence: The pathogen occurs throughout the world.

T. saginata can grow to a length of up to 10 meters. It consists of an anterior portion (scolex) followed by numerous segments (proglottids). The posterior portion contains uteri with up to 100 000 eggs (▶ E).

Pathogenesis (host cycle): Taenia eggs are deposited on grassland in waste water or feces, where cattle, the intermediate hosts, ingest them with grass. In the bovine small bowel, the hexacanths or oncospheres emerge from the eggs and migrate into the wall of the bowel. They enter the striated muscle via the bloodstream. In the musculature, they encyst and mature within three months to the cysticercus stage, which can cause infection. The parasite is transferred to its primary human host by consumption of rare beef containing the parasite in its cysticercus stage. The cysticercus stage of the parasite extends its scolex when it enters the human small bowel. This allows it to attach to the mucosa, where it grows into an adult tapeworm.

Pathogen identification: includes the cysticercus stage (cysticercus bovis), a vesicle the size of a pea with a scolex (▶ F).

✛ Clinical presentation: About 25 % of all infections are asymptomatic. Symptoms include vomiting, abdominal pain, ravenous hunger, and weight loss.

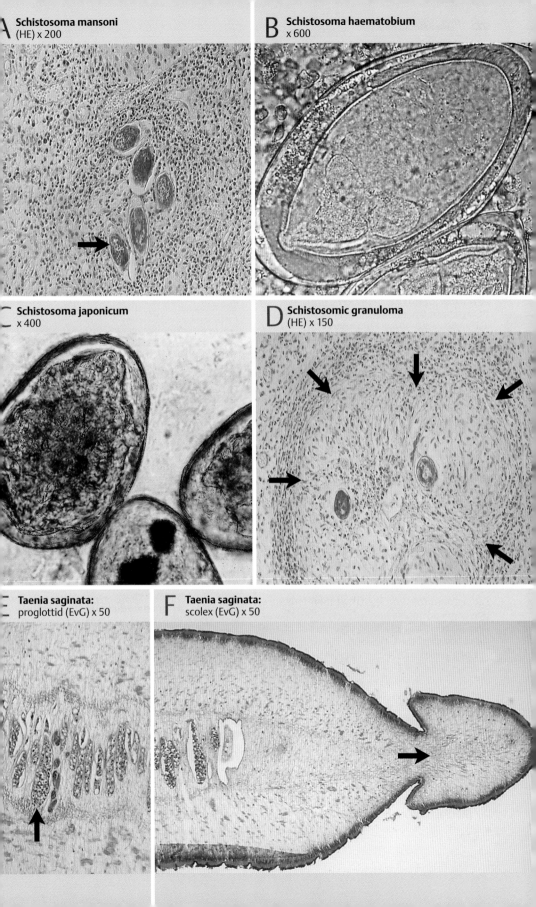

A Schistosoma mansoni (HE) x 200

B Schistosoma haematobium x 600

C Schistosoma japonicum x 400

D Schistosomic granuloma (HE) x 150

E Taenia saginata: proglottid (EvG) x 50

F Taenia saginata: scolex (EvG) x 50

▬ Taenia solium

Synonym: Pork tapeworm.

Pathogen that causes cysticercosis.

Rarely, humans (an intermediate host of the pork tapeworm) may contract cysticercosis as a result of infection with the cysticercus stage of parasite.

Pathogenesis (host cycle): Infection occurs by ingesting undercooked pork containing the parasite in its cysticercus stage. In the human small bowel, the tapeworm eggs hatch but do not normally cause pathologic changes. In rare cases involving fecal contamination of food, the larvae penetrate the wall of the bowel and migrate to the skeletal and cardiac muscle (and occasionally the lung, liver, and brain as well) by hematogenous dissemination. The parasite manifests itself in these tissues as larvae the size of millet grains (cysticercosis).

Pathogen identification: includes whitish hardened nodules measuring 3–10 mm and detectable by veterinary meat inspection (the parasite in its cysticercus stage; ► A) as well as proglottids in the stool.

✚ **Clinical presentation:** Symptoms include ravenous hunger, loss of appetite, abdominal pain, and anal itching.
Complications (neural cysticercosis): Brain infestation manifests itself in clustered, cystic parasite structures (► B) that spread into the subarachnoid space.

☺ **Prominent patient:** Pharaoh Akhenaton or Amenophis IV of Egypt (1362–1356 BC), who may be regarded as having laid the foundation of monotheism.

▬ Echinococcus granulosus

Synonym: Canine tapeworm (adult form: 3–6 mm in length).

Pathogen that causes echinococcosis (hydatid disease).

Humans are intermediate hosts, not the definitive hosts.

Pathogenesis (host cycle): Using their four suction cups and double hooked scolex, these parasites attach themselves to the mucosa of the small bowel by the thousands. The worms consist of a scolex and 4–5 proglottids containing testes and ovaries. One of these segments drops off every two weeks, releasing over 500 eggs that are excreted into the external environment in feces. Herbivores such as sheep ingest these eggs while grazing. The eggs hatch in the duodenum, releasing invasive larvae (oncospheres) equipped with two pairs of hooks that invade the lacteal vessels and branches of the portal vein. Lodging primarily in the liver, they mature to a second cystic larval form (hydatid or Echinococcus hydatidosus). Brood capsules containing thousands of embryonic tapeworms (proscolices) develop from their inner germinal cell layer. The hydatids with their pathogenic scolices enter the definitive host when a carnivore such as a dog eats the carcass or offal of an infected herbivore such as a sheep or goat. Close contact with infected dogs can cause the eggs of E. granulosus to be passed to humans, where the hydatids develop primarily in the liver and lungs.

Pathogen identification: includes a hydatid wall of homogeneous eosinophilic cuticula with hooked scolices on the interior surface. Echinococcus hooks are shaped the antlers of a two-point buck (► C2, D).

✚ **Clinical presentation and morphology:** In a few cases, *E. hydatidosus* remains latent or spontaneous regression occurs with calcification (p. 134). These hydatids contain a sediment of dead scolices and granular calcification (hydatid sand). The hydatids grow slowly and may remain asymptomatic for years. *Echinococcosis of the liver* (occurring in 60% of all cases) involves displacement symptoms (► E). *Echinococcosis of the lung* (occurring in 20% of all cases) involves coughing, dyspnea, and bronchial penetration (the hydatid fluid has a salty taste). Where pleural penetration occurs, air entering the pleural space can lead to pulmonary collapse (pneumothorax). *Echinococcosis of bone* (occurring in 2% of all cases) leads to spontaneous fractures where long bones are involved. Vertebral involvement may lead to gibbus (extreme kyphosis) with paraplegia.

▬ Echinococcus multilocularis

Synonym: fox tapeworm.

Pathogen that causes alveolar echinococcosis.

Occurrence: The pathogen is endemic only in certain regions of Europe, including southern Germany, Austria, Switzerland, and the Balkans. Humans are intermediate hosts.

Pathogenesis (host cycle): The fox, the definitive host, excretes eggs in its feces. These are then ingested by small rodents such as field mice that serve as intermediate hosts. Multiple small, densely packed cysts containing infectious scolices (E. alveolaris) develop and proliferate in the entrails of these animals, which are prey for the fox. Human infestation occurs incidentally, such as in hunters skinning infected foxes. These cases lead to infestation of the liver and alveolar echinococcosis (► F; infestation of the gallbladder).

✚ **Clinical presentation:** Patients present with a mass in or around the liver.

A **Taenia solium:** (skeletal muscle) cysticercus stage

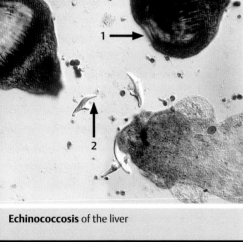

B **Cysticercus stage** (HE) x 7

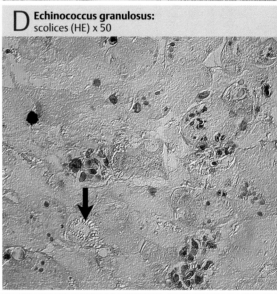

C **Echinococcus granulosus:** scolices (HE) x 25

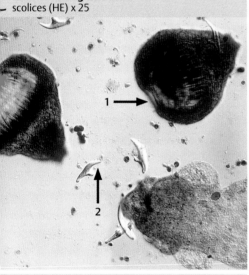

D **Echinococcus granulosus:** scolices (HE) x 50

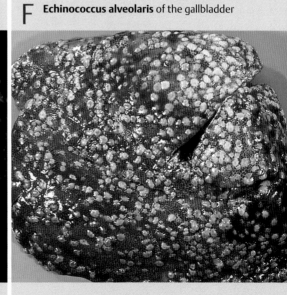

E **Echinococcosis** of the liver

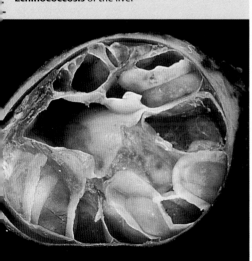

F **Echinococcus alveolaris** of the gallbladder

Nematodes

■ Enterobius vermicularis

Synonym: pinworm.
Occurrence: worldwide.

Textbook example of the world's most common transmissible disease.

Pathogen that causes oxyuriasis.

Pathogenesis (host cycle): Adult worms live in the mucosa of the large bowel (primarily in the cecum and appendix). After mating, the pregnant female migrates out of the host's anus at night and deposits its eggs on the perianal skin. This causes itching; the patient scratches the area and subsequently ingests the eggs as a result of oral contact with the fingers.

Pathogen identification: The parasite is round in cross section (▶A1) with an eosinophilic outer membrane and spiked (alae; ▶A2).

✚ **Clinical presentation and morphology:** The parasite is usually an incidental finding following appendectomy for acute appendicitis.

■ Wuchereria bancrofti

Pathogen that causes filariasis in the form of parasitic lymphatic edema, leading to elephantiasis.

The pathogen is a thread-like nematode occurring primarily in tropical and subtropical regions.

Pathogenesis (host cycle): A mosquito is the intermediate host. The infectious larvae mature within the insect and are passed to humans by mosquito bites. The pathogens colonize the lymph vessels and lymph nodes, where they develop into sexually mature nematodes. These organisms cause chronic obstructive lymphangitis that successively leads to obstruction of lymph drainage with distension of the lymph vessels upstream of the stenoses.

Pathogen identification: includes a worm measuring slightly less than 0.2 mm (▶B1) visible in cross section in the lymph vessel (▶B2). It exhibits an outer cuticula, two inner uteri with microfilaria and an intestine.

✚ **Clinical presentation and morphology:** Filariasis involves obstructive lymphangitis and lymph edema (p. 246) primarily in the lower extremities. This leads to tissue sclerosis and distension of the lower extremity that resembles an elephant's foot (elephantiasis).

■ Trichinella spiralis

Pathogen that causes trichinosis.

Occurrence: ubiquitous.

Sources of infection include all carnivorous and omnivorous animals such as domestic pigs, wild boars, dogs, foxes, badgers, rats, and bears.

Pathogenesis (host cycle): The pathogen is ingested with meat contaminated with larval cysts. The male parasites measuring approximately 1.5 mm and females measuring approximately 4 mm hatch in the small bowel, where they initially penetrate the intestinal wall and then temporarily return to the intestinal lumen. These organisms become sexually mature and mate within about one week. The fertilized females remain viable and able to reproduce for about four weeks. During this period, they give birth to about 1000 larvae measuring about 100 μm each and detectable by veterinary meat inspection. The larvae are then transported to the skeletal and cardiac muscle via the thoracic duct and circulatory system. There the spiral larvae encyst (▶C) and may survive for up to 30 years. The next carnivore serves as a host for reproduction.

Pathogen identification: includes a spiral worm (▶C, D1) surrounded by an ovoid hyaline capsule (▶D2) that leads to regressive calcification.

✚ **Clinical presentation and morphology:** Symptoms include febrile muscle pain, dangerous myocarditis, and blood eosinophilia.

❗ **Note:** Trichinosis is diagnosed by muscle biopsy obtained from a particularly painful site. Consumption of bear meat that is cured without cooking involves a high risk of infection.

In summary, we may conclude that both host and pathogen fight hard to ensure their survival. Some pathogens either attack the genome and trigger the death of the host cell, or they alter its genome in such a manner that the host cell can no longer die and must continue to reproduce the pathogen indefinitely. Occasionally this conflict between host and pathogen takes place in helpless embryonic tissue, wreaking havoc with the coordination of highly time-sensitive design plans.

The following section systematically examines these derangements that affect the transmission and execution of the body's design plans: hereditary disorders and developmental anomalies.

▼—
▼

A **Oxyuria** (appendix)
(HE) x 50

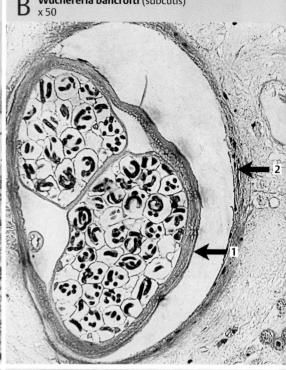

B **Wuchereria bancrofti** (subcutis)
x 50

C **Trichinella spiralis** (crush preparation)
x 10

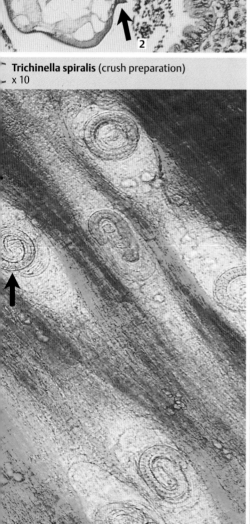

D **Trichinella spiralis** (skeletal muscle)
(HE) x 10

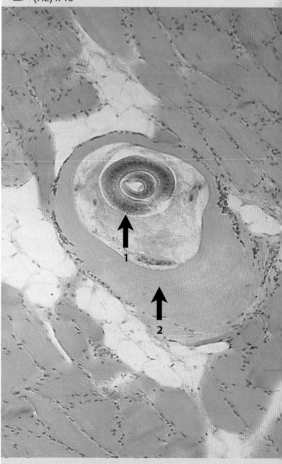

―――――― **Summary** ――――――

Hereditary disorders are diseases that are attributable to genetic defects.

▶ **Mutations** are permanent alterations of genetic material. A mutation may occur without any discernible cause (spontaneous mutations) or may be induced by exogenous influences (mutagens). Mutagens include ionizing radiation (ultraviolet, x-ray, or gamma radiation), chemical substances, (DNA or RNA analogs, alkylating agents, etc.), viruses and other microorganisms. Mutations can occur at any level in the structural hierarchy of elements comprising human genetic material. Defects at the chromosome and gene levels are clinically significant. Mutations can also occur in body cells (somatic mutations) or germinal cells (germ-line mutation). Somatic mutations are not inheritable. However, they play an important role in aging (p. 124) and in the development of cancer. In contrast, generative mutations can be inherited. Mutations result in the synthesis of an altered gene product that often leads to an altered phenotype. In extreme cases, the mutation may have no consequences whatsoever (occult mutation) or may directly cause death (lethal mutation).

▶ **Constitutional gene defects** are invariably present in every cell of the body as they were either inherited from a parent or were newly created in the fertilized ovum (zygote).

▶ **Non-constitutional Acquired gene defects** appear at some point in life in an individual cell and are subsequently passed on to daughter cells. Newly occurring genetic defects figure prominently in the development of tumors.

▶ **Gametic disorders** are associated with aberrations of the normal chromosome series that are visible under the light microscope (▶ A, p. 289). Numeric aberrations are deviations in the number of chromosomes from normal; structural aberrations are deviations in the structure of an individual chromosome that are visible under the light microscope. Such chromosome aberrations may be used to identify developmental anomalies in prenatal cell biopsies.

Numeric chromosome aberrations are common. They are attributable to nondisjunction of a sex chromosome or autosome (any chromosome other than the sex chromosomes) during meiosis of an ovum or, less often, a sperm cell.

― *Aneuploidy* (p. 8) is an abnormal number of chromosomes in a cell which is not an exact multiple of the haploid number.

― *Triploidy* is a tripling of the complete haploid set in all cells of the body due to double fertilization of the ovum by two sperm cells (paternal cause) or due to failure of the reduction of the chromosome set (with the release of the polar body) in the ovum (maternal cause).

― *Trisomy* is the presence of three of a certain chromosome in an otherwise normal (diploid) set due to nondisjunction of a chromosome pair during meiosis and mitosis. This results in cells with 47 chromosomes instead of 46.

― *Polysomy* is the presence of multiple copies of a certain chromosome in an otherwise normal set.

― *Monosomy* is the lack of one chromosome from a certain homologous pair or the lack of one sex chromosome in an otherwise normal cell as a result of nondisjunction. Autosomal monosomy does not permit normal embryonic development, whereas an embryo with monosomy of a sex chromosome will be viable.

Structural chromosome aberrations are changes in chromosome structure that are visible under the light microscope. They may occur on the long chromatid (q) or the short chromatid (p). Individual segments of the chromosome are often lost (deletions, **del**) or added (duplication or amplification). Segments may also be located in a different position (inversion, **inv**, or translocation, **t**). Too many of the genes located on the affected chromosome segment (+) or too few (–) will disrupt the genetic balance.

― *Unbalanced chromosome aberrations* occur as a result of fractures of one or more chromosomes that are repaired incorrectly or not at all, with the result that individual chromosome segments may be present once or may repeat. The risk of such chromosome aberrations increases with maternal age.

― *Balanced chromosome aberrations* are produced by the action of mutagens. In these cases, the entire complement of genetic material is present. However, some of it is distributed incorrectly on the individual chromosomes.

Monogenic hereditary disorders are caused by a mutation of a specific gene. These disorders exhibit an autosomal dominant or recessive inheritance pattern, or an X-linked dominant or recessive inheritance pattern.

Multifactorial hereditary disorders involve polygenic inheritance and result from the unfavorable interplay of genetic makeup and a series of environmental factors.

Mitochondrial hereditary disorders involve a mutation of mitochondrial DNA and are only passed on by the mother. The inheritance of these disorders does not follow Mendel's laws.

Chromosomal Disorders

General definition: These are disorders or developmental anomalies characterized by an aberration, visible under the light microscope, of the normal chromosome set or chromosome structure in one or both gametes and/or the zygote (gametopathies).

✚ **General clinical presentation** of *chromosomal disorders:*
Chromosome aberrations are detectable in over 50% of all spontaneous abortions occurring up to the 20th week of pregnancy. Their specific incidence is as follows:
- Trisomies: 50%
- XO-Status: 20%
- Triploidy: 15%
- Tetraploidy: 5%
Only a small proportion of zygotes with chromosome aberrations mature. The following percentages of fetuses with these disorders are born live:
- Trisomy 21: 25%
- Trisomy 18: 5%
- Trisomy 13: 1.5%
- XO-Status: 1.5%
Chromosome aberrations are particularly common among patients with these afflictions:
- Abnormal sexual development: 30%
- Primary amenorrhea: 25%
- Developmental anomalies, mental retardation: 25%
- Patients with spontaneous abortions: 5%
- Sterility: 2%

Autosomal aberrations and sex chromosome aberrations are differentiated, depending on the type of chromosome involved. Chromosome lesions are either numeric or structural:
— *Numeric aberrations* involve an alteration of the genome due to a deviation in the number of chromosomes.
— *Structural aberrations* involve an alteration in the genome due to a structural deviation in an individual chromosome that is visible under the light microscope.

Autosomal Aberrations

Pathogenetic principles:
— *Triploidy* is the most common chromosomal disorder. Here, the cells receive a triple set of chromosomes instead of the normal diploid set. This additional genome is the result of one of two processes.
   — A paternal cause is common and involves double fertilization of an ovum by two sperm cells.
   — A maternal cause involves fertilization of an ovum whose polar body was not released in meiosis.

— *Trisomy* is the most common nonfatal chromosomal disorder. Here, there are three copies of a certain chromosome in an otherwise normal set. This is due to nondisjunction of the two homologous chromosomes during maternal meiosis (the most common cause) or paternal meiosis. The result is an ovum with either one chromosome too many (positive variant or trisomy) or one too few (negative variant or monosomy). Cells with the negative variant are not viable. Triploidy results where a sperm cell with the normal haploid number fertilizes an ovum with the positive variant.

❗ **Note:** The *viability of trisomic zygotes* depends on chromosome size. Fetal death occurs earlier and more frequently, the larger the affected autosome is. Trisomy 21 has the best prognosis for survival as it involves the smallest autosome.

General morphology: Carriers of autosomal aberrations exhibit typical characteristics:
— *Low birth weight* with retarded development and general immaturity;
— *Multiple deformities,* primarily in the craniofacial region, hands, and feet;
— *Internal developmental anomalies,* primarily including the heart, kidneys, and gastrointestinal tract;
— *Functional disabilities,* including mental retardation and muscular hypotony and hypertony;
— *Fetal death;* autosomal aberrations are lethal to the fetus in 70–80% of pregnancies in which they occur.

Numeric Autosomal Aberrations

■ Triploidy

Definition: Chromosomal disorder due to derangement of the ovum during fertilization.

Pathogenetic principle: See p. 287.

Morphology: The disorder usually produces an early spontaneous abortion in which an embryo is absent or present only in its rudimentary stages. The placenta (► A) exhibits distended, edematous, poorly vascularized, myxoid cystic villi that are largely covered by hyperplastic trophoblasts (partial hydatiform mole; ► B).

■ Trisomy 21 (Down Syndrome)

Definition: This syndrome results from trisomy of chromosome 21 and is characterized by a triad of symptoms:
— Epicanthal folds ("mongolism");
— Mental retardation;
— Malformations.

Pathogenesis: The disorder is caused by nondisjunction of the two homologous chromosomes 21 during meiosis (principle: see p. 287). The probability of this event increases with maternal age. The nondisjunction affects gene locus 21q21–22, which encodes the β-amyloid protein (p. 50).

✚ **Clinical presentation and morphology:** Chromosome 21 is the smallest autosome, which means that trisomy 21 has the best prognosis of all trisomies. The disorder may be *diagnosed before birth* by amniocentesis and cytogenetic studies.
– *Facial malformations* include epicanthal folds, widely spaced eyes (hypertelorism; ► C, D) in an oblique cat-like position, and a large furrowed tongue (macroglossia).
– *Hands:* They exhibit simian creases (► C) and short, stubby fingers (brachydactyly), and a foreshortened and deflected little finger (clinodactyly).
– *Cerebral* symptoms include mental retardation and presenile dementia.
– *Musculature:* It is hypotonic; joints can be hyperextended and a distinct pot belly (► C) is present.
– *Immunologic* symptoms include reduced immunity and a small thymus (with cystic dysplasia of the Hassall corpuscles). Patients have an increased risk of leukemia (p. 358).

■ Trisomy 18 (Edwards Syndrome)

Definition: This syndrome results from trisomy of chromosome 18.

Pathogenesis: The disorder is caused by nondisjunction (p. 287).

✚ **Clinical presentation and morphology:** Life expectancy is approximately three months.
– *Craniofacial dysplasia* includes micrognathia (abnormal smallness of the upper jaw), a short neck, low-set malformed ears (► E), preauricular appendages, unilateral cleft lip and palate, and a long narrow cranium (dolichocephaly).
– *Skeletal malformations* include radial aplasia, camptodactyly (crossed, flexed fingers), and a foreshortened dorsiflexed great toe.

– *Obligatory cardiopathy* includes ventricular septum defect and valvular defects.
– *Intestinal malformations* include diaphragmatic hernias.
– *Renal malformations* include a single, fused horseshoe kidney.

■ Trisomy 13 (Patau Syndrome)

Definition: This syndrome results from trisomy of chromosome 13.

Pathogenesis: See p. 287.

✚ **Clinical presentation and morphology:** Life expectancy is approximately 50–100 days.
– *Facial dysplasia* includes bilateral cleft lip and palate, microphthalmos, coloboma, microtia, hypertelorism (widely-spaced eyes).
– *Cerebral* symptoms include absence of the olfactory bulb (rhinencephalon) and fusion of the frontal lobes (holoprosencephaly).
– *Internal malformations* include cystic kidneys, urogenital deformities, and cardiac defects (septum defects).
– *Polydactyly* (supernumerary fingers; ► F) is present.
– Infants also have *rocker-bottom feet.*

Structural Autosomal Aberrations

General definition: Clinical syndromes resulting from loss or addition of a segmental band, a segment, or a chromosome within the autosome.

■ Deletion Syndrome
Cri du Chat Syndrome

Definition: The syndrome is caused by partial deletion of the short chromatid of chromosome 5 (del5p).

✚ **Clinical presentation and morphology:**
– *Facial symptoms* include widely-spaced eyes, epicanthal folds, and broad-based nose, micrognathia, and low-set ears.
– *Cerebral symptoms* include microcephalus and mental retardation.
– *Vocal symptoms* include a weak voice resembling a cat's cry (hence the French name), presumably due to laryngeal hypoplasia.

De Grouchy Syndrome

Definition: The syndrome is caused by partial deletion of the long chromatid of chromosome 18 (del18q).

✚ **Clinical presentation and morphology:**
– *Facial symptoms* include ptosis of the eyelids, saddle nose, and projecting ears.
– *Cerebral symptoms* include microcephalus and mental retardation.
– *Sensory organ symptoms* include atresia of the auditory canal and atrophy of the optic nerve.

■ Microdeletion Syndromes

Definition: Small partial aneuploidies (often in the form of a microdeletion) that are barely detectable or undetectable in cytogenetic studies.

✚ **Clinical symptoms** include circumscribed dysplasia, developmental anomalies, tendency to develop tumors (increased risk of carcinoma), and mental retardation.

A **Triploidy:** partial hydatiform mole

B **Triploidy:** partial hydatiform mole (HE) x 50

C **Trisomy 21**

D **Trisomy 21:** facial features

E **Trisomy 18:** facial features

F **Trisomy 13:** polydactyly

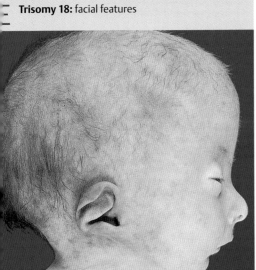

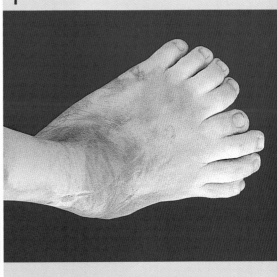

■ Microdeletion Syndromes (Continued)

░ Retinoblastoma Syndrome

Definition: Malignant intraocular tumor of the neural retina resulting from loss of segment 14 on the long chromatid of chromosome 13.

Pathogenesis: A congenital chromosome defect del(13q14) leads to mutation of the retinoblastoma tumor suppressor-gene (RB1; p. 324). Only the presence of a second defect of the RB1 gene (a "second hit") will result in a genetically determined bilateral retinoblastoma and predispose the patient to developing secondary tumors (see below).

╋ **Clinical presentation and morphology:**
Initial tumor (retinoblastoma): Arising from the retina, this is the most common malignant tumor in small children (▶ B1). Growth may be exophytic, with the tumor extending into the vitreous body and subretinal space, or endophytic into the retina, optic nerve, and meninges. The tumor blocks the pupil's aperture, creating a "cat's eye" amaurosis (▶ A) and causing blindness.
Histologic findings include small "blue" tumor cells with little cytoplasm arranged in a rosette (▶ B2). *Tumor growth* is rapid, leading to tumor necroses with radiodense calcifications. Metastases develop rapidly.
Secondary tumors occur several years after the initial tumor manifests itself. Patients tend to develop pineal gland blastomas and/or malignant bone tumors such as osteosarcomas or Ewing sarcomas.

░ WAGR Syndrome

Definition: Hereditary syndrome caused by loss of segment 13 on the short chromatid of chromosome 11. This is characterized by a quartet of symptoms that includes **W**ilms' tumor (nephroblastoma; ▶ C), **A**niridia, **G**enital anomalies, and mental **R**etardation.

Pathogenesis: A congenital chromosome defect del(11p13,15) leads to mutation of the WT1 and WT2 genes (Wilms' tumor suppressor gene; p. 324).

╋ **Clinical presentation and morphology:** *Wilms tumor* is the most common malignant renal tumor in children. *Histologic findings* include an embryonic mixed-cell tumor of the kidney consisting of three components:
- The *epithelial component* has primitive formations of tubular tumor cells (▶ D1) and glomeruloid tumor cells.
- The *blastemic component* is a hypercellular mass of undifferentiated tumor cells with little cytoplasm (▶ D2).
- The *mesenchymal component* contains fibrous myxoid tissue (▶ D3), some of which contain rhabdomyosarcoma elements.
Tumor growth is rapid, with necroses.
Metastases occur late by hematogenous dissemination.

Sex Chromosome Aberrations

General pathogenesis: These aberrations may be numeric and/or structural. They typically become clinically significant only at puberty, manifesting themselves in gonadal dysfunction, abnormal stature, and psychopathy with deficient intelligence.

■ Klinefelter's Syndrome

Definition: Chromosome aberration: 47, XXY.

╋ **Clinical presentation and morphology:**
- *Gender phenotype:* Patients are phenotypic males, sex chromatin-positive, and may be eunuchoid. They typically exhibit hypospadia and small testes with tubular dysgenesis manifested as hyalinized tubules (▶ E1), and Leydig cell hyperplasia (▶ E2).
- *Fertility:* Patients are sterile due to azoospermia or oligospermia.
- *Diagnosis:* Increased gonadotropin and estrogen in the urine with subnormal 17-ketosteroid and reduced levels of pregnanediol, estrone, and estradiol excretion.

■ XYY Syndrome

Definition: Chromosome aberration: 47, XYY.

╋ **Clinical presentation and morphology:**
- *Gender phenotype:* Patients are phenotypic males.
- *Stature:* Patients are tall.
- *Organ lesions* include renal agenesis, acne, and varices.
- Patients' *social behavior* is usually characterized by aggressive brutality.
- *Fertility* is normal to slightly reduced.

■ Turner's Syndrome

Definition: Chromosome aberration: 45, XO.

Pathogenesis: The disorder is usually caused by nondisjunction of the paternal gamete, leading to lack of a paternal X or Y chromosome (see p. 287).

╋ **Clinical presentation and morphology:**
- *Gender phenotype:* Patients are phenotypic females with rudimentary ovaries, leading to primary amenorrhea, failure of breast development, and a low hairline on the back of the neck.
- *Stature:* Patients are short.
- *Vascular lesions:* stenosis of the aortic isthmus, congenital lymphedema on the dorsum of the hands and feet, and webbing of the neck.
- *Fertility:* Patients are sterile.

Chromosome Breakage Syndromes

Definition and pathogenesis: These include inherited autosomal recessive disorders in which fragility of the DNA is increased due to one or more of these chromosome changes:
- Increased switching of sister chromatids (▶ F, G);
- Chromatid and chromosome fractures;
- Defective DNA repair enzymes (see p. 6).

╋ **Clinical presentation and morphology:**
Xeroderma pigmentosum (p. 6): ultraviolet radiation causes skin tumors as early as in adolescence.
Ataxia telangiectasia (p. 190): ultraviolet radiation and x-rays cause leukemia and malignant lymphomas.
Fanconi's anemia: mitomycin and psoralen produce anemia.
Bloom's syndrome: ultraviolet radiation causes skin telangiectasia and malignant lymphomas.

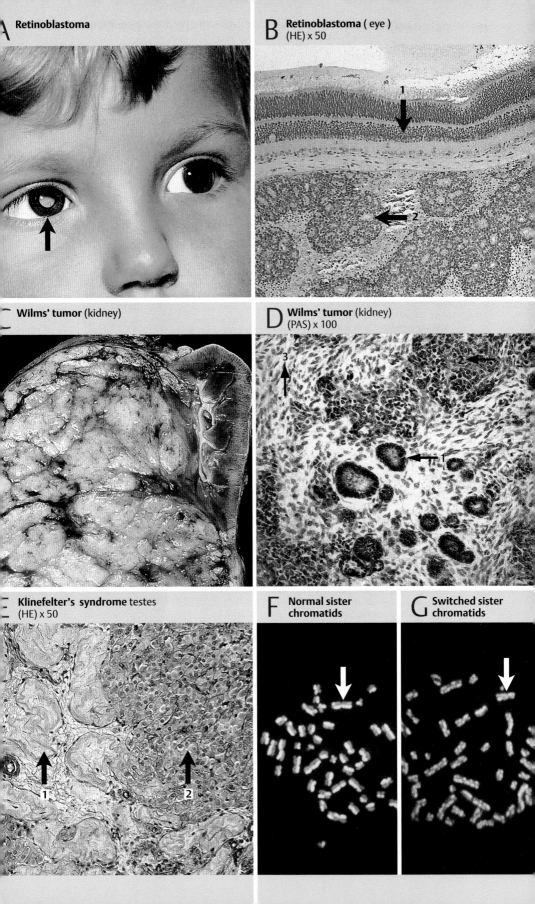

A Retinoblastoma

B Retinoblastoma (eye)
(HE) x 50

C Wilms' tumor (kidney)

D Wilms' tumor (kidney)
(PAS) x 100

E Klinefelter's syndrome testes
(HE) x 50

F Normal sister chromatids

G Switched sister chromatids

Single-Gene Disorders

General definition: These rare disorders are attributable to mutation of a certain gene without chromosomal defects visible under the light microscope. They are inherited according to mendelian principles, and their clinical manifestations are also determined by the penetrance and expressivity of the respective gene.

Autosomal Dominant Inheritance

Definition and pathogenesis: A single abnormal gene (allele) on a single chromosome in a heterozygous individual is sufficient to cause a hereditary disorder.

> **Note:** The *rule of thumb for clinical manifestation* of genetic disease is as follows:
> - *Pattern of inheritance:* Carriers transmit the abnormal gene (allele) to half of their offspring.
> - *Incidence by gender* is equal in males and females.
> - *Incidence by generation:* Carriers with manifest genetic disease can occur in every generation insofar as the disorder does not impair fertility.
> - *Familial variation:* The disorder's severity varies among carriers within a family group. Cases exist in which the respective gene does not affect all carriers (incomplete penetrance).
> - *Risk to offspring:* There is no increased risk for the children of a carrier's unaffected offspring.
> - *Most severe disease:* The homozygous dominant form involves severe pathology and leads to premature death. The same applies to carriers as a result of new mutations, with the result that the disease is not passed on.
> - *Parents as carriers:* When both parents are carriers, their offspring have a 75% chance of developing the disease.
> - *Age of manifestation:* The disorder often first manifests itself in adulthood.

Examples:
- *Adult polycystic kidney disease* (Potter type III) involves bilateral cystic kidneys due to impaired tubular morphogenesis, which is induced by mutations of the PKD-genes (= polycystic kidney disease).
- *Type II hyperlipoproteinemia* (p. 51).

Autosomal Recessive Inheritance

Definition and pathogenesis: For a hereditary disorder to manifest itself, the abnormal gene (allele) must be present on both autosomes; i.e., disease occurs only in a homozygous individual.

> **Note:** The *rule of thumb for clinical manifestation* of genetic disease is as follows:
> - *Pattern of inheritance:* Twenty-five percent of the offspring of a carrier develop the disease as homozygous carriers; 50% are clinically healthy heterozygous carriers, and 25% are healthy homozygous non-carriers. The incidence by gender is equal in males and females.
> - The patient's parents are obligatory carriers and usually clinically normal (heterozygous). They often have a common ancestor with the genetic disease.

> - *Relatives:* The patient's siblings are often the only other affected individuals in the same family group.
> - *Marriage of carriers:* Marriages among blood relatives who are carriers produce homozygous recessive offspring who invariably develop the disorder.

X-Linked Dominant Inheritance

Definition and pathogenesis: In these hereditary disorders, only the gene of one X chromosome need be affected. The dominant allele is active in every cell of the male (hemizygous individual); according to Lyon's hypothesis (see below), it is only active in some of the cells of the female.

> **+ Clinical consequences:** The course of the disorder is more severe in males than in females, and many male fetuses die in utero. All offspring of those males surviving to adulthood will develop the disease. Affected females will have equal numbers of diseased and healthy offspring.

X-Linked Recessive Inheritance

Definition and pathogenesis: For a hereditary disorder to manifest itself clinically, the abnormal gene (allele) must be present on both X chromosomes. In a heterozygous female, the normal gene on one X chromosome can almost completely obscure the disease trait on the other X chromosome and produce a clinically normal individual. This compensatory mechanism is absent in males, who have only one X chromosome.

> **Note:** *Lyon's hypothesis* maintains that in women only one X chromosome is genetically fully active. Early in the female's embryonic life, the paternal X chromosome is randomly inactivated in some of the cells and the maternal X chromosome in others. The respective inactivation is irreversible and applies to all daughter cells that stem from that original cell. This produces a 1:1 mosaic of expression for paternal and maternal alleles on the X chromosome.

> **Note:** The *rule of thumb for clinical manifestation* of these genetic disorders is as follows:
> - *Incidence by gender:* Males develop symptoms; females generally do not.
> - *Pattern of inheritance:* Clinically normal carrier mothers transmit the pathogenic gene to half of their sons. All sons of affected fathers develop the disease; all daughters are carriers.
> - *Cause of manifestation in women* is a random occurrence in which the X chromosome bearing the abnormal allele is active in the majority of cells. Causes include loss of the X chromosome or a homozygous state.

Example: hemophilia A (p. 402).

> **Note:** The *rule of thumb for inheritance* is: structural anomalies generally follow a dominant pattern of inheritance, whereas metabolic anomalies generally follow a recessive pattern.

19

Hereditary Disorders

Multifactorial Hereditary Disorders

General definition: Occurring more frequently in some families than in others, these disorders result from the unfavorable interplay of environmental factors and genetic makeup.

Pathogenesis: Several pairs of genes are invariably involved in creating the genetic constitution that triggers the disease. The individual genes involved in the disorder often have an additive effect and are transmitted according to mendelian principles.

Polygenic inherited traits include:
- habitus;
- stature;
- artistic abilities;
- skin and hair color;
- body weight;
- capability of glucose metabolism;
- blood pressure;
- intelligence;
- minor malformations (p. 304).

> **Note:** The rule of thumb for clinical manifestation is as follows:
> - *Risk of repetition with one affected parent* for each additional child is 2–5%.
> - *Risk of repetition with affected relatives*: For each additional child, the risk of repetition is 10–15% where two immediate relatives (parent or sibling) are affected.
> - *Relative risk of developing the disease.* It varies with the genetic proximity of the relationship, decreasing where more remote relatives are affected.
> - *Gender-related risk* of manifestation: Various multifactorial disorders manifest themselves more frequently in one gender than in the other.

With most multifactorial disorders such as obesity, diabetes mellitus, hypertension, dementia, or malformations, the difference between normal and abnormal may be gradual and difficult to identify. In such cases, threshold values are used to define the border between healthy and pathologic conditions.

> **Note:** In multifactorial disorders, malformations are extremes of the normal distribution Bell curve and lack sharp demarcation from the normal range.

Mitochondrial Hereditary Disorders

General definition: These are disorders that arise due to mutations in mitochondrial DNA.

Pathogenesis: The mutation occurs in the second genome (the mitochondrial genome) and is transmitted according to the principles of cytoplasmic inheritance described below.

An ovum receives several thousand mitochondria whereas a sperm cell has comparatively few mitochondria in its tail, which do not penetrate the ovum during fertilization. This means that a mitochondrial DNA mutation that produces a mitochondrial hereditary disorder is not inherited according to Mendel's laws; an affected mother passes it to all of her children, who all develop the disease. The net effect is that all sons and daughters are carriers of the mutation but only the daughters pass the disease on their offspring.

> ✚ **Clinical presentation:** Mitochondrial DNA encodes a few key enzymes involved in oxidative metabolism. Mutations cause mitochondrial hereditary disorders (p. 20).
> The mitochondrial hereditary disorders primarily manifest themselves in dysfunction of tissue rich in mitochondria. Several types of tissue may be affected and are listed here in decreasing order of disease incidence.
> - *Brain:* damage to astrocytes and ganglia leads to encephalopathies that tend to produce epilepsy; patients are no longer able to stand and require assistance. Optic neuropathy leads to blindness.
> - *Type I skeletal muscle fibers* may be affected, producing myopathy.
> - *Damage to the cells of the islets of Langerhans* leads to mitochondrial diabetes mellitus (p. 78) with neurologic symptoms.

> **Note:** Mitochondrial hereditary disorders are not inherited according to Mendel's laws.

Summary

Normal development requires extensive intercellular communication, involving understanding the signals sent by others and maintaining a speed and spatial pattern of growth appropriate to the surrounding tissue. Both genetic defects and noxious environmental agents can impair this intercellular communication. Appropriate compensatory mechanisms can produce a broad degree of variation in individuals' outward appearance or phenotype. The distribution of characteristics among all possible phenotypes follows a bell curve. Characteristics of a certain phenotype that lie outside this normal degree of variation are referred to as developmental anomalies.

With respect to causal pathogenesis, we may differentiate several component processes in early ontogeny that interact to produce a phenotype typical of the species.

▶ **Cell proliferation** in ontogeny and in subsequent regeneration in postnatal life is regulated by a number of genes. These include proto-oncogenes and the growth factors they encode as well as their adversaries, the tumor suppressor genes.

▶ **Cell determination and differentiation**: This term includes the steps in the functional specialization of a cell. Insofar as they produce visible morpho-

logic changes, these steps are referred to as differentiation. This process involves the precisely coordinated action of suppressor genes, pattern-regulating genes, and proto-oncogenes. It becomes apparent that at any one time in the process of developmental growth, only a few genetic factors determine whether a tumor, a deformity, or both will develop.

▶ **Cell migration**: To migrate to the proper site, the various differentiated cells make of use a motor in the form of intrinsic ameboid motion, a starting signal in the form of growth factors, orientation aids in the form of the extracellular matrix, and a reception committee in the form of cell adhesion molecules. After cell migration, the individual tissues contact each other. In a process known as induction, they can mutually influence each other and form organ structures according to a pattern. This in turn requires regulatory genes and also leads to fusion processes.

▶ **Cell death (apoptosis):** An important part of development growth is the orderly elimination of cells over time and at certain sites in a coordinated process. This is effected by programmed cell death or apoptosis.

In a nutshell, this chapter on malformations is really about proliferation and differentiation.

Basic Teratologic Terminology

Gametopathy: Malformation resulting from chromosome lesions in the ovum or sperm cell.

Blastopathy: Mailformation resulting from disturbance of blastogenesis (during the first 16–18 days of pregnancy).

Embryopathy: Deformity resulting from disturbance of embryonic development (during the third–8th week of pregnancy).

Fetopathy: Deformity resulting from disturbance of fetal development (from the 9th week of pregnancy until birth).

Embryotoxic and fetotoxic injury: Any exogenous disturbance, ranging from reversible injury to lethal injury.

Teratogenic injury: Embryotoxic and fetotoxic injuries that manifest themselves as disturbed morphogenesis.

Teratologic determination period: The period in which a teratogenic agent must act in the sensitive phase of organ or tissue development in order to cause a certain pattern of injury. The causative agent may be either an intrinsic (i.e., genetic) factor or an extrinsic (i.e., environmental) factor. As the sensitive phase of organ development often lasts only a few days, the resulting defect often allows one to conclude when the injury occurred. This sensitive phase occurs at different times for the various organ primordia. Some exogenous tera-

togenic agents prefer certain organ primordia (organotropism).

■ **Malformation** is a morphologic change in one or more organs occurring during intrauterine development that lies beyond the normal range of variation in the species. Teratogenesis and tumorigenesis are closely related. Malignant tumors occur more frequently in association with malformations (especially dysontogenetic tumors in early childhood).

■ **Anomalies** are morphologic deviations that are not sharply distinguished from the normal range of variation, for example hypertelorism.

■ **Dysplasia** is a generalized or locally occurring microscopic textural disturbance that only reaches its final degree of severity after puberty, for example skeletal dysplasia.

> **Note:** A malformation is a morphologic change in one or more organs occurring during intrauterine development that lies beyond the range of variation typical of the species.

General Etiology

■ **Genetic causes (p. 286).**

■ **Exogenous causes:**

There are several noxious environmental agents that can cause injury during embryonic development and often even during the fetal phase. These agents cause injury to both genetically normal and genetically predisposed individuals and include:

— *High doses of ionizing radiation;*
— *Cytostatic agents* such as aminopterin;
— *Pharmaceuticals* such as thalidomide;
— *Alcohol abuse;*
— *Viruses* such as rubeola and cytomegalovirus;
— *Bacteria* such as Listeria and Treponema;
— *Protozoans* such as Toxoplasma gondii.

Factors affecting intrauterine development: These factors do not cause embryopathy in the strict sense, but they can severely disrupt fetal development. Such factors include:

— *Enzyme disorders* such as maternal phenylketonuria;
— *Metabolic disorders* such as maternal diabetes mellitus;
— Maternal *hypervitaminosis A;*
— Disturbed *estrogen and progesterone* regulation in mother;
— *Immune reactions against the fetus* such as blood group incompatibility;
— *Pre-eclampsia;*
— *Amniotic transplacental infections.*

General Causal Pathogenesis

With fertilization, the ovum receives its full complement of genetic material and development of the individual (ontogeny) begins according to the genetic plan. This plan is implemented by means of several processes:

— Cell proliferation (increase in the cell population by mitosis);
— Cell determination and differentiation;
— Cell migration;
— Cell death (generally apoptosis).

Cell Proliferation

Physiology: Cell proliferation occurs in these stages:

— **Signal reception:** A ligand (growth factor) binds to "its" receptor on the cell membrane.
— **Signal transduction:** Limited activation of growth factor receptors activates signal-transducing proteins on the inside of the cell membrane (mitogen-activated protein kinase cascade).
— **Signal transmission:** The proliferation signal is passed to the cell nucleus by cytoplasmic second messenger substances.
— **Signal implementation:** Induction and activation of nuclear regulatory factors initiate DNA transcription, resulting in cell division.

The individual steps in proliferation are regulated by cell contact mechanisms and proliferation stimulators, inhibitors, and modulators.

■ Cell Contact Mechanisms

Definition: These are "adhesive proteins" (cell adhesion molecules) which they use for orientation in tissue. They belong to the supergene families and fulfill several functions.

— **Selectins** bind a cell to others not of the same type without Ca^2. This allows cells of other types to be removed, resulting in cell selection.
— **Cadherins,** components of the cellular adhesion organelles (desmosomes), allow a cell to bind to others of the same type without Ca^2. This causes cells to find each other and remain in contact, forming an epithelial organ tissue. Desmosomes are part of the epithelial cell-to-cell communication system. Interrupting the contact to an adjacent cell permits mitosis and proliferation; re-establishing contact with adjacent cells terminates proliferation. This is known as contact inhibition of proliferation.
— **Integrins** bind the cells to the collagen of the basement membrane or the fibronectin of the extracellular matrix. This anchors cells in the connective-tissue matrix.

■ Proliferation Stimulators

Definition: These are factors that generate and/or forward proliferation signals to the protein machinery of the cell nucleus in the process of signal transduction. They include c-onc and growth factors.

▥ **Proto-oncogene** (c-onc)

Definition: Collective term of normal gene sequences whose gene products contribute to regulating proliferation processes. When abnormally activated, they can transform the cells into malignant cells (p. 118, 322).

The c-onc control reception of the signal on the "contacted" cell, transformation of the signal in its cytoplasm, and implementation of the signal in its cell nucleus.

Depending whether they are located on or within the cell, the c-onc act in the following ways:

— *Class I includes* ligands in the form of the peptide hormone, and c-onc products EGF (epidermal growth factor) and PDGF (platelet-derived growth factor).
— *Class II includes* membrane-bound or intracytoplasmic *receptors* (c-*erb* B and c-*erb* A, respectively). Usually these include tyrosine kinases in the cytoplasmic receptor domains and the gene product of the c-onc.
— *Class III includes second messenger substances,* intracellular signal-transducing substances in the form of protein kinases (c-*src*) or membrane-bound GTP-binding oncoproteins (such as the *ras* oncoprotein family).
— *Class IV includes transcription factors* that modulate the activity of the transcription machinery and in so doing control the activity of the growth factors.
— *Class V includes apoptosis control factors.* The mitochondrial c-onc *bcl*-2 inhibits apoptosis (p. 128, 132).

⫶⫶ Growth Factors

Definition: Collective term of mitogenic peptide hormones that promote:

— *Receptor-mediated proliferation* and
— *Cell differentiation and motility.* In the latter case, a cell can only divide by mitosis after first having broken off contact with adjacent cells under the influence of a scatter factor.

Growth factors are produced by *autocrine secretion* or *paracrine secretion:*

— *Autocrine secretion*: The growth fator is created by a cell also possessing the respective growth factor receptor. Limited autocrine secretion occurs during embryogene sis and tissue regeneration; continuous autocrine secretion occurs in tumor growth.
— *Paracrine secretion*: The growth factor is produced by a cell not itself responding to the substance. This is the typical type of growth factor secretion.

■ Proliferation Inhibitors

Definition: Collective term for inhibitors proliferation at certain critical points of the cellular cycle. These substances include

— *Antagonistic growth factors* such as TGF-β and TGF-α and
— *Suppressor genes* (anti-oncogenes) such as p53, RB1, and WT1 (p. 324). These suppressor genes promote cellular differentiation and in so doing also inhibit cellular autonomy and tumor development (hence the synonym tumor suppressor genes).

■ Proliferation Modulators

Homeobox Genes

Definition: Genes that have conserved an evolutionary sequence of base pairs (homeobox) that can give rise to a certain pattern of growth in tissue as a result of asymmetric cell division.

Expression of the HOX genes is controlled in part by their own gene products, the HOX proteins, and in part by the growth factor.
HOX genes encode transcription factors with an amplifying effect and a diminishing effect. Depending on the pattern of expression, they provide the cell with a "memory" of its position. The cell "remembers" its original address and determination throughout an unlimited number of cell divisions. This causes a cell group to change its rostral-caudal, posterior-anterior, and proximal-distal growth gradients, resulting in asymmetry and a specific growth pattern.

✚ **Clinical Presentation:** Defective expression of the HOX genes leads to malformations in organs and their innervation patterns. An example is: *Neuronal colonic dysplasia* in which involves failure of the sympathetic nerve fibers to branch into the wall of the colon. The inhibitory effect of the sympathetic nerves on the myenteric plexus is absent, and the affected segment of the colon remains in spastic contraction.

Cell Determination and Differentiation

■ Cell Determination

Definition: Not accompanied by any morphologic or biochemical changes, this is the process by which cells become committed to a specific course of subsequent development. The cell and its daughter cells "remember" that developmental decision that was made.

■ Cell Differentiation

Definition: This is process of specialization in which a cell is prepared for a particular task. It may or may not involve noticeable biochemical and/or morphologic changes.

The essential stage of differentiation involves two processes.

— One is the expression of *differentiation genes* such as HLA molecules, adhesion molecules, and a cytoskeleton.
— The other is the expression and secretion of *extracellular anchoring proteins* such as fibronectin and laminin that bind the cell to the extracellular matrix.

Cell Migration

Definition: Orderly movement of cells of various determinations to programmed locations at programmed times to produce a specific pattern of tissue.

To migrate, the cells require a "motor," a "starting signal," a "map" with information about the path and direction, and a "homing device."

— The *migration motor* is the cell's intrinsic ameboid motion.
— The *migration starting signal* is given by diffusible substances such as growth factors.
— The *migration map:* provided by the extracellular matrix for the movement of all migrating cell systems. This matrix forms the roads guiding the migrating cells in the desired direction.
— The *migration homing device* consists of specific adhesion proteins on the surface of the cell. With the aid of these cellular adhesion molecules, migrating cells of the same type are able to find each other at the target site. These cells then bond together to form tissue patterns.

Apoptosis (Cell Death)

Definition: Programmed cell death (apoptosis; p. 128) occurs diffusely or locally in the form of zones of apoptosis (► A, B).

The cellular necrosis program is adapted to normal embryogenesis by cell-to-cell communication and by mitochondrial proto-oncogene (*bcl*-2). Cells producing signal substances can send their messenger substances to the target cells via the extracellular matrix of bloodstream after being stimulated by differentiation genes.

Apoptosis has several effects on developmental growth:

— *Division in the blastemas of the extremities:* An example of a typical defect is syndactyly in which the fused fingers or toes fail to divide (► C).
— *Fusion of initially paired blastemas:* An example of a typical defect is failed fusion of the sternum in which the two sternal primordia persist as separate structures, resulting in a split sternum.
— *Regression of embryonic structures:* Example of a typical defect is Meckel's diverticulum, in which the vitelline duct persists, resulting in a diverticulum or outward bulging of the small bowel approximately 50–100 cm proximal to the ileocecal valve (► D). This often occurs with heterotopic gastric mucosa (► E1) in the topical mucosa of the small bowel (► E2). This can result in an ectopic gastric ulcer.

Apoptotic tear in the buccopharyngeal membrane
(SEM) x 500

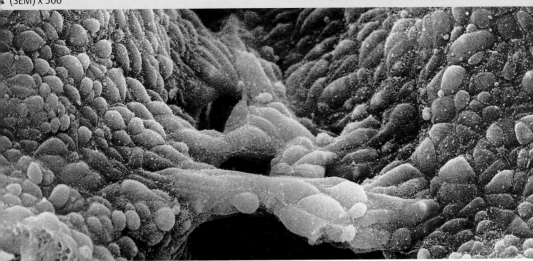

Zones of apoptosis in the blastemas of the
extremities

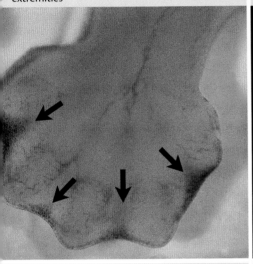

C **Syndactyly** between second and third toes
and fourth and fifth toes

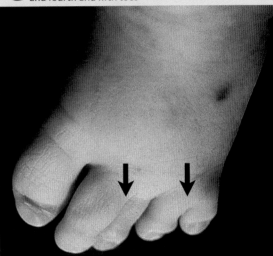

D **Meckel's diverticulum**

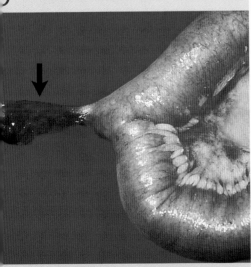

E **Meckel's diverticulum**
(HE) x 50

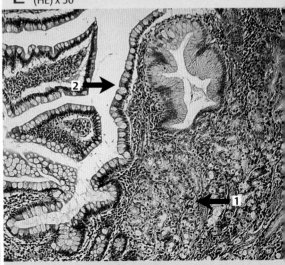

Blastopathies

Definition: See p. 294.

General pathogenesis: During blastogenesis, the developing embryo is completely unprotected against pathogens and is highly sensitive to injury from endogenous and exogenous causes. In most cases, the embryo dies as a result of such influences, triggering an early spontaneous abortion. In other cases, the remaining cells regenerate according to their prospective capacity. Where the separated mass of cells is sufficiently large, two or more independent fetuses will arise from one zygote.

> **Note:** *Isolated malformation:* It refers to a single malformed fetus that is not conjoined with another fetus, single malformation refers to a malformation of an organ or part of the body within a fetus.

Conjoined Twins-Malformations

General pathogenesis: These result from disruption of the division process in the blastoderm during blastogenesis.

Several different types of conjoined twins will result according to the symmetry of the separated cell masses and their regenerative capacity.

■ Complete Symmetrical Double Malformations

Pathogenetic mechanisms include incomplete separation of the cell masses or fusion of two primitive strips during gastrulation. This produces two complete fetuses conjoined at a certain location. The individual parts of such twins are mirrored along the plane of adhesion (► A, B).

Several types of conjoined twins are differentiated according to the location of the adhesion:
— *Xiphopagus* refers to conjoined sterna.
— *Thoracopagus* refers to conjoined chests (► A, B).
— *Cephalopagus* refers to conjoined heads.
— *Pygopagus* refers to conjoined sacra or coccyges.
— *Ischiopagus* refers to conjoined pelvises.
— *Chorioangiopagus* refers to normal identical twins with conjoined placental vessels.

☺ **Prominent Patients**
The original Siamese twins (thoracopagi; ► A) were Chang and Eng Bunker (1811–1874). Each married and they fathered a total of 11 children.

■ Incomplete Symmetrical Double Malformations

Pathogenesis: Incomplete cleavage produces two incompletely separated cell masses, and the twin cranial or caudal sections of the body vary in their further development. This leads to conjoined twins with two heads, two thoraxes, or two abdomens.

Several types of such conjoined twins are differentiated according to the part of the body doubled:
— *Monocephalus diprosopus* exhibits twin faces (a Janus malformation exhibits two faces in opposite directions).
— *Dicephalus* exhibits two heads and usually two legs (dipus) and two, three, or four arms (di-, tri-, or tetrabrachius).
— *Dipygus* exhibits doubling of the lower half of the body.

■ "Parasitic" Asymmetrical Double Malformations

Pathogenesis: Incomplete separation of the cell masses leads to development of two fetuses with widely varying degrees of development that are conjoined at a certain location.
— The *autosite* is a nearly normal twin.
— The *parasite* is a rudimentary twin that exhibits tissues bordering on teratomas (embryonic tumors) in the region conjoined with the autosite.

The resulting malformation is described as:
— An *epignathus* where the parasite is conjoined at the lower jaw;
— A *sacral parasite* where the parasite is joined in the sacral region.

☺ **Clinical Record:** The largest number of multiple births included 15 babies (10 girls and 5 boys), delivered by caesarean section, by a 35-year-old mother in Rome, Italy, on July 22, 1971.

Feto-fetal Transfusion Syndrome

Definition and pathogenesis: In monochorionic diamniotic twin placentation, vascular anastomoses are present in umbilical cord (► C). These anastomoses have no functional effect where both fetuses have equal cardiac output. In the presence of acute circulatory insufficiency of one fetus, the temporarily stronger fetus will pump its blood into the circulatory system of the weaker one.
— The *recipient*, the larger twin (► D1), suffers hypervolemic shock (p. 392; ► E1);
— The *donor*, the smaller twin with anemia (► D2), suffers hypovolemic shock (p. 392; ► E2). This leads to death of both twins.

The "original" Siamese twins

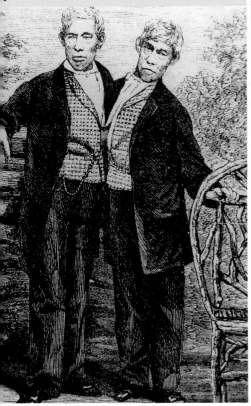

B Cephalothoracopagi

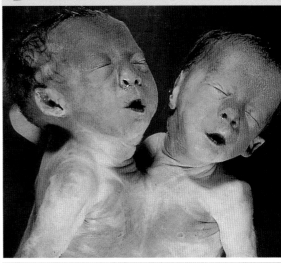

C Feto–fetal transfusion syndrome
(radiograph of placenta)

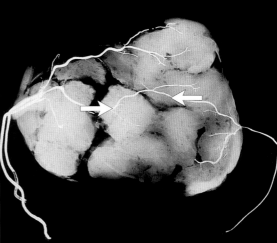

D Feto-fetal transfusion syndrome (twins)

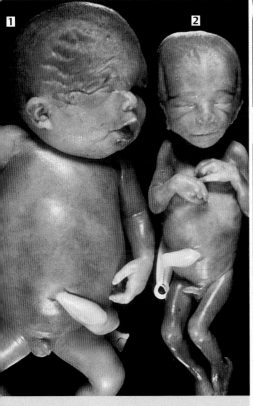

1   2

E Feto-fetal transfusion syndrome (twins)

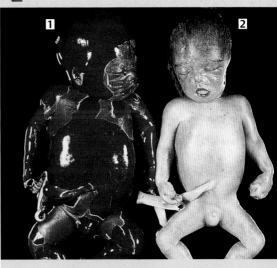

1   2

Embryopathies

Definition: See p. 294.

General pathogenesis: In the embryonic phase, the cells descended from the earlier daughter cells have differentiated and are no longer pluripotential. This means that abnormal development will no longer result in double formations but will only produce individuals with single or multiple malformations.

Several types of errors in morphogenesis may be differentiated according to the specific causative mechanism:
— *Malformation* in the strict sense is where an intrinsic error in the primordium leads to a genetically determined morphologic defect in an organ, part of an organ, or part of the body. This defect may take the form of inhibited development, hyperplasia, or heteroplasia.
— *Disruption* is where secondary exogenous damage to an intact embryo leads to a morphologic anomaly in an organ, part of an organ, or part of the body.
— *Deformation* is where local mechanical forces *in utero* lead to an anomaly in an organ, part of an organ, or part of the body with respect to morphology, size, or position. An *example* is hypoplasia of the lung in oligohydramnios or Potter sequence (p. 302).

Morphogenetic Forms of Embryopathy

Isolated (Single) Malformations

■ **Supernumerary Malformations** are malformations in which an organ or part of the body is present in excess.

Examples:
— Polydactyly (supernumerary fingers)
— Doubling of the renal pelvis, ureter, and uterus.

■ **Fusion Malformations** are malformations resulting from failed separation of organs or tissues.

Examples:
— Hypodactyly (missing fingers) due to fusion of the finger primordia;
— Cyclopia due to fusion of the optic primordia;
— Holoprosencephaly due to fusion of the frontal lobes of the brain.

■ **Failures of dorsal Fusion (Dysraphia)** may occur along the posterior embryonic fusion lines, leading to cleft posterior structures.

Examples include defects in neural tube formation such as spina bifida (cleft spine), failed fusion of the lumbar or coccygeal spine (▶ A).

■ **Failures of ventral Fusion** may occur along the anterior embryonic fusion lines, leading to cleft anterior structures along the midline.

Examples include:
— Cleft lip and palate;
— Ectopia cordis (cleft sternum with exposure of the heart);
— Thoracogastroschisis (combined fissure of the chest and abdomen with exposure of the viscera; p. 305, ▶ D);

— Omphalocele (herniation of the viscera into a thin membranous sac);
— Exstrophy of the bladder (anterior fissure of the lower abdomen and bladder with diverticulum of the bladder).

■ **Agenesis** is the absence of an organ or part of the body due to absence of its primordium.

Example: unilateral left renal agenesis, in which the left adrenal gland assumes a coronal position (▶ E).

■ **Aplasia** is the absence of an organ or part of the body due to failure of a rudimentary primordium to develop.

Example: renal aplasia.

■ **Hypoplasia** is abnormally small size of an organ or part of the body due to premature cessation of growth.

Example: renal hypoplasia.

■ **Atresia** is the absence of a physiologic ostium or the lumen of a hollow organ.

Example: anal atresia (absence of the anus; ▶ B).

■ **Stenosis** is abnormal narrowing of an ostium or the lumen of a hollow organ.

Example: stenosis of the aortic isthmus (narrowing of the isthmus of the thoracic aorta, i.e., the segment between left subclavian artery and the junction with the ductus arteriosus, which is usually obliterated).

■ **Vestige** refers to persisting rudimentary parts of organs that normally regress during intrauterine development.

Example: Meckel's diverticulum of the small bowel in the presence of a partially persisting vitelline duct (p. 296).

■ **Hamartia** is localized developmental disturbance of a tissue structure derived from a germ layer.

Example: cavernous hemangioma (▶ C), a common, usually subcapsular tumor in the liver of blood spaces resembling the corpus cavernosum (▶ D).

■ **Chorista** is ectopic differentiated tissue that has become displaced into the tissue of another germ layer.

Example: ectopic germ of the adrenal cortex.

■ **Cysts** are hollow spaces with an epithelial lining that arise due to excessive proliferation of epithelium of retention of substances that would otherwise be released from inner or outer surfaces.

Example: cystic kidney occurring in type III oligohydramnion or Potter's sequence (▶ F).

■ **Atavism** is the recurrence of primitive phylogenetic morphology.

Example: is polymastia (occurrence of more than two breasts).

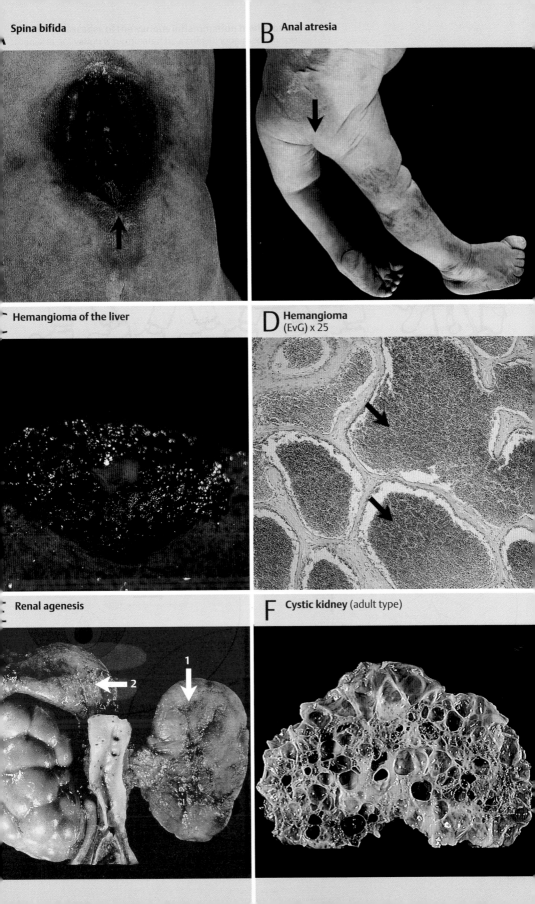

A Spina bifida

B Anal atresia

Hemangioma of the liver

D Hemangioma (EvG) x 25

Renal agenesis

1
2

F Cystic kidney (adult type)

Multiple Malformations

Definition: These are a series of malformations that can occur in an individual at random, independently of one another, or in certain combinations sharing a common cause or pathogenetic interdependence.

■ **Field Defects** are groups of malformations that arise due to disturbances in a certain field of embryonic development. Their cause may be of a primary nature (a defective primordium) or a secondary nature (a disruption).

✚ **Clinical example:** *Holoprosencephaly* is a combined facial and cerebral malformation involving failure of separation of the cerebral hemispheres in the forebrain and arhinencephalia. The most severe form of these groups of malformations is cyclopia (▶ A), characterized by a single central eye and a nose-like stump of skin (proboscis) superior to the eye.

■ **Sequence** refers to a pattern of multiple malformations occurring as a cascade as a result of a single primary or secondary developmental disturbance.

✚ **Clinical example:** *Oligohydramnios sequence (Potter's sequence)* is a multifactorial pattern of injury involving renal agenesis, urethral obstruction, and loss of amniotic fluid. This leads to *uniform injury* (oligohydramnios) that in turn causes *disruptions* (amnion nodosum, fetal compression, and pulmonary hypoplasia) that combine to form a typical teratologic phenotype.
Common characteristics of all oligohydramnios sequences include:
- *facial dysmorphism* (▶ C) with folds inferior to the eyelids, a small chin, a parrot's beak nose, and prominent earlobes;
- *thoracic deformity* (narrow box-like chest);
- *hand and foot deformations* due to caudal regression of the distal trunk. Extreme variants of this include
- *sirenomelia* (▶ B) with a single leg-like extremity and
- *complete caudal regression* (▶ E).

■ **Syndrome** refers to pattern of multiple malformations that occur as a result of a common primary or secondary disturbance in more than one field of embryonic development.
Example: Down's syndrome.

■ **Congenital disorder** refers to an anomaly due to an inherited disposition that is present at birth and exhibits conditioned progression and a tendency to worsen.
Example: hereditary glycogenosis.

Etiologic Forms of Embryopathy

■ **Radiation Embryopathy**

Pathogenesis: The phase of greatest sensitivity to radiation extends from the 5th to 13th week of pregnancy. The resulting injury to the embryo depends on the radiation dose.

✚ **Clinical presentation and morphology:** Infants exhibit microcephaly, mental retardation, eye damage, short stature, and occasionally skeletal deformities.

■ **Diabetic Embryopathy**

Definition: Embryopathy that occurs in poorly controlled or untreated maternal diabetes mellitus (in 3–12% of all cases) associated with intestinal atresia, heart defects, polydactyly, and clubfoot (p. 78).

■ **Thalidomide Embryopathy**

Definition: Typical malformation syndrome primarily occurring in the form of limb abnormalities following intake of thalidomide.

Pathogenesis: Even a single dose of 100–300 mg of thalidomide taken between the 25th and 44th days after conception produces severe defects.

✚ **Clinical presentation and morphology:**
Limb abnormalities include
- *agenesis or hypogenesis.* In their least severe form these include hypoplasia of the thenar eminence and thumb and radial hypoplasia or aplasia; in their most severe form, phocomelia with absence of the peripheral radial rays or amelia (▶ D). Symptoms also include
- *supernumerary structures* such as three phalanges in the thumb.

Craniofacial malformations:
- *Auricular defects* include anotia (absence of the outer ear), often in association with deafness and cranial nerve damage.
- *Ocular defects* include coloboma due to failure of fusion of the embryonic optic cup and microphthalmos.
- *Dental anomalies* may also be present.
Organ malformations include defects of the heart, major vessels, and lungs as well as esophageal, duodenal, intestinal, and anal atresia.

■ **Congenital Rubella Syndrome:** See p. 240.

Cyclopia

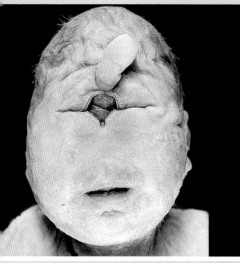

Face in oligohydramnios sequence

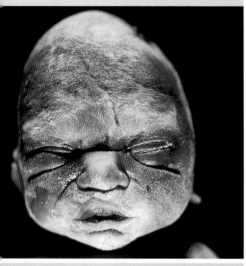

Phocomelia

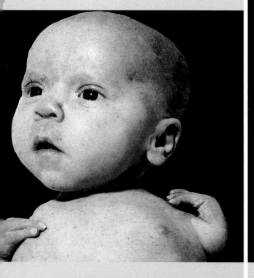

B **Potter's sequence:** sirenomelia

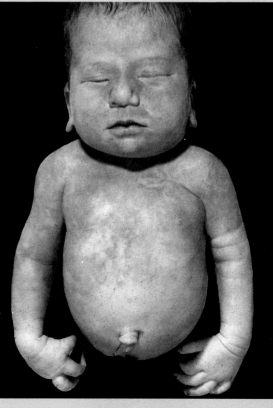

E **Potter's sequence:** complete caudal regression

■ Embryofetal Alcohol Syndrome

Definition: Alcohol-associated syndrome involving at least five of these criteria:
— *Maternal alcohol abuse;*
— *Intrauterine hypotrophy* leading to low birth weight;
— *Failure to thrive:* reduced growth after birth and slow weight gain;
— *Microcephalus;*
— *Motor and mental retardation* with subsequent motor hyperactivity (hyperactive child syndrome).
— *Characteristic face* (► A) with epicanthal folds, drooping eyelids (ptosis), foreshortened nose, nasolabial folds, and small chin (microgenia).

■ Amniotic Band Syndrome

Textbook example of an extreme form of mechanically induced developmental anomalies.

Definition: This is a sequence of disruptions caused by cords and sheets of tissue adhesions between the fetal membranes and the embryo.

Pathogenesis: The sequence begins with a rupture of the amniotic sac insofar as the amniotic sac and chorion are not conjoined. This causes the embryo to prolapse fully or partially into the chorionic cavity, giving rise to a variety of adhesions (► C3) between structures such as the head (► C1) and placenta (► C2). These adhesions ensnare and constrain the embryo and subject it to traction, impairing the development of the affected organ fields and leading to deformities of organs (such as the ear; ► C5) and/or extremities (► C4).

The *morphology* of the impairment malformations depends on the position and severity of the adhesions.
— *Craniofacial defects* many include
— anencephaly,
— encephalocele (► B) in which the occipital bone is absent and the brain displaces into a hernial sac (cele).
— *Oral and facial deformities* may be present in the form of cleft lip and palate.
— *Abdominal wall defects* may include thoracogastroschisis with displacement of the heart (► D1), lung (► D2), and intestine (► D3).
— *Amputations of extremities* may also occur.

■ Teratogenesis and Tumorigenesis

General pathogenesis: Teratogenesis and tumorigenesis are merely two different stages in the intrauterine response to disrupting influences. A cell or tissue can develop one of the several lesions, depending on its differentiation and on the stage of development in which a genetic or exogenous insult becomes fully effective.
— Insults in *an early stage of development* produce a malformation.
— Insults at *a later stage of development* produce combinations of malformations and tumors (p.382).
— Insults in *the fetal and postpartum stage of development* produce tumors.

Example: A persisting subcapsular renal blastema is tissue from which a tumor may develop.

■ Multifactorial Malformations

Pathogenesis: A number of malformations occur due to the interplay of several teratogenic noxious agents and/or genetic and exogenous factors. Such multifactorial malformations include:
— Defects in neural tube formation;
— Malformations of the extremities;
— Impaired sexual differentiation;
— Torsional anomalies of the bowel;
— Cardiovascular defects.

Embryofetal alcohol syndrome

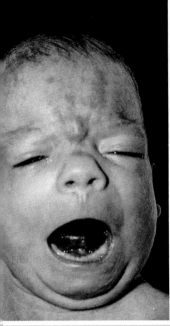

B Encephalocele

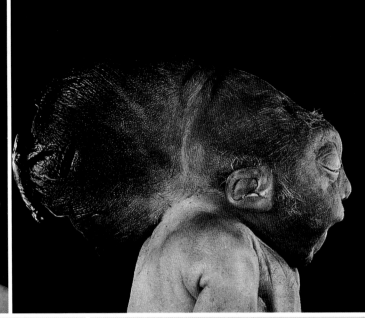

Amniotic band syndrome

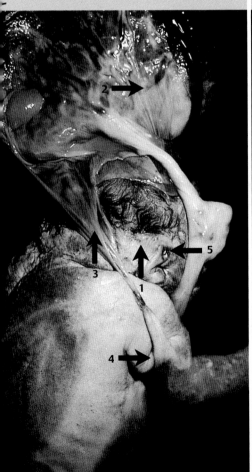

D Thoracogastroschisis

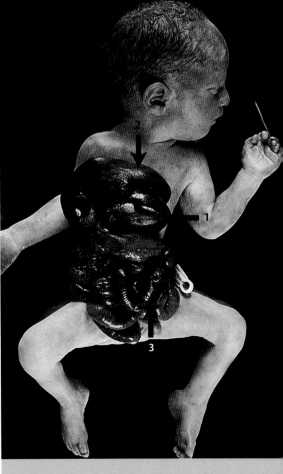

Fetopathies

Physiology: Tissues and organs that were present in rudimentary form in the embryo grow and mature during the fetal period. The hemopoietic and circulatory systems are now fully functional.

General Definition: See p. 294.

General etiology: At this stage, a noxious agent will no longer produce disease in the entire fetoplacental complex. Fetopathy is nearly exclusively attributable to exogenous causes (primarily infection). Because the fetus' inflammatory defenses are still rudimentary (p. 220), infection produces characteristic focal damage with dysfunction after the defect heals.

■ **Diabetic Fetopathy** See p. 80; this manifests itself in a pasty, obese appearance of the fetus (► A).

■ **Cytomegalovirus Fetopathy**

Pathogenesis: See p. 248.

✚ **Clinical presentation and morphology:**
The disease can affect all organs. Typical symptoms include
- *Cytomegalovirus encephalitis* with necrotizing inflammation, focal liquefaction with calcifications.
- *Microcephalus:* Surviving fetuses develop *microcephaly* with granular ependymitis and
- *Obstructive hydrocephalus* with periventricular calcifications, leading to spastic paralysis.

■ **Listerial Fetopathy**

Pathogenesis: See p. 256.

✚ **Clinical presentation and morphology:**
- *Infant septic granulomatosis:* septic dissemination of the pathogen leads to multiple initial necroses. Later it produces histiocytic and epithelioid mixed-cell granulomas the size of a pinhead (p. 256) primarily in the shoulders, back, lungs, and liver (► B).
- *Listerial encephalitis* is characterized by focal necroses primarily in the pons and medulla oblongata.

❗ **Note:** *Listerial granulomas* occur at perivascular locations due to their hematogenic origin.

■ **Fetal Toxoplasmosis**

Pathogenesis: See p. 276.

✚ **Clinical presentation and morphology:**
- *Toxoplasma encephalitis* is characterized by ubiquitous miliary granulomas (► C) of adventitial cells, astrocytes, microglial cells, plasma cells, and eosinophils whose centers contain cellular detritus. Coagulation necrosis occurs with calcification (► D), and Toxoplasma pseudocysts (p. 277; ► D1) are present.
- *Obstructive hydrocephalus* is present.
- *Toxoplasma chorioretinitis* occurs with eosinophils and immature blood cells.

■ **Congenital Syphilis**

Pathogenesis: See p. 262. The path of infection is exclusively transplacental.

▥ **Fetal syphilis** leads to fetal death or manifest maceration.

▥ **Early infant syphilis** involves bullous separation of the skin over a large area (neonatal pemphigus).

▥ **Late infant syphilis** involves fibrotic organ inflammation.

✚ **Clinical presentation and morphology:**
- *"Flint stone" liver:* Interstitial fibrosis (► E) press the liver cell structures apart (► E2); interspersed with this are granulomas containing lymphocytes and histiocytes (miliary syphilomas; ► E3). Isolated hemopoietic foci are also present.
- *Pneumonia alba:* Interstitial pneumonia with a white cut surface containing lymphocytes, histiocytes, and plasma cells is present.
- *Syphilitic osteochondritis* involves widening of the epiphyseal growth plates that resists maceration and is due to ineffective cartilage resorption. This results in direct pericellular calcification of cartilage in the form of a lattice of calcification (► F).

▥ **Childhood syphilis:** Patients who survive the infection develop decaying ulcerous gummas in the skeletal system, mucous membranes, skin, liver, lymph nodes of the neck, and brain.

✚ **Clinical presentation and morphology:**
- *Hutchinson's incisors:* A typical barrel-shaped deformity of the upper incisors occurs.
- *Saber shins* result from syphilitic osteochondritis.
- *Saddle nose:* The nose is depressed due to gummatous destruction of the nasal skeleton.

❗ **Note:** *Hutchinson's triad* includes
1. parenchymatous keratitis of the eye,
2. 8th nerve deafness, and
3. Hutchinson's incisors.

In summary, the process of development proceeds in these stages:
- Blastemic cells are not yet differentiated.
- This leads to cell migration.
- This in turn leads successively to cell proliferation and cell differentiation.

We encounter these same stages in regeneration and tumor growth. For this reason, it is often difficult to draw the line between ontogeny and tumorigenesis. Regeneration and tumorigenesis are discussed in the next section.

20

Congenital Malformations

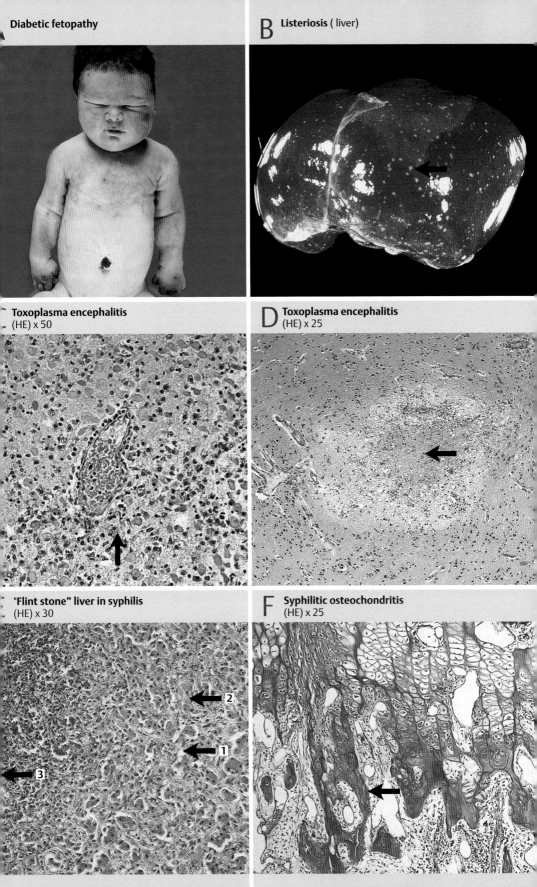

Diabetic fetopathy

B **Listeriosis** (liver)

Toxoplasma encephalitis
(HE) x 50

D **Toxoplasma encephalitis**
(HE) x 25

"Flint stone" liver in syphilis
(HE) x 30

F **Syphilitic osteochondritis**
(HE) x 25

"Mending" Tissue Damage
Tissue Repair

Summary

This section examines the subject of proliferation and differentiation discussed in the previous chapter on congenital malformations from a biologic standpoint. Specifically, we will discuss the reversal of differentiation, proliferation, and differentiation that occurs when lost tissue is replaced.

▶ **Regeneration**: Tissue is replaced according to the same principles that regulate growth and differentiation during ontogeny. These include the cell contact mechanisms and proto-oncogenes, growth factors, and suppressor genes. These factors enable the body to repair a tissue defect either completely with the original tissue or with substitute tissue. This process may be observed in wound healing. In a certain sense, wound healing is an alternate type of injury-induced inflammation that begins with an exudative inflammatory reaction and either heals immediately (by first intention) or, in the case of larger defects, becomes a granulating inflammatory reaction that eventually heals and leaves behind scar tissue (healing by second intention). This process of wound healing also applies in slightly modified form to the healing of bone fractures and wounds in organs.

▶ **Metaplasia**: Recurrent tissue injuries result in adaptive modification of tissue differentiation. This means that the original tissue becomes transformed into "sturdier" tissue exhibiting distinct differentiation. Such a process of metaplasia can be triggered by the stem cells or by differentiated tissue cells.

▶ **Heteroplasia**: Tissue injuries occasionally cause migration of mature tissue to a different location where it develops into a tumor-like lesion after healing.

▶ **Tumor-like lesions**: Tissue injury can cause focal overshooting of the regeneration process, creating a tumor-like growth that is reversible after the triggering stimulus is withdrawn. This makes it clear that regeneration can develop into tumorigenesis and vice versa.

Tissue Repair

General definition: Tissue repair refers to replacement of lost tissue.

The regenerative capability of an organ decreases with the age and size of the tissue defect. There are also topographic differences in a tissue's regenerative capability (good regeneration at the craniocaudal poles). Two physiologic processes enable normal organs and tissues to maintain a constant mass.

Generation of new cells is achieved by regulating cell proliferation; the body uses factors that stimulate or inhibit proliferation to adapt to specific requirements.

Elimination of cells is achieved by regulating programmed cell death (apoptosis; p. 128, 132).

Physiology: Cells of postnatal human tissue may be classified as belonging to one of several compartments according to their mitotic capability, maturity, and functional competence.

— *Stem-cell compartment:*
  Biologic function: maintaining the existence of a tissue. It consists of pluripotential cells capable of mitosis (intermitotic cells). Some of these are transferred to the proliferation compartment by the action of mobilization factors and therefore from the G_0 to G_1 phase of the cell cycle. The rest of the cells remain in the stem-cell compartment in the G_0 phase, where they occasionally are recognizable as a germinative layer of cells.

— *Proliferation compartment:*
  Biologic function: ensuring rapid supply of cells. It consists of intermitotic cells with a short generation interval. This results in coordinated cell proliferation, which in turn leads to successive differentiation.

— *Differentiation compartment:*
  Biologic function: developing mature tissue.

— *Function compartment:*
  Biologic function: ensuring the function of the tissue. It consists of mature cells capable of mitosis (postmitotic cells) arranged in a configuration typical of the specific organ or tissue.

— *Elimination compartment:*
  Biologic function: eliminating old damaged cells by apoptosis (p. 128, 132).

Note: A tissue's differentiation capability is inversely proportional to its regeneration ability.

Several types of tissue may be identified according to whether proliferation or function predominates.

Labile tissue:

Biologic function: Such tissue consists of loosely aggregated cells of various differentiations and minimal adaptability. It is highly sensitive to sublethal injury and is readily able to regenerate.

Due to its high cell turnover, the size of the proliferation compartment in this tissue is adapted to its elimination compartment. These tissues most frequently give rise to "genetic errors" that result in tumors.

Occurrence: hemopoietic and lymphopoietic system and cutaneous and mucosal epithelia.

Quiescent tissue:

Biologic function: This tissue is a complex structure of cells with high longevity having a low physiologic rate of cell elimination and proliferation. This leads to a high rate of metabolic performance and/or functional reliability. The tissue is highly adaptable. Sublethal cell injury results in hypertrophy and hyperplasia; lethal cell injury triggers tissue regeneration.

This tissue consists of cells potentially capable of mitosis (reversibly postmitotic cells). Under physiologic conditions, its proliferation and differentiation compartments are accordingly small and the function compartment large.

Occurrence:
— Liver and renal epithelia
— Exocrine and endocrine epithelia
— Connective and supporting tissue
— Smooth muscle cells

Permanent tissue:

Biologic function: This tissue is a highly complex structure of cells with high longevity having a low physiologic rate of cell elimination and no proliferation, giving it the level of functional reliability required for critical life functions. The tissue is highly adaptable. Sublethal cell injury results in volumetric hypertrophy; lethal cell injury (primarily ischemia) leads to numeric atrophy but not tissue regeneration.

This tissue consists of cells incapable of mitosis (irreversibly postmitotic cells). Accordingly, they contain neither a proliferation compartment nor a differentiation compartment; they consist solely of a very large function compartment and small elimination compartment.

Occurrence: ganglion cells of the central nervous system and striated muscle.

> **Note:** Malignant tumors of *labile tissues* are the most common forms of cancer.
>
> - Epidermis → skin cancer.
> - Bronchial mucosa → lung cancer.
> - Intestinal mucosa → cancer of the bowel.
> - Cervical mucosa → cervical cancer.
> - Hemopoietic tissue → leucemias.

> **Note:** The incidence of tumor in a tissue is proportional to its proliferation rate. One *exception* is the *mucosa of the small intestine*, which has a high proliferation rate and a low incidence of carcinoma.

> **Note:** Malignant tumors of quiescent (or stable) tissue are among the rarer forms of cancer.

The mechanisms listed below control the replacement of lost cell material in the regeneration process. They also play a key role in tissue proliferation during ontogeny.

Regulatory Mechanisms

Physiology: Replacement of lost cell material in the repair process is regulated by mechanisms similar to those that regulate tissue proliferation in ontogeny (p. 295).

Cell contact mechanisms: For reparative proliferation to compensate for loss of tissue, the cells capable of mitosis must first be released from the tissue structure and migrate into the tissue defect that is to be closed. This is effected by scatter factors, which also function as migration factors and regulate cell migration.

Proliferation factors: Depending on the specific organ and tissue, these include certain hormones (sex hormones), vitamins (A, B_{12}, and folic acid), proto-oncogenes (p. 295, 322), and the growth factors (p. 296, 321).

Proliferation inhibitors: These substances diminish the effect of growth factors and proto-oncogenes. Some of them are actually antagonists of the proto-oncogenes (anti-oncogenes and suppressor genes; p. 296, 324). Some of them function as differentiation factors and promote cell maturation.

> **Note:** *Tissue repair* is regulated by the same mechanisms as ontogeny and tumor growth.

Physiologic Regeneration

Definition: Replacement of cells or tissues during the course of normal "wear and tear."

■ **Solitary regeneration:** Replacement of a type of cell or tissue at one time only during the life of the individual.

Example: Replacement of deciduous teeth by permanent dentition.

■ **Cyclical regeneration:** Regeneration of a tissue at certain specified interval.

Example: Regeneration of the endometrium after menstruation.

■ **Permanent regeneration:** In many tissues, tissue death and replacement is a continuous process (as in molting tissue). This also applies to tissue with reversibly postmitotic cells. However, it is not as apparent in these tissues due to the longevity of the cells they contain.

Example: epithelium of the intestinal mucosa.

Pathologic Regeneration

General definition: Closure of defects caused by cell injury in a cell system or tissue.

Complete Regeneration

Definition: Generation of new tissue-specific cells to close a defect and restore the original tissue architecture.

Pathogenesis: Regeneration is only possible under these conditions:
- The defect occurs in molting tissue or stable tissue.
- Damage is limited to organ-specific cells.
- The integrity of the epithelial basement membrane and/or the perivascular connective tissue forming the original stromal structure is preserved.

Example: Regeneration of the amputated left claw of a molting crayfish (▶ A, B).

Incomplete Regeneration

Definition: Closure of tissue defects with by means of replacement tissue.

Occurrence: wounds and large areas of necrosis.

Pathogenesis: Such regeneration occurs under these conditions:
- There is destruction of irreversibly postmitotic cells in permanent tissue.
- The defect extends to the basement membrane and the stromal structure.

Example: wound healing.

Wound Healing

Definition: Closure of a discontinuity in tissue associated with a loss of substance (wound) by generation of replacement tissue (initially granulation tissue, later scar tissue).

Etiologic factors include:
- *trauma* (such a cut);
- *ischemia* (such as an infarction);
- *inflammation* (such as an abscess).

Pathogenesis (▶ C):
- *Wound* results in bleeding.
- *Temporary closure* is brought about by blood coagulation, leading to hemostasis.
- *Mediators are generated* by necrosis at the edge of the wound. These mediators lead to
- *exudation,* in which increased vascular permeability (p. 196) produces a wound exudate and edema at the edge of the wound, thus cleaning the wound bed. The mediators also trigger
- *chemotaxis* (p. 200), attracting granulocytes and later macrophages to the site. Mediators also trigger

- *infection defenses* and initiate clearing of the necrosis.
- *Proliferation signals:* Thrombocytes and histiocytes generate growth factors (platelet-derived growth factor or PDGF and macrophage-derived growth factor or MDGF) for fibroblasts and endothelial cells →
- *Granulation tissue forms* as a result. A mesenchyme rich in capillaries (p. 224) grows from the edge of the wound, accompanied by numerous fibroblasts →
- *Scar tissue* then forms. The fibroblasts mature and produce connective tissue rich in collagen fibers →
- *Definitive closure* of the wound is the result.

Healing of a Skin Wound

■ Types of Wound Healing

Three clinical types of wound healing are distinguished.

Healing by First Intention

Pathogenesis: Where the clean undamaged edges of the wound are approximated, the wound will close directly without formation of granulation tissue.

Healing Under a Scab

Pathogenesis: A fibrinous scab covers what is usually a minor superficial skin defect. This prevents the wound from drying out and forms a barrier against infection. The scab separates once the healed defect beneath it has re-epithelialized.

Healing by Second Intention

Pathogenesis: Where a tissue defect separates the edges of the wound (such as in a laceration and contusion), a temporary covering of granulation tissue bridges the defect until it is replaced by scar tissue.

All three forms of skin wound healing involve the phases described in the next section.

Review: Refer to the section on exudative and granulating inflammation (p. 196, 226).

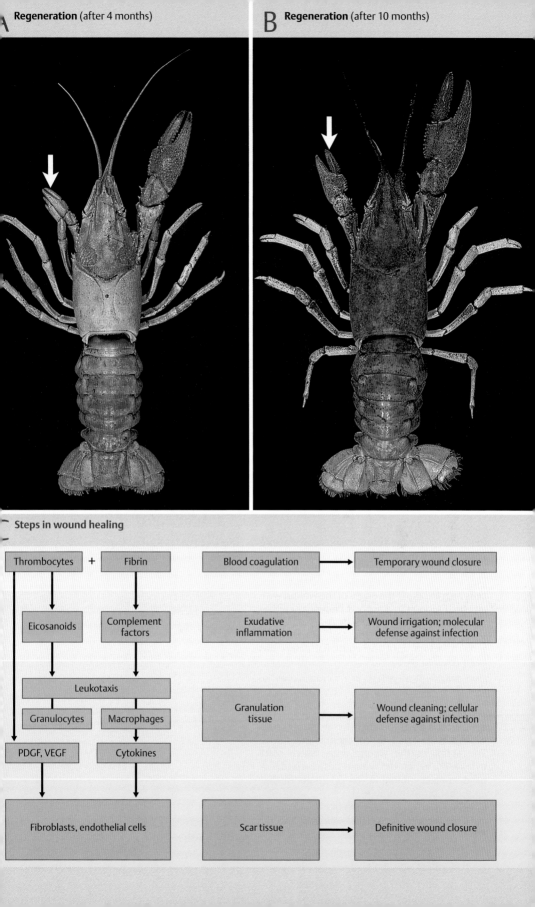

A **Regeneration** (after 4 months)

B **Regeneration** (after 10 months)

Steps in wound healing

Thrombocytes	+	Fibrin

Eicosanoids	Complement factors

Leukotaxis

Granulocytes	Macrophages

PDGF, VEGF	Cytokines

Fibroblasts, endothelial cells

Blood coagulation	→ Temporary wound closure
Exudative inflammation	→ Wound irrigation; molecular defense against infection
Granulation tissue	→ Wound cleaning; cellular defense against infection
Scar tissue	→ Definitive wound closure

■ Phases of Wound Healing

▨ Inflammatory Phase: Tissue injury involves a defect with compromised vascular structures. The fibrogen in the resulting serofibrinous wound secretion coagulates in the wound, which is rich in thrombokinase, and forms a scab (▶ A, E).

Short scenario: temporary wound closure.

The tissue damage triggers an alterative exudative inflammation reaction in its vicinity, then → local generation of inflammation mediators (p. 202), then → hyperemia in wound margin, then → edema of wound margin, and → excretion of a serofibrinous exudate with immunoglobulins into the wound bed.

Short scenario: Wound cleansing with a molecular defense against infection.

▨ Resorption Phase: Neutrophilic granulocytes migrate into the wound's vicinity after 6 hours, and histiocytes and lymphocytes do so after 12 hours (▶ B). The result: the annihilation, dismemberment, and removal of the pathogens and elimination of tissue detritus.

Short scenario: cellular "waste disposal service" resisting infection on a cellular level.

▨ Proliferative Phase: At the end of the inflammatory phase (after about 3 days), granulation tissue rich in capillaries with numerous fibroblasts (▶ C) develops under the influence of thrombocytic and macrophagic growth factors (TGF-β, PDGF, and VEGF; p. 320).

Short scenario: These factors act as a "road building crew".

The capillaries and fibroblasts of this tissue extend into the wound area. Fibroblasts at the edges of the wound emit scatter factors that release epidermal cells from the epithelial tissue into which they are integrated. These epidermal cells migrate along the edges of the wound with ameboid motion in a process known as epithelial migration. They proliferate (▶ F) under the influence of thrombocytic and macrophagic growth factors until the epithelial defect has been covered (▶ G).

Short scenario: These cells act as a "tarpaulin cover" to close the wound.

▨ Repair Phase: Once the tissue defect has been closed by granulation tissue, strong connective tissue rich in collagen fibers forms. This stabilizes the wound area, which scars over (▶ D). When the wound has re-epithelialized, contact inhibition (p. 321) halts further epithelial proliferation (▶ H).

Short scenario: This represents definitive wound closure, and the inflammatory cells of the "work crew" leave the site.

❗ Note: The *principles of epidermal wound healing:*
– Epithelial reserve cells differentiate.
– Epithelial cells migrate to the wound.
– They then proliferate.
– Further proliferation after closure is suppressed.

❗ Note: All wound healing involves an inflammatory reaction even in the absence of infection.

✚ Complications of skin wound healing:
These may be attributed to several predisposing factors:
– Contamination of the wound by foreign bodies;
– Diabetes mellitus;
– Hypercortisolism (p. 122)
– Ischemic and coagulation disorders;
– Proliferation inhibition (cytostasis or age).

Wound rupture usually follows infection of the wound.

Seroma occurs when a larger cavity in the vicinity of the wound fills with blood, serum, and lymph, impairing wound healing.

Traumatic epidermal cysts result from the spread of germinative epidermal cells into the deep plane of the wound.

Granulomas: Foreign-body granulomas form around nonabsorbable foreign bodies such as particles of glove powder and suture material and lipophage granulomas around necrotic fatty tissue (p. 236).

Exuberant granulation or "proud flesh" is a condition in which more granulation tissue is formed than is required to bridge the defect. This results impaired wound healing. This condition occurs primarily in the gingivae as a granulomatous epulis and in the skin as a telangiectatic epulis.

Keloid refers to a hypertrophic scar that extends beyond the skin adjacent to the wound. This complication is more common in blacks than in whites. Some cultures exploit the formation of keloids to create decorative ritual scars. A simple *hypertrophic scar* as distinct from a keloid does not extend beyond the wound.

Chronic wounds may result from:
– Tissue sequestra in the wound area;
– Pre-existing scar;
– Tuberculosis;
– Radiation;
– Neurologic damage.
Secondary tumor development is possible.

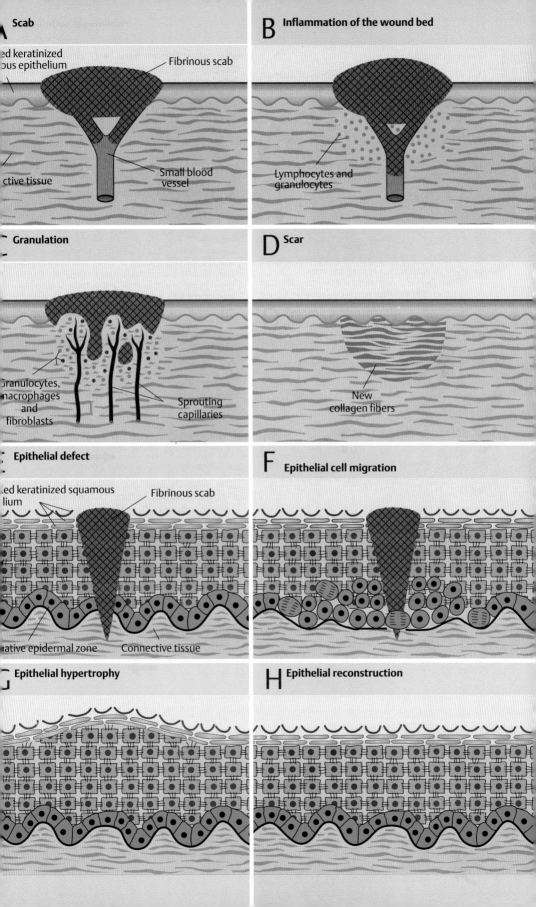

A Scab

Ked keratinized
ous epithelium

Fibrinous scab

ctive tissue

Small blood
vessel

B Inflammation of the wound bed

Lymphocytes and
granulocytes

C Granulation

Granulocytes,
macrophages
and
fibroblasts

Sprouting
capillaries

D Scar

New
collagen fibers

E Epithelial defect

Ked keratinized squamous
lium

Fibrinous scab

ative epidermal zone

Connective tissue

F Epithelial cell migration

G Epithelial hypertrophy

H Epithelial reconstruction

Fracture Healing

Definition: Fractures are complete or incomplete interruptions in the continuity of bone (incomplete fractures include greenstick fractures).

Once the edges of the wound (in this case the fragments) are approximated as in a skin wound, such a "bone wound" heals by either first or second intention. Accordingly, one differentiates between primary and secondary fracture healing.

■ Healing by First Intention

General definition: Healing of a fracture without formation a callus where there is a gap of less than 1 mm between the fragments.

Fracture healing may assume one of two forms, depending on the approximation of the fragments.
— *Contact healing* occurs where the two fragments are in direct contact. The existing osteons (▶ A2, B2) drill through the ends of the fragments perpendicular to the plane of the fracture like termites (▶ A1, B1).
— *Healing across a fracture gap* occurs when the gap between the two fragments is less than 1 mm. A capillary-rich mesenchyme grows into the narrow fracture gap, initially forming a plate of lamellar bone parallel to the plane of the fracture. Later this is replaced by osteons (▶ C2) aligned perpendicular to the fracture gap (▶ C1).

■ Healing by Second Intention

Definition: Healing of a fracture across a gap measuring several millimeters with formation a fracture callus (temporary replacement tissue).

▥ Phases of Fracture Healing (▶ E–H)

Fracture hematoma: The fracture causes bleeding between the fragments (▶ E). A narrow band of tissue along the margins of the fragments becomes necrotic, which widens the fracture gap.

Connective tissue callus: A mesenchyme rich in capillaries extends out from the surrounding soft tissue into the fracture hematoma. This results in proliferation of fibroblasts in the vicinity of the fracture. The gap fills with connective tissue, forming a temporary callus (▶ F).

Bony callus: Woven bone (▶ G) develops from this highly vascularized new connective tissue. Over time, this is transformed into lamellar bone that forms the definitive bony callus (▶ D, H).

One distinguishes between periosteal, intermediate, and endosteal calluses, depending on their location and tissue of origin.

✚ Complications of fractures:
Posttraumatic osteomyelitis involves bacterial infestation of the fracture hematoma. Occurring primarily in open fractures, this results in inflammation of the bone marrow that spreads to the bone and periosteum.
Pseudarthrosis (false joint) occurs when the fragments are not immobilized during the healing process. Here the connective tissue callus fails to become transformed into an initial bony callus, and the fragments remain mobile with respect to each other.
Exuberant callus involves failure of the periosteal callus to regress after healing. This can occur in isolated cases, especially in the presence of fistulas secondary to osteomyelitis.

❗ Note: Fractures are classified as either *traumatic* (occurring as a result of trauma) or *pathologic* (occurring secondary to insufficient trauma). A tumor should always be excluded in the later case.

Wound Healing in Internal Organs

■ Reversibly Postmitotic Cells:

Here, wounds heal according to the normal principle of wound healing. Tissue repair begins in the organ-specific cells and begins in the stromal cells only a few days later. The vascular connective tissue in defect is destroyed, preventing regeneration. The defect is therefore filled with scar tissue.

■ Irreversibly Postmitotic Cells:

Repair of these tissues, which include skeletal and cardiac muscle, consists almost exclusively of connective tissue scarring.

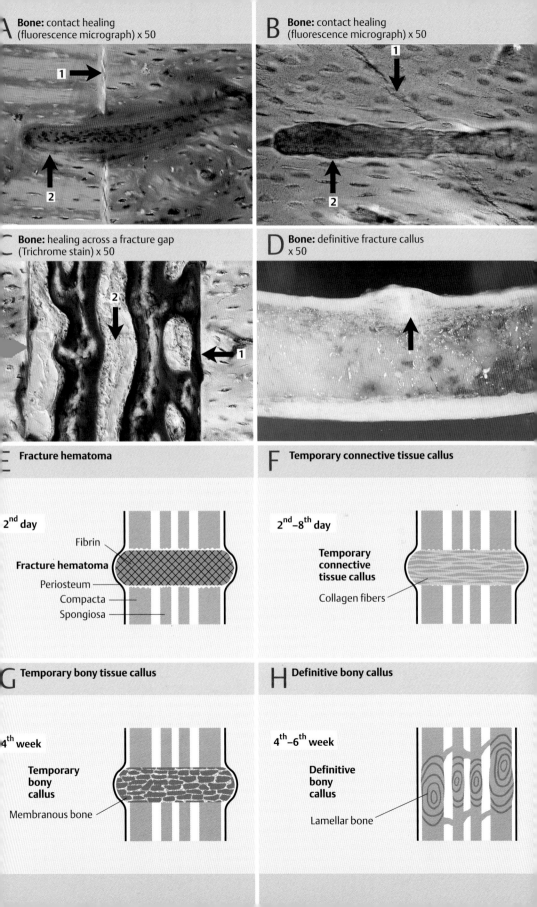

A **Bone:** contact healing (fluorescence micrograph) x 50

B **Bone:** contact healing (fluorescence micrograph) x 50

C **Bone:** healing across a fracture gap (Trichrome stain) x 50

D **Bone:** definitive fracture callus x 50

E **Fracture hematoma**

2nd day

Fibrin

Fracture hematoma

Periosteum

Compacta

Spongiosa

F **Temporary connective tissue callus**

2nd–8th day

Temporary connective tissue callus

Collagen fibers

G **Temporary bony tissue callus**

4th week

Temporary bony callus

Membranous bone

H **Definitive bony callus**

4th–6th week

Definitive bony callus

Lamellar bone

Wound Healing in the Central Nervous System

■ Open Brain Injuries

Definition: Brain injury involving traumatic division of the dura (laceration) and exposure to the outside.

Pathogenesis: A penetrating injury causes subarachnoidal bleeding with perifocal medullary edema with no contrecoup lesion (see below). This injury poses an increased risk of infection.

Morphology: Focal liquefaction of the brain tissue (liquefactive necrosis) is present. Macrophages phagocytize the tissue detritus within two days (free lipids produce lipophages; bleeding produces siderophages), and a brownish yellow area of resorption begins to form. The proliferation of glia, capillaries, and fibroblasts, resulting in formation of a glial fascial dural scar, follows:

✚ **Complications:**
Perifocal cerebral edema results in increased intracranial pressure that can produce compressive neuropathy.
Early meningitis (purulent meningitis) can produce several sequelae:
– *Diffuse purulent medullary inflammation* can lead to demarcation by granulation tissue, producing a cerebral abscess.
– *Purulent ependymitis* (purulent inflammation of the ventricular wall) may occur secondary to or independently of cerebral abscess. This leads to collapse of the ventricular wall.
– *Internal pyocephalus* (intraventricular suppuration) leads to purulent obstruction of the aqueduct and obstructive hydrocephalus.
Cerebrospinal fluid fistula may occur in frontal trauma.
Late meningitis can occur secondary to CSF fistula several months after the trauma and lead to a late abscess.
Epilepsy can result from dural scars.

■ Closed Brain Injuries

Definition: Brain injury without division of the dura (cerebral contusion).

Pathogenesis: Blunt cranial trauma, such as a blow or fall, transmits kinetic energy to the brain, producing a coup injury. The brain then strikes the opposite inner surface of the skull, producing a contrecoup injury. This primarily occurs in the crests of the gyri (► A) in the form of bleeding and liquefactive necrosis. Tissue detritus is removed as in an open injury. This results in wedge-shaped defects in the crests of the gyri with a glial scar and thickening of the leptomeninx with brown discoloration due to deposits of hemosiderin (► B).

✚ **Complications:**
Epilepsy can result from dural scars.
Perifocal cerebral edema may result (p. 428).
Apallic syndrome is a chronic condition lasting several months in which necrosis, edema, and bleeding in the cerebral medulla result in suspension of cerebral cortical function. The condition is characterized by coma and paralysis in which the brainstem centers remain intact and functional.
Epidural hematoma (► E) is a circumscribed hemorrhage between the skull and the intact dura caused by rupture of the medial meningeal artery. This results in gradual compression of the brain due to increased intracranial pressure after a brief asymptomatic interval.
Subdural hematoma (► C, D) is a hemorrhage occurring between the intact dura and arachnoid primarily caused by rupture of bridging veins. Several forms are distinguished according to their specific etiology.
– *Acute subdural hematoma* occurs immediately after craniocerebral trauma and is characterized by brain compression.
– *Chronic subdural hematoma* involves slight bleeding following minor trauma. This triggers organization by granulation tissue, which may remain clinically occult for a long period before the onset of brain compression symptoms.
– *Hemorrhagic pachymeningitis* is bilateral chronic subdural hematoma from microhemorrhages that occur in the absence of obvious trauma. The cause of the disorder is not known but may possibly be attributable to hypervitaminosis B.

■ Wound Healing in Peripheral Nerves

(Regeneration of the axon of peripheral nerves)

Pathogenesis: Traumatic interruption of the axon triggers proliferation from the proximal stump of the nerve. Where the original nerve sheath of Schwann cells is intact, the axons will regenerate along it and re-establish contact with the terminal organ.

✚ **Complications:**
Scar neuromas can develop where the axons proliferating from the proximal stump of the divided nerve fail to establish contact with the original nerve sheath. This leads to bulbs of axonal scar tissue that form very painful nodules (► F1). Granulomas may occasionally develop around foreign bodies that have entered the wound (► F2).

❗ **Note:** Brain trauma without a macroscopic lesion is a *cerebral concussion;* trauma that involves a macroscopic lesion is a *cerebral contusion.*

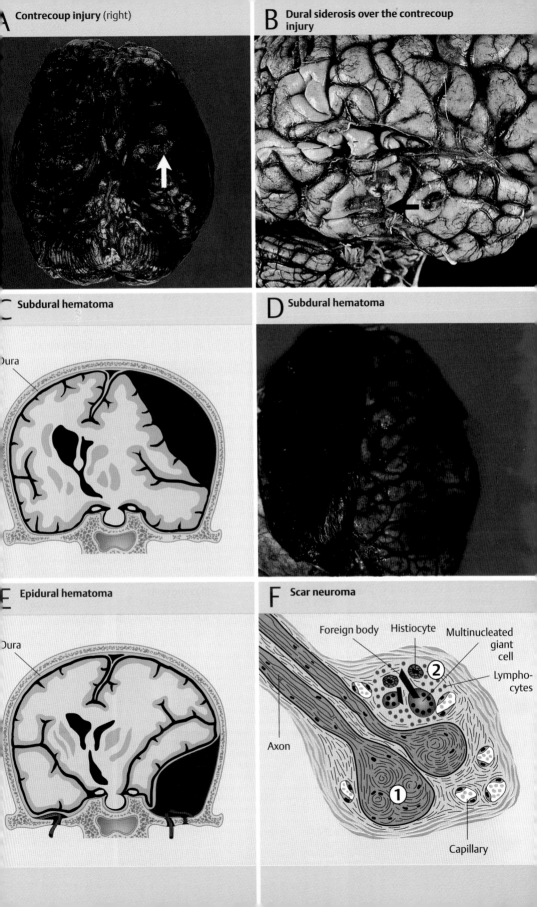

A Contrecoup injury (right)

B Dural siderosis over the contrecoup injury

C Subdural hematoma

Dura

D Subdural hematoma

E Epidural hematoma

Dura

F Scar neuroma

Foreign body · Histiocyte · Multinucleated giant cell

②

Lympho-cytes

Axon

①

Capillary

Metaplasia

General definition: Transformation of a certain type of differentiated tissue into another type of differentiated tissue.

General pathogenesis: There are three ways in which metaplasia can occur:
- *Stem-cell metaplasia* occurs where labile tissue is subjected to chronic injury. Its pluripotential reserve cells are transformed into tissue with greater resistance to physical and chemical influences. In the process they lose some of their original function.
- *Direct metaplasia* occurs where differentiated cells are transformed into differentiated cells of another type without cell division.
- *Indirect metaplasia* is rare and occurs where differentiated cells proliferate and first pass through a transitional stage before they are transformed into differentiated cells of another type.

Epithelial Metaplasia

■ Squamous Metaplasia

▨ **Ciliated Respiratory Epithelium (► B1):**

Chronic sinus bronchitis causes hyperplasia of the goblet cells (► A). This in turn results in thickening of the mucous layer to protect the epithelium. Persistent inflammation leads to squamous metaplasia, as squamous epithelium is more resistant to noxious agents (► B2).

▨ **Stratified Columnar Epithelium:** Chronic cervicitis and cholecystitis leads to squamous metaplasia.

▨ **Glandular Columnar Epithelium:** Chronic inflammation and/or increased estrogen levels lead to squamous metaplasia of the glandular columnar epithelium primarily in the endometrium and prostate (► C).

▨ **Urothelium:** Chronic urocystitis (especially urolithiasis, p. 138; schistosomiasis, p. 280) leads to squamous metaplasia.

■ Intestinal Metaplasia

Chronic gastritis leads to gastric mucosal metaplasia with development of small bowel characteristics such as a brush border (alkali phosphatase, microvilli), goblet cells and granular cells of Paneth (► D).

■ Urothelial Metaplasia

This involves the transformation of prostatic columnar epithelium close to the urethra into urothelium.

Mesenchymal Metaplasia

- *Compression* transforms the mesenchyma into hyaline cartilage.
- *Strain* transforms the mesenchyma into tendon tissue.
- *Elastic deformation* ossifies the mesenchyma.

> **Note:** Metaplasia is not necessarily precancerous. However, it can develop into an optionally precancerous condition in the presence of a persistent noxious agent.

Heteroplasia

General definition: Occurrence of non-neoplastic tissue at a location where it does not normally occur, either in a heterotopia or as a result of tissue dissemination.

Heterotopia

Definition: Displacement of tissue early in ontogeny to an abnormal location (choristoma).

➕ Occurrence:
- *Pancreatic tissue* may occur in the stomach or in Meckel diverticula.
- *Gastric mucosa* may occur in the esophagus or in Meckel diverticula (p. 296).
- *Central nervous system tissue* (► E1) with expression of glial proteins (► F1) may occur in the nasal mucosa beneath the respiratory epithelium (► E2, F2). This is known as a nasal glioma.

Tissue Displacement

Definition: This is a collective term for traumatic or iatrogenic displacement of tissue.

➕ Occurrence:
- *Cholesteatoma* occurs in an inflammatory eardrum injury. Squamous epithelium of the external auditory canal is displaced into the middle ear where it encysts, leading to compressive atrophy.
- *Endometriosis* involves displacement of endometrial glandular tissue together with cytogenic stroma into the myometrium, ovary, or peritoneum.
- *Traumatic epidermal cysts* may occur following traumatic displacement of epidermis into the subcutaneous tissue (this may occur in the volar and plantar regions).

Repair of tissue injury begins with pluripotential reserve cells. These cells must dedifferentiate to the extent that they can temporarily dissociate themselves from tissue structures and divide. The next chapter describes what happens when these dissociated cells "forget" their molecular reintegration program.

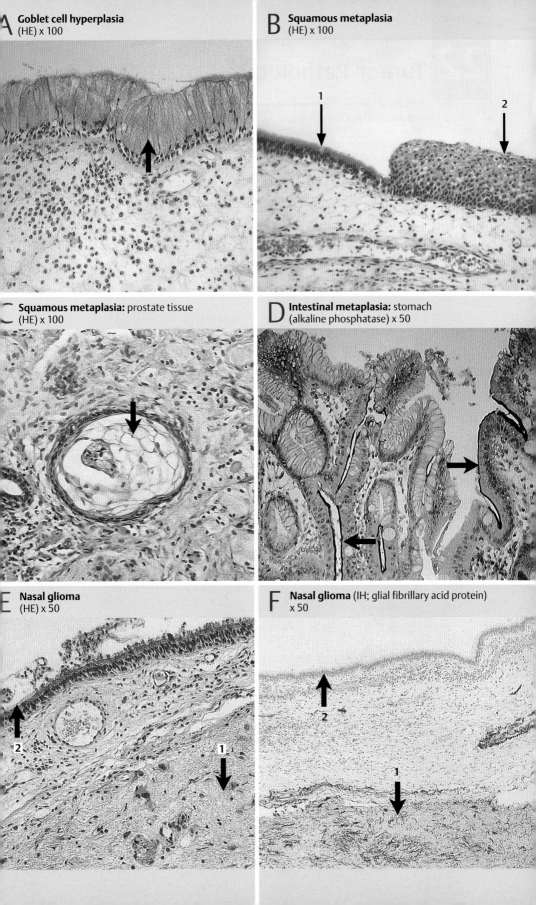

A Goblet cell hyperplasia
(HE) x 100

B Squamous metaplasia
(HE) x 100

1

2

C Squamous metaplasia: prostate tissue
(HE) x 100

D Intestinal metaplasia: stomach
(alkaline phosphatase) x 50

E Nasal glioma
(HE) x 50

2

1

F Nasal glioma (IH; glial fibrillary acid protein)
x 50

2

1

Summary

▶ **Causal tumorigenesis**: Most tumors arise from division of a mother cell in which mutation causes inadequate activation of proto-oncogenes and often genes regulating development, together with the inactivation of tumor suppressor genes and differentiation genes that regulate developmental growth and tissue repair. This explains why a tumor is characterized by unregulated proliferation, with resulting tissue growth, and by unregulated differentiation, with resulting anomalous tissue patterns. Tumor cells therefore become alienated from normal cells, although the immune system usually fails to recognize them as "foreign" and eliminate them. Once a component has broken free of the original chromosomal structure, further losses of information regulating cellular development occur. This means that an initial tumorous development triggered by *chemical, viral,* or *physical* agents will perpetuate itself, and a tumor will begin to take shape.

▶ **Formal tumorigenesis**: Every tumor begins as a circumscribed lesion. During progression of the tumor, the individual tumor cells, and therefore all their progeny, lose differentiation characteristics so that the communication among them breaks down and there is nothing more to hold them in a cohesive aggregate structure. Tumor tissue "goes to seed" and its appearance changes. Tumor cells proliferate like weeds and begin to inundate themselves and the surrounding normal tissue. At the same time, clumps of tumor cells may seed and crop up at remote locations in the body. For this to occur, the new tissue substrate must be compatible with the tumor cells. Referred to as metastasis, this process of tumor seeding usually occurs through the blood or lymph vessels. From a clinical standpoint, it is the most serious tumor complication and marks an ominous turning point in the course of the tumor disorder. Tumor complications also include the paraneoplastic syndromes, which are usually attributable to the fact that the protein machinery of the tumor cells synthesizes "nonsense" proteins or proteins that act as antigens.

▶ **Tumor classification**: Deranged proliferation and differentiation characterize the growth and appearance of a tumor. Therefore, a tumor's morphology provides information about its origin and its biologic behavior. Histologic evaluation of a tumor provides the basis for the therapy concept used in treating it.

General Definition of "Tumor"

Synonym: neoplasia.

A tumor is an abnormal mass of tissue resulting from autonomous, progressive, excessive proliferation of body cells not integrated into normal tissue.

Exception: Postpartum choriocarcinoma is a malignant tumor of placental trophoblasts which are the child's own cells.

> ⚠ **Note:** *"Tumor" in the original wider sense* denotes any circumscribed increase in volume of a tissue (a swelling).

Several types of tumors are differentiated according to their biologic behavior or malignancy status.

Benign Tumors

These are limited circumscribed tumors that do not metastasize into other regions of the body, do not recur after resection, and do not have a fatal outcome.

> ⚠ **Note:** Two exceptions: A tumor occurring in an *unfavorable anatomic location* that causes compressive destruction of vital structures. For example, benign pituitary tumors cause compressive atrophy of glandular tissue. A tumor with *excessive hormone production* that can cause fatal metabolic derangements. For example, an islet cell adenoma of the pancreas causes hyperinsulinism.

Malignant Tumors

These are ill-defined tumors that invade surrounding tissue and can metastasize into other regions of the body, recur after resection, and invariably lead to a fatal outcome if left untreated.

> ⚠ **Note:** Several terms are used in referring to *malignant tumors:*
> - *Cancer* is the common term for all malignant tumors.
> - *Carcinoma* is the common term for malignant epithelial tumors.
> - *Sarcoma* is the common term for malignant nonepithelial tumors.
> - *Solid tumors* are circumscribed tumors such as carcinomas and sarcomas.
> - *Non-solid tumors* are systemic autonomous proliferations of noncohesive individual cells, such as occur in leukemias (p. 358).

Tumors of Limited Malignancy

These include epithelial and nonepithelial tumors that invade and destroy surrounding tissue but rarely if ever metastasize.

Tumor-like Lesions

These are neoplasms that tend to regress spontaneously and completely.

Causal Tumorigenesis

Review of proliferation: see also congenital malformation (p. 94) and tissue repair (p. 308).

Cancer is a genetic disorder that arises from a single body cell (monoclonal disorder). In humans and other animals, it may be triggered by noxious chemical, viral, and physical agents with mutagenic effects. Cells acquire several characteristics during the course of this disease.

— *Defects in the DNA-repair* mechanism cause an accumulation of DNA defects, one of which can affect the proliferation signalling genes.
— *Unrestrained growth:* Unregulated activation of growth-inducing genes (oncogenes) and ineffectiveness of growth-inhibiting genes (tumor suppressor genes) leads to excessive, chaotic, and ruthlessly proliferative tissue growth.
— *Cellular immortality:* Genetic defects affecting apoptosis and the retardation of programmed cell death by re-expressing of telomerase (p. 71) lead to uninhibited inter- and intracellular proliferation.
— *Lack of integration into tissue:* Defective differentiation genes lead in turn to defective intercellular communication and communication between cells and the extracellular matrix. This means that tumor cells are poorly integrated into cohesive cellular aggregates and into the extracellular matrix.
— *Alienation:* Defective differentiation genes lead to false "self" characteristics that deceive the immune system, which overlooks alienated tumor cells.
— *Cellular "vagrancy":* Disturbed regulation of the formation of mobility factors and abnormal activation of these factors causes cells to migrate in the body.

These tumor characteristics are attributable to dysfunction of:
— DNA repair
— Communication factors
— Cell death regulators
— Proliferation regulators
— Differentiation factors
— Immune factors

Disturbed DNA repair

Those genes responsible for DNA repair (p.6) are also called *caretaker genes*. Their defects are based on a germ line mutation that only takes effect when both alleles are defective. The initial result is genetic instability (p.290), which affects primarily tumor suppressor and oncogenes, leaving unrestrained proliferation and immortalization of the affected cells in its wake.

Examples of caretaker gene defects:
— **Nucleotide excision repair** (p. 290) in xeroderma pigmentosum, ataxia teleangiectatica, Bloom's syndrome, Fanconi's anemia.
— **DNA mismatch repair:** in hereditary nonpolyosis colon cancer (p. 380).

> **Note:** Because they cannot repair radiation damage, tumors with defective caretaker genes are radiocurable.

Disturbed Cellular Communication

Normal cells stop growing as soon as they come into contact with each other; this is known as contact inhibition. After this occurs, they attach themselves to the adjacent cells by means of cellular adhesion molecules (p.295). They communicate with these cells and from orderly patterns of tissue. With tumor cells, this intercellular communication is interrupted by defective expression of differentiation genes. This is why tumor cells rarely if ever form tissue patterns, exhibit destructive "antisocial" growth, and leave the cellular aggregate.

Proliferation Disinhibition

Damage to the genome disrupts the normal expression of genes regulating the growth and differentiation of affected cells:
— **HOX genes** lead to reactivation of genes that are normally active only during the embryonic phase.
— **Growth factors** (GF) lead to uncontrolled secretion and action and therefore to deranged growth.
— **Oncogenes** alter the signal transmission causing proliferation with their gene products (see below).
— **Suppressor genes:** The ineffectiveness or absence of suppressor genes that would otherwise suppress cell proliferation and promote cell differentiation (see below).

■ Growth Factors

Definition: See p. 296.

Pathogenetic function: Growth factors occur only in small concentrations in normal postnatal tissue. Hyperfunction of these factors contributes significantly to the development of tumors.

Growth factor hyperfunction is usually attributable either to:
— *Autocrine secretion* (in which the target cell is the producing cell) or to
— *Over expression* of a growth factor gene resulting in excessive growth factor production.

Growth factor hyperfunction has several consequences typically encountered in tumors:

— **Disruption of intercellular communication:** Tumor cells talk to themselves in the sense that they create scatter factors by autocrine secretion. These form a functional complex ("motility factor") with the receptor of the oncogene c-*met*.
— **Cell motility** causes tumor cells to leave the cellular aggregate and to divide; the daughter cells migrate away from one another.
— **Tissue invasion** occurs with the aid of proteases (tissue metalloproteinase) on the tumor cell surface.
— **A permanent proliferation signal** results from abnormal quantities and types of receptors and/or excessive generation of growth factor.

■ **Proto-oncogenes**

Definition: See p. 295.

Pathogenetic function (▶ A): There are two mechanisms by which the physiologic proto-oncogenes (c-onc) are transformed into cancer-causing oncogenes.

Structural alteration of a proto-oncogene may occur in one of two ways:

A *single-point mutation* (▶ D1) of a c-onc allele with substitution of a nucleotide causes synthesis of an abnormal protein or oncoprotein. Because the proto-oncogenes are dominant, mutation of only a single c-onc allele is sufficient to cause this change.
Translocation of a proto-oncogene (▶ D2) with rearrangement of the genetic material.

Disturbed regulation of c-onc expression can transform a proto-oncogene into an oncogene by:
— *Translocation* of a proto-oncogene on to another chromosome and integration into a remote gene locus with a high degree of transcription activity leads to over-expression of the proto-oncogene. A genetic rearrangement at this point will then result in an altered gene structure; this in turn results in a modified gene product and an abnormal oncoprotein.
— *Gene amplification* (▶ D3) may result from autocrine secretion (p. 296; ▶ D4) or invasion by a highly expressive retrovirus in the vicinity of the proto-oncogene's locus (▶ D5). In these cases, the controlling gene no longer has any influence; the gene copies are replaced, leading to overproduction of oncoproteins.

The proto-oncogenes have the following functions that can promote the development and progression of a tumor when they are deranged.

▓ **Growth Factors:** These may be encoded by certain proto-oncogenes (▶ A), i.e, c-*sis* encodes platelet-derived growth factor; c-*int*-2 and c-*hst* encode fibroblast growth factors.

Continuous proliferation may be triggered by over expression of a growth factor or autocrine secretion of the growth factor.

▓ **Growth Factor Receptors:** These are transmembrane proteins that react with tyrosine kinase on their cytoplasmic part; ▶ A, B. They are encoded by certain proto-oncogenes such as c-*erb B2* (▶ B), c-*fms*, and c-*met*.

Continuous proliferation may be triggered by:
— *Over-expression;*
— *Point mutation* of the growth factor receptor, resulting in long-term binding of the growth factor and activation of the receptor with growth factor binding due to permanent activation of tyrosine kinase;
— *Autocrine secretion.*

▓ **Signal-Transducing Proteins:** The gene products of several oncogenes mimic the function of signal transducers. This leads to deranged proliferation.

Examples:
— **C-src** is located on the membrane at the desmosome and acts as a tyrosine-specific protein kinase. This accelerates the cycle of cell division and activates cytoskeletal proteins such as vinculin by phosphorylation.
  In a c-src mutation, vinculin undergoes excessive phosphorylation. This leads to disintegration of the cytoskeleton and disrupts intercellular communication and communication between the cell and the extracellular matrix. This results in cell proliferation that continues without regard to the contact inhibition in normal tissue.
— **C-ras:** Normally activated *ras* protein is a G or regulator protein that binds guanine triphosphate (GTP) and generates the second messenger substance c-AMP via adenylate cyclase. It is inactivated by its own GTPase activity. In a c-*ras* mutation, the G protein loses its GTPase activity, continuously producing second messenger substance for proliferation.
— **C-mos** and **c-mil** encode serine-threonine-specific protein kinases. The residual serine or threonine are transferred to corresponding target proteins, and c-AMP and Ca^2 ions are generated as second messenger substances. A c-*mos* or c-*mil* mutation results in continuous production of second messenger substance for proliferation.

▓ **Nuclear Regulation Factors:** A few proto-oncogenes in the cell nucleus control the replication machinery and in so doing regulate the cell's growth and differentiation.

Examples:
— **C-myc, c-myb, c-jun, c-fos** (▶ C) and **c-rel** are transcription activators. A mutation of these proto-oncogenes leads to continuous proliferation.
— **C-erb A** encodes the thyroxin receptors and is a transcription inactivator (gene repressor). It leads to termination of the cell division so that the cell can differentiate. A mutation of this proto-oncogene leads to continuous proliferation and inability to differentiate.

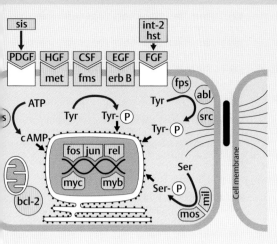

Proto-oncogenes:

c-abl = Abelson leukemia in mice
c-bcl = B-cell lymphoma
v-erb = erythroblastosis
v-fos = FBJ osteosarcoma in mice
v-fps = Fujinami PRCII sarcoma in birds
c-hst = human stomach tumor
c-int = onc causing breast cancer in mice,
         activated by insertion
v-jun = avian sarcoma virus, gene 17
         (junana = Japanese 17)
c-met = methyl-nitroso guanidine
         treated human sarcoma
v-mil = Avian Mill Hill 2 retrovirus
v-mos = Molony sarcoma in mice
v-myc = myelocytomatosis
v-myb = Avian myeloblastosis
v-ras = Kirsten sarcoma in rats
v-rel = Avian reticuloendotheliosis
v-src = Rous sarcoma
v-sis = simian sarcoma

Growth factors:

CSF =
colony stimulating
factor

EGF =
epidermal growth
factor

FGF =
fibroblast growth
factor

HGF =
hepatocyte growth
factor

PDGF =
platelet derived
growth factor

B **c-erb B2**
(IH) x 600

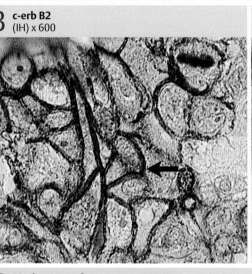

C **c-fos**
(IH) x 600

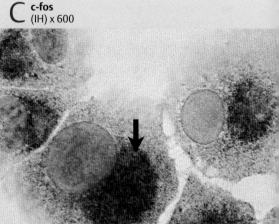

D **Mechanisms of oncogene activation**

Single-point mutation

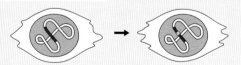

Translocation

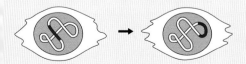

3 Amplification

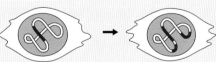

4 Autocrine secretion

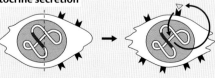

5 Viral insertion

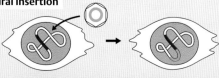

Disturbed Cell Death

Genes, such as *bax* and *bcl*-2, regulate cell death (p. 128) according to the functional requirements of a tissue. This occurs when *bcl*-2 functions antiapoptotically, by preventing cytochrome-c release and by blocking the activation factor Apaf-1, whereas *bax* causes cytochrome-c release by membrane perforation. If these mechanisms are deranged in non-postmitotic (divisible) cells, they accumulate within the tissue, forming a tumor. Another mechanism introducing apoptosis is the age-dependent shortening of telomeres (p. 124), which is prevented in germ cells by a telomerase.

Examples thereof:
— Bcl-2 overexpressed in follicular B-cell lymphomas due to translocation.
— Malignant tumors express telomerase, thereby becoming immortal.

Tumor Suppressor Genes

Synonym: anti-oncogenes

Definition: Collective term for genes whose products physiologically inhibit cell proliferation, promote cell differentiation, and also suppress certain steps in tumorigenesis and metastasis.

A single copy of such a tumor suppressor gene is sufficient to maintain control over growth. Therefore the defect only becomes apparent where both alleles are affected, i.e., in a recessive mutation (loss of heterozygosity).

Pathogenesis: The function of these genes can be blocked by single-point mutation, deletion, or association with viral or endogenous proteins. They can be categorized functionally as:
— "Gatekeeper" genes that directly regulate tumorigenesis by inhibiting its growth or by promoting their death. They are rate-limiting for tumor initiation
— Other suppressor genes whose inactivation leads to tumor progression.

The next section examines the role of those most thoroughly-researched tumor suppressor genes.

Retinoblastoma Gene

This gene (= RB-gene) was discovered in retinoblastoma, a malignant retinal tumor (p. 290).

RB-gene: The product of this gene binds transcription factors, inhibiting the expression of genes that control the transition from the G1 phase to the S phase in the cell cycle. This inhibits mitosis.

RB-gene inactivation occurs in extremely aggressive rapidly proliferating carcinomas (breast carcinomas, small-cell bronchogenic carcinomas, and glioblastomas) and sarcomas (osteosarcoma).

Wilms' Tumor Genes

These genes (= WT-genes) were discovered in Wilms' tumor or nephroblastoma, a malignant renal tumor (p. 290).

WT-1 gene: The product of this gene inhibits the transcription of a mitogen[1]. In this manner, it promotes differentiation of the embryonic primordium of the kidney and inhibits adjacent genes such as IGF-2[2] that control initiation of the cell cycle.

WT-2 gene: This gene regulates proliferation.

WT-gene inactivation: A Wilms' tumor is frequently associated with congenital malformations of the kidney in the form of simultaneous occurrence of medullary tissue, cortical tissue, and nephroblastoma nodules (▶ C).

p53 Tumor Suppressor Gene

p53 gene: The product of this gene arrests the cell in the G1 phase in the event of DNA damage, giving it the opportunity to repair the DNA. Where this is unsuccessful, p53 initiates apoptosis in the respective cell.

p53 inactivation may occur as a result of mutation. Mutated *p53* protein inactivation promotes tumor development. Its gene product is broken down more slowly than normal protein, leading to intranuclear accumulation of *p53* protein (▶ A).
This occurs in acquired somatic mutations in many tumors and in constitutional mutations in members of families with a history of familial cancer.
The gene may also be inactivated by association with viral proteins or endogenous proteins.

Neurofibromatosis Genes

These genes (= NF-genes) were discovered in tumors occurring in generalized neurofibromatosis (p. 368).

NF-1 gene: The product of this gene is a GTPase activator (neurofibromin) that interrupts the signal effect of the *ras* protein.

NF-1-Inactivation: Congenital mutation of an NF-1 allele leads to multiple proliferations of melanocytes (café au lait macules; ▶ B) and tumors in the form of neurofibromas, primarily occurring in the skin (▶ D) and peripheral nerves (▶ F) and consisting of wave-like arrangements of Schwann cells expressing S-100 (▶ p. 327, F) in a loose fibrous stroma (p. 368).

NF-2-Inactivation: Loss of both NF-1 alleles (together with p53 mutations) leads to neurogenic sarcomas.

NF-2 gene: This gene encodes a protein associated with the cytoskeleton (*merlin*).

NF-2 allele defect → acoustic neurinoma.

Adenomatous Polyposis Coli Gene

This gene (= APC-gene) was discovered in tumors in adenomatous polyposis of the colon (p. 380).

APC gene: The product of this gene regulates the progression of the cells in the differentiation and apoptosis pool via the microtubules. It inactivates the T-cell transcription factor Tcf by binding to the β-catenin signal transducing molecule. This results in proliferation inhibition.

---

[1] Early growth response-1-protein
[2] IGF-2 = insulin-like growth factor

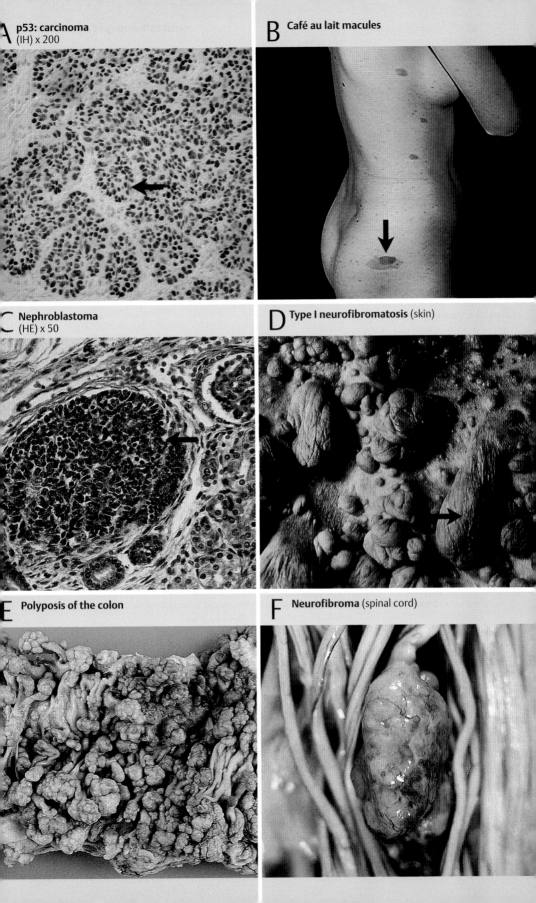

A p53: carcinoma
(IH) x 200

B Café au lait macules

C Nephroblastoma
(HE) x 50

D Type I neurofibromatosis (skin)

E Polyposis of the colon

F Neurofibroma (spinal cord)

APC-Inactivation: Congenital mutation of an APC allele leads to familial polyposis the colon (► E; p. 368).

Loss of both APC alleles: The mutated gene no longer inactivates the β-catenin via serine threonine kinase; instead it forms a stable complex with it. This results in continuous proliferation, leading to disorders like colorectal carcinoma and other tumors such as malignant melanoma (p. 366).

Tumor Immunology

Physiology: The immune system's main task is to eliminate invading foreign organisms and, presumably, tumor cells that have become foreign. The latter statement postulates an underlying mechanism known as immune surveillance that is thought to function as follows. Mutations continually produce body cells with abnormal antigens (tumor antigens). Cytotoxic T cells recognize these cells as "foreign" and destroy them.

Tumor Antigens

Cancer cells form two types of antigens.

Tumor-specific antigens occur in certain tumors (usually experimentally induced tumors) and not in normal cells; they can trigger a humoral or cellular immune reaction. Autoreactive antibodies formed against them or cytotoxic lymphocytes also attack other endogenous antigens, triggering cell destruction in remote body tissues and leading to what is known as paraneoplastic syndrome (p. 350).

Tumor-associated antigens occur in tumors and in normal cells. These include oncofetal and differentiation antigens.

■ Oncofetal Antigens

Definition: These are surface antigens that are hardly ever expressed after the fetal period but can occur again in larger quantities in immature tumors.

These antigens are not specific to any one tumor and do not trigger a tumor suppressive immune reaction. These are the most common ones:
— *α-Fetoprotein* (AFP) is a glycoprotein detectable in serum and liver cells (► A). It is expressed in hepatocellular carcinoma (p. 322) and yolk sac tumor[1] (► B), which release AFP into serum.
— *Carcinoembryonic antigen* (CEA) is a glycoprotein of the immunoglobulin superfamily. It is expressed in fetal intestinal tissue and again in gastrointestinal tumors (► C), which release CEA into serum.
— *Chorionic gonadotropin* (β-HCG) is a glycoprotein that suppresses T cells. It is expressed in chorionic cells and again in choriocarcinoma[2] cells (► D) and in aggressive carcinomas of the gastrointestinal tract, respiratory tract, and breast, which release β-HCG into serum.

■ Differentiation Antigens

Definition: These are membrane antigens that regulate intercellular communication and therefore the interaction of cells. These antigens are also expressed by tumor cells, some of them in altered form.

In addition to the clusters of differentiation of the leukocytes, these antigens include:
— *prostate-specific antigen* (PSA), detectable in the prostate gland and in prostate tumors (p. 374), and
— *S-100 antigen*, which controls the cell cycle and binds Ca^2. S-100 is detectable in Schwann cells (► F), melanocytes, melanomas (p. 366), tumors of the neural crest, lipocytes (p. 356), and in liposarcomas.

Tumor Immunity

Most tumor disorders involve immune reactions to a certain extent.
— *Humoral immune reactions:* Antibodies against tumor-associated surface antigens occur as part of the immune response to tumors. In a few cases, they inhibit tumor growth to a certain extent, or kill tumors by antibody-dependent cellular cytotoxicity. However, they often have just the opposite effect: They cover tumor-specific antigens, masking them for cytotoxic T cells, which then do not kill them.
— *Cell-mediated immunity:* The T-cell system can destroy tumor cells after detecting the tumor-specific antigen. Tumor cells may be destroyed
    — *Directly* by cytotoxic effector cells, and
    — *Indirectly* by release of certain cytokines (IL-2 and TNF-α) which transforms macrophages into "tumor eaters" and activates natural killer cells. This leads to an inflammatory reaction with formation of epithelioid granulomas in the contributory lymph nodes of a tumor, creating a sarcoid-like lesion and destroying some of the tumor cells.

However, immune surveillance usually fails for these reasons:
— *Lack of immunity:* The tumor cells' tumor-specific antigens exhibit insufficient immunogenicity.
— *Lack of T-cell clones:* The body's immune system tolerates tumor antigens because of the absence of an appropriate tumor-induced T-cell clone.
— *T-cell inefficiency:* The cytotoxic effector cells fail to detect the tumor antigen due to either ineffective HLA expression or because peeled-off tumor antigens block their antigen receptors (HLA molecules).

> **Note:** Solid tumors do not occur without perifocal inflammation.

---

[1] A yolk sac tumor is a malignant germinal epithelial tumor that mimics yolk sac structures in the form of thin tumorous strands with a flattened cubical epithelial covering in a glandular, papillary, or glomeruloid arrangement, in edematous, mesh-like, intermediate tissue that resembles the yolk sac mesenchyma.

[2] A choriocarcinoma is a highly malignant tumor of proliferating trophoblastic epithelium in the form of (a) syncytial multinucleated chorial giant cells and (b) mononuclear trophoblastic tumor cells that invade, destroy, and proliferate in maternal tissue.

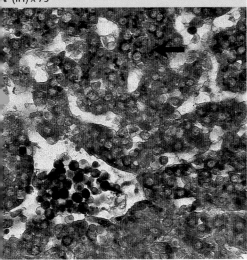

AFP: fetal liver
(IH) x 75

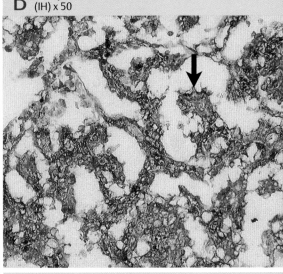

AFP: yolk sac tumor
(IH) x 50

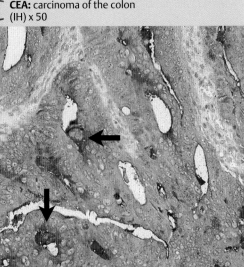

CEA: carcinoma of the colon
(IH) x 50

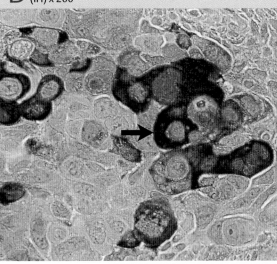

β-HCG: choriocarcinoma
(IH) x 200

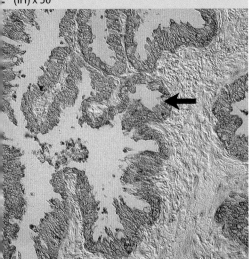

PSA: normal prostate
(IH) x 50

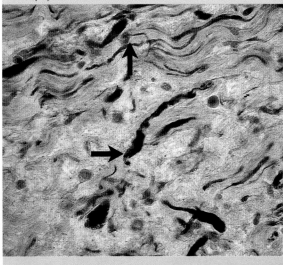

S-100: neurofibroma
(IH) x 75

Chemical Tumorigenesis

Definition: Chemical carcinogens are substances that cause cancer.

The most important carcinogens are listed below:
— *Polycyclic aromatic hydrocarbons* such as benzpyrene and benzanthracene occur in tar, soot, and cigarette smoke and cause bronchogenic carcinoma.
— *Halogenated hydrocarbons* such as vinyl chloride occur in the PVC processing industry and cause angiosarcomas of the liver (p. 334).
— *Nitrosamines* are common in the environment and are ingested with food. They cause gastrointestinal tumors.
— *Aromatic amines* occur in the dye manufacturing and cause carcinoma of the urinary bladder (aniline cancer).
— *Mycotic toxins* such as aflatoxins are produced by fungi such as mildew and primarily in moist grain silos. They cause hepatocellular carcinoma (p. 332).
— *Pyrrolizidine alkaloids* occur in herbs, seasonings (nutmeg), vegetables (peas and beans), and certain types of tea (coltsfoot, maté). They cause hepatocellular carcinoma (p. 332).

Two types of carcinogens are differentiated according to their point of attack.
— *Genotoxic carcinogens* cause genetic mutations in specific tests, such as the Ames test for bacterial mutagenicity[1].
— *Non-genotoxic carcinogens* usually sabotage intercellular communication. The affected cell becomes independent of it environment and begins to proliferate. This means that non-genotoxic carcinogens promote the growth of tumors but do not trigger their development.

Stages of Carcinogenesis

The process by which a carcinogen transforms cells into tumor cells involves the following stages (► A):

■ **Initiation:** A chemical carcinogen is first rendered bioactive or transformed into its active carcinogenic form in organ tissue (► A1, B), usually by enzyme action. This interacts with the cellular DNA, producing genetic damage and cell necrosis (► A2). As long as this injury has not been passed on to the daughter cells, it can still be repaired by DNA repair enzymes and is directly proportional to the carcinogen dose.

Two potencies of carcinogens are differentiated:

Complete carcinogens cause malignant transformation of the target cell without the aid of other cofactors;

incomplete carcinogens cause malignant transformation of the target cell only with the aid of other cofactors.

The various carcinogens influence each other's effects in one of two ways. Complete and incomplete carcinogens can have an additive effect, whereas the effect of a weak carcinogen can be significantly enhanced by cofactors.

■ **Promotion:** This is the process that triggers the proliferation of initiating cells, causing the genetic error to become established in daughter cells and producing dysplasia (p. 340; ► A3, C) with polyploid cells.

■ **Latency:** This follows promotion and varies in duration.

■ **Progression:** This is the first step in tumor development and involves irreversible transition from a single preneoplastic cell to a neoplastic cell. This neoplastic cell becomes the mother cell of a proliferating cell clone (clonal expansion). This clone grows into a macroscopically visible tumor nodule (► A4) that is initially benign and later malignant (► A5; hepatocellular carcinoma or wide complexes of tumor cells, ► D1, without liver sinus and with bile thrombi, ► D2; see also p. 332).

■ **Metastasis** (p. 346): With increasing progression, the transformed cells lose their surface differentiation antigens and with them their cohesiveness. Cells leave the primary cell mass, migrate, and colonize other tissues and organs, where they form secondary tumors (metastases).

---

[1] In the Ames test, Salmonella with an easily deranged single-point mutation at the histidine locus are unable to synthesize histidine. Exposure to a carcinogen causes them to mutate back and regain the ability to synthesize histidine. The quantity of reverting organisms is proportional to the carcinogenic effect.

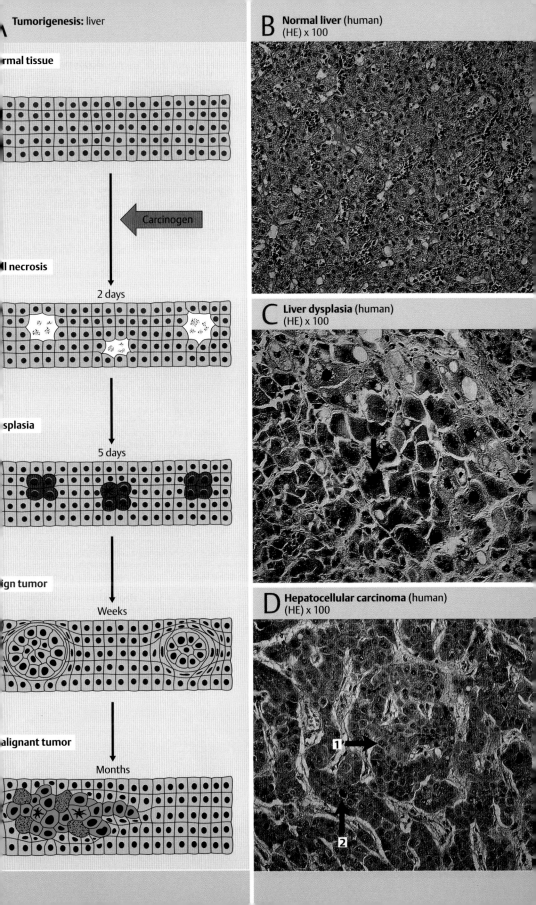

A Tumorigenesis: liver

Normal tissue

Carcinogen

Cell necrosis

2 days

Dysplasia

5 days

Benign tumor

Weeks

Malignant tumor

Months

B Normal liver (human)
(HE) x 100

C Liver dysplasia (human)
(HE) x 100

D Hepatocellular carcinoma (human)
(HE) x 100

1'

2

Metabolic Carcinogen Activation

A carcinogen is activated in a cascade of processes (▶ A).

— A ***parent carcinogen*** (▶ A1) is the "starting" product of a carcinogen. It is rarely active in this form.

— A ***proximate carcinogen*** (▶ A2) results when the initial carcinogen is transformed into a stable intermediate form by microsomal mixed function oxidases containing cytochrome P 450.

— An ***ultimate carcinogen*** (▶ A3) results when proximate carcinogens spontaneously dissociate into reactive activation products. These ultimate carcinogens have one characteristic in common: they possess one electrophilic molecular region with which they can bond to nucleophilic groups of cellular macromolecules such as DNA, RNA, and proteins.

DNA interference: The electrophilic reaction groups of chemical carcinogens occur either as
— *small molecules* in the form of alkylated substances such as CH_3^+ (▶ A3), or:
— *very large molecules*, known as "bulky adducts" with DNA bases. These adducts adhere to the DNA like bubble gum and impair its function.

A variety of alkylating agents can be broken down to produce the same ultimate carcinogen.

Nucleophilic positions at the purine and pyrimidine bases are also alkylated in the DNA in addition to the phosphate groups of the nucleic acid structure. This forms a bridging hydrogen bond between complementary DNA bases, causing defective boding during DNA replication (▶ B, C) and transcription.

The "molecular policeman" protein *p53* (p. 324) becomes active at this point. The cell has a chance to repair the DNA damage with alkyl transferase. Failure of this DNA repair results in a point mutation. Where cell proliferation is intense and there are numerous DNA defects, the DNA sequence may occasionally be "miscopied," producing a point mutation of a proto-oncogene. This transforms it into an oncogene and leads to deranged proliferation.

Organ and Species Specificity

Chemical carcinogens are highly specific. This is reflected in the fact that certain carcinogens only affect certain species of animals and then only cause tumors in certain organs. This also applies to carcinogens that cause disease in humans.

Several factors determine the organ and species specificity of a carcinogen.
— The ***stage of development*** of an individual determines a tissue's content of mixed function oxidases required for activation.
— The ***activity of the mixed function oxidase system*** depends on individual predisposition and on the organ.
— ***How the substance is supplied*** is a factor applying primarily to carcinogens that rapidly and locally dissociate into their active form and to those that are detoxified by the liver.
— The ***cumulative dose*** (what dose over what period of time) is important.
— The ***promoter*** may exhibit a certain organ specificity.
— ***Gender*** is important, as the receptors present in target tissue (such as gonads) increase their receptivity for a chemical carcinogen.

Chemical carcinogens cause genetic damage that affects certain organs and tissues in proportion to their dose. In contrast, tumor-producing viruses specifically alter with host genome via certain genes and gene products. They either activate the proliferation machinery or deactivate the mechanisms that retard proliferation. This is a genetically programmed survival strategy of tumor-producing viruses.

Carcinogens: activation cascade

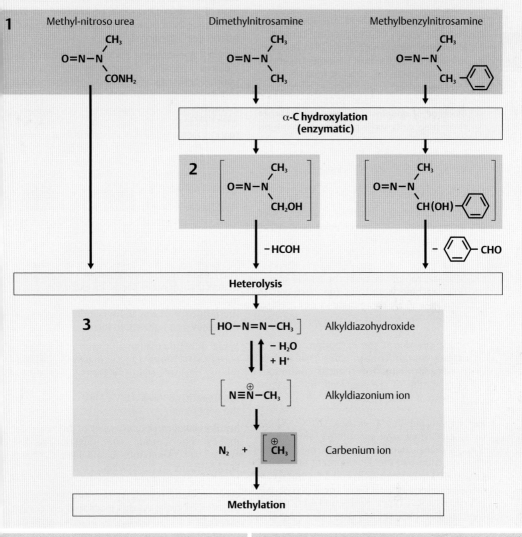

1

Methyl-nitroso urea

$$O=N-N\begin{array}{c}CH_3\\\\CONH_2\end{array}$$

Dimethylnitrosamine

$$O=N-N\begin{array}{c}CH_3\\\\CH_3\end{array}$$

Methylbenzylnitrosamine

$$O=N-N\begin{array}{c}CH_3\\\\CH_3\end{array}$$

α-C hydroxylation (enzymatic)

2

$$\left[O=N-N\begin{array}{c}CH_3\\\\CH_2OH\end{array}\right]$$

$$\left[O=N-N\begin{array}{c}CH_3\\\\CH(OH)\end{array}\right]$$

$-$ HCOH

$-$ CHO

Heterolysis

3

$[HO-N=N-CH_3]$ Alkyldiazohydroxide

$-H_2O$
$+H^+$

$[N\equiv\overset{\oplus}{N}-CH_3]$ Alkyldiazonium ion

N_2 + $[\overset{\oplus}{CH_3}]$ Carbenium ion

Methylation

B **Normal matching:** guanine → cytosine

Cytosine   Guanine

C **Defective matching:** methylguanine → thymine

Thymine O^6-Methylguanine

22

Tumor Pathology

Viral Tumorigenesis

General pathogenesis: There are several mechanisms by which viruses produce tumors.
— *Insertional mutagenesis:* Viral DNA becomes integrated into the host genome, triggering over expression by adjacent host genes.
— *Viral oncogenes* (v-onc): Viruses contain oncogenes that are usually mutated.
— *Blockage of apoptosis:* Viruses immortalize their host cells with proteins that inhibit apoptosis.
— *Immunosuppression:* Viruses suppress the body's immune defenses.

DNA Tumor Viruses

General pathogenesis: The DNA tumor viruses are incorporated into the host cell genome by instable or stable insertion.
— *Instable insertion* is most common. The DNA viruses have certain genes whose encoded products rapidly activate the cell's replication machinery, causing the host cell to form new virus components until it is exhausted. The *result* is a lytic cycle of infection.
— *Stable insertion* is the exception. The DNA viruses contain control genes that encode the oncoproteins. The *result* is continuous proliferation of the host cell, the survival strategy of these viruses.

■ **Human papilloma viruses** (HPV): These cause epidermal viral acanthoma (skin warts) and laryngeal papillomas (► A) in humans. They contribute to the development of cervical carcinomas in women (► B) and anogenital carcinomas in homosexual men. The high risk papilloma viruses (types 16, 18, and 31) contain the transforming genes E7 and E6.
— *E7* bonds to the *Rb* suppressor gene, causing a loss of control over the cell cycle with continuous proliferation.
— *E6* bonds to and inactivates the *p53* suppressor gene, leading to tolerance of DNA errors and tumor progression.

■ **Adenoviruses:** Adenoviruses (especially types 12, 18, and 31) are highly tumorigenic in humans and other mammals. They contain the transforming genes E1A and E1B.
E1A: His gene product bonds to the gene products of cellular *RB* and *p53* suppressor genes and to a nuclear transcription factor.
E1B: His gene product bonds to the gene products of cellular *RB* and *p53* suppressor genes.

This interaction between viral oncoproteins and intrinsic cellular proteins inhibits apoptosis. This suppresses apoptosis in infected cells, enabling them to survive. Other results are continuous proliferation, which inhibits differentiation.

■ **Epstein-Barr Virus** (EBV): This infects human B lymphocytes and is involved in the pathogenesis of Burkitt's lymphoma and nasopharyngeal carcinoma.

Burkitt's lymphoma is endemic in malarial regions of Africa. It is caused by the following pathogenetic cascade: Malarial infection leads to B-cell proliferation with generation of high quantities of immunoglobulin. Superinfection with EBV leads to production of a viral transformation factor (LMP-1). This results in expression of *bcl*-2, which blocks apoptosis and renders the B cells immortal. It also disrupts intercellular communication, resulting in loss of contact inhibition.

This has several consequences. The immortalized cells proliferate continuously. During the course of this continuous proliferation, chromosomes break apart at the heavy and light chain locus of the immunoglobulins (► C). This results in translocation of chromosomal material to another locus in exchange for c-*myc*. The c-*myc* infiltrates the genome under the influence of the transcriptional activity of the heavy and light chain locus.

Result: A highly malignant tumor of B lymphoblasts (► D1) with typical macrophages containing nuclear detritus (► D2).

■ **Hepatitis B Virus** (HBV): HBV contributes to the genesis of

hepatocellular carcinoma as part of the following pathogenetic cascade: HBV infection successively leads to hepatitis B and liver cirrhosis. HBV contains an HBx protein coding sequence that becomes integrated into the gene of a cell cycle regulator (cyclin A), resulting in over expression of cyclin A. This leads to regenerative proliferation of hepatocytes and to increased receptivity to alimentary carcinogens such as aflatoxin (p. 328).

This has several consequences. The continuous proliferation of certain genes such as the *p53* suppressor gene and their tendency to mutate result in deranged growth with proliferations of abnormal cells (► E) colocalized with HBs antigens (► F). This subsequently leads to impaired differentiation. *Result:* A hepatocellular carcinoma.

Note: In contrast to the retroviral oncoproteins, the DNA viral oncoproteins in the eukaryotic cells **do not** have a homologue.

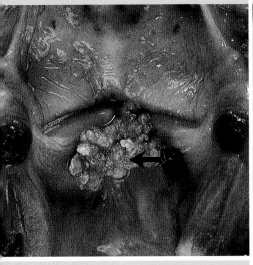

A Laryngeal papillomatosis

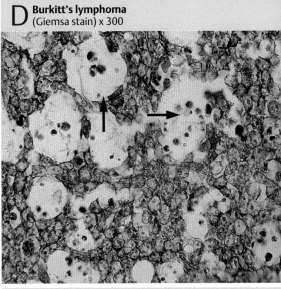

B Cervical carcinoma

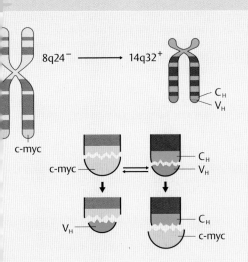

C 8 → 14 translocation

8q24⁻ → 14q32⁺

C_H
V_H

c-myc

c-myc

C_H
V_H

V_H
C_H

C_H
c-myc

D Burkitt's lymphoma
(Giemsa stain) x 300

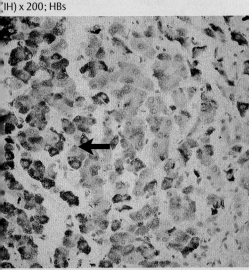

E HBV: liver
(IH) x 200; HBs

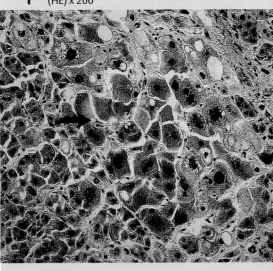

F Initial hepatocellular carcinoma
(HE) x 200

RNA Tumor Viruses

Synonym: oncornaviruses.

These viruses cause leukemia (p. 358), malignant lymphomas (p. 362), and sarcomas in birds, mice, hamsters, and cats. The human T-cell leukemia viruses (HTLV) cause disease in humans (p. 244).

The genome of the RNA tumor viruses consists of linear single-stranded RNA. It contains the following three structural genes:
— *Group-specific antigen gene* encodes an RNA-associated core protein.
— *Polymerase gene* carries the information for reverse transcriptase.
— *Envelope gene:* His product is a viral envelope protein that determines the virus's host specificity.

The start and stop signal for the transcription program of viral structure genes are identical RNA sequences in the form of long terminal repeat (LTR) sequences on both ends of the viral genome.

RNA tumor virus can infect a cell in three different ways:
— *Noncytocidal infection* causes the host cell to replicate and release numerous viral particles but does not kill it.
— *Latent infection* may occur.
— *Transforming infection* leads to tumor.

Two groups of RNA tumor viruses are differentiated:
— *Moderately carcinogenic retroviruses* have a complete retroviral genome.
— *Highly carcinogenic retroviruses* have a deficient retroviral genome with an additional control gene (v-onc). They can only reproduce within the cell with the aid of "helper viruses". They induce tumor within a few weeks.

These v-onc are proto-oncogenes or portions of proto-oncogenes that the virus has "stolen" on its way through an infected host cell. Introduction of a v-onc into the genome of the virus usually results in damage to or deletion of a viral structural gene.

After being assimilated by a retrovirus, a c-onc can be converted into an oncogene in one of two ways.
— *Structural change* may occur due modification of the c-onc sequence or fusion with a viral structural gene.
— *Over-expression* may occur where a c-onc comes under the control of the virus's highly expressive long terminal repeat sequences.

> **Note:** Every v-onc in an RNA tumor virus corresponds to a cellular counterpart (c-onc) in the eukaryotic cells.

Physical Tumorigenesis

■ Ionizing Radiation

Pathogenesis: Particulate radiation ionizes the water in affected cells (p. 152). This results in the formation of radicals and peroxides that lead to fracture and cross-linkage of DNA strands. Point mutations occur where DNA repair is unsuccessful. Uncontrolled proliferation occurs where this mutation affects a c-onc.

Example: Thorotrast, a radiographic contrast medium formerly used, contained thorium as a source of α-radiation (► A) and led to retention of radionuclides in the reticuloendothelial system of the liver. This treatment induced several tumors after a latency period of 20–40 years. These included *angiosarcomas* (► C) arising from proliferative cavernous vessels (► E1) and lined with an atypical endothelium, and *bile duct and hepatocellular carcinomas.*

■ Ultraviolet Radiation

Pathogenesis: Sunlight contains ultraviolet B radiation, which only penetrates superficially. This causes formation of DNA thymine dimers in the basal epidermis. Point mutations occur in a c-onc where DNA repair is unsuccessful. This results in uncontrolled proliferation (see ionization).

Results include squamous cell carcinoma and/or malignant melanocyte tumors and basal cell carcinomas (p. 384).

■ Foreign Bodies

Some foreign bodies act as carcinogens.
— *Asbestos* (p. 142): Inhalation of asbestos dust (► B) leads to chronic inflammation, mesothelioma, and lung cancer.
— *Bivalent metals* such as nickel cause mutation of the *p53* suppressor gene, leading to malignant connective tissue tumors (sarcomas).
— *Schistosoma haematobium* (► D; p. 280): Infestation leads to chronic inflammation of the bladder (urocystitis). The resulting chronic tissue repair stimulus leads to carcinoma of the bladder.
— *Clonorchis sinensis* (oriental liver fluke; ► F1). The larvae of the pathogen enter the bloodstream via the skin, and from there they enter the bile ducts (► F2). Here the parasite matures, causing chronic inflammation of the infested bile ducts (cholangitis). The resulting chronic tissue repair stimulus leads to carcinoma of the bile duct.

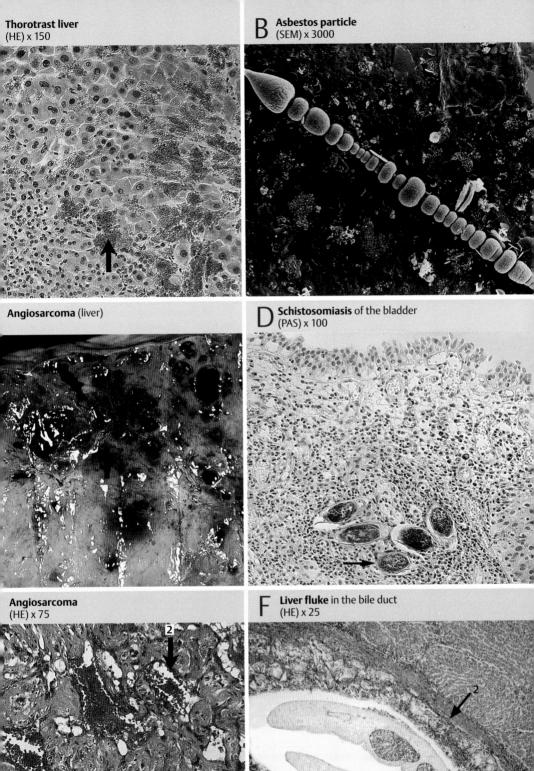

Thorotrast liver
(HE) x 150

B **Asbestos particle**
(SEM) x 3000

Angiosarcoma (liver)

D **Schistosomiasis** of the bladder
(PAS) x 100

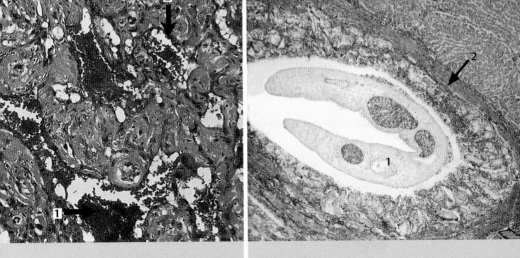

Angiosarcoma
(HE) x 75

F **Liver fluke** in the bile duct
(HE) x 25

Human Tumorigenesis

Predisposition

Only the predisposition to tumor disorders is hereditary.

A number of processes may accentuate such a predisposition.
— *Defective suppressor* and/or *differentiation genes* during embryogenesis lead to dysontogenetic tumors (p. 382).
— *genome instability syndrome* with defective DNS repair, leading to mutation of the genes controlling proliferation and differentiation (p. 6).
— *Negative variance of the mixed function oxidases* that detoxify carcinogens lead to accumulation of carcinogens in the body.
— *Susceptibility to addiction* can lead to nicotine and/or alcohol dependence and accumulation of carcinogens.
— *Genetic immune deficiency syndromes* (p. 188) involve deficient immune surveillance.

Such a predisposition to cancer leads to the development of multiple tumors in multiple organs and tissues and occurs in certain families as a genetically determined tumor syndrome. Here are two examples:
— *Muir-Torre syndrome* involving a "caretaker" gene mutation (MLH1, MSH2 = mismatch repair); leads to gastrointestinal and genitourinary tumors, skin tumors, and breast cancer (▶ A, breast cancer in twins).
— *Li-Fraumeni cancer syndrome* involves a mutation of the *p53* suppressor gene. This leads to early cancer as well as sarcomas, carcinoma of the adrenal cortex, bronchogenic carcinoma (p. 378), colorectal carcinoma (p. 379), gliomas (p. 368), leukemia, and lymphomas.

> **Note:** The *rule of thumb for predisposition to cancer* is that multiple carcinomas occurring before the fifth decade of life suggest a familial predisposition, usually with autosomal dominant inheritance.

Hormonal Factors

These are involved in the processes of proliferation and differentiation for a number of reasons.
— Hormones use the same or similar receptors as growth factors.
— Hormones induce the expression of growth factors or apoptosis receptors.
— Hormones generate the same second messenger substances as certain proto-oncogenes.

Consequence: an imbalance between acute hormone supply, receptor supply, and hormone effect leads to abnormal proliferation and to tumor.

> **Note:** With respect to *tumors and hormones,*
> - *breast and prostate carcinoma* can be treated with sex hormone antagonists.
> - *Endometrial carcinoma* can be induced with estrogens.

Age

■ Senile tumors:

A tumor is the result of a summation of genetic damage acquired during a latency period. Often threshold values are only exceeded in advanced age. As a result, the peak age for cancer in humans lies between 55 and 75 years.

■ Childhood tumors:

Embryonic and fetal organs are highly sensitive to chemical carcinogens. These can induce tumors *in utero*. The resulting impairment of differentiation leads to dysontogenetic tumors (p. 382).

Nutritional Factors and Drug Use

■ Nutritional Fats:
Increased intake of fat leads to elevated secretion of bile acids that can be changed into carcinogens by intestinal bacteria. This increases the risk of colorectal carcinoma (p. 380).

■ High Nutritional Fiber Intake:
This decreases the risk of carcinoma of the colon.

■ Alcohol Abuse (▶ B):
Alcoholic beverages, especially distilled fruit spirits, contain nitrosamines (from putrefactive substances). Ethanol interferes with the mixed function oxidase system especially in the liver, impairing its detoxification of carcinogens. This leads to cytotoxicity and hypovitaminosis (especially of vitamin A). This interferes with repair of the squamous epithelium and leads to esophageal carcinoma.

■ Cigarette Smoke (▶ C):
Smoke contains substances such as benzpyrene and nitrosamine that cause *p53* mutation that leads to bronchogenic carcinoma (p. 378).

Environmental Factors

These factors lead to increased incidence of certain tumors in specific geographical locations.
— *Stomach cancer* is ten times as common in Japan than in Western industrialized countries.
— *Esophageal cancer* is more common in the Asian "esophageal cancer belt" extending from Belarus to eastern China.
— *Skin cancer,* especially melanomas and basal cell carcinomas (p. 336, 384), occur more often among the descendants of fair-haired Celtic immigrants in northern Australia, where there is increased exposure to ultraviolet radiation.
— *Cervical cancer* is rare among women whose partners are circumcised; apparently smegma is at least conducive to its induction.

Familial mammary carcinoma in twins

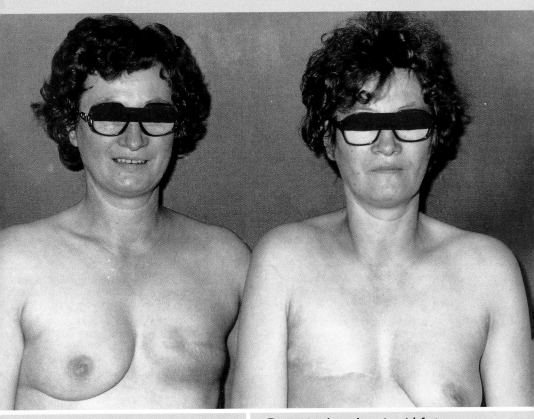

Alcohol dependence is a risk factor

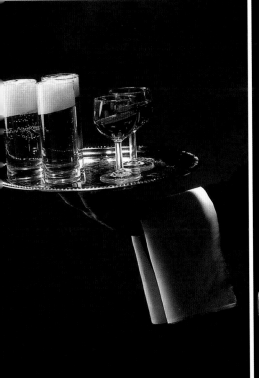

C **Nicotine dependence is a risk factor**

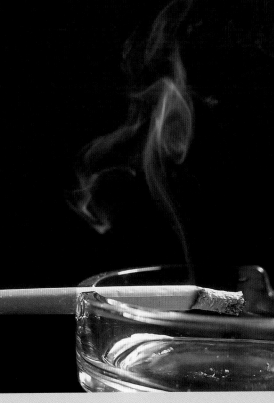

Genetic Changes

A causative chemical, viral, or physical agent can be identified in only a few cases of cancer in humans. Previous studies have now made it possible to combine the various genetic changes leading to a malignant tumor into a multi-stage model.

■ **Susceptibility Genes:** Some patients exhibit a familial predisposition to develop tumors (often accompanied by congenital malformations). This is caused by defects in genes regulating differentiation, the enzyme system that detoxifies carcinogens, and DNA repair.

Result: a patient receptive to carcinogens.

■ **Tumor Promotion:** Many substances, among them pharmaceuticals such as barbiturates, can increase the tumorigenic effect of a noxious agent.

Result: abnormal cell proliferation.

■ **Oncogene Activation:** At some point a point mutation occurs on a single proto-oncogene in a single cell (the mother cell). If this also occurs in the other allele (commonly referred to as a second hit), the proto-oncogene becomes an oncogene as a result of continuous function or overproduction (over-expression). The proliferation signal is no longer counteracted, and the mother cell becomes a monoclonal tumor cell family.

Result: hyperplasia (p. 118).

■ **Defective Apoptosis**

This occurs as a result of:
– Mutation of suppressor genes such as *p53*;
– Blockage of suppressor genes such as *p53*;
– Blockage of the apoptosis mechanism by viral proteins;
– Re-expression of telomerase (p. 71).

This results in a genetically altered cell that becomes immortal and acts as a proliferative perpetual-motion machine.

Result: atypical hyperplasia in which growth is still characterized by intercellular cohesion.

■ **Defects in Differentiation Genes:** The stages that now follow occur as a result of "accidents caused by excessive speed of cell division." This results in the loss of additional alleles that encode the detection molecules on a cell, with the effect that intercellular communication is disrupted. The primary cellular mass loses its cohesion, and with it the contact inhibition of cell division. This leads to uncontrolled proliferation of tumor cells that crowd each other out (▶ A, B).

Result: destructive growth characterized by loss of intercellular cohesion, an "accident caused by brake failure" in the form of unchecked cell division.

■ **Defects in Metastasis-Suppressor Genes:** Finally, defects occur in those genes that guarantee the cell differentiation that inhibits metastasis. The tumor cells also produce factors with which they set themselves in motion (mobility factors; p. 312). This results in uncontrolled cell migration.

Result: the seeding of tumor cells into other organs and tissues – "hit and run accidents".

■ **Defective Immune Surveillance** (p. 326): It is usually difficult for these continuously proliferating tumor cells to survive. They must compete with other cells for nutrients and are vulnerable to the snares of immune surveillance. This results in a process of natural selection that favors those tumor cells that have degenerated to the point that they can withstand any internal deficit or external attack.

Result: tumor cells best characterized as "antisocial survival experts".

■ **Resistance to Therapy:** The degeneration of tumor cells leads to expression of genes that resist pharmaceuticals and the mutation of genes that control apoptosis. Apoptosis therefore fails to occur secondary to treatment with cytostatic agents and radiation therapy.

Result: the development of tumor subfamilies that do not respond to treatment.

The following section examines the morphologic processes that influence the development of a tumor.

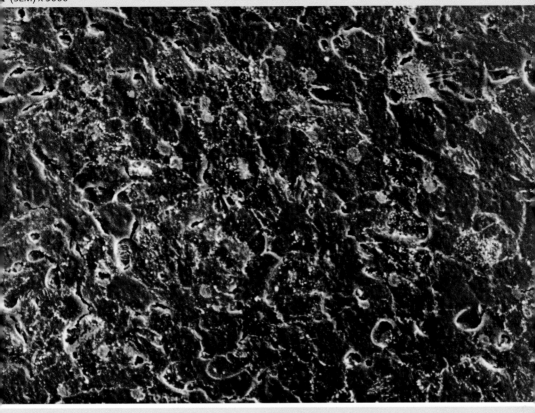

Normal keratinocytes (cell culture)
(SEM) x 5000

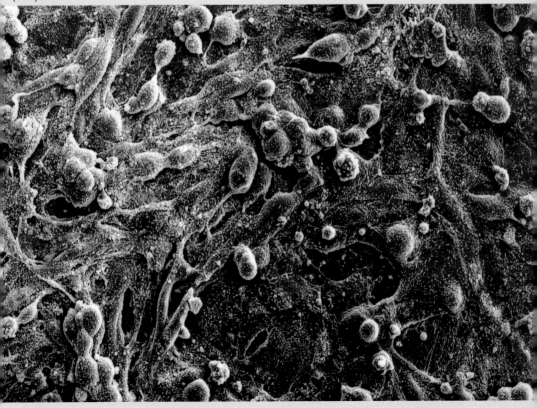

Tumorous keratinocytes (cell culture)
(SEM) x 5000

Formal Tumorigenesis

Precursors and Early Stages

A neoplastic tissue proliferation develops into a malignant tumor in several stages. At times it is difficult to draw a clear morphologic distinction between benign and malignant tumors, as the transition between the two stages cannot always be clearly defined. Such tumors are often referred to as *borderline tumors*.

Yet in certain types of tissue the precursors of cancer are well-defined *precancerous lesions* and/or pass through a noninvasive intermediate form (*carcinoma in situ*) into an invasive form. In certain organs such as the stomach and uterus, detection of carcinomas in the early stages of infiltration (*early cancer*) is possible, with a particularly good prognosis.

The precursors and early stages of cancer are discussed separately in the following section because of their specific prognostic significance.

Precancerosis

General definition: These are tissue changes with an increased statistical risk of malignancy.

General pathogenesis: Precancerous lesions may arise as a result of congenital cell characteristics or acquired tissue characteristics.
— A *precancerous condition* is one that predisposes the patient to a precancerous malady, i.e., xeroderma pigmentosum (p. 6).
— A *precancerous lesion* is an acquired tissue change such as actinic keratosis (p. 150).

These precancerous conditions may exhibit varying biologic behavior. Some become malignant tumors only occasionally and only after a prolonged period of time ("facultatively"). Others become malignant tumors often and within a short time ("obligatorily").

General morphology of the most common precancerous tissue changes is illustrated below. Several histologic forms may be distinguished according to the specific tissue.

■ Leukoplakia

Definition: This is a white patch of altered superficial epithelium that cannot be wiped off (▶ C1, D).

Histologic findings include focal squamous tissue changes characterized by:
— *Hyperkeratosis,* increased cornification with formation of nonnucleated cornified scales;
— *Parakeratosis,* excessively rapid cornification with formation of nucleated cornified scales (▶ B1);
— *Basal cell hyperplasia* (▶ B2, C2);
— *Inflammation,* lymphocytic infiltration of the stroma (not necessarily present).

The *prognosis* is favorable. Concurrent presence of dysplasia represents a precancerous condition.

Intraepithelial Neoplasia (= Dysplasia)

Definition: This refers to reversible histologic deviation of epithelial tissue from normal (▶ A) with deranged differentiation but controlled proliferation. It is a precancerous lesion.

Histologic findings include cells that exhibit marked variability in the nuclear size (pleomorphism) and mitoses with loss of functional epithelial orientation (loss of polarity; ▶ A, B1). The *prognosis* is favorable.

Carcinoma in Situ

Definition and morphology: Severe epithelial atypia (for example in the squamous epithelium) and loss of polarity are present with an intact basement membrane (▶ E1) and histologic findings of noninvasive carcinoma (▶ E2, F). The *prognosis* is favorable.

Microinvasive Carcinoma

Definition and morphology: Early form of carcinoma (primarily of the cervix uteri) that penetrates the basement membrane and invades tissue to a maximum depth of 3–5 mm. The *prognosis* is favorable.

Transformation of a cell into a cancer cell produces unequivocal evidence in the cell itself and its nucleus that is of diagnostic value. These signs are discussed in the next section.

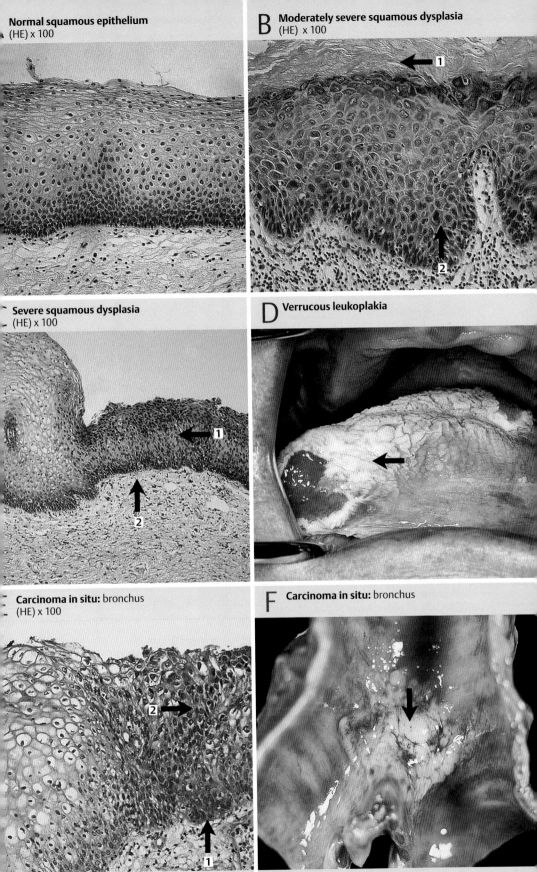

Normal squamous epithelium
(HE) x 100

B **Moderately severe squamous dysplasia**
(HE) x 100

Severe squamous dysplasia
(HE) x 100

D **Verrucous leukoplakia**

Carcinoma in situ: bronchus
(HE) x 100

F **Carcinoma in situ: bronchus**

Cellular and Nuclear Changes

Cellular Changes

■ **Anaplasia:** Malignant tumors synthesize defective extracellular matrix proteins (fibronectin and laminin) and cell adhesion proteins. This results in the loss of normal intercellular and cell-to-matrix communication. The cells lose their identity and are barely able to adhere together in cohesive tissue patterns. They leave their customary location and settle elsewhere.

■ **Biochemical Convergence:** The organelles in all malignant tumor cells are rarified, and the ratio of nucleus to cytoplasm is shifted in favor of the nucleus. Consequently, anaplastic tumors arising from different tissues tend to simplify their metabolism and covert to anaerobic glycolysis. In doing so, they assume functional and ultrastructural characteristics of embryonic cells such as oncofetal organelles (p. 12).

Nuclear Changes

Recapitulation: See description of nuclear changes (p. 10).

General morphology: The cells of a malignant tumor contain mitotically active nuclei of varying size (polymorphism) and with varying chromatin content (polychromasia) that exhibit stout nucleoli (▶ A). Occasionally, they are also multinucleated (▶ B).

These nuclear changes are an important criterion for malignancy and are due to the changes in DNA content and/or chromosome material described below.

■ DNA Content of Tumor Cells

▧ **Benign Tumors** consist of cells with diploid and occasionally tetraploid DNA content.

▧ **Malignant Tumors** consist of cells with incomplete sets of chromosomes and abnormal DNA values. These are both higher than the normal diploid DNA value and exhibit a wider range of variation than in nonmalignant cells (aneuploidy).

■ Chromosome Aberrations

These are typical of a malignant transformation and invariably involve loss of genes, often referred to as a genetic "domino effect" or "cytogenetic noise".

▧ Primary Aberrations

These may occur in two different variations.

— *Germ cell mutations* are mutations that are already present in a zygote (either inherited from one parent or a new mutation) and are therefore congenital.

— *Somatic mutations* only occur later in a single cell of the body.

Such mutations impair the function of proto-oncogenes and tumor suppressor genes and lead to continuous proliferation.

▧ Secondary Aberrations

Additional chromosome material is either lost after a primary aberration (gene deletion leads to aneuploidy) and/or implanted into a different chromosome where chromosome fractures are present. This is known as chromosome translocation. The result is a loss of suppressor and/or differentiation genes, which successively leads to uncontrolled proliferation and loss of differentiation.

▧ Tertiary Aberrations

Additional chromosome aberrations occur in rapidly proliferating tumor cells in the final stage of the tumor. These lead to a loss of metastasis suppressors and therefore to metastasis.

Examples:
— *Philadelphia chromosome* (▶ C): In the illustration, the long segment on chromosome 22 has broken off and translocated to chromosome 9. This affects the c-*abl* proto-oncogene (tyrosine kinase; gene locus 9q34), which becomes an active oncogene. C-*abl* physiologically regulates the growth of pluripotential hemopoietic bone marrow stem cells. The 9→22 translocation recombines the c-*abl* gene with the *bcr* oncogene at gene locus 22q11, which is coded for a GTPase-activating protein. This produces a newly constituted gene that transcribes an abnormal *bcr-abl* RNA, resulting in synthesis of an abnormal oncoprotein (*bcr-abl* protein). This in turn leads to a continuous proliferation signal. The *result* is chronic and also acute myelogenous leukemia (p. 360).
— *B-cell lymphomas* are caused by specific translocations in what is known as the pre-B phase of lymphocytic development. These translocations involve rearrangement of the genes for immunoglobulins. The enzyme recombinase erroneously joins together two immunoglobulin genes and proto-oncogenes like c-*myc*. This turns the proto-oncogene into an oncogene, leading to a continuous proliferation signal for B lymphocytes. This *results* in B-cell lymphomas.

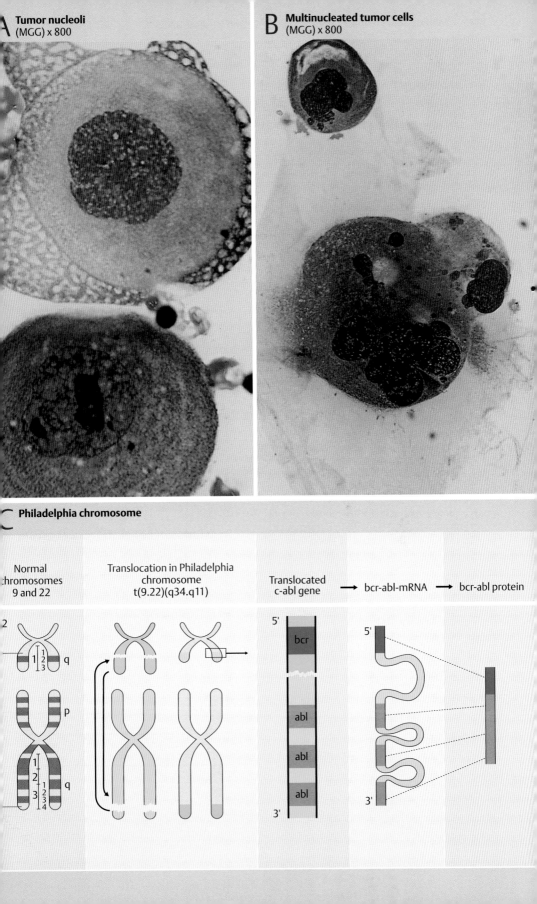

A Tumor nucleoli
(MGG) x 800

B Multinucleated tumor cells
(MGG) x 800

C Philadelphia chromosome

Normal chromosomes 9 and 22	Translocation in Philadelphia chromosome t(9.22)(q34.q11)	Translocated c-abl gene	→ bcr-abl-mRNA → bcr-abl protein

22

1
1
2
3
q

p

1
2
3
1
2
3
4
q

5'
bcr

abl

abl

abl
3'

5'

3'

Tumor Angiogenesis

Every tumor makes use of the existing vascular network at least to a certain extent. This leads to qualitative and quantitative changes in the affected portion of the vascular network. The tumor also utilizes several factors to develop its own vascular system.

— **Tumor-associated angiogenic factors** such as fibroblast growth factors (bFGF, VEGF) attract and stimulate proliferation of endothelial cells, and their proteolytic action leads to branching of capillary endothelia.
— **Non-tumor angiogenic factors** such as tumor necrosis factor (TNF-α) from macrophages leads to proliferation and migration (branching) of capillary endothelia.

This results in profound localized vascular changes in the vicinity of malignant tumors characterized by four distinct angiographic symptoms.

— **Inhomogeneous vascular network:** Tumor growth outstrips the growth of the tumor vascular network, which is functionally overtaxed. This means that the margin of the tumor has better vascular supply than the center.
— **Variations in vascular diameter:** Tumor growth greatly distends the existing vascular network and the increased tissue pressure compresses it.
— **Abrupt changes in vascular direction:** The tumor's vascular network does not exhibit a symmetric structure, but a chaotic pattern of irregular branches.
— **Abrupt termination of vascular structures:** Occurring as a result of necrosis and arteriovenous shunts, these vascular irregularities result in the reversal of blood flow and hemostasis.

Tumor Dissemination

A benign tumor remains within its tissue of origin and cannot extend across long distances into other organs. In contrast, the spread of malignant tumors exhibits the following four characteristics (see also p. 350):

— **Infiltration:** The tumor cells penetrate the surrounding tissue (► A).
— **Invasion:** The tumor cells penetrate lymph and blood vessels (► B).
— **Tissue destruction** occurs in the vicinity of the tumor as a result (► C).
— **Metastasis:** Tumor cells colonize other tissues far from the original tumor site.

This abnormal tumor cell behavior in tissue aggregates is due to four pathogenetic causes.

— **Loss of thigmotaxis** (thigmo = greek touch; taxis = movement): Tumor cells navigate using certain proteins of the extracellular matrix (laminin, fibronectin), and propagate along certain tissue structures such as nerve sheaths (► D) and collagen fibers (► E).

— **Loss of contact inhibition:** As soon as normal cells come into contact with each other, they cease to migrate or divide. This is known as contact inhibition. The termination signal initiating this inhibition is received by surface structures such as adhesion molecules (integrins, cadherins). These structures transmit the signal via second messenger substances to the cell nucleus, which controls proliferation. The impaired transmission of this termination signal in malignant tumor cells interrupts intercellular communication, causing tumor cells to continue to proliferate to the extent that they kill each other off.

— **Loss of intercellular cohesion:** Tumor cells leave their cellular aggregate for two reasons.
   — Tumor cells repel each other because of their negative surface charge produced by the carboxyl groups of their membrane-bound sialic acid.
   — Loss of adhesion occurs due to the mutation of certain suppressor genes. These genes change the adhesion molecules and result in loss of intercellular cohesion (► F).

— **Loss of cellular "staying put":** Tumor cells either secrete proteases, or force the host cells to do so. Involved therein are cysteine, serin-, and metalloproteinases, which dissolve primarily those epithelial and vascular basement membranes containing collagen. These proteases are restrained by tissue inhibitors of metalloproteases, a factor absent in invasive tumors. In the final stage, the tumor cells up-regulate tumor cell migration factors like HGF, and exit the primary cellular mass, aided by migration-furthering extracellar matrix cleavage products.

The following section takes a closer look at metastasis as part of tumor dissemination.

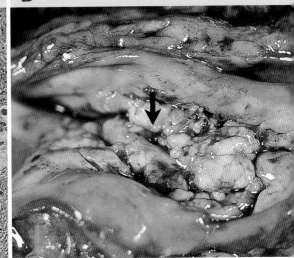

A **Muscle infiltration:** prostate carcinoma
(HE) x 200

B **Penetration of the vena cava:** renal carcinoma

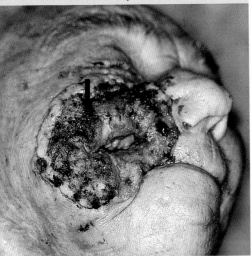

C **Tissue destruction:**
carcinoma of the maxillary sinus

D **Invasion of a nerve sheath:** carcinoma
(HE) x 100

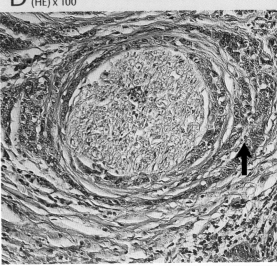

E **Thigmotaxis** along collagen fibers (carcinoma)
(HE) x 100

F **Cellular discohesion:** mucinous carcinoma
(PAS) x 250

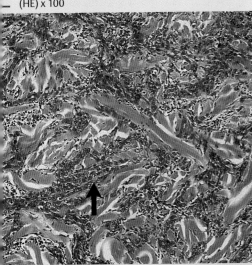

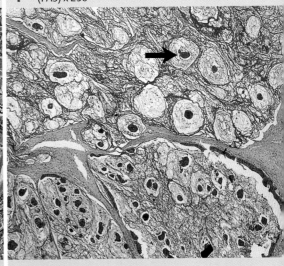

Metastasis

Definition: Dissemination of tumor cells from one part of the body to another remote location, where they establish themselves and grow into secondary tumors.

> **Note:** *Metastasis* in a wider sense refers to the spread of any disease process from one part of the body to another.

Pathogenesis involves the interaction of several processes:

— **Loss of metastasis-suppressor genes:** Metastasis is prevented by metastasis suppressor genes. The encoded products of these genes have several functions.
  — *Cadherins* promote intercellular adhesion.
  — *Tissue inhibitors of metalloproteinase (TIMP)* prevent tumor cells from using metalloproteinases to breach the barrier of the vascular basement membrane.
  — *pNM23* (nonmetastatic gene 23): The product of this gene has to do with nucleoside diphosphate kinase activity. Its role in metastasis is unclear.
  These genes only cease to function in the latter stages of neoplastic disease.

— **Loss of cohesion:** At the beginning of metastasis, the tumor cells lose genes that encode the adhesion molecules (integrins) that cling to proteins of the extracellular matrix (collagen, laminin, and fibronectin) and those that encode the cell's "adhesive" receptors that match the matrix proteins.

— **Cell motility** is brought about by intrinsic factors in the tumor.

— **Intravasation and extravasation:** Under the influence of certain growth factors, tumor cells secrete proteolytic enzymes that degrade the extracellular matrix (p. 344). This allows tumors cells to migrate through the vessel wall into the lumen of the vessel and to later leave the vessel and re-enter tissue (see leukocyte transmigration, p. 200).

— **Circumvention of immune surveillance:** This is achieved by reduced expression of HLA self-recognition molecules on the surface of the tumor cell and by the tumor cell acquiring a fibrin coating in the blood vessel (tumor embolus).

— **Colonization:** Tumor cells colonize certain organs because they detect organ-specific adhesion molecules and because of the presence of a target address on the surface of the tumor cell in the form of lectins.

According to the "soil and seed" concept, the respective "seeds" (tumor cells) are matched to the "soil" (the organ or tissue). This explains why metastases are rarely found in the spleen or skeletal muscle and why prostate, kidney, thyroid, and breast carcinomas frequently metastasize into bone.

— **Latent tumor cells:** Isolated tumor cells may colonize an organ or tissue and remain latent for 10–20 years. Aggressive growth may then occur for unknown reasons, leading to late metastases (for example in breast cancer).

> **Note:** Symptoms of bone metastases include:
> – Bone pain;
> – Pathologic fractures;
> – Compression of the spinal cord.

◼ Lymphatic Metastasis

Definition: Dissemination of tumor cells via the lymphatic system.

Formal pathogenesis: Lymphatic metastasis follows one of three patterns.

— **Tumorous lymphangiosis:** Tumor cells that separate from the margin of a tumor usually initially invade lymph vessels (which lack a basement membrane). Then the tumor cells usually migrate through the vascular wall within 24 hours. Where the flow in the respective lymph vessel is conducive to it, tumor cells may even proliferate within the lymph vessels and grow along them (▶ A, B, C1).

Several forms of tumorous lymphangiosis are distinguished according to the primary neoplasia.
  — *Carcinomatous lymphangiosis* involves a carcinoma as the primary neoplasm (▶ A, B).
  — *Sarcomatous lymphangiosis* involves a sarcoma as the primary neoplasm.
  — *Blastomatous lymphangiosis* involves a blastoma as the primary neoplasm.

— **Lymph-node metastasis:** Tumor cells usually spread to the next lymph node (▶ C3). There, they initially seed the marginal sinus (▶ C2, D) and later overrun the entire lymph node (▶ E). This eventually leads to a rupture of the capsule with proliferation of the tumor beyond the confines of the capsule and invasion of neighboring blood vessels.

— **Remote metastases:** From the initial infestation of a lymph node, tumor cells spread into the immediate downstream nodes and later to more remote nodes. They can then enter the venous bloodstream via the thoracic duct.

Example: Lymph node metastasis of a primary carcinoma of the palate (▶ F).

> **Note:** The *rule for metastases* is that carcinomas primarily spread via lymphatic metastases and sarcomas primarily via hematogenous metastases.

A **Carcinomatous lymphangiosis:** skin (HE) x 100

B **Carcinomatous lymphangiosis:** pleura

C **Carcinomatous lymphangiosis:** lymph nodes (HE) x 25

D **Micrometastases:** lymph nodes (HE) x 50

E **Lymph node metastasis**

F **Metastasis:** cervical lymph node

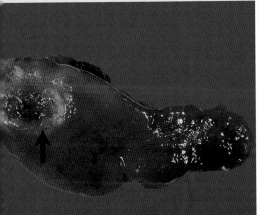
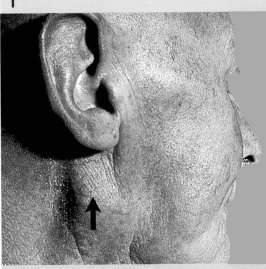

■ Hematogenous Metastasis

Definition: Dissemination of tumor cells via the bloodstream, leading to metastatic disease.

Formal pathogenesis: There are three stages in hematogenous metastasis:
— *Invasion phase:* Most tumor cells pass from the lymph system into the bloodstream. There most of them are destroyed within 24 hours.
— *Embolus phase:* In circulation, tumor cells aggregate in clumps (► B1) and surround themselves with a coat of fibrin (► B2), forming a tumor embolus that lodges in precapillary arterioles.
— *Implantation phase:* As time passes, individual tumor cells break out of the embolus and pass through the postcapillary venules. Where they encounter appropriate adhesion factors, these tumor cells adhere to the endothelial surface of organ vessels. They then extravasate and invade the organ tissue. The invading tumor cells establish their own vascular system and develop into secondary tumors.

> **Note:** Sarcomas, follicular carcinomas of the thyroid, and renal cell carcinomas tend to exhibit early hematogenous metastasis.

There are four basic patterns of hematogenous metastasis (► A).

▦ Lung Pattern

A primary tumor located in the *lung* initially spreads via the pulmonary veins. From there, tumor cells spread to the left heart, and the tumor can colonize any of the organs supplied by the extrapulmonary vessels (► A1).

▦ Liver Pattern

A primary tumor located in the *liver* initially spreads via the hepatic veins. From there, tumor cells spread to the right heart, lungs, and left heart. From there, the tumor can colonize any of the organs supplied by the extrapulmonary vessels (► A2).

▦ Vena Cava Pattern

Here, the primary tumor is located in the area drained by the *superior or inferior vena cava* (such as a kidney, bone, or thyroid tumor). The tumor cells initially spread to the right heart and can colonize the lung (► A3).

▦ Portal Vein Pattern

A primary tumor located in the *intestine* initially spreads via the portal vein to the liver, where it metastasizes. From there, tumor cells spread via the hepatic veins and vena cava to the lung (► A4) in the same manner as the liver pattern.

■ Cavitary Metastasis

Tumor cells invade a body cavity such as the pleura, peritoneum, pericardium, subarachnoid space, or tendon sheath. From there, they spread within the respective cavity and colonize it with one or more metastases. Manifestations of such metastatic disease include:
— Pleural carcinosis/sarcomatosis (► D);
— Peritoneal carcinosis/sarcomatosis (► C);
— Pericardial carcinosis/sarcomatosis (► E);

> **Note:** A hemorrhagic pleural or peritoneal effusion suggests carcinoma.

■ Canalicular Metastasis

This refers to metastasis within a duct system lined with epithelial tissue. *Occurrences* of this rare pattern of metastasis include:
— Breast carcinoma via the lactiferous ducts;
— Carcinoma of the gallbladder via the bile ducts;
— Carcinoma of the bladder via the ureter.

■ Inoculated Metastases

Invasive diagnostic and surgical procedures such as biopsy and exudate aspiration (p. 2) can lead to iatrogenic dissemination of tumor cells along the wound canal of the biopsy.

> **Note:** Despite the frequency of fine-needle aspirations, inoculated metastases remain rare.

A Hematogenous metastasis

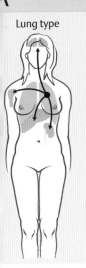
Lung type

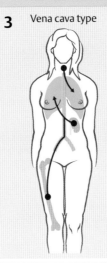
2 Liver type

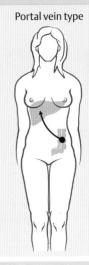
3 Vena cava type

4 Portal vein type

B Tumor embolism
(HE) x 100

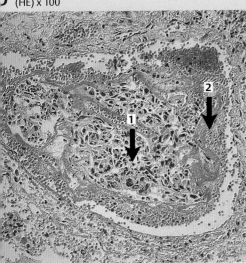

C Peritoneal carcinosis: metastatic rectal carcinoma

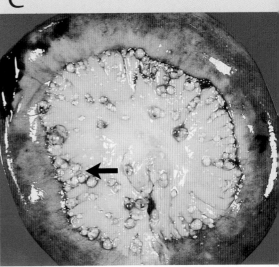

D Pleural sarcomatosis:
metastatic sarcoma of the uterus

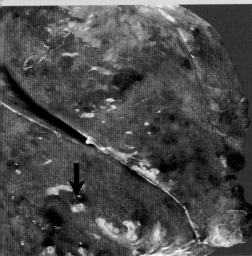

E Pericardial sarcomatosis:
metastatic sarcoma of the uterus

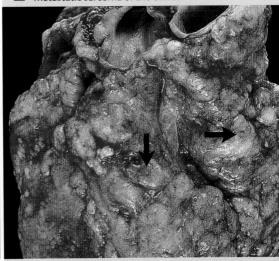

Characteristics of benign and malignant tumors (see also p. 344)

	Benign tumors	**Malignant tumors**
Growth	Slow with – *Expansion, displacement* – *Compression* → Compressive atrophy of surrounding tissue	Rapid with – *Destruction* – *Infiltration* (▶ D) – *Thigmotaxis* – *Vascular invasion* – *Metastases*
Size	Increases slowly; tumor may become very large ("knapsack tumor"; ▶ B)	Increases rapidly
Capsule	Present; tumor can be surgically "enucleated" from capsule due to compression of local stroma	Partially or entirely absent; tumor frequently recurs after resection
Maneuverability	maneuverable	non-maneuverable
Histologic findings	Usually a perfect image of the histologic mother tissue with a low mitosis count and absence of necrosis	Primitive image of the histologic mother tissue with a high mitosis count and necrosis
Variability of cell size	Cellular and nuclear isomorphism (cells and nuclei of largely the same size)	Cellular and nuclear polymorphism (cells and nuclei of varying size)
DNA content	Nuclear euploidy (uniform coloration of nuclei) with the exception of endocrine tumors, which exhibit nuclear polyploidy	Nuclear aneuploidy, polyploidy, and polychromasia (varying coloration of nuclei)
Ratio of nucleus to cytoplasm	Normal	Nuclei predominate
Nucleoli	Invisible or small and round	Enlarged and irregular
Clinical course	Usually clinically asymptomatic except for compression symptoms; do not recur or metastasize	Produce a wide range of late symptoms; frequently recur and metastasize

Tumor Regression

Pathogenesis: Regressive changes in a malignant tumor, and occasionally in a benign one, are attributable to the following mechanisms:

— Rapid tumor growth;
— An insufficient vascular network;
— Immune system intervention.

Characteristic morphologic findings occur in central regression of a tumor.

— *Necroses* may be spontaneous or iatrogenic.
— *Spontaneous hemorrhages* may occur due to tumor necrosis or therapy.
— *Scarring* may occur, producing crater-like retraction of the surrounding tissue. Superficial liver metastases produce a typical "cancer crater" (▶ A).
— *Dystrophic calcification* occurs in patients with certain tumors (see below), where tumor clusters calcify into concrements resembling grains of sand ("psammomatous" calcification).

> **Note:** Psammomatous calcification is typical of papillary ovarian carcinomas, papillary thyroid carcinomas, and meningiomas.

Sequelae of Tumor Regression

■ **Remission:** The tumor may regress under chemotherapy and/or radiation therapy.

■ **Complete remission:** Extensive chemotherapy and/or radiation therapy may completely destroy the tumor to the extent that no tumor tissue is detectable.

■ **Spontaneous remission:** This refers to the complete disappearance of a malignant tumor (a) in the absence of treatment or (b) under treatment whose efficacy has yet to be demonstrated.

Possible causes of such "self-healing" may include re-establishment of (a) apoptosis or (b) differentiation. For example, a neuroblastoma may differentiate into a ganglioneuroblastoma, that in turn becomes a ganglioneuroma (p. 382).

■ **Recurrence:** This refers to the reappearance of a tumor following resection or complete remission.

Depending on the type and differentiation of the tumor, the patient's immune status, and the success of therapy, recurrence may be early or late.

— *Early recurrence* involves compromised immune defenses; the tumor reappears after a few months, usually in the same place (local recurrence).
— *Late recurrence* involves good immune defenses; the tumor reappears only after a period of years, usually in a different place (remote recurrence).

A Cancer "crater": liver metastases

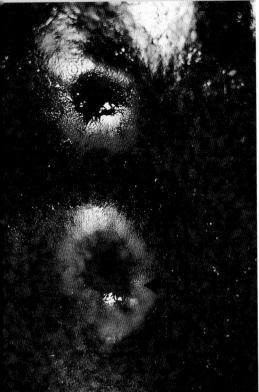

B "Knapsack" tumor: lipoma

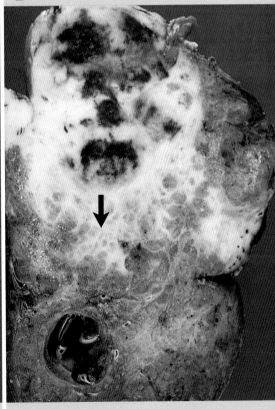

C Enucleated fibroadenoma of the breast

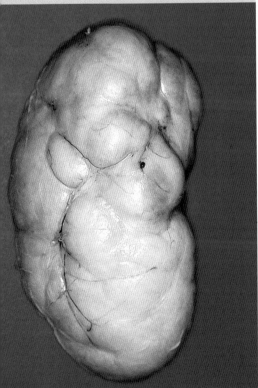

D Tumor infiltration (thyroid carcinoma)

Tumor Complications

The lesions described below complicate the simple growth of the tumor. The combination of such lesions with tumor expansion and metastasis constitute neoplastic disease that extends beyond the tumor as such.

Local Complications

■ **Stenosis:** Tumors can lead to several compression syndromes.

— *Expansion* of the tumor compresses the surrounding tissue (▶ A) and causes stenosis in hollow organs (▶ A2, compression of the small bowel by a mesenterial liposarcoma; p. 356). Complications may include difficulties in swallowing, impaired micturition, disruption of intestinal motility, and also increased intracranial pressure (p. 428).

— *Infiltration* of the tumor can cause congestion in a hollow organ. Complications may include prestenotic dilation of the duct, stasis and congestion of secretions or excretions, and bacterial infestation of the congested area.

■ **Circulatory Disruption:** Tumor growth that compromises or infiltrates vascular structures produces a variety of lesions.

— *Obstruction of venous drainage* is common and successively leads to varicose changes in the walls of the veins and thrombosis.

— *Vascular thrombosis* may result from vascular stenosis and/or substances produced by the tumor itself that promote coagulation.

— *Bleeding* due to erosion of vascular structures may lead to spitting of blood from the lungs or bronchi (hemoptysis), vomiting of blood (hematemesis), passage of bloody stools (melena), blood in the urine (hematuria), acyclic bleeding from the uterus (metrorrhagia), and hemorrhagic effusions (▶ B).

■ **Tumor Necrosis** (▶ C): occurs as a result of the interplay of several factors. These include:

— Thrombotic arterial obstruction;
— Vascular compression by the tumor;
— Twisting of the tumor pedicle;
— Cytokines (macrophagic TNF-α);
— Aggressive tumor therapy.

✚ **Complications of tumor necrosis:**
– *Ulceration* of the inner or outer body surface may occur, primarily in gastrointestinal, skin, and breast cancer (▶ D).
– *Perforation* of the tumor necrosis may occur into hollow organs or through the surface of the skin (▶ E).
– *Fistulas* may form that communicate with adjacent organs.

■ **Disruption of Organ Function:** occurs especially in tumors that not only mechanically alter the organ parenchyma and its supporting tissue but also destroy them.

Particularly susceptible tissues include:
— Neurovascular structures;
— Urinary tract,
— Intestinal tract;
— Skeletal system, where bone tumors can cause pathologic fractures (▶ F).

Systemic Complications

Advanced neoplastic disease regularly produces four types of systemic lesions.

■ **Tumor Metastases** (see above): occasionally occur even in the early phases of neoplastic disease.

■ **Cancer Cachexia:** involves weight loss in cancer patients. Causes include:
— *Impaired swallowing* due to the tumor;
— *Impaired digestion* due to the tumor;
— *Generation of TNF-α* by macrophages stimulated by tumor-associated antigens.
— *Generation of leptin* (fat-cell hormone; p. 84). This results in loss of appetite (anorexia), reduced intake of nutrients, decreased body fat, and increased energy consumption.

■ **Tumor Anemia:** produces the characteristic pale skin of cancer patients. It is due to several factors, including:
— Blood loss due to internal bleeding;
— Lack of substances that promote maturation of blood cells;
— Autoreactive antibodies against erythrocytes;
— Displacement of bone marrow by tumorous infiltrates.

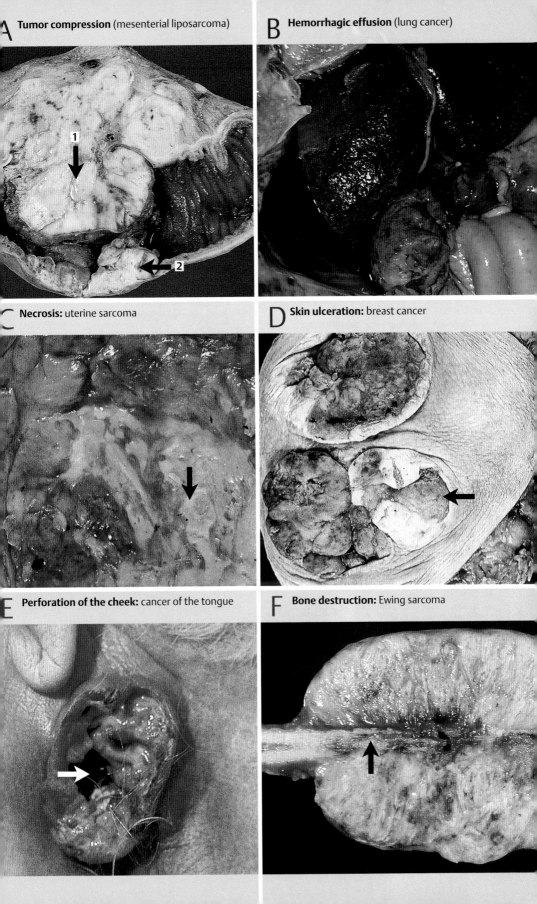

A Tumor compression (mesenterial liposarcoma)

B Hemorrhagic effusion (lung cancer)

C Necrosis: uterine sarcoma

D Skin ulceration: breast cancer

E Perforation of the cheek: cancer of the tongue

F Bone destruction: Ewing sarcoma

■ Paraneoplastic Syndromes

Definition: Collective term for a group of generalized pathologic manifestations that are not attributable to the local effects of a tumor but are linked to the existence of a tumor and can regress after the tumor has been removed.

Pathogenesis: Often unclear.

— *Cell destruction* occurs due to formation of autoreactive antibodies against tumor antigens and "self" antigens and as a result of apoptosis caused by certain tumor proteins.
— *Dysfunction* results from synthesis of peptides with endocrine and enzymatic effects.

▥ Endocrinopathies

General pathogenesis: Tumors synthesize ectopic hormones of substances similar to hormones. The most important forms are as follows:

— *Cushing's syndrome* is caused by formation of ACTH and occurs in patients with bronchial cancer.
— *Flush's syndrome* is caused by formation of serotonin and leads to facial erythema, diarrhea, colic, and bronchospasm.
It occurs in patients with bronchial or ileal carcinoid (p. 384).

— *Schwartz-Bartter's syndrome* is caused by formation of proteins resembling ADH and leads to hyponatremia.
It occurs in patients with small cell bronchogenic carcinoma (p. 378).

— *Hypercalcemia syndrome* is caused by formation of parathormone-like protein.
It occurs in patients with squamous cell bronchogenic carcinoma or renal cell carcinomas.

▥ Nerve and Muscle Syndromes

Pathogenesis: Nerve cells and/or muscle fibers are destroyed by autoimmune processes and by tumor-induced apoptosis. The most important forms are as follows:

— *Myasthenia gravis* occurs in patients with thymus tumors (thymomas).
— *Limbic encephalopathy* occurs in patients with small cell bronchogenic carcinoma.
— *Degeneration of the cerebellar cortex* occurs in patients with small cell bronchogenic carcinoma, breast cancer, or ovarian carcinoma.

▥ Vascular and Hematologic Changes

Pathogenesis of the most important forms is described in the following section.

— *Hemolysis:* The tumor synthesizes cytotoxic substances and/or autoreactive antibodies, damaging the bone marrow and leading to hemolytic anemia.
This occurs in patients with leukemias or Hodgkin's disease's lymphoma (p. 362).

— *Erythrocyte proliferation:* The tumor synthesizes substances that stimulate erythropoiesis (erythropoietin), leading to polyglobulism (an overabundance of erythrocytes).
This occurs in patients with renal cell carcinoma.

— *Leukocyte proliferation:* The tumor synthesizes substances that stimulate myelopoiesis, leading to a leukemoid reaction.
This occurs in patients with stomach cancer or large cell bronchogenic carcinoma.

— *Macroscopic coagulopathy:* The tumor synthesizes thromboplastic substances that lead to thrombosis (p. 404).
This occurs in patients with pancreatic or adenoid carcinomas.

— *Disseminated intravascular coagulation* (p. 402): The tumor synthesizes thromboplastic and fibrinolytic substances that consume the clotting factors.
This occurs in patients with leukemias.

> **Note:** Coagulopathy is characterized by thrombotic vascular occlusion (primarily in the lung), whereas disseminated intravascular coagulation is characterized by hyalin microthrombi (primarily in the microvasculature of the lung).

▥ Dermatologic Disorders

— *Acanthosis nigricans* manifests itself as thickening of the skin with clearly discernible papillary lines, hyperpigmentation, and wart-like papillomas.
It occurs in patients with stomach cancer or squamous cell bronchogenic carcinoma.

— *Bazex's syndrome* (paraneoplastic acrokeratosis) manifests itself as reddish purple plaques of calcification on the hands, feet, nose, and ears.
It occurs in patients with carcinoma of the tongue or tonsils.

— *Erythema gyratum repens* is a rare skin rash resembling zebra stripes that changes daily.
It occurs in patients with various carcinomas.

— *Hypertrichosis lanuginosa* is a rare manifestation involving excessive growth of the head and body hair.
It occurs in patients with various carcinomas.

This concludes the discussion of the processes that explain the biologic behavior of a tumor. The following section examines the general criteria used in classifying and evaluating tumors, and presents the most important forms of tumors.

Tumor Classification

Current methods of tumor classification attempt to identify the tumor according to its tissue of origin (type), the extent its spread (stage), and its level of differentiation (grade).

Staging: The stage of neoplastic disease is defined according to three criteria. Together, they comprise what is known internationally as the *TNM system.*
- **T** refers to local **t**umor growth.
- **N** refers to spread to regional lymph **n**odes.
- **M** refers to distant **m**etastasis.

Several prefixes are used to provide additional information.
- TNM refers to initial clinical and radiologic staging.
- pTNM refers to postoperative or pathologic staging.
- yTNM refers staging following chemotherapy.
- rTMN refers staging in the presence of recurrent cancer.

Grading: This involves histologic evaluation of the extent to which a tumor corresponds to its tissue of origin.
- **G1** indicates a high degree of differentiation (low malignancy).
- **G2** indicates a moderate degree of differentiation (moderate malignancy).
- **G3** indicates a low degree of differentiation (high malignancy).
- **G4** indicates no differentiation (very high malignancy, indicating an anaplastic tumor).

> **Rule of thumb:** The less differentiated a tumor is, the greater its malignancy, the more rapid its growth (mitosis count). Its sensitivity to radiation and spontaneous rate of necrosis will also be correspondingly high.

Typing: Tumors are classified as follows according to their tissue of origin (see below):
- Benign nonepithelial tumors;
- Malignant nonepithelial tumors;
- Benign epithelial tumors;
- Malignant epithelial tumors.

Nonepithelial Tumors

General Definitions

Mesenchymal Tumors

These tumors consist of tissues that originate in the middle germ layer or mesoderm, primarily from the pluripotential supporting tissue of the embryo (mesenchyma). This definition applies to tumors of connective tissue, supporting tissue, and muscle.

> **Exceptions:**
> - Tumors of the kidney, adrenal cortex, and mesothelia can develop an epithelial tissue pattern.
> - Cells of the hemopoietic and lymphopoietic systems are derived from mesoderm. However, they do not form a distinct group of tumors.
> - Schwann cell and melanocytic tumors, which are derived from ectodermal tissue, form mesenchymal patterns of growth.

For this reason, the World Health Organization introduced the definition of an additional tumor group, soft tissue tumors.

Soft Tissue Tumors

This is a collective term for nonepithelial tumors that arise exclusively from cells of nonskeletal tissue including peripheral nerve tissue.

> **Exceptions:**
> The following tumors *are not* considered soft tissue tumors:
> - Tumors of the macrophage system and tumors of the hemopoietic and lymphopoietic systems;
> - Tumors of supporting tissue such as bone and glia;
> - Melanocytic tumors.

Benign Nonepithelial Tumors

General morphology: These tumors exhibit striking similarity to their physiologic tissue of origin. For this reason, the names of these neoplasms include the tissue of origin with the suffix "-oma" (for example, a tumor of fatty tissue is a lipoma).

> ✚ **Clinical presentation:** These tumors grow slowly and can become very large.

Malignant Nonepithelial Tumors

General morphology: Because of fleshy appearance of their cut surface, these tumors are known as sarcomas (from Greek *sarx*, flesh).

> ✚ **Clinical presentation:** These tumors grow rapidly with extensive tissue destruction and produce primarily hematogenous metastases.

> **Rule of thumb:** In *grading sarcomas,* malignancy increases with decreasing similarity to the tissue of origin, and in direct proportion to the mitosis count (10 or more mitoses in the visual field at 40-power magnification), and the extent of tumor necroses.

Fibrous Tumors

■ Fibroma

Occurrence: Ubiquitous and common.

Definition and morphology: Benign, nodular, fibrous tumor. Depending on their collagen content, fibromas are referred to as hard or soft (fibroma molle).

■ Fibrosarcoma

Occurrence: Rare, found primarily in the lower extremities.

Definition: Malignant, metastasizing fibrous tumor.

Histologic findings include spindle-shaped and polymorphic tumor cells in a "herring bone" pattern.

Immunohistochemical findings include tumor cells with a cytoskeleton containing vimentin.
The *prognosis* is generally unfavorable and depends on the tumor stage and extent of its spread.

Muscle Tumors

■ Leiomyomas

Occurrence: These common tumors usually occur in groups in the uterus (► A), intestinal tract, and vascular walls.

Definition: A benign spherical tumor composed of mature smooth muscle cells (► A).

Histologic findings include a swirling pattern of interwoven tumor cells (► B) with cigar-shaped nuclei. Each tumor cell (smooth muscle cell) has a "sock" of basement membrane wrapped around it. Regressive changes such as hyalinization, calcification, and/or ossification may be present. However, no necrosis will occur.

■ Leiomyosarcoma

Occurrence: This rare tumor occurs in the retroperitoneum and, rarely, in the uterus (► C).

Definition: A malignant nodular tumor composed of immature smooth muscle cells.

Histologic findings generally resemble a hypercellular leiomyoma often with only slight cellular polymorphism (► D) but with mitoses (over 10 mitoses per 10 visual fields at ×40 magnification). Necroses are usually present as well (► C).

Immunohistochemical findings include tumor cells with a cytoskeleton containing actin.
The *prognosis* depends on the tumor stage.

■ Rhabdomyoma

Occurrence: This very rare tumor occurs primarily in the heart.

Definition: Benign tumor of mature striated muscle cells.

Histologic findings include "spider cells" (polygonal spider-like tumor cells with vacuolar cytoplasm (containing glycogen), some of which exhibit striations.

■ Rhabdomyosarcoma

Occurrence: This rare tumor occurs in the head and neck region and genitals in infants and in the extremities in adults.

Definition: A group of highly malignant tumors of embryonic striated muscle tissue.

Histologic findings include stellate and spindle-shaped polymorphic tumor cells with striations in cytoplasmic tails ("tadpole cells"). Regressive change include necroses.

Immunohistochemical findings include tumor cells with a cytoskeleton containing desmin and myosin.
The *prognosis* is very poor.

Tumors of Fatty Tissue

■ Lipoma

Occurrence: This tumor is found in subcutaneous and submucosal tissue, Rarely, it may also occur at intramuscular sites, and these tumors tend to recur. It is the most common benign mesenchymal tumor.

Definition: Benign solid tumor of mature tumor cells (adipocytes) that store fat in a single vacuole.

Histologic findings perfectly mimic fatty tissue but with the connective tissue organizing it into the lobular structure typical of fatty tissue.

■ Liposarcoma

Occurrence: This tumor is found in the thigh (► E), back, and retroperitoneum.

Definition: Malignant soft yellowish tumor (► E) of fat cell precursors (preadipocytes).

Histologic findings: Fat is stored in multiple vacuoles (► F) in the cytoplasm and nucleus of the tumor cell, creating a typical scalloped nucleus. Regressive changes include necroses and myxoid degeneration of the stroma. In its extreme form, this manifests itself as a myxoid liposarcoma.

■ **Myxoid Liposarcoma** is a liposarcoma in which myxoid stroma predominates. It exhibits proliferation of plexiform capillaries, which produce a histologic pattern resembling crow's feet.

Immunohistochemical findings in all liposarcomas include tumor cells that express S-100 antigen.
The *prognosis* is often favorable, although the tumor recurs.

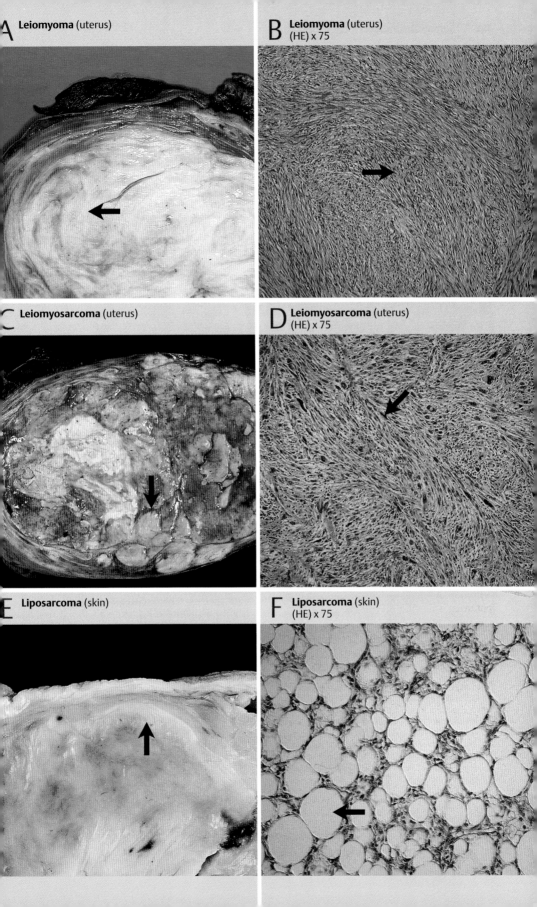

A Leiomyoma (uterus)

B Leiomyoma (uterus) (HE) x 75

C Leiomyosarcoma (uterus)

D Leiomyosarcoma (uterus) (HE) x 75

E Liposarcoma (skin)

F Liposarcoma (skin) (HE) x 75

Cartilage Tumors

■ Chondroma

Occurrence: The tumor occurs within the bones of the hands and feet.

An osteochondroma is a neoplasm arising as cartilage-capped bony outgrowth on a skeletal bone.

Definition and morphology: A benign tumor of mature chondrocytes that perfectly mimics hyaline cartilage.

> **Note:** *Pelvic chondromas* are often malignant.

■ Chondrosarcoma

Occurrence: The tumor arises in the pelvis or in long cortical bones such as the humerus, tibia (► A), and femur (► C).

Definition and morphology: This is a slow-growing malignant tumor arising from chondrocyte precursors, some of which develop into bizarre giant cells (► E), and exhibiting some of the characteristics of hyaline cartilage (► E). Regressive changes include necrosis, bleeding, and osteolysis.

Bone Tumors

■ Osteoma

Occurrence: The tumor arises primarily in bones that develop from the desmocranium.

Definition and morphology: This benign tumor arising from osteocytes perfectly mimics cancellous lamellar bone with a fibrous fatty medulla. It exhibits slowly expansive growth (► B = osteoid-osteoma).

■ Osteosarcoma

Occurrence: This tumor is found primarily in long bones in adolescents (► D). It is the most common malignant tumor of the skeletal system.

Definition: A highly malignant sarcoma of pluripotential osteocyte precursors.

Histologic findings include sarcomatous stromal tissue with polymorphic cells (► F1) with an uncalcified tumor osteoid (► F2) and disorganized tumorous cancellous tissue.

Tumor cells secrete cytokines and growth factors. One of the following types of osteosarcoma will occur, depending on the specific substance secreted:
- **Proliferation of osteoblasts** successively leads to bone remodeling and an osteoplastic osteosarcoma.
- **Proliferation of osteoclasts** successively leads to dissolution of bone and an osteolytic osteosarcoma.
- **Proliferation of capillaries** leads to a telangiectatic osteosarcoma.

Leukemias

Definition: Autonomous systemic proliferation of hematopoietic or lymphopoietic stem cells in the form of a non-solid tumor.

Several types may be distinguished according to biologic and clinical criteria:
- **Myelogenous leukemia** arises from pluripotential hemopoietic stem cells.
- **Lymphatic leukemia** arises from pluripotential lymphatic stem cells.
- **Acute leukemias** involve a high rate of proliferation without differentiation; their clinical course is rapid.
- **Chronic leukemias** involve a low rate of proliferation of immortal cells with good differentiation; their clinical course is slow.
- **Aleukemic leukemias** exhibit an absence of tumor cells in the peripheral blood.
- **Leukemic leukemias** are characterized by abundant tumor cells in the peripheral blood (as the redundant term suggests).
- **Chronic myeloproliferative disorders** involve neoplasia of pluripotential myeloid stem cells (hemopoietic bone marrow stem cells). There are several such disorders.

- *Chronic myelogenous leukemia* is primarily characterized by leukemic neoplastic granulopoiesis.
- *Essential thrombocythemia* involves generation of neoplastic megakaryocytes.
- *Polycythemia vera* primarily involves proliferation of neoplastic erythrocytes and granulocytes and generation of neoplastic megakaryocytes.
- *Primary myelofibrosis* involves leukemic neoplastic myelopoiesis and production of growth factors that stimulate fibroblasts and leads to fibrous obliteration of the bone marrow.
- *Chronic proliferative lymphatic disease* involves neoplasia of T and B stem cells. One such disorder is *chronic lymphatic leukemia.*

Depending on which homing receptors are formed, these neoplasms colonize several different tissues including
- Lymph nodes (*nodal lymphomas*),
- Intestinal mucosa (*lymphomas of mucosa-associated lymphoid tissue or MALT*), and
- Skin (*cutaneous lymphomas*).

Etiologic factors include ionizing radiation, chemical carcinogens such as benzol, and viruses such as HTLV-1 and HTLV-2.

Pathogenetic chain reaction: Etiologic factors lead to a fracture at a gene locus that is subject to somatic recombination during cell differentiation (these primarily include the loci for light and heavy immunoglobulin chains and the T-cell receptor). The resulting translocation of genetic material to loci of proliferation or differentiation genes leads to deranged genetic regulation and generation of a leukemic cell clone that displaces normal hemopoiesis. The result is a lack of leukocytes, erythrocytes, and thrombocytes.

> **✚ Clinical result:** Anemia, leukopenia with susceptibility to infection, and thrombopenia accompanied by a tendency to hemorrhage.

A Chondrosarcoma

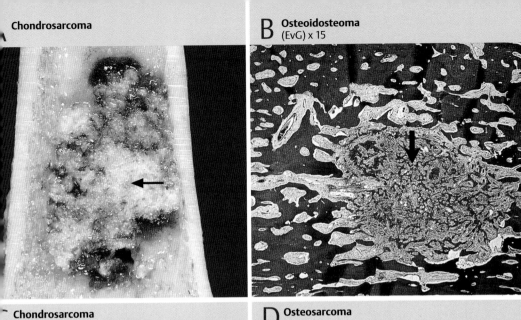

B Osteoidosteoma
(EvG) x 15

Chondrosarcoma

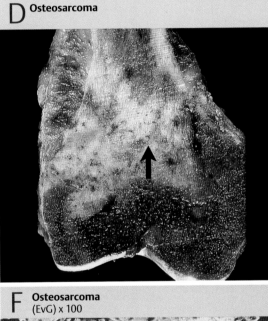

D Osteosarcoma

Chondrosarcoma
(HE) x 100

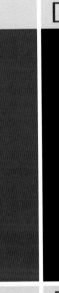

F Osteosarcoma
(EvG) x 100

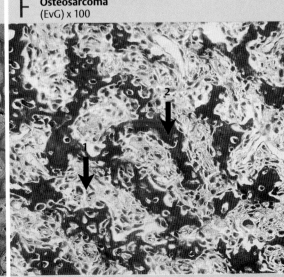

22

Tumor Pathology

■ Acute Myelogenous Leukemia

Occurrence: The disorder is more common in adults than in children.

Definition: Collective term for diseases of a stem-cell clone that lacks the ability to mature.

Acute myelogenous leukemia (AML) involves one or more of these cellular elements:
— *Myeloblasts* (cytoplasm containing peroxidase and chloracetate esterase);
— *Monocytopoiesis elements* (cytoplasm containing α-naphthyl acetate esterase);
— *Erythrocytopoiesis elements.*

Acute myelogenous leukemia is classified according to the differentiation and maturity of the leukemia cells.

Morphology:
— *Bone marrow* is glossy dark red with ill-defined grayish leukemic foci that displace all three types of hemopoietic cells.
— *Leucemic hiatus:* Abnormal hematologic findings in peripheral blood include immature cells derived from the neoplastic stem-cell clone along with non-neoplastic stem cells.
— *Liver:* It is slightly enlarged due to the presence of diffuse nondestructive infiltrate between the trabeculae.
— *Spleen:* It is moderately enlarged due to the presence of diffuse infiltrate displacing the follicles.
— *Lymph nodes* exhibit minimal involvement.

✚ **Clinical presentation:** Complete remission can be achieved in younger patients with high-dosage chemotherapy and transplants of bone marrow stem cells.

■ Chronic Myelogenous Leukemia (CML)

Occurrence: The disorder manifests itself from the fourth to sixth decade of life.

Definition: Disease of a stem-cell clone that retains the ability to mature.

Chronic myelogenous leukemia (CML) involves *myelopoiesis elements.*

Morphology:
— *Bone marrow* is glossy dark red (► A) with grayish-white leukemic foci 1 mm in diameter with displacement symptoms (see above).
— *Liver:* It exhibits massive hepatomegaly due to the presence of diffuse parenchymal infiltrate.
— *Spleen:* It exhibits massive diffuse infiltrate and extramedullary bleeding. This results in splenomegaly and anemic splenic infarctions from vascular stenoses caused by leukemia cells.
— *Lymph nodes* are enlarged due to infiltrate (► B1) between the follicles (► B2).

✚ **Clinical presentation:** After a clinical course of several years, the disorder accelerates and precipitates a refractory crisis with blast cells.

■ Acute Lymphoblastic Leukemia

Synonym: acute lymphoblastic lymphoma.

Occurrence: The disorder primarily manifests itself in small children up to the age of four.

Definition: Clonal proliferation of lymphatic precursor cells that lack the ability to mature.

Acute lymphoblastic leukemia (ALL) involves *lymphoblasts* with PAS-positive cytoplasm.

Morphology:
— *Bone marrow* exhibits grayish-white leukemic infiltrates with displacement symptoms (see above).
— *Liver:* It exhibits hepatomegaly due to nondestructive infiltrate in the portal field.
— *Spleen:* It exhibits splenomegaly due to diffuse infiltrate that displaces the follicles.
— *Lymph nodes* are enlarged due to diffuse infiltrate (lymphadenia).
— *Central nervous system:* It exhibits diffuse meningeal infiltration that leads to leukemic meningeal disease, a source of subsequent recurrence following chemotherapy.

✚ **Clinical presentation:** Stable complete remission may be achieved by chemotherapy only in small children.

■ Chronic Lymphocytic Leukemia (CLL)

Occurrence: The disease occurs in the sixth decade of life and is far more common in men than in women.

Definition: Clonal proliferation of precursors of lymphatic B and T cells with a "rigid" morphologic and phenotypical pattern of maturation of the leukemic cells.

Chronic lymphocytic leukemia (CLL) involves *mature B lymphocytes (rarely T lymphocytes).*

Morphology:
— *Bone marrow* exhibits diffuse and focal grayish-red coloration with displacement of the myeloid cells containing chloracetate esterase (► E1) by leukemia cells (► E2).
— *Liver:* It exhibits hepatomegaly due to infiltrate in the portal field.
— *Spleen:* It exhibits diffuse and partially micronodular infiltrate that leads to splenomegaly.
— *Systemic lymph nodes* exhibit diffuse infiltrate that successively leads to lymphadenosis (► F) and leukemic lymphoma (see below).

✚ **Clinical presentation:** After an uneventful clinical course of several years of observation, the disorder takes on an aggressive form (lymphoma).

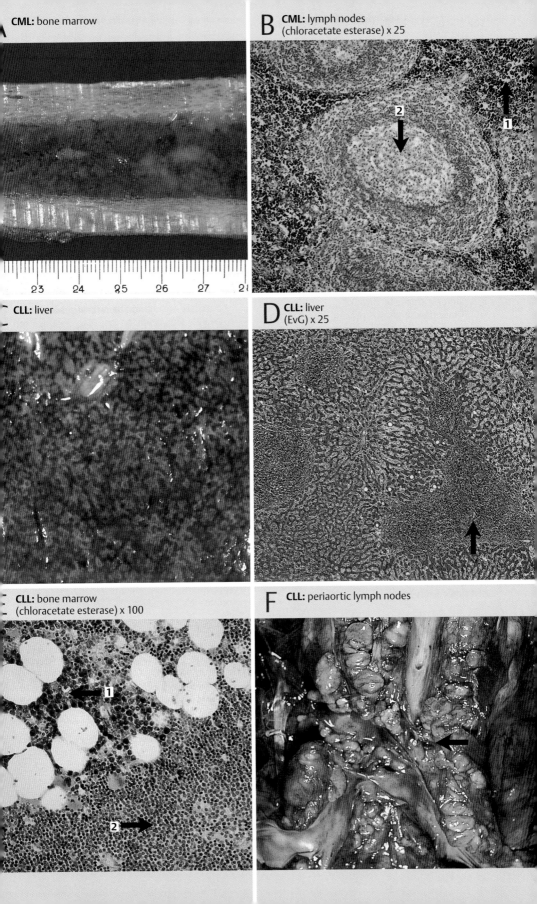

CML: bone marrow

B CML: lymph nodes
(chloracetate esterase) x 25

CLL: liver

D CLL: liver
(EvG) x 25

CLL: bone marrow
(chloracetate esterase) x 100

F CLL: periaortic lymph nodes

Malignant Lymphoma

Definition: Collective term for malignant primary neoplasms arising from lymphatic cells.

Lymphomas are classified as Hodgkin's lymphomas or non-Hodgkin's lymphomas. They are also classified according to their location inside or outside lymph nodes and according to their malignancy status. Less malignant forms primarily develop from lymphocytes; more malignant forms primarily develop from blast cells.

■ Hodgkin's Lymphomas

Synonym: Malignant lymphogranulomatosis.

Definition: A morphologic disease entity involving heterogenous neoplasms usually derived from a few pathognomonic blast cells (Hodgkin cells and Reed-Sternberg cells) and accompanied by inflammation.

Morphologic characteristics:
— *Tumor blast cells* are present in two forms. *Hodgkin cells* (► A) are blast cells that express CD30 and exhibit a large bean-shaped nucleus and a nucleolus nearly the size of a lymphocyte nucleus.
Reed-Sternberg cells are giant cells that express CD30 and are formed by fusion of several Hodgkin cells.
— *Inflammatory infiltrate:* It contains T cells, B cells, neutrophils, eosinophils, histiocytes, and fibroblasts.

Macroscopy: The lymph nodes in Hodgkin's disease appear extremely enlarged. Their cut section has a nodular, fishmeat-like appearance, often with necrosis. Depending on the stage of the tumor, whitish tumorous nodules measuring up to 2 cm may be present in the spleen (► D). The cut section has the appearance of coarsely ground sausage filling. The liver is covered with infiltrated lymphomas.

Histologic Subtypes

▦ Lymphocyte Predominance Type

Occurrence: The disorder occurs in the cervical region during the third and sixth decades of life. Men are affected more often than women.
— *Nodular subtype:* It is classified as a B-cell lymphoma. In rare cases, the disorder can progress to a large B-cell lymphoma.
— *Diffuse subtype:* It can progress to mixed cellularity Hodgkin's disease.

— *Tumor cells* include a few "popcorn cells" (small Hodgkin cells with a popcorn-like scalloped nucleus) and isolated Reed-Sternberg cells.
— *Inflammatory infiltrate* includes large numbers of B lymphocytes.

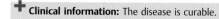 **Clinical information:** The disease is curable.

▦ Nodular Sclerosis Type

Occurrence: The disorder occurs in the mediastinum above the age of 30. Men are affected more often than women.

— *Tumor cells* include a few Hodgkin cells and a few Reed-Sternberg cells exhibiting cytoplasmic shrinkage due to fixation (lacunar cells; ► E, F1).
— *Inflammatory infiltrate* includes T lymphocytes, a few neutrophils and eosinophils, necrosis and bands of sclerotic scar tissue (► F2). This leads to nodular organization of the lymph nodes.

✚ **Clinical information:** The disease is curable; it may also progress to large cell B-cell lymphoma.

▦ Mixed Cellularity Type

Occurrence: The disorder occurs in the cervical and abdominal region in the second to seventh decade of life. Men are affected more often than women.

— *Tumor cells* include many classic Hodgkin cells and Reed-Sternberg cells (► G).
— *Inflammatory infiltrate* includes many T lymphocytes and many neutrophils and eosinophils. Many of focal necrosis and scarring are present.

✚ **Clinical information:** The prognosis is poor.

▦ Lymphocyte-Depletion Type

Occurrence: The disorder occurs in the abdomen in the fourth to eighth decade of life. Men are affected more often than women.

— *Tumor cells* include large quantities of Hodgkin cells and Reed-Sternberg cells with pronounced nuclear polymorphism (hence the synonym Hodgkin's sarcoma).
— *Inflammatory infiltrate* includes a few T lymphocytes and hardly any neutrophils or eosinophils.

✚ **Clinical presentation:** The prognosis is very poor. This often occurs as the final stage of mixed cellularity Hodgkin's disease.

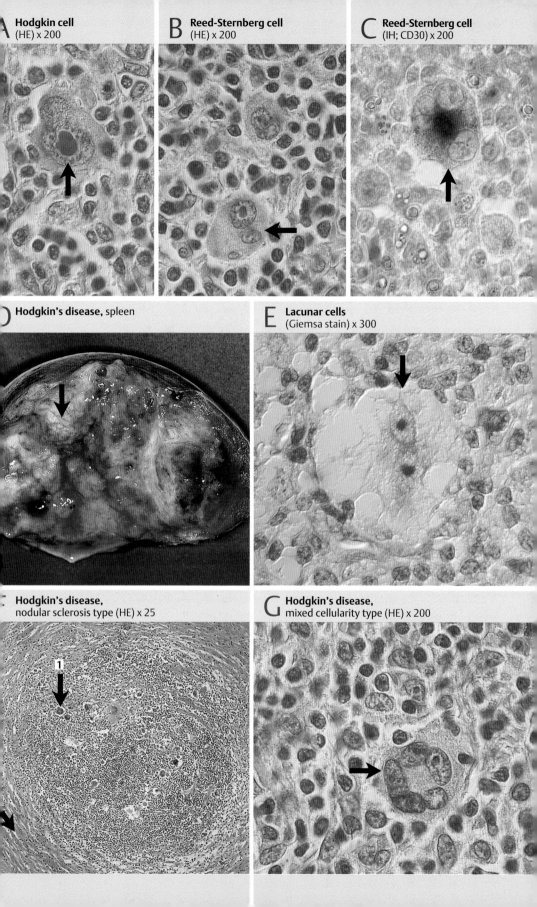

A Hodgkin cell
(HE) x 200

B Reed-Sternberg cell
(HE) x 200

C Reed-Sternberg cell
(IH; CD30) x 200

D Hodgkin's disease, spleen

E Lacunar cells
(Giemsa stain) x 300

F Hodgkin's disease,
nodular sclerosis type (HE) x 25

G Hodgkin's disease,
mixed cellularity type (HE) x 200

■ Non-Hodgkin's Lymphomas

Definition: These entities represent a heterogeneous group of neoplasms arising from B cells, T cells, or histiocytes.

Depending on which homing receptors are expressed, non-Hodgkin's lymphomas (NHL) exhibit the following patterns of tissue colonization.

— *Nodal non-Hodgkin's lymphomas* only colonize and expand in lymph nodes.
— *Extranodal non-Hodgkin's lymphomas* colonize other lymphatic organs such as the thymus, spleen, bone marrow, and mucosa-associated lymphoid tissue (MALT) and other tissues of other organs (primarily the liver and skin).

Morphologic characteristics:
— *Immunohistochemical findings* include CD20+ (B-cell marker) in B-cell NHL and CD3 (T-cell marker) in T-cell NHL.
— *Organotropy:* Nodal or extranodal manifestation and dissemination may be present.
— *Release into the bloodstream* leads to acute lymphoblastic or chronic lymphocytic leukemia.

Morphology: Often only lymph nodes in certain regions are affected, although occasionally all lymph nodes appear pulpy and enlarged.

The most common non-Hodgkin's lymphomas are described below.

▦ Follicular Lymphoma

Definition: NHL composed of follicular center B-lymphocytes

Pathogenesis: By a translocation the apoptosis-blocking bcl-2-gene on chromosome 18 is juxtaposed to the IgH-gene on chromosome 14; giving the tumor cells a survival advantage.

Morphology: The nodal architecture is destroyed by neoplastic follicles (► E, F, G), which extend into the perinodal tissue. The cells are differentiated into centrocytes and centroblasts.

▦ Mantle Cell Lymphoma

Definition: Progressive NHL of virgin B-cells of mantle zone or primary follicles.

Pathogenesis: By a translocation, the cell cyclus-regulating cyclin-D1 gene on chromosome 11 is juxtaposed to the Ig-promotor on chromosome 14, giving tumor cells a proliferative advantage.

Morphology: The tumor cells surround residual reactive germinal centers.

▦ Extranodal Marginal Zone B-Cell Lymphoma of MALT-Type

Definition: Slowly growing NHL showing histologic homology with the normal lymphoid tissue occurring in various mucosal and extranodal sites.

Pathogenesis of gastric MALT-Lymphoma: Helicobacter pylori-induced chronic gastritis perpetuates and interferes with the apoptotic loss of proliferated lymphocytes. They invade the gastric epithelia (= lymphoepithelial lesions). NHL-regression after antibiosis.

▦ Diffuse Large Cell B-Cell Lymphoma

Definition: Aggressive, rapidly growing NHL composed of large "blasts".

Pathogenesis: Heterogenous NHL-group either de-novo or from pre-existent NHL.

Morphology: The tumor cells reveal a broad cytoplasmic rim and contain small or prominent central nucleoli. Necrosis is common. Sclerosis occurs.

▦ Plasmacytoma

Definition: NHL of B-cell clones resembling plasma cells (► B). The disorder manifests itself in two forms.

— *Solitary plasmacytoma* (= solitary myeloma) as osseous "punched-out lesions" (► A) or extraossous lesion (better prognosis);
— *Multiple myeloma* as multicentric lesion (worse prognosis).

Tumor characteristics: The tumor generates immunoglobulins primarily in the form of IgG and/or its light chains (► C) that are stored within the cytoplasm as Russell bodies ((p. 12) and released into the blood. This produces several clinical sequelae:

— *Bence-Jones proteinuria*: Immunoglobulin light chains are excreted via the kidneys, leading to proteinuria.
— *"Myeloma kidney"*: The accumulation of such proteins harms the tubules (►D1) and creates tubular casts that obstruct the tubuli and induce a peritubular inflammation with histiocytic giant cells (►D2). Result: enlarged pale kidney.
— *Amyloidosis* (see p.48).
— *Hypercalcemia* due to osteolytic bone destruction.

▦ Burkitt-Lymphoma

Definition: In equatorial Africa endemic, highly aggressive B-cell NHL.

Pathogenesis: The c-myc on chromosome 8 is translocated to the Ig heavy or light chain gene on chromsosome 14, 2 or 22, and allows the tumor cells to proliferate permanently.

Morphology: NHL composed of mitotic active medium-sized cells with multiple nucleoli. Frequent apoptotic bodies phagocytised by macrophages ("starry sky appearance") are observed (see fig. 332 D).

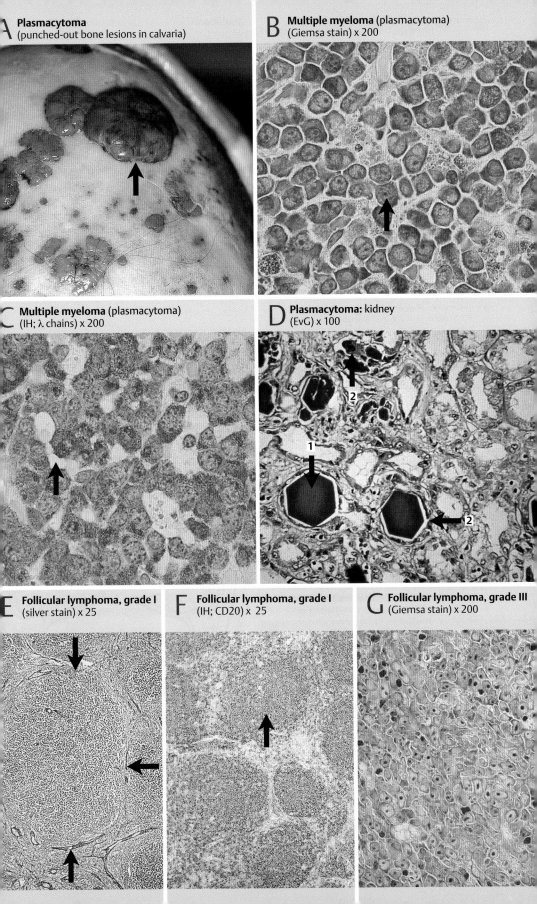

A **Plasmacytoma**
(punched-out bone lesions in calvaria)

B **Multiple myeloma** (plasmacytoma)
(Giemsa stain) x 200

C **Multiple myeloma** (plasmacytoma)
(IH; λ chains) x 200

D **Plasmacytoma:** kidney
(EvG) x 100

E **Follicular lymphoma, grade I**
(silver stain) x 25

F **Follicular lymphoma, grade I**
(IH; CD20) x 25

G **Follicular lymphoma, grade III**
(Giemsa stain) x 200

Melanocytic Tumors

> **Note:** *General immunohistochemical findings* include expression of S100 antigen and HMB-45 antigen. Melanocytic tumors are derived from neuroectodermal tissue.

■ Melanocytic Nevi

Synonyms: pigmented nevus, mole.

Definition: Tumor of modified melanocytes (nevus cells).

The melanocytic nevi are classified according to their location and cytologic features.

▒ Acquired Melanocytic Nevus

This dark brown, slightly raised, sharply demarcated skin lesion measuring several millimeters is composed of aggregates or "nests" of oval melanocytes. Several types are differentiated according to their position.
— *Junctional nevi* occur in children at the junction between dermis and epidermis (► A).
— *Compound nevi* occur in young adults. Nests of melanocytes form "droplets" extending deep into the dermis and diminish in size as they mature (vertical maturation).
— *Intradermal nevi* occur in adults. They exhibit nests of melanocytes in the dermis that are not in contact with the epidermis. These nevi regress, producing fibrosis.

▒ Congenital Melanocytic Nevi

These nevi are present at birth. Histologic findings are identical to acquired nevi, although the lesions themselves are usually larger and covered with hair.

Special forms of nevocellular nevi:
— *Spindle and epithelioid cell nevi* occur in children and young adults. These benign tumors consist of epithelioid and spindle melanocytes (usually without melanin) and are histologically similar to malignant melanomas.
— *Blue nevi* can occur at different ages. The solitary lesion is a flat, blue or black tumor of melanin-containing spindle melanocytes interwoven with the fascicular structure of the dermis.
— *Dysplastic nevi* occur in young adults. These are multiple brownish tumors measuring up to 1 cm and consisting of variably polymorphic melanocytes. These lesions have an increased rate of malignant degeneration and can become malignant melanomas.

■ Malignant Melanoma

Definition: A highly malignant tumor in the skin or mucosa adjacent to the skin.

Pathogenetic factors include susceptibility genes (p. 338), β-catenin mutation (p. 324), and exposure to ultraviolet radiation (p. 150).

Malignant melanomas may exhibit *radial* or *vertical* patterns of growth.

Radial growth melanomas include superficial spreading melanomas and lentigo maligna melanomas.

Superficially-spreading melanomas can occur anywhere but on the volar surfaces of the hands or feet, most often on the back in men and in the calves in women.

Morphologic findings include a flat, brownish, irregularly colored tumor (► C) in which nests of melanocytes extend in and along the epidermis (► D).

Lentigo maligna melanomas occur in skin damaged by ultraviolet radiation (especially in the face), where they develop from lentigo maligna, a precancerous lesion (► E).

Morphologic findings include a flat, brownish pale, irregularly colored, ill-defined tumor (► E) extending as bands of atypical cells in and along the basal layer of the epidermis in the presence of a deficient basement (► F).

Vertical growth melanomas include nodular melanomas.

Nodular melanomas can occur anywhere.

Morphologic findings include primarily vertical spread of raised nodular tumor tissue, usually dark brown, consisting of atypical melanocytes, some of which are pigmented (► B).

> **Note:** The *prognosis for melanoma* depends on the depth of the lesion; the deeper the penetration, the worse the prognosis.

Brain Tumors

■ Gliomas

General definition: Tumor arising from astrocytes, oligodendrocytes, ependymal cells, and plexus epithelial cells.

General morphology: These tumors often exhibit a radial grouping of cell nuclei. The term *rosette* is used to refer to such a grouping around a nonvascular lumen. A radial arrangement of nuclei around a vascular structure or a virtual center is referred to as a *pseudorosette*.

> **Note:** *Gliomas* present with the following general clinical features:
> – The *tumor is ill-defined* due to its infiltrative growth into the tissue of the brain.
> – *Systemic metastases are extremely rare.*
> – The *tumor often distorts the topography of the brain.*
> – Complications include *death from increased intracranial pressure.*

> **Note:** *Gliomas are diagnosed* by immunohistochemical findings of expressed GFAP (an acidic glial fiber protein).

The next section examines the following gliomas:
– astrocytomas;
– glioblastomas;
– oligodendrogliomas.

Junctional nevus
(HE) x 25

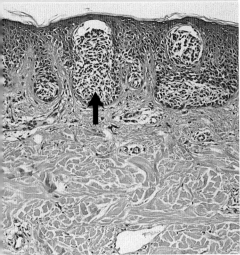

Nodular malignant melanoma
(HE) x 10

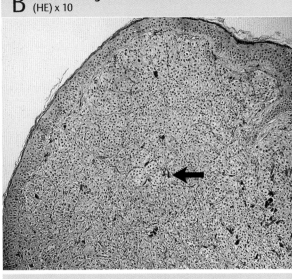

Superficial spreading melanoma

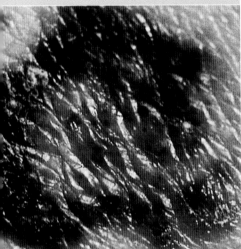

Superficial spreading melanoma
(HE) x 100

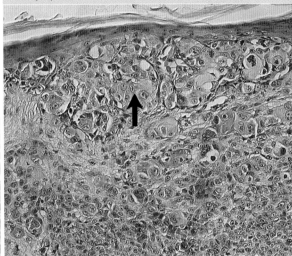

Lentigo maligna

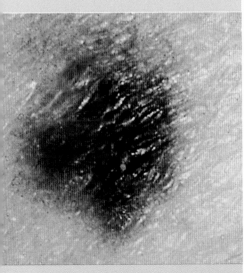

Lentigo maligna melanoma in situ
(IH; HMB-45) x 25

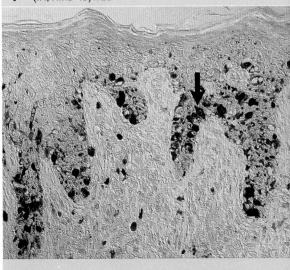

Astrocytomas

General definition: Astrocytic tumors of varying malignancy.

— *Pilocytic astrocytoma*

Occurrence: cerebellum, third ventricle, brain stem, and cerebrum (rare).
Age of manifestation: children and adolescents.

Definition: benign glioma.
Morphology: This firm, nodular tumor exhibits long, thin, hairlike cytoplasmic processes. Typical findings include Rosenthal fibers, in the form of elongated cytoplasmic processes with aggregates of glial fibers (▶ A).

➕ **Clinical presentation:** The prognosis is good; recurrences are rare.

— *Gemistocytic astrocytoma*

Occurrence: cerebrum.
Age of manifestation: adults.

Definition: low-grade glioma.
Morphology: This ill-defined tumor consists of astrocytic tumor cells with stout process and cytoplasmic accumulation of GFAP (▶ B).

➕ **Clinical presentation:** The tumor grows slowly. It tends to recur and evolve into less differentiated forms.

Glioblastoma

Occurrence: The tumor occurs in adulthood, in the cerebrum with a butterfly pattern of contralateral expansion.

Definition: Highly malignant glioma.
Morphology: Ill-defined tumor with a brightly colored cut surface:
- *Yellow coloration* is indicative of fatty degeneration with bands of necrosis (▶ D), leading to cystic disintegration.
- *Red discoloration* occurs due to bleeding from necroses and an abundance of glomeruloid vascularization as a result of tumor growth factor (EGF).
- *The pulpy appearance* of the tumor is due to its hypercellularity with multinucleated giant cells (▶ E) and oval polymorphic spindle cells.

➕ **Clinical presentation:** Patients exhibit symptoms of apoplexy. The prognosis is very poor.

Oligodendroglioma

Occurrence: cerebrum.
Age of manifestation: adults.

Definition: Slowly growing tumor arising from oligodendrocytes.
Morphology: Ill-defined tumor of small, densely packed tumor cells (exhibiting a dark nucleus in bright cytoplasm) that creates a honeycomb pattern. Signs of regression include bleeding, cysts, and calcification.

➕ **Clinical presentation:** Patients exhibit symptoms of epilepsy. The tumor tends to evolve into less differentiated forms.

■ Nerve Sheath Tumors

General definition: Tumors arising from the sheath cells or craniospinal nerves.

Schwannoma

Occurrence: A solitary lesion may be present (primarily in the cerebellopontine angle, i.e., an acoustic neuroma), or the tumor may occur as multiple lesions in type 2 neurofibromatosis (p. 324).

Definition and morphology: Benign soft tumor in the form of a bulbous expansion usually occurring in a peripheral nerve as a result of proliferation of Schwann cells and perineural fibroblasts. The cut surface of the tumor is grayish-white.
Histologic findings include spindle-shaped tumor cells in a loose fibrous mesh, some of which exhibit an arrangement resembling schools of fish with parallel nuclei (▶ C).

➕ **Clinical presentation:** Symptoms depend on the location. Tumor in the acoustic nerve leads to unilateral hearing loss; tumor in a nerve root leads to paraplegia.

Neurofibroma

Occurrence: A solitary lesion may be present, or the tumor may occur as multiple lesions in type 1 neurofibromatosis (p. 324).

Definition and morphology: Benign encapsulated Schwann-cell tumor arising from craniospinal and peripheral nerves. The cut surface of the tumor is whitish-yellow.
Histologic findings include spindle-shaped tumor cells in a loose, undulating, fibrous mesh.
Immunohistochemical findings of all nerve sheath tumors include expression of S-100 antigen.

■ Meningioma

Occurrence: margin of the sphenoid and falx cerebri.
Age of manifestation: adults; the tumor is more common in men than in women.

Definition: Benign arachnoid cell tumor (▶ F).
Morphology: Spherical or lobulated tumor consisting of spindle-shaped tumor cells (meningothelial cells of the arachnoid) that tend to assume an arrangement resembling the layers of an onion (▶ G). The tumor is located between the soft meninges (▶ F), successively leading to formation of a capsule and reactive hyperostosis of the skull.

Immunohistochemical findings include double expression of vimentin and desmoplakin.
The most common growth patterns are meningothelial and fibroblastic meningioma.
- *Psammomatous meningioma* exhibits dense epithelial clusters of tumors cells forming numerous corpuscles resembling the layers of an onion, leading to "psammomatous" calcification (p. 136).
- *Fibroblastic meningioma* exhibits chains and swirls of tumor cells rich in collagen fibers with few onion-like corpuscles.

➕ **Clinical presentation:** *Sporadic meningiomas* are usually solitary; *meningiomas associated with type 1 neurofibromatosis* occur as multiple lesions.

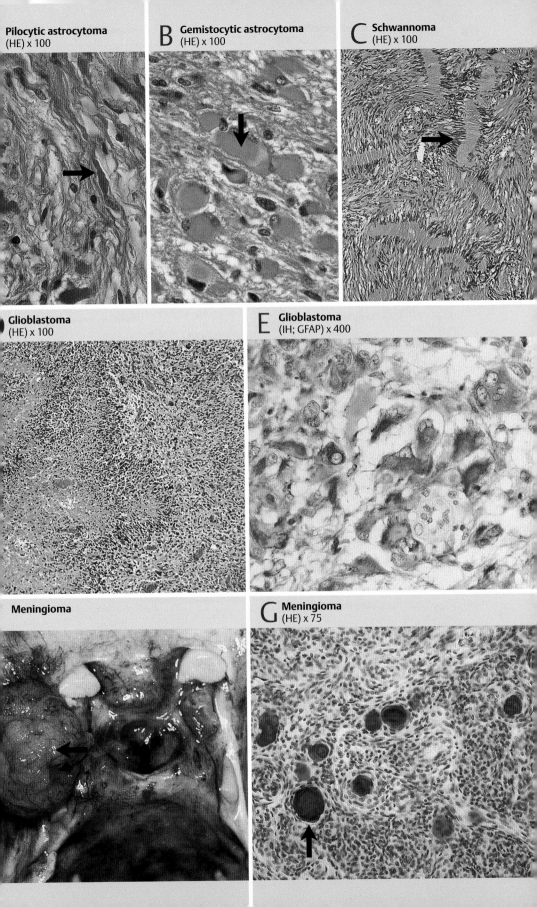

Pilocytic astrocytoma
(HE) x 100

B Gemistocytic astrocytoma
(HE) x 100

C Schwannoma
(HE) x 100

Glioblastoma
(HE) x 100

E Glioblastoma
(IH; GFAP) x 400

Meningioma

G Meningioma
(HE) x 75

Benign Epithelial Tumors

General definition: Tumors of the superficial or glandular epithelia.

These tumors assume the form of either papillomas or adenomas, depending on whether the tumor epithelium develops branching or tubular folds.

Papillomas

Definition: Broad-based superficial tumor of branching villous vascular stroma covered by neoplastic epithelium. Two forms are differentiated according to the predominant direction of growth:

— *Exophytic papillomas* are the commonest form. The tumor (► A1) primarily grows above the plane of the epithelial surface (► A2).
— *Endophytic papillomas* are rare. Here, the tumor primarily grows beneath the surface of the epithelium as an inverted papilloma and remains largely covered by the epithelium. These tumors exhibit a smooth surface and can mimic an invasive malignancy. *Caution* is advised, as endophytic papillomas tend to recur.

Note: A *polyp* is defined as any pediculate projection on the surface of the skin or a mucous membrane. This specifically includes non-neoplastic growths.

Several types of papillomas are differentiated according to the epithelium from which they arise.

■ Basal Cell Papilloma

Synonym: seborrheic keratosis.

Occurrence: Trunk, arms, and face in older patients.

Morphology: Cap-like epidermal projection of a villous layer of acanthocytes growing into the deep plane and exhibiting scaly keratinized epithelium extending into the projecting papillae. This leads to formation of dome-like keratinized projections.

■ Mucosal Papilloma

Occurrence: Oral cavity, nose (there occasionally as an inverted form), nasopharynx, and larynx.

Morphology: The tumor is a branching growth of columnar or squamous epithelium (► E).

■ Papilloma of Glandular Excretory Ducts

Occurrence: exocrine glands and breast.

Morphology: These tumors resemble mucosal papillomas. As in the corresponding adenomas, immunohistochemical tests for actin can be used to demonstrate the myoepithelium (► C, breast).

■ Urothelial Papilloma

Occurrence: The tumors often occur a multiple lesions in the urinary tract and are potential precancerous lesions.

The tumor tissue is easily injured because of its exposure to the flow of urine. This leads to microhematuria.

Morphology: The tumor consists of a branching villous proliferation of urothelium about seven cells thick with a highly vascularized stroma.

Note: All *glandular and mucosal papillomas* should be regarded as potentially precancerous lesions.

Adenomas

Definition: Tumor arising from glandular, parenchymal, or mucosal epithelium and consisting of proliferative epithelial folds or tubules in or on a stroma. Stasis of secretion leads to development of chambers.

Several types of adenomas are differentiated according to the epithelium from which they arise.

■ Solid Adenoma

Occurrence: glandular organs.

Morphology: The lesion is a nodular tumor with proliferation of glandular epithelium (► B1) in a stroma. It is sharply demarcated from its surrounding tissue of origin and exhibits a smooth surface with a fibrous tumor capsule (► B2).

■ Tubular Adenoma

Occurrence: primarily in the intestinal tract.

Morphology: The lesion is generally a pediculate, superficially smooth tumor nodule of proliferating epithelial tubules (a mucosal polyp) in the lumen of a hollow organ.

Example: appendiceal adenoma (► D).

■ Villous Adenoma

Occurrence: primarily in the intestinal tract.

Morphology: The lesion is generally a broad-based tumor of epithelial villi on a highly vascularized stroma that projects into the lumen of a hollow organ. Its villous surface is easily injured, resulting in bleeding.

■ Cystadenoma

Occurrence: primarily in the ovaries and salivary glands.

Morphology: This ballooning tumor consists of epithelium that forms a hollow cavity due to stasis of a secretion. It has a smooth surface.

■ Fibroadenoma

Occurrence: primarily in the breast (► F).

Morphology: The lesion is a smooth nodular tumor of epithelial tubules (► F1) that become compressed and folded as the stroma proliferates (► F2).

Papilloma of a lactiferous duct
(HE) x 25

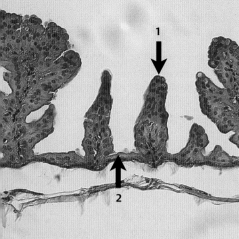

B Solid adenoma
(HE) x 50

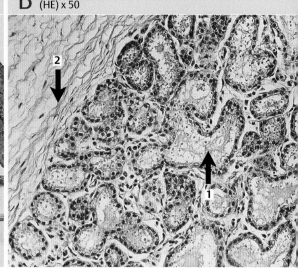

Adenoma of a lactiferous duct
(IH; actin) x 50

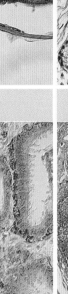

D Appendiceal adenoma
(HE) x 15

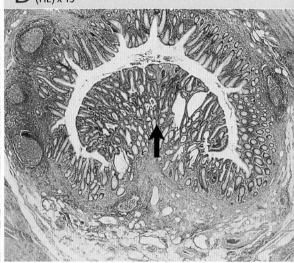

Squamous cell papilloma
(HE) x 25

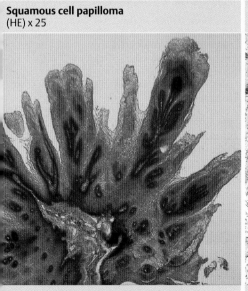

F Fibroadenoma
(HE) x 25

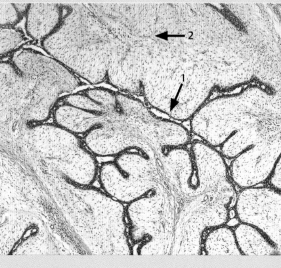

Malignant Epithelial Tumors

Several types of malignant epithelial tumors are differentiated according to their growth pattern, tendency to develop necrosis, and stroma.

— *Papillary carcinomas* resemble papillomas but have a larger surface area.
— *Polypoid carcinomas* resemble benign polyps but usually measure larger than 2 cm.
— *Ulcerated carcinomas* exhibit central necrosis that has created an ulcerated crater surrounded by a ring-like wall.
— *Cystic carcinomas* arise due to malignant degeneration of cystadenomas.
— *Scirrhous carcinomas* exhibit stromal proliferation around the tumor villi. This leads to diffuse tumor growth.
— *Medullary carcinomas* are soft pulpy tumors with little stroma that are reminiscent of bone marrow.
— *Multicentric carcinomas* develop simultaneously at several sites in the epithelium of origin.

Squamous Cell Carcinoma

Definition: A collective term for carcinomas that mimic squamous epithelium, exhibiting filamentous eosinophilic cytoplasm, sharply demarcated cell borders, and often keratinization.

Tissue patterns in a squamous cell carcinoma range between two extremes according to the degree of differentiation of the tumor.

■ **Highly Differentiated Forms:** exhibit layers of cells that tend to keratinize and form cornified clumps that are layered like an onion (► A, B).

■ **Undifferentiated Forms:** are polymorphic carcinomas with a high mitosis count that usually do not keratinize.

— *Spindle-cell squamous carcinoma* is a *special histologic form.* These tumors are undifferentiated squamous cell carcinomas exhibiting pronounced stroma and spindle-shaped deformation of the tumor cells. This produces a pattern of growth that resembles a sarcoma. The prognosis is poor.

☺ **Prominent patient:** Sigmund Freud (1856–1939), Austrian psychiatrist, died of the sequelae of a squamous cell carcinoma of the larynx.

Adenocarcinoma

Definition: Collective term for carcinomas of the mucosa or exocrine or endocrine glandular epithelium with formation of lumina within the tumor cell complex or lumina within the tumor cells themselves in the form of inner surfaces.

Several types may be identified according to their degree of differentiation and mucin secretion.

■ **Highly Differentiated Forms**

▦ **Acinic Carcinoma:** The epithelium of the carcinoma exhibits a histologic tissue pattern resembling a glandular acinus.

▦ **Tubular Carcinoma:** The carcinoma mimics glandular tubules. These tubules lie "back-to-back" due to slight stromal reaction (► C).

■ **Moderately Differentiated Forms**

▦ **Cribriform Carcinoma:** The epithelium of the carcinoma exhibits a "gland in a gland" pattern resembling a sieve (► D).

Examples include several prostate carcinomas (p. 374) and adenoid cystic carcinoma (► D).

▦ **Papillary Carcinoma:** The epithelium of the carcinoma folds to form a tumor papilla.

Examples include bronchial, thyroid, and ovarian carcinoma (► E).

■ **Mucigenous Carcinomas**

Several types of mucin-producing carcinomas are differentiated according to the quantity of mucin produced and where it is deposited.

— *Cystadenocarcinomas* secrete massive amounts of mucin, creating a cavity in the tumor tissue.
— *Tubular carcinomas* excrete mucin into the tumor tubules.
— *Mucinous carcinomas* produce massive amounts of mucin in the glandular acini of the tumor. This causes the acini to burst, creating extracellular deposits of a mucin and giving the cut section of the tumor a glassy, transparent appearance.
— *Signet-ring cell carcinomas* are undifferentiated carcinomas characterized by loss of intercellular cohesion with massive vacuolar accumulations of mucin in all the cells of the tumor. This produces a typical "signet ring" cellular deformation with peripheral displacement of the nucleus.
— *Solid carcinomas with mucinous single-cells* are undifferentiated carcinomas characterized by intercellular cohesion. These tumors exhibit small amounts of intracellular mucin in isolated tumor cells without significant cellular deformation.

Urothelial Carcinoma

Definition: Collective term for malignant carcinoma of the urinary tract.

Two forms are differentiated:

■ **Papillary Urothelial Carcinomas:** These are anaplastic or invasive carcinomas with a urothelial thickness of at least seven layers of cells. These carcinomas form a macroscopic fringe (► F).

■ **Solid Urothelial Carcinomas:** These are predominantly solid, often ulcerated carcinomas that project mushroom-like into the lumen. They are anaplastic and invasive tumors.

The next section examines the most common carcinomas of specific organs.

Squamous cell carcinoma
(HE) x 75

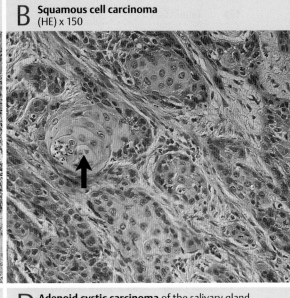

B **Squamous cell carcinoma**
(HE) x 150

Tubular adenocarcinoma
(HE) x 75

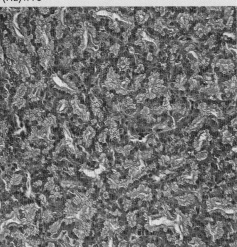

D **Adenoid cystic carcinoma** of the salivary gland
(HE) x 75

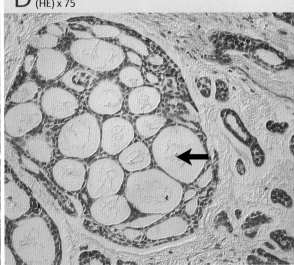

Papillary ovarian carcinoma
(HE) x 75

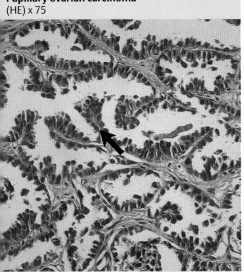

F **Papillary carcinoma** of the bladder

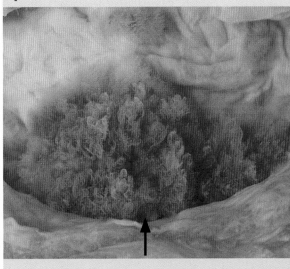

Carcinomas of Specific Organs

■ Prostatic Carcinomas

Definition: Collective term for all carcinomas of the prostate gland.

The most common location of the lesion is in the posterior peripheral portions of the gland; the peak incidence is over 70 years of age.

Pathogenesis: Prostatic carcinomas are usually multicentric adenocarcinomas that arise as the result of the following genetic defects.

— **Loss of heterozygosity in suppressor genes** *1p, 8p, 10q,* and *BRCA1*[1] leads to tumor progression and loss of differentiation.
— **Oncogene activation:** in the presence of an excess of androgen in tissue with increased density of androgen receptors. This leads to over-expression of *c-erb B2* with excessive formation of epithelial growth factor receptors. This in turn results in continuous proliferation.
— **Loss of the anti-metastasis gene** occurs. Deletions in the α-catenin gene and reduced E-cadherin expression result in lack of cell-to-cell adhesion in the prostatic epithelium, promoting invasion by prostatic carcinoma.

Morphology: Most prostatic carcinomas arise as multicentric lesions from the peripheral portions of the gland and are therefore detectable by rectal digital palpation. The tumor initially spreads within the prostate. Periurethral spread only occurs later (► F), and the resulting obstruction of the urethra is a late symptom. This leads to urine retention with hypertrophy of the wall of the bladder and development of "trabeculated bladder".

Macroscopic examination reveals a pulpy yellowish, usually homogeneous tumor (► F).

Histologic tumor grades: Prostatic carcinomas are generally adenocarcinomas with varying degrees of malignancy.

— **Prostatic intraepithelial neoplasia** (PIN) is a preinvasive neoplasm with an atypical epithelium several cells in width (► A1) exhibiting enlarged cell nuclei and nucleoli. The neoplasm is present within pre-existing prostatic glandular structures (► A2).
— **G1 carcinomas** are slowly growing prostatic carcinomas exhibiting tubules of single-cell thickness with light cytoplasm. The tumorous glands often lie close together without significant amounts of interposed stroma. These are referred to as "back-to-back" gland formation (► B).

— **G2 carcinomas** are cribriform prostatic carcinomas that exhibit "gland-in-a-gland" structures (► C) and form a pattern resembling a sieve. The nucleoli are enlarged. The tumor's growth is discontinuous, and it invades nerve sheaths. The sieve-like pattern is often retained in the metastases. Characteristic *cytologic findings* in the tumor glands include a roughly concentric, sheaf-like arrangement of cells (► D).
— **G3 carcinomas** exhibit rapid growth characterized by loss of cytocohesivity. The tumor cells often lie isolated and widely disseminated within the pre-existing prostatic stroma. There is barely a trace of a glandular pattern of growth.

The larger the carcinoma, the more widely varied will be the mixture of histologic tumor patterns it exhibits.

Metastases

— *Early lymphatic metastases* primarily occur in the regional pelvic lymph nodes.
— *Late hematogenous metastases* are of the vena cava type and are osteoplastic. These metastases occur primarily in the lower spine, sacrum, and pelvis as a result of the tumor's osteoblastic growth factor. Metastases may then occur in the lung.

pTNM Classification

— **pT1:** Clinically unapparent carcinoma as an incidental histologic finding.
— **pT2:** Palpable carcinoma confined within the prostate.
— **pT3:** Carcinoma extends through the prostate capsule and/or infiltrates the seminal vesicle.
— **pT4:** Carcinoma invades adjacent structures other than the seminal vesicle.

☺ **Prominent patient:** François Mitterand (1916–1996), former French President.

Note: The *clinical aspects of prostatic carcinoma:*
– An increased serum level of prostate-specific antigen (PSA; p. 326) may be attributable to carcinoma (► F).
– Abnormal findings upon rectal digital palpation are then confirmed by fine-needle biopsy and cytologic and histologic studies.
– Anti-androgen therapy is then initiated.

Note:
– *Prostatic carcinoma* arises in the peripheral portions of the gland. It exhibits centripetal growth and produces late symptoms.
– *Prostatic hyperplasia* arises in the central portions of the gland. It exhibits centrifugal growth and produces early symptoms such as urine retention.

----
[1] *BRCA* = breast cancer antigen, p. 376.

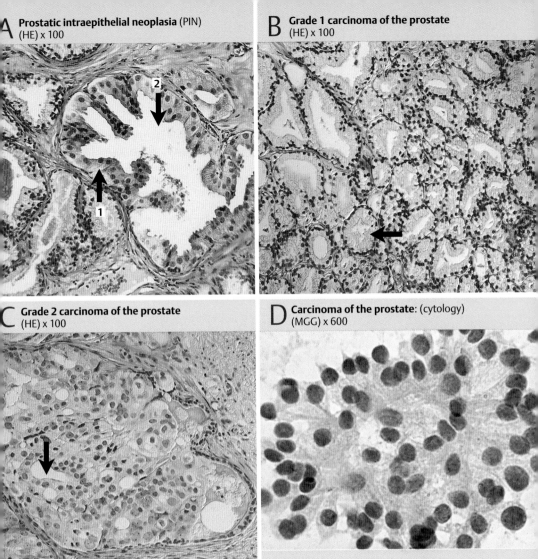

A Prostatic intraepithelial neoplasia (PIN)
(HE) x 100

1

2

B Grade 1 carcinoma of the prostate
(HE) x 100

C Grade 2 carcinoma of the prostate
(HE) x 100

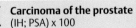

D Carcinoma of the prostate: (cytology)
(MGG) x 600

E Carcinoma of the prostate
(IH; PSA) x 100

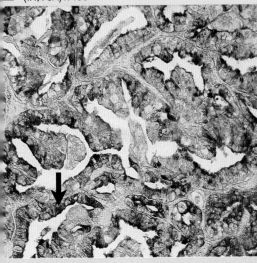

F Carcinoma of the prostate

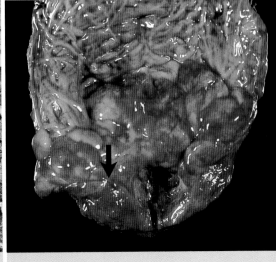

■ Carcinoma of the Breast

Definition: Collective term for all carcinomas of the breast gland (breast cancer).

The most common location of the lesion is in the upper outer quadrant.

Predisposing factors include:
— *Family history* that includes a mother with breast cancer;
— *Menstrual cycles:* early menarche and late menopause;
— *Gravidity:* nulliparity or early primipara;
— *Nutritional factors,* such as diet high in fat and animal proteins;
— *A history of breast disease,* including proliferative mastopathy with atypia (which can be difficult to distinguish from carcinoma), carcinoma in the contralateral breast, and prior ovarian carcinoma.

Pathogenesis: The tumor arises as the cumulative result of the following genetic defects.
— **Loss of heterozygosity in the susceptibility genes** BRCA[1]. These are transcription factors that normally function as suppressor genes. Loss of an allele and mutation lead to early occurrence of breast and ovarian carcinoma.
— **Suppressor genes** *p53* and *RB* are inactivated.
— **Oncogenes** *c-ras, c-myc,* and *c-erb-B2* are activated, leading to continuous proliferation due to an excessive supply of estrogen in the tissue.

Histologic Tumor Types

▦ Ductal Carcinoma (70% of all cases)

Histogenesis: Carcinoma arises from the epithelium of the lactiferous ducts, often as a multifocal lesion.
— **Ductal carcinoma in situ** (► A1) is a tumor that initially spreads only within the lactiferous ducts, which are surrounded by a myoepithelium containing actin (► A2). Within the ducts, the tumor issue disintegrates and develops central calcifying necroses that appear as radiographic "microcalcifications" in mammograms. The tumor detritus can be expressed from the duct like the contents of a blackhead. This is known as a comedocarcinoma.
— **Invasive ductal carcinoma** is a tumor that penetrates the basement membrane with duct-like epithelial strands several cells in width (► B), stromal proliferation (scirrhous carcinoma), and microcalcification.

▦ Lobular Carcinoma

Histogenesis: Carcinoma arises from the lobular terminal ducts (acini), usually as multifocal lesions.
— **Lobular carcinoma in situ** often arises as bilateral multicentric lesions. The tumor often initially spreads only within the lobules, and may do so for years (► C). This leads

successively to stasis of secretions and calcification.
— **Invasive lobular carcinoma** penetrates the basement membrane, producing strands of tumor tissue one cell in width (► D) along collagen fibers with tumor-induced stromal proliferation (scirrhous carcinoma).

Less malignant forms of carcinoma of the breast are rare and occur primarily in older women (exception: tubular carcinoma).
— **Tubular carcinomas** exhibit a purely tubular ductal proliferation one cell in width.
— **Papillary carcinomas** (p. 372).
— **Mucinous carcinomas** produce and deposit excessive amounts of mucin.
— **Medullary carcinomas** (p. 372) exhibit a pulpy tumor tissue with massive quantities of inflammatory infiltrate containing lymphocytes and plasma cells.

Growth patterns of all carcinomas of the breast are as follows:
— **Vertical inward growth** leads to infiltration of the pectoralis.
— **Vertical outward growth** leads to infiltration of the skin (► E), which may include retraction of the nipple, and to skin ulceration.
— **Horizontal lymphatic growth** leads to widespread dissemination in the cutaneous lymphatics, and can lead to lymphedema and thickening of the skin known as *peau d'orange.*
— **Horizontal epidermal growth** in a ductal carcinoma close to the nipple with affinity for skin (► F) results in infiltration of the skin by tumor cells. This produces an eczematoid lesion (Paget's disease of the nipple).

pTNM Classification of all breast carcinomas:
— *pT1:* Breast carcinoma measuring 2 cm or less.
— *pT2:* Breast carcinoma measuring between 2 and 5 cm.
— *pT3:* Breast carcinoma larger than 5 cm.
— *pT4:* Breast carcinoma with invasion of the chest wall and skin.

Note: The *therapeutic approach for breast carcinoma* involves immunohistochemical studies to determine the estrogen and progesterone receptor status and subsequent anti-estrogen therapy.

Note: *Breast carcinoma is diagnosed* as follows:
- Mammographic microcalcifications suggest but *are not unequivocal evidence* of breast carcinoma.
- Biopsy provides definitive histologic proof. Therefore the rule of thumb in the presence of suspected breast carcinoma is: "when in doubt, take it out."

Note: A "breast lump" may be due to one of several causes, including:
- fibrous cystic benign mastopathy;
- fatty tissue necrosis;
- benign fibroadenoma;
- breast carcinoma.

---

[1] *BRCA* = breast cancer antigen (BRCA1 and 2).

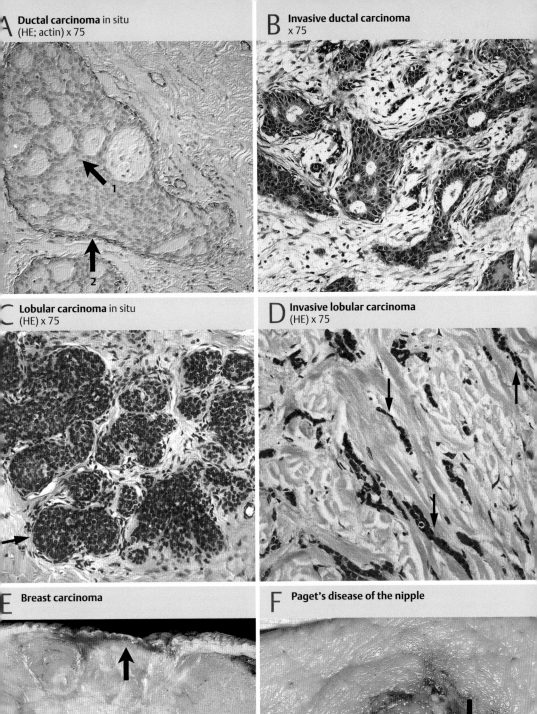

A **Ductal carcinoma** in situ
(HE; actin) × 75

B **Invasive ductal carcinoma**
× 75

C **Lobular carcinoma** in situ
(HE) × 75

D **Invasive lobular carcinoma**
(HE) × 75

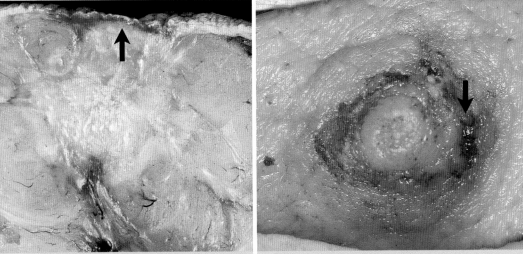

E **Breast carcinoma**

F **Paget's disease of the nipple**

■ Lung Carcinoma

Definition: Collective term for highly malignant carcinomas of the bronchial or of the bronchiolo-alveolar epilthelia, or of the neuroendocrine cells.

Predisposing factors:
— **Cigarette smoking** is the most common factor (p. 336).
— **Occupational hazards** involving inhalation of noxious agents (rare), radioactive dusts such as in uranium mining, gases from coking plants, silicates, asbestos, chromates, and nickel.

Pathogenesis: Exposure to the noxious agent leads to chronic bronchitis. This in turn triggers malignant transformation of a pluripotential endodermal stem cell (hence the increased incidence of paraneoplastic syndromes; p. 352) as the result of the following genetic defects.
— **Loss of heterozygosity in differentiation gene** 3p.
— **Suppressor genes** p53 and RB are inactivated.
— **Oncogenes** c-ras and c-myc are activated.
— **Anti-metastasis gene** loss (p. 346).

Topographic tumor types:
— **Diffuse type** is rare and exhibits a pattern of dissemination resembling pneumonia.
— **Central type** is a common form that arises in the vicinity of the hilum with macroscopic involvement of a bronchus. This then leads to bronchial obstruction and secondary pneumonia (► C).
— **Peripheral type** is characterized by lack of macroscopic involvement of a bronchus (► E).
— **Pancoast tumor** represents a *special form of bronchogenic carcinoma.* Here, a bronchogenic carcinoma at the tip of the lung penetrates the chest wall. The cancer then spreads into the brachial plexus and the cervical thoracic sympathetic nerves, producing Horner syndrome (miosis, ptosis, and enophthalmos).

Histologic Tumor Types

Squamous Cell Carcinoma

Occurrence: Primarily as central carcinomas, these tumors account for 40% of all bronchogenic carcinomas are more common in men than women.

Macroscopic appearance: The tumor is a pulpy, grayish-white carcinoma that usually arises at bronchial bifurcations (► A). Tumor growth is initially exophytic and ulcerative. Tumor cells designamate, and cytologic studies confirm their presence in sputum. Later, the growth of the carcinoma becomes invasive and leads to stenosis (► C).

Histologic findings include squamous cell carcinomas with varying degrees of tissue differentiation and well-defined cell borders (intercellular bridges) and eosinophilic cytoplasm due to production of keratin, enlarged nucleoli and occasionally, keratin pearls.

✚ Therapeutic principle: "Knife and Ray"-tumors are treated by total surgical removal and postoperative radiation therapy. Advanced tumors are treated with adjunctive chemotherapy.

Small Cell Carcinoma

Occurrence: Known as "smoker's cancer," these highly malignant tumors primarily occur as central carcinomas. They account for 15% of all bronchogenic carcinomas and are equally distributed among men and women.

Macroscopic appearance: The tumor exhibits a finger-like pattern of growth at an early stage, extending into the peribronchial and perivascular connective tissue. Necrosis and metastases occur at an early stage.

Histologic findings include an unstructured mass of small cells with hyperchromatic nuclei and a residual degree of neuroectodermal differentiation (► B). As a result, immunohistochemical findings include expression of synaptophysin. The weak nucleoskeleton of these cells makes their nuclei very vulnerable (leading to crush artifacts), and the cells dent each other. *Cytology:* "nuclear molding".

✚ Therapeutic principle: "Drug-Ray-Knife"-tumors are treated first by chemotherapy, and then by radiation therapy. Early small cell carcinoma ("limited disease") is treated by initial radiation therapy to reduce tumor size and control lymph nodes, followed by secondary surgical removal. The cranium is treated with radiation therapy as prophylaxis against metastasis.

Adenocarcinomas

Occurrence: Primarily occurring as peripheral carcinomas (and rarely as diffuse carcinomas), these tumors account for 10% of all lung carcinomas. They are equally distributed among men and women.

Morphologic findings include a round, pulpy lung carcinoma with necroses.

Histologic findings include a bronchogenic carcinoma usually consisting solely of glandular cell complexes (► D1). Such a tumor with squamous cell components may be referred to as an adenosquamous carcinoma (► D2).

Bronchioalveolar carcinoma is a *special form of adenocarcinoma.* A rare carcinoma, the tumor cells grow diffusely into the bronchides and alveoles and cover them like wallpaper (► F).

✚ Therapeutic principle: Treatment is identical to squamous cell carcinoma.

Large Cell Carcinoma

Occurrence: Tumors arise in the periphery and account for 10% of all bronchogenic carcinomas. They are more common in men than in women.

Morphologic findings: a round, pulpy bronchogenic carcinoma with necroses.

Histologic findings: tumor complexes characterized by cytocohesivity, and consisting of undifferentiated, polymorphic cells with abundant cytoplasm and prominent nucleoli.

✚ Therapeutic principle: Treatment is identical to squamous cell carcinoma.

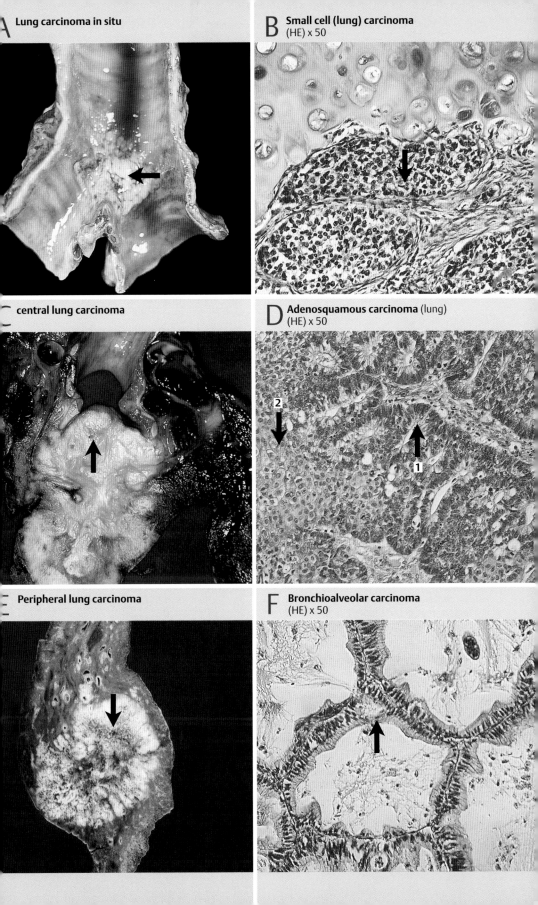

A Lung carcinoma in situ

B Small cell (lung) carcinoma (HE) x 50

C central lung carcinoma

D Adenosquamous carcinoma (lung) (HE) x 50

E Peripheral lung carcinoma

F Bronchioalveolar carcinoma (HE) x 50

■ Colorectal Carcinoma

Occurrence: This is the most common carcinoma of the intestinal tract. The peak incidence is between 60–70 years, and the tumor is more common in men than in women.

Definition: Collective term for carcinomas of the mucosa of the colon.

Predisposing factors (p. 336) include:
— *Precancerous condition,* such as ulcerative colitis lasting more than 10 years, Crohn's disease lasting more than 10 years, Lynch's syndrome (hereditary nonpolyposis colon carcinoma or HNPCC) with multiple synchronous and/or metachronous extraintestinal tumors and secondary colorectal carcinoma;
— *Precancerous lesions,* such as several colorectal adenomas, familial adenomatous polyposis coli with over 100 adenomas (► A), and synchronous and/or metachronous secondary tumors.
— *Nutritional factors,* such as diet low in plant fiber and high in fat and refined carbohydrates.

Pathogenesis: Malignant transformation of stem cells of the colorectal mucosa occurs as the collective effect of the following genetic defects.
— *Loss of heterozygosity in the susceptibility gene* makes the mucosa sensitive to nutritional factors leading to formation of adenomas.
— *Mutation of caretaker genes* such as *hMSH2* and *hMLH1* leads to tolerance of mismatched pairs of DNA bases.
— *Defects in gatekeeper genes,* specifically in the *APC* gene (p. 338) and *p53* gene lead to DNA defects that are not repaired by cell division.
— *Oncogenes* such as *c-ras, c-er B,* and *c-myc* are activated, producing a continuously proliferating adenoma.
— *Differentiation genes* such as the *DCC* gene (p. 324) are defective, leading to malignant degeneration of the adenoma into an invasive colorectal carcinoma.
— *Nonmetastatic gene* such as pNM23 are defective, leading to metastatic colorectal carcinoma.

Macroscopic Types of Colorectal Carcinoma
— *Polypoid exophytic type* generally has a favorable prognosis.
— *Ulcerating type* exhibits central tumor necrosis (► E). The prognosis depends on the depth of invasion.
— *Diffuse infiltrating type* exhibits diffuse endophytic growth, usually with minimal differentiation. The prognosis is poor.

Histologic types of colorectal carcinoma: These tumors (► B) produce varying quantities of mucin.

---

[1] DCC = deleted in colon cancer; its gene product is a cell adhesion molecule (N-CAM) of the integrin family.
[2] CEA = carcinoembryonic antigen.

Mucinous Carcinoma is a rare colorectal carcinoma producing excessive amounts of mucin stored in extracellular deposits (► D). As these lake-like deposits increase in size, they displace the mucin-producing cells to the periphery and give the cut section of the tumor a gelatinous appearance.

Mucigenous Adenocarcinomas are common tumors. The cells of these differentiated colorectal carcinomas secrete mucin into the lumen of the tumorous gland.

Signet-Ring Cell Carcinomas are rare, slightly differentiated colorectal carcinomas with growth characterized by loss of cytocohesivity. Isolated tumor cells appear diffusely disseminated in tissue and store mucin in cytoplasmic vacuoles. These cells exhibit characteristic signet ring compression of the nucleus (► F).

Metastases of Colorectal Carcinomas
— *Lymphatic metastasis* occurs via the pericolonic and periaortal lymph nodes to the thoracic duct and from there to the supraclavicular lymph nodes.
— *Hematogenous metastasis* follows the vena cava pattern in rectal carcinoma and the portal vein pattern in colonic carcinoma. Later, hematogenous metastases may follow the liver pattern of dissemination.

pTNM Classification of all colorectal carcinomas:
— *pT1:* Tumor invades the submucosa.
— *pT2:* Tumor invades the muscularis propria.
— *pT3:* Tumor invades the subserosa and farther.
— *pT4:* Tumor invades other adjacent organs.

✚ Common symptoms of colorectal carcinomas:
– *Bleeding* due to highly vascularized tumor tissue, susceptibility of the tumor tissue to injury from feces, and ulceration due to necrosis.
– *Obstruction syndromes* occur with irregular bowel function, constipation, and diarrhea.
– *Unexpected passing of feces* instead of flatulence is typical of rectal carcinoma.

❗ Note: *Colorectal carcinoma diagnosis:*
– Immunohistochemical findings include expression of CEA[1].
– Serum CEA secretion is a parameter of the clinical course of the carcinoma (p. 326).
– Clinical findings include fresh or occult blood in the stool.
– Biopsy confirms the tumor; 75% of all colorectal carcinomas occur in the rectum and sigmoid. They may be demonstrated by colonoscopy or digital palpation.

☺ Prominent patients:
French composer Claude Debussy (1862–1918) and former US President Ronald Reagan.

A Colorectal polyposis

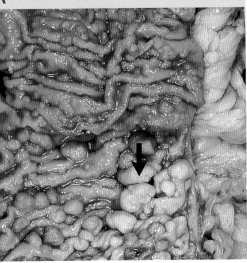

B Adenocarcinoma of the colon
(PAS) x 100

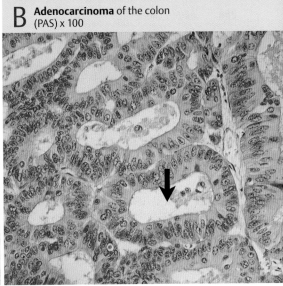

C Adenocarcinoma of the colon

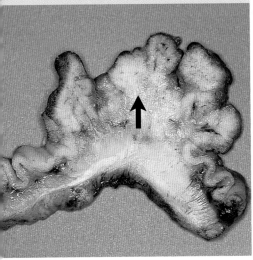

D Mucinous carcinoma of the colon
(PAS) x 50

E Ulcerating carcinoma of the colon

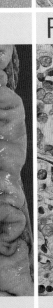

F Signet-ring cell carcinoma of the colon
(HE) x 100

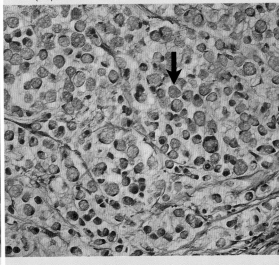

Dysontogenetic Tumors

General definition: Tumor arising from hetero-topic embryonic tissue that became displaced from its original location during embryonic de-velopment and was therefore unable to develop further.

Several types of tumors are differentiated according to the stage of development at which the heterotopic em-bryonic tissue remains frozen.

Teratoma

Occurrence: These tumors account for 30% of all tumors in the newborn and occur primarily in the gonads (espe-cially in young boys) and less often in the mid-line of the mediastinum (especially in young adults), in the retro-peritoneum, and within the cranium. Sacrococcygeal teratomas (occurring especially in girls) are usually pre-sent before birth.

General definition: The tumor consists of pluri-potential cells exhibiting a disorderly mixture of differentiated tissue from all three germ layers. *Histogenesis:* The tumors are derived from un-fertilized germ cells.

Teratomas are classified as mature or immature, de-pending on the degree of differentiation of the tissue that forms the tumor.

■ Mature Teratoma

Definition: Benign cystic tumor exhibited ma-ture tissue from all three germ layers.
— *Ovarian dermoid cysts* represent a special form of teratoma. These benign, sharply de-marcated, cystic tumors contain hair and sebum. Differentiated tissues such as seba-ceous glands, hair follicles (► A), squamous epithelium (► C1), teeth (► A2), cartilage, bone, and nerve tissue may be found within the walls of these cysts. Thyroid tissue (► C2) is also present on occasion.

■ Immature Teratoma

Occurrence: These tumors are found primarily in the go-nads where they occur most often in young boys. Rarely, they occur in the mid-line of the mediastinum, in the retroperitoneum, and within the cranium.

Definition: This malignant solid or small cystic tumor consists of minimally differentiated epithelial or mesenchymal tissues in the form of ciliated epithelium (► E1), hyaline cartilage (► E2), and bone (► E3).

Embryonal Tumors (Blastomas)

General definition: These are highly malignant tumors of undifferentiated cells of an organ pri-mordium that are no longer pluripotential.

Pathogenesis: The tumor arises during embryo-nic development and usually manifests itself in early childhood.

■ Neuroblastoma (► B, D, F)

Occurrence: The tumor usually occurs in the adrenal me-dulla, less often in the sympathetic chain.

Definition: This lesion is a malignant tumor of the sympathetic nervous system that forms ca-techolamine.

Morphologic findings include a grayish-red, pul-py tumor of small cells with little cytoplasm that occasionally form pseudorosettes. Second-ary maturation of the tumor cells to ganglion cells may occur, successively resulting in gang-lioneuroblastoma, ganglioneuroma. Sponta-neous remissions are possible (p. 350).

Metastasis occurs early via hematogenous dissemina-tion and follows the vena cava pattern.

■ Medulloblastoma

Definition: This highly malignant lesion is the most common tumor of the cerebellum in chil-dren. It consists of undifferentiated cells in a pseudorosette pattern.

Metastasis occurs via dissemination through the cere-brospinal fluid to the cerebrum and spinal cord.
Complications include hydrocephalus due to occlusion.

■ Retinoblastoma (p. 324)

■ Nephroblastoma (p. 324)

Embryonal Tumors Arising from Vestigial Tissue

■ Ameloblastoma

Definition: This semimalignant, locally invasive tumor of the jaw arises from vestiges of the odontogenic epithelium.

Morphology: see p. 384.

■ Craniopharyngioma

Definition: This semimalignant, locally invasive tumor arises from vestiges of the embryonic structures involved in the development of the anterior pituitary (pituitary diverticulum or pouch of Rathke).

Morphology: see p. 384.

■ Chordoma

Definition: This semimalignant, locally invasive tumor arises from vestiges of the notochord.

Morphology: see p. 384.

■ Mesodermal Mixed Tumor

Definition: This tumor consists of pluripotential vestiges of the paramesonephric ducts from which the uterovaginal tract develops.

✚ General clinical presentation: Embryonal tu-mors arising from vestigial tissue are usually non-me-tastasizing malignant tumors (p. 384) that are locally invasive and tend to recur. Metastases are exception-ally rare.

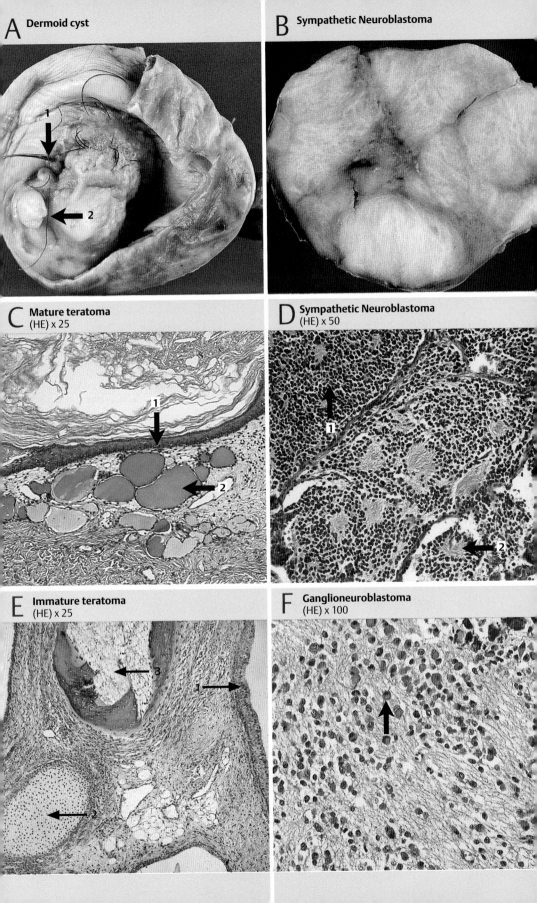

A Dermoid cyst

B Sympathetic Neuroblastoma

C Mature teratoma
(HE) x 25

D Sympathetic Neuroblastoma
(HE) x 50

E Immature teratoma
(HE) x 25

F Ganglioneuroblastoma
(HE) x 100

Semimalignant Tumors

Definition: These are destructive, locally invasive tumors that rarely if ever metastasize.

■ Basal Cell Carcinoma

Definition: A semimalignant, locally invasive skin tumor of basaloid epidermal cells.

Pathogenesis: See p. 6, 334, and 336.

Morphology: The tumor arises from the basal layer of the epidermis as a roughly conical nodular arrangement of minimally polymorphic cells. The peripheral epithelial layer exhibits radial palisades (▶ B1) interspersed with tumor-induced stroma (▶ B2). This stroma may contain inflammatory infiltrate.

Patterns of Growth:

▦ Nodular Ulcerous Type

Occurrence: The tumor arises primarily in the face.

This tumor exhibits an exophytic pattern of growth with primarily solid complexes of tumor cells. It infiltrates and penetrates the epidermis, producing local areas of necrosis. The resulting ulceration of the skin (▶ A) produces what was once referred to as "rodent ulcers" where the lesion is surrounded by reactive stroma.

▦ Multicentric Type

Occurrence: The tumor arises primarily on the trunk.

The tumor exhibits superficially invasive growth, spreading horizontally in a discontinuous pattern along tumor-induced stroma.

✚ **Clinical presentation:** The tumor requires extensive excision with a margin of normal tissue.

▦ Sclerosing Type

Occurrence: The tumor arises in skin exposed to sunlight.

Here, the tumor-induced stroma dominates, producing cleft, compressed cords of tumor cells.

✚ **Clinical presentation:** This tumor is highly invasive and tends to recur, requiring extensive excision with a margin of normal tissue.

■ Carcinoid Appendix

Definition: Semimalignant tumor of the dispersed neuroendocrine system in the appendix.

Morphology: This yellowish white tumor is rarely larger than 1 cm. It fills the entire lumen of the appendix and invades the mesoappendix. The tumor consists of lobular arrangements of nodules of minimally polymorphic tumor cells (▶ C).

Immunohistochemical findings include expression of chromogranin (▶ D).

✚ **Clinical presentation:** Metastases are exceptionally rare. The tumor produces serotonin but because this is catabolized in the liver, carcinoid flush does not occur (p. 354).

❗ **Note:** The term *dispersed neuroendocrine system* refers to neuroendocrine cells that do not form a cohesive macroscopic organ but are dispersed throughout the body as isolated cells or in small groups.

❗ **Note:** The term *carcinoid tumor* refers to *all* tumors of the dispersed neuroendocrine system.

❗ **Note:** *Carcinoid tumors of the ileum and bronchi* are more common than carcinoid tumors of the appendix. However, they are better described as invasive low-grade neuroendocrine carcinomas.

■ Ameloblastoma

Occurrence: The tumor arises in the jaw and is far more common in men than in women.

Definition: see p. 382.

Morphology: The tumor lacks a capsule of connective tissue. It grows in a polycystic pattern and invades the medulla space of the mandible.

Histologic findings include a tumor consisting of complexes of columnar epithelium that form a peripheral palisade bordering the stroma and merge in the center with a reticulum resembling odontogenic pulpa. The tumor forms either an insular epithelial pattern (follicular type) or a net-like pattern of communicating strands (reticular type; ▶ E).

■ Chordoma

Occurrence: The tumor arises from the base of the skull (clivus) and in the spine.

Definition: see p. 382.

Morphology: The tumor exhibits plant-like, large vesicular, isomorphic tumor cells arranged in large lobules in a mucinous substance (▶ F).

■ Craniopharyngioma

Occurrence: The tumor arises in the pituitary.

Definition: see p. 382.

Morphology: The tumor consists primarily of squamous epithelium with communicating reticular epithelial strands. It exhibits the palisade-like epithelial arrangement seen in basal cell carcinomas and the open reticular pattern of epithelium seen in ameloblastomas.

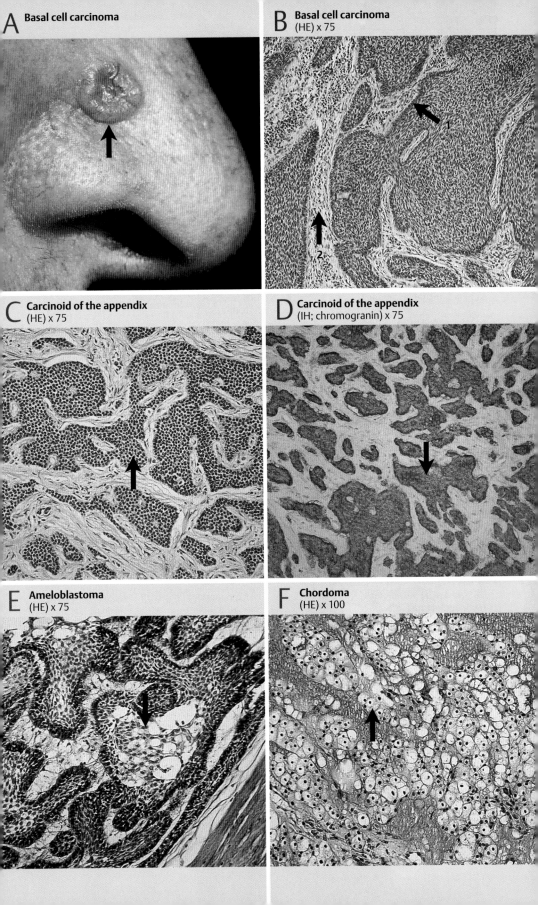

A Basal cell carcinoma

B Basal cell carcinoma
(HE) x 75

C Carcinoid of the appendix
(HE) x 75

D Carcinoid of the appendix
(IH; chromogranin) x 75

E Ameloblastoma
(HE) x 75

F Chordoma
(HE) x 100

From the "Autobahn" to a "Dead-end"

Generalized Circulatory Disorders

Summary

A hierarchical control system regulates blood circulation. Disturbances in this system that result in excessive or insufficient blood flow pose a risk for the body.

▶ **Arterial hypertension**: The kidney is integrated into the arterial system in such a manner that it can control blood pressure according to its own requirements, which optimizes its blood filtration function. This is reflected in the fact that increased blood pressure is the general response to renal disorders that exceed a certain degree of damage (renal hypertension). However, the pathogenesis of most hypertension disorders is complex and not fully understood, as is the case with essential hypertension. Only a few types of hypertension are attributable to endocrine, neurologic, or cardiovascular causes.

▶ **Pulmonary hypertension** refers to increased blood pressure in the pulmonary arteries. It can occur as an idiopathic disorder or secondary to changes in the parenchyma of the lung. As is generally true of hypertension disorders, it manifests itself in vascular lesions. The capacity of the right ventricle of the heart to respond to pulmonary hypertension with muscular hypertrophy limits life expectancy.

▶ **Portal hypertension** is attributable to impaired drainage via the portal vein. This condition is a regular complication of scarring of the hepatic parenchyma. The severity of the condition is limited by vascular bypasses that develop around the congested area drained by the portal vein. These vessels initially develop varices and can rupture.

▶ **Shock** is systemic hypotension in the form of generalized cardiovascular collapse with critical hypoperfusion of vital organs. The key pathogenetic feature of shock is the progressive breakdown in circulatory regulation. This begins with the failure of initial reflex compensatory mechanisms such as increasing cardiac output and diverting blood flow from nonessential areas in the circulatory system. Finally, there is total loss of control over the microvasculature. This results in activation of the clotting system with formation of microthrombi, which can often lead to fatal disseminated intravascular coagulation with generalized bleeding.

▶ **Bleeding** may result from local vascular injuries either within the microvasculature or in larger vessels, or it may result from a ubiquitous vascular or coagulation defect (hemorrhagic diathesis).

Arterial Hypertension

General definition: This disorder consists of protracted, abnormally high arterial blood pressure defined as systolic pressure exceeding 140 mmHg and diastolic pressure exceeding 90 mmHg.

Essential Hypertension

Textbook example of a multifactorial disorder exhibiting polygenic inheritance.

Definition: Arterial hypertension in which all known causes of high blood pressure have been ruled out.

Pathogenetic mechanisms:
— *Genetic factors:* The animal model for this disorder involves breeds of rats that exhibit two congenital forms of hypertension, a neural form due to sympathetic hyperactivity and a renal form due to defective excretion of sodium.
— *Defective excretion of sodium* occurs. However, the causes and underlying mechanism are not known.
— *Stress factors* such as emotional and psychological conflicts can trigger hypertension. This stimulates vascular baroreceptors, decreasing the sensitivity of the cerebral cortex and pain sensitivity. Arterial hypertension is therefore a "learnable" strategy for coping with stress.
— *Deregulation of the renin-angiotensin-aldosterone system* occurs. However, the causes and underlying mechanism are not known.

Renal Hypertension

Definition: Arterial hypertension due to:

— *hypertension in the renal parenchyma* with parenchymal shrinkage or
— *renovascular hypertension* with extrarenal and intrarenal arterial stenosis.

Pathophysiology:

The *classic animal model:* Goldblatt kidney:
— *One-kidney model* (▶ A), removal of one kidney and arterial stenosis in the remaining kidney (▶ A) leads to reduced vascular supply and reduction in the renal parenchyma capable of diuresis. This in turn leads to retention of sodium and water and causes hypervolemia. The result is hypervolemic hypertension.
— *Two-kidney model* (▶ B), unilateral renal arterial stenosis with an intact contralateral kidney leads to unilateral renal ischemia (p. 69). The ischemic kidney generates increased quantities of renin and therefore angiotensin II as well. The result is hypertension due to vascular resistance.
   Later, aldosterone secreted by the adrenal cortex leads to retention of sodium and water and causes hypervolemia. The result is hypervolemic hypertension.

☺ **Prominent patients** with essential hypertension: Russian revolutionary V. I. Lenin (1870–1924). Former US president Franklin D. Roosevelt (1882–1945).

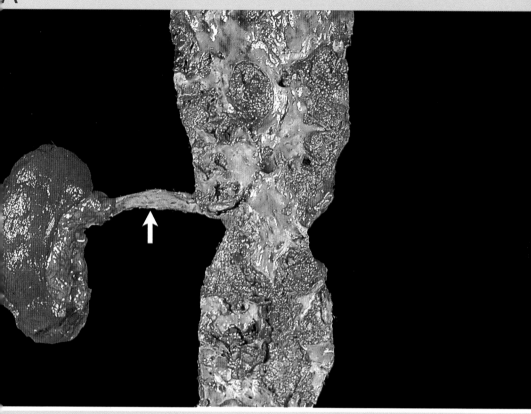

A Goldblatt kidney: single kidney with arterial stenosis in the absence of a second kidney

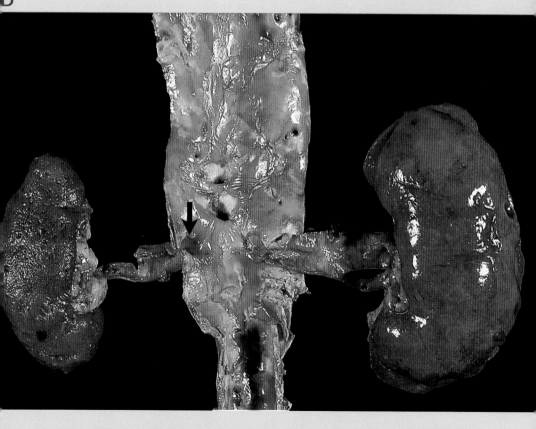

B Goldblatt kidney: unilateral renal arterial stenosis with an intact contralateral kidney

■ Renovascular Hypertension

Etiologic factors include constriction of the lumen of the renal artery by 70% due to:
— *Arteriosclerosis* of the renal artery;
— *Incomplete thrombosis* of the renal artery;
— *Fibromuscular dysplasia* of the renal arteries;
— *Cystic degeneration of aortic media* (p. 60) involving the renal artery;
— *Compression of the kidney* by a tumor or due to shrinkage of the renal capsule with an intact contralateral kidney.

Pathogenesis follows Goldblatt's two-kidney model (p. 386).

■ Renoparenchymal Hypertension

Etiologic factors include:
— *Bilateral shrinkage of the renal parenchyma* and
— *Unilateral shrinkage of the renal parenchyma* with arterial stenosis in glomerulonephritis, pyelonephritis, hydronephrosis (atrophy of the renal parenchyma due to retention of urine), or arteriosclerosis.

Pathogenesis follows Goldblatt's single-kidney model (p. 386).

Endocrinal Hypertension

Definition: This rare type of arterial hypertension is caused by a primary disorder of certain endocrine organs or by a high dose of a certain hormone.

Etiologic factors:
— **Pheochromocytoma**
    Definition: This is a tumor of the adrenal medulla or the paraganglia (► A) that is usually benign.
    Morphology: A yellowish-brown tumor displaces the adrenal cortices (► A). The tumor consists of large cells arranged in configurations that resemble bales of cells ("Zellballen") (► B). Their slightly basophilic cytoplasm contains neuroendocrine granulae, and they have hyperchromatic polyploid nuclei.
    Immunohistochemical findings include expression of chromogranin (► C).
    Complications: The tumor occasionally produces adrenaline and/or noradrenaline. This results in arterial hypertension with paroxysmal hypertensive crises that cause death.
— **Primary aldosteronism** (Conn's syndrome; p. 122).
— **Cushing's syndrome** (p. 122).

Cardiovascular Hypertension

Definition: This arterial hypertension is caused by a pathogenic cardiovascular change.

Etiologic factor:
— *Reduced elasticity* of the major vessels and
— *Valvular defects* with reflux, both of which lead to hypertension.

Neurologic Hypertension

Definition: This extremely rare type of arterial hypertension results from the failure of peripheral or central blood pressure regulators.

Two pathogenetic forms exist.
— *Hypertension* occurs as a result of failure of blood pressure receptors in the carotid sinus secondary to traumatic, inflammatory, or sclerotic lesions.
— *Cerebral hypertension* occurs as a result of traumatic or inflammatory damage to the brain stem or diencephalon.

Sequelae of Arterial Hypertension

■ Hypertensive Cardiac Hypertrophy

▥ **Hypervolemic Hypertension:** Increased stroke volume initially leads to dilatation and subsequently to left ventricular hypertrophy (p. 116).

Result: A (primary) eccentric hypertrophy of the left ventricle (eccentric hypertrophy = dilative).

▥ **Resistance Hypertension:** Increased ejection initially leads to adaptive left ventricular hypertrophy.

Result: A (primary) concentric hypertrophy of the left ventricle (concentric hypertrophy = non-dilative).

Chronically increased ejection resistance leads to further ventricular hypertrophy. The heart then exceeds the critical threshold weight of 500 g, resulting in an imbalance between the mass of the myocardium and its capillary supply network. This leads to superimposed ventricular dilation.

Result: (secondary) eccentric hypertrophy of the left ventricle.

■ Hypertensive Arteriopathy

Physiology: Normally the smooth muscle cells of the media are arranged in opposing spirals. This allows the media to convert the physiologic compressive load into a tensile load.

Where normal intravascular pressure is exceeded, the muscle spirals are extended and the length of the vessel is increased. Macroscopic findings include tortuous vascular structures. The resulting compressive load is primarily borne by the myocytes of the vascular wall media. This triggers reactive expression of growth factor, transforming the myocytes into "fiber generators." The result is concentric progressive fibrotic reinforcement of the arterial wall extending from the intima (► D1, E1) to the media (► D2, E2), eventually leading to fibrotic arteriosclerosis.

Result: Arterial stenosis that leads to secondary hypertension due to increased vascular resistance, resulting in self-perpetuating hypertension.
Complications include massive hypertensive cerebrovascular hemorrhages (p. 398).

> **Note:** Hypertensive vascular disease may be diagnosed *in vivo* in the retinal vessels of the fundus of the eye.

> **Note:** Left ventricular insufficiency with cardiac pulmonary edema is a sign of hypertension with a poor prognosis.

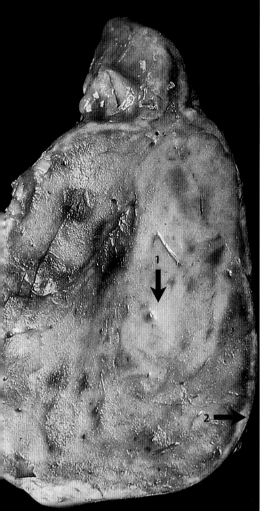

A Pheochromocytoma

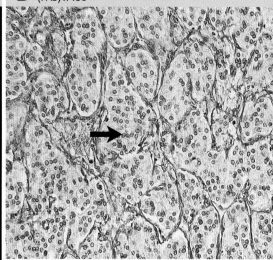

B Pheochromocytoma (Zellballen pattern)
(PAS) x 150

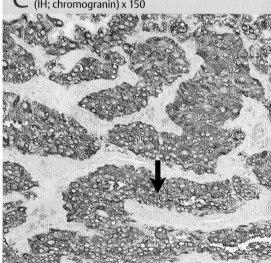

C Pheochromocytoma
(IH; chromogranin) x 150

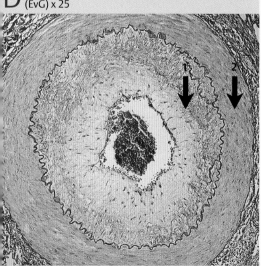

D Hypertensive arteriopathy
(EvG) x 25

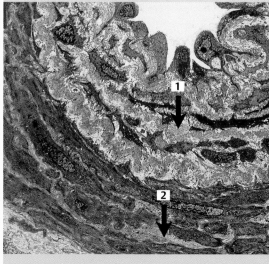

E Hypertensive arteriopathy
(TEM) x 2000

Pulmonary Hypertension

Definition: Chronically increased pulmonary arterial pressure at rest in excess of 30/15 mmHg.

> **Note:** There are several *criteria for excluding pulmonary hypertension.* The increased vascular resistance triggering the hypertension must not be attributable to these mechanisms
>
> – left ventricular insufficiency;
> – shunts between the pulmonary and extrapulmonary vessels;
> – increased vascular pressure in the pulmonary veins.

■ Primary Pulmonary Hypertension

Definition: Pulmonary hypertension of uncertain etiology.

Morphology:
– **Elastic pulmonary arteries** exhibit punctate lipid deposits and calcification (► A) as in general arteriosclerosis (i.e., pulmonary arteriosclerosis).
– **Muscular pulmonary arteries** initially exhibit concentric intimal fibrosis (► C). Later, nodular proliferations of myocytes and structures resembling angiomas (capillary masses that mimic neoplasms; ► E) in the intima of minor muscular arteries. These are often accompanied by areas of myocyte necrosis in the walls of the pulmonary arteries with a secondary inflammatory reaction.

> ✚ **Clinical presentation:** This rare disorder is far more common in women than in men. Its peak incidence is between the ages of 20 and 30.

■ Secondary Pulmonary Hypertension

Definition: Pulmonary hypertension with an established etiology. This disorder occurs in three forms.

▦ Vasorestrictive Pulmonary Hypertension

Pathogenesis: Several processes restrict the cross-section of the pulmonary artery and reduce the parenchyma of the lung. These include:

– Destructive pulmonary infection;
– Proteolytic destruction of the lung;
– Pulmonary fibrosis (► B) and/or scarring;
– Pneumectomy (surgical removal of one lung).

These processes reduce the overall cross section of the pulmonary flow tract and cause vascular obstruction by involving the remaining pulmonary vessels in the disease process. This is complicated by reflex constriction of the small tributary pulmonary arteries (von Euler-Liljestrand reflex), which leads to alveolar hypoxia (p. 22).

▦ Vaso-obstructive Pulmonary Hypertension

Pathogenesis: Several mechanisms combine to reduce the overall cross-section of the pulmonary vessels by more than half. These include:

– Recurrent multiple peripheral pulmonary embolisms (► D; p. 410);
– Primary inflammation of the pulmonary arteries with secondary thrombotic occlusion;
– Involvement of the vascular bed in a primary inflammation of the parenchyma of the lung with secondary stenosis.

▦ Vasoconstrictive Pulmonary Hypertension

Pathogenesis: A drop in the partial pressure of oxygen Pa_{O2} or in the quotient of Pa_{O2}/Pa_{CO2} leads to reflex constriction of the minor pulmonary arteries. This produces pulmonary hypertension due to vascular resistance in the presence of the following conditions:

– Stenosis in the tracheobronchial system;
– Restricted mobility of the chest;
– Restricted lung compliance of lung tissue;
– Reduced oxygen content of inhaled air.

Sequelae of Pulmonary Hypertension

■ Chronic Cor Pulmonale

WHO definition: Right ventricular hypertrophy (not insufficiency) as a result of disease that impairs the function and/or structure of the lung.

Pathogenesis: Chronically increased pressure in the pulmonary vessels leads to increased right ventricular output, which over time produces concentric hypertrophy of the right ventricle. Chronically increased ejection resistance will eventually cause the right ventricle to exceed the critical threshold weight of 80 g, resulting in an imbalance between the mass of the myocardium and its capillary supply network. This leads to dilation of the myocardium.

Result: Eccentric hypertrophy of the right ventricle (cor pulmonale; ► F).

■ Hypertensive Pulmonary Vascular Disease

See also primary pulmonary hypertension.

> **Note:** Dilation is a morphologic correlate of *heart failure.*

> **Note:** Sequelae of *left heart failure* include engorgement of the pulmonary circulatory system via the left atrium. This congestion produces alveolar pulmonary edema.
> Duration of left heart failure may be long, persisting several days.

> **Note:** Sequelae of *right heart failure* include engorgement of the systemic vessels (such as the cervical and hepatic veins). This congestion leads to congestive induration and atrophy and cardiac edemas. Total right heart failure is usually of short duration and leads to sudden cardiac death.

A Pulmonary arteriosclerosis grade I

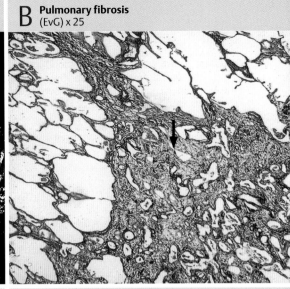

B Pulmonary fibrosis (EvG) x 25

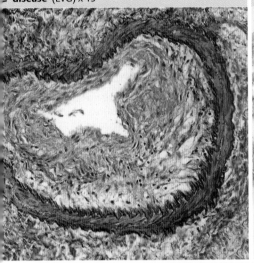

Hypertensive pulmonary vascular disease (EvG) x 15

D Pulmonary microembolism (PAS) x 25

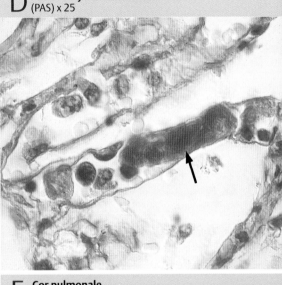

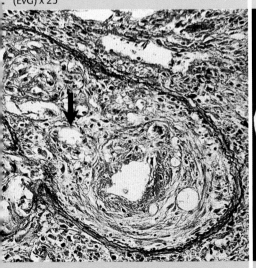

Hypertensive pulmonary vascular disease grade II (EvG) x 25

F Cor pulmonale

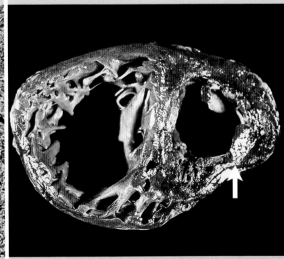

Portal Hypertension

Definition: Chronically increased blood pressure in the portal venous system due to any type of drainage impairment. The disorder is most often caused by cirrhosis of the liver (p. 42).

Pathogenesis: Several mechanisms can lead to portal hypertension:

Intrahepatic block is due to:
— Cirrhosis of the liver (p. 42).
  Here, destruction of the lobular parenchymal structure occurs due to:
  — Impaired drainage from the hepatic parenchyma via the central veins;
  — Impaired drainage into the parenchyma from the portal regions;
  — Collateral intrahepatic circulation through anastomoses between the portal vein and other veins and arteries.
— Echinococcosis of the liver (p. 282).

Posthepatic block: It is rare but can occur due to *impaired drainage of the hepatic veins* as a result of right heart failure (see previous section) or hepatic venous thrombosis (Budd-Chiari syndrome and venous occlusive disease).

Extrahepatic block: It is rare but can due to *occlusion of the portal vein* as a result of portal vein thrombosis or compression of the portal vein in the presence of an abdominal mass.

Sequelae of Portal Hypertension

■ Development of Collateral Circulation

Synonym: portosystemic shunts.

▥ Esophageal Varices

Definition: The most common type of collateral circulation in portal hypertension forms as a result of abnormal dilation of the periesophageal venous plexus in the distal esophagus.

Pathogenetic chain reaction: Engorgement of the gastric veins with portal blood in turn leads to engorgement of the submucosal veins of the fundus of the stomach and distal esophagus (► A). This causes a reversal of flow with the venous blood draining through the azygos vein into the superior vena cava (anastomosis between the portal vein and vena cava).

> ✚ **Complications:** Engorged submucosal veins are prone to injury due to their exposed position. Large chunks of food are sufficient to cause ruptured varices (► B), which can lead to fatal bleeding.

▥ Caput Medusae

Definition: Varicose subcutaneous veins lead to the umbilicus in portal hypertension (► C).

Pathogenetic chain reaction: Engorgement of the portal vein causes the umbilical vein in the round ligament of the liver to reopen (cirsomphalos). The blood then drains into the superior and inferior vena cava.

> ❗ **Note:** *Hemorrhoids are not related to portal hypertension.* The cavernous body of the rectum is supplied by arteries and drains through venous plexuses. In portal hypertension, the venous pressure is too low to cause engorgement of the cavernous body of the rectum.

■ Congenitive Splenomegaly

Definition: Enlargement of the spleen due to engorgement with venous blood as a result of:

— Cirrhosis of the liver (common);
— Splenic vein thrombosis (rare);
— Extrahepatic portal vein thrombosis (rare).

Pathogenesis: Engorgement of the spleen with venous blood causes congestive splenomegaly (the organ may weigh up to 1000 g; ► D, E) with hyperplasia of the splenic sinus and plexus with reactive fibrosis (► G) but unchanged follicles (► F2). This results in dense layering of the sinus endothelium, leading to a splenic "fibroadenia" (► G). Another consequence is focal extravasation of blood into the spleen, resulting in focal deposits of hemosiderin (p. 106) with calcification and scarring in the form of Gandy-Gamma nodules (► F1).

> ❗ **Note:** *Complications of splenomegaly* generally include an increase in the rate at which cellular components are removed from circulating blood in the spleen (hypersplenism), resulting in anemia.

■ Ascites

Definition: Accumulation of serous protein-containing fluid in the peritoneal sac with portal hypertension.

Pathogenesis: Portal hypertension is thought to have the following consequences (see edema, p. 424):
— Increased hydrostatic pressure in the peritoneum leads to transudation (p. 424).
— Hepatic lymph production increases.
— Oncotic pressure is decreased as the result of hyperalbuminemia (hepatic synthesis is disturbed).
— Slowed blood flow in the prehepatic flow tract successively leads to secondary hyperaldosteronism (p. 122), renal sodium and water retention, and hypervolemia.

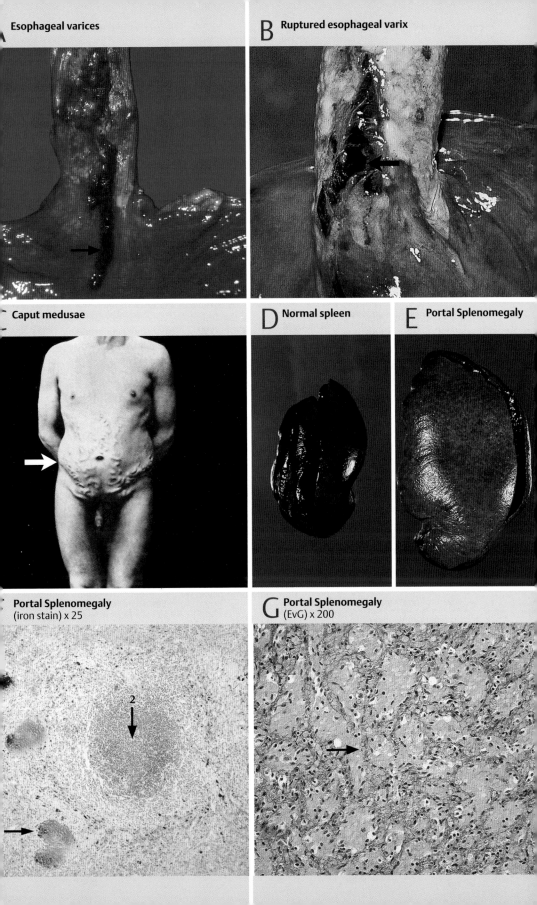

A Esophageal varices

B Ruptured esophageal varix

C Caput medusae

D Normal spleen

E Portal Splenomegaly

F Portal Splenomegaly (iron stain) x 25

G Portal Splenomegaly (EvG) x 200

Shock

Textbook example of the disease process that is most often fatal.

Recapitulation: See "Changes in Microcirculation" (p. 196).

General definition: Acute generalized cardiovascular collapse with critical loss of microvascular blood supply in vital organs and progressive ischemic hypoxidosis.

Pathogenetic Forms of Shock

■ Cardiogenic Shock (common)

Occurrence: Rupture or an aortic aneurysm or of the myocardium, myocardial infarction, or cardiac arrhythmia.

These conditions lead to reduced cardiac output and/or absolute hypovolemia. Both of these in turn lead to loss of microvascular blood supply.

■ Hypovolemic Shock (common)

Occurrence:
- Intraoperative or traumatic blood loss;
- Blood plasma loss due to a burn or crush injury;
- Water loss in cholera (p. 262), diabetic coma, or acute addisonian crisis (p. 112).

These events lead to absolute hypovolemia.

■ Septic Shock (common)

Occurrence: Bacterial sepsis (p. 222) can produce endotoxic shock, and burns can cause shock due to burn toxins.

Toxic endothelial injury leads to loss of microvascular blood supply relative hypovolemia.

■ Anaphylactic Shock (rare)

Occurrence: systemic anaphylaxis (p. 168).

This condition leads to generalized release of vasoactive substances. That in turn causes loss of microvascular blood supply, which results in relative hypovolemia.

■ Endocrine Shock (very rare)

Occurrence:
- Total pituitary and adrenal failure.
- Insulin shock (insulin overdose) bcauses metabolic disruption and hypovolemia that in turn lead to a compensatory adrenergic vasomotor response.
- Adrenalin shock in pheochromocytoma (p. 388) causes massive vasoconstriction.

These conditions lead to relative hypovolemia and/or tissue injury.

■ Neurogenic Shock (extremely rare)

Occurrence: Peripheral or central vasomotor injury results in decreased vascular tone, causing blood to pool in the microvasculature.

This condition leads to relative hypovolemia.

Hemodynamic Forms of Shock

■ Hyperdynamic Shock Syndrome

Pathogenetic chain reaction: Shock leads to increased sympathetic nerve activity. This in turn activates the renin-angiotensin-aldosterone system, triggering an increase in cardiac output and restoring normal blood pressure. This creates a *situation in the microvasculature* (► B) in which the precapillary arterioles are constricted and the arteriovenous anastomoses are open.

The *result* is slowed blood flow, which leads to aggregation of erythrocytes into sludge.

■ Hypodynamic Shock Syndrome

▥ Reversible Stage of Shock

Pathogenetic chain reaction: Shock with decreased cardiac output triggers a sympathetic adrenergic reaction with release of adrenaline and vasopressors. This creates a

situation in the microvasculature in which the arterioles in the flow tracts containing α-receptors, such as the skin, musculature, kidneys, and the area supplied by the splanchnic nerves are constricted, whereas blood flow is not constricted in the flow tracts containing β-receptors, such as the brain and heart.

Result: Blood circulation is effectively concentrated in the central regions of the body.

▥ Irreversible Stage of Shock

Pathogenetic chain reaction: In the late stage of shock, acidic cellular metabolites block the effect of catecholamines on the myocytes of the vascular walls. This creates the following *situation in the microvasculature:*
- The arterioles are dilated where venules are constricted. This increases vascular filtration pressure.
- Serum is then pressed into the interstitium, increasing hematocrit levels and worsening the hypovolemia.
- Blood flow slows, leading to erythrocyte sludge formation that in turn causes endothelial necrosis.
- Thrombocyte aggregation occurs.
- Clotting factors are released.
- The clotting cascade is activated.

Result: Clotting factors (p. 402) are consumed. This leads to generation of hyaline microthrombi, which primarily lodge in the microvasculature of the lung.

> **Note:** The Shwartzman-Sanarelli reaction (► A) is a classic animal model for shock with depletion of clotting factors (see disseminated intravascular coagulation, p. 402).
> - *Initial injection of endotoxin* causes endothelial and thrombocytic damage and triggers complement activation via the alternate pathway. This activates (a) the fibrinolysis system and (b) clotting factors with formation of fibrin, leading to fibrin phagocytosis by the RES.
> - *A second injection* 24 hours later again leads to fibrin formation. However, the fibrin is no longer phagocytized by the reticuloendothelial system, resulting in an RES blockade (p. 26). Microthrombi form, and the condition progresses to disseminated intravascular coagulation (p. 402), which leads to shock.

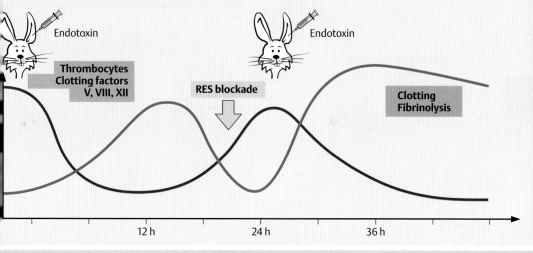

Shwartzman-Sanarelli phenomenon
(model for shock with disseminated intravascular coagulation)

Endotoxin

Endotoxin

Thrombocytes
Clotting factors
V, VIII, XII

RES blockade

Clotting
Fibrinolysis

12 h   24 h   36 h

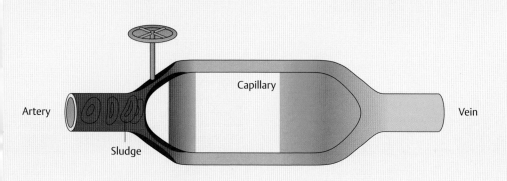

Hypodynamic shock

Artery

Capillary

Vein

Sludge

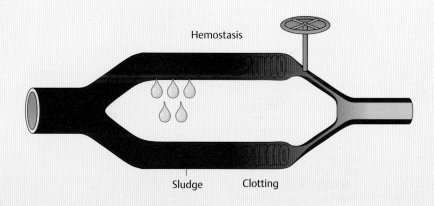

Hypodynamic shock

Hemostasis

Sludge   Clotting

> **Note:** "Shock organs" include the lung, kidney, liver, and interstitium. Hyaline microthrombi produce an effect equivalent to shock.

> **Note:** General clinical symptoms in shock include pallor, clammy skin, cold digits, collapsed superficial veins, arterial hypotension, impaired consciousness, and acute kidney failure.

Sequelae of Shock

■ Shock Lung (very common)

Textbook example of the most common manifestation of shock.

Pathogenesis:

— *Early phase* (1–6 days):
  Principle: Activation of mediators leads to exudative alveolitis.

  Shock activates the classic inflammation mediators (p. 202). This has several consequences.
    — Exudative alveolitis (diffuse alveolar injury syndrome, p. 40) leads to interstitial pulmonary edema (▶ A, B).
    — This attracts and activates leukocytes in the pulmonary microvasculature, resulting in the release of proteases.
    — This in turn activates mediators (p. 203), resulting in a self-perpetuating spiral of inflammation.
    — Toxic O_2 and N_2 metabolites are generated.
  Result: The destruction of the alveolar endothelial and epithelial layer. Fibrinous exudate also spreads over the alveolar surface; artificial respiration causes it to coalesce into a dense hyaline membrane (▶ C).

— *Late phase* (after 6 days):
  Principle: Exudative alveolitis progresses to sclerosing alveolitis.
  Perfusion and ventilation of the lungs are limited by progressive fibrosis of the interstitial tissue and excessive epithelial tissue repair.
  Result: adult respiratory distress syndrome (ARDS, p. 40).

■ Shock Kidney (common)

Pathogenesis: Two forms of renal insufficiency are differentiated:
— Kidney failure can occur due to *functional exclusion* of the kidneys from blood circulation, or
— As a result of *microthrombotic congestion* of the arterioles and glomerular vessels (▶ D).

Both cases cause renal ischemia. This reduces the activity of the ion pumps, resulting in swelling of the tubular epithelium in the form of apical cellular edema (p. 32). Edema in turn causes congestion of the tubules. The high-energy substrates are then lacking when re-perfusion occurs. Cells therefore become flooded with Ca^2. This damages the tubules and causes sequestration of the apical cell vesicles, leading to tubular congestion.

Histologic findings include kidneys with "wide tubules" (p. 33).

Macroscopic characteristics include a pale renal cortex due to renal ischemia and cyanotic medulla due to delayed venous drainage (▶ E).

Result: Acute kidney failure.

■ Shock Hepatopathy (common)

Pathogenesis: Microthrombi (occurring in 30% of all cases) and/or ischemia lead to necrosis.

Result: Necrosis of individual cells and/or necrotic areas in the middle lobe of the liver (▶ F).

■ Shock Pancreatopathy (common)

Pathogenesis: Ischemic acinar necrosis leads to autodigestion.

Result: Acute pancreatitis with focal areas of intra-parenchymal fatty necrosis (p. 132).

■ Shock Endocarditis (7–10% of all cases)

Pathogenesis: In the presence of disseminated intravascular coagulation, the circulating thrombocyte aggregates accumulate like warts on the existing endothelial defects on the edges of the mitral and/or aortic valves.

Result: Verrucous endocarditis.

■ Shock Enteropathy (less common)

Pathogenesis: Microthrombi (p. 406) and/or greatly reduced perfusion of the bowel causes hemorrhagic mucosal erosions. These lead to fibrinous exudation on the surface of the erosions.

Result: Ischemic pseudomembranous enteropathy (p. 208).

■ Shock Encephalopathy (rare)

Pathogenesis: Ischemia due to protected hypotension leads to tissue necrosis.

Results: Cerebral purpura (punctate microhemorrhages in the brain) and focal areas of medullary necrosis or symmetric hemorrhagic infarctions.

■ Shock Endocrinopathy (very rare)

Pathogenesis: The disorder is caused by shock-induced microthrombi and capillary damage in endocrine organs.

Results: Adrenal necrosis in the setting of meningococcal sepsis (Waterhouse-Friderichsen syndrome; p. 216) and pituitary necrosis in the setting of toxemia of pregnancy (Sheehan syndrome; ▶ G).

☺ **Prominent patient:** Jesus of Nazareth died of shock in about 30 A.D.
Scourging (whipping) caused electrolyte loss and hypovolemia, precipitating the hyperdynamic phase of hypovolemic shock.
Crucifixion in orthostatic or erect posture led to the hypodynamic phase of hypovolemic shock; death resulted from right heart failure.

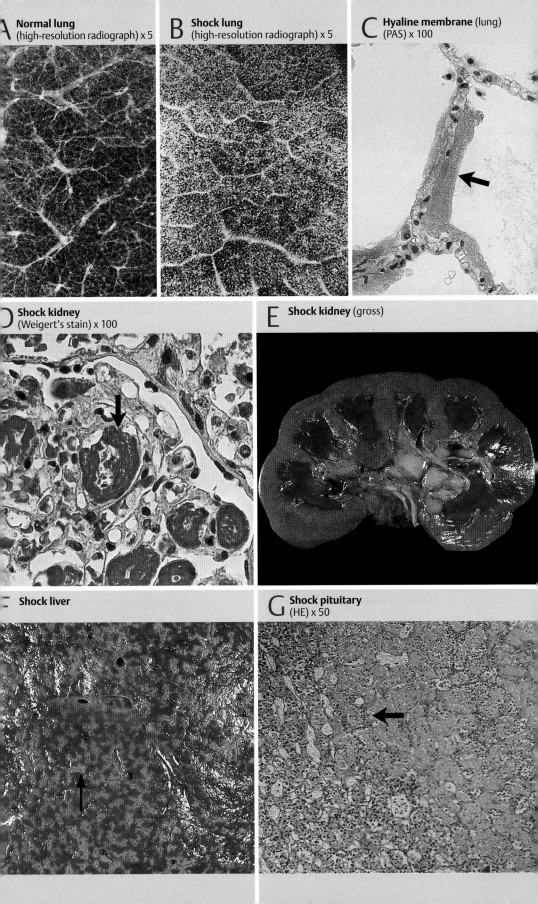

A Normal lung
(high-resolution radiograph) x 5

B Shock lung
(high-resolution radiograph) x 5

C Hyaline membrane (lung)
(PAS) x 100

D Shock kidney
(Weigert's stain) x 100

E Shock kidney (gross)

F Shock liver

G Shock pituitary
(HE) x 50

Hemorrhage

Synonym: bleeding.

General definition: The escape of whole blood out of the cardiovascular system to the surface of the body or into body tissues or cavities.

Bleeding Through Ruptures (common)

Definition: Bleeding through ruptures occurring as a result of the inability of a vascular wall or the wall of the heart to withstand forces acting upon it (such as tensile or compressive forces).

Pathogenesis and sequelae: Two basic mechanisms can cause the wall of the vessel or heart to give way under internal pressure: weakening of the wall and over-stretching.

■ Weakening of the Vessel Wall

may occur due to several causes:
— A *textural defect* may be present in the vessel.
  — *Cerebral aneurysms:* a congenital defect in the arterial circle of the cerebrum produces a berry aneurysm (► A; p. 62). In middle age, this can rupture due to weakness of the vessel wall, leading to fatal massive cerebral hemorrhage (► B).
  — *Scurvy* involves acquired weakness of the vessel walls as a result of deficient collagen synthesis caused by vitamin C deficiency (p. 38).

— Vascular *inflammation* can occur
  — *Syphilitic aortitis* (p. 58),
  — *Polyarteritis nodosa* (p. 58).

— Vascular *sclerosis* can occur
  — *Arteriosclerotic aneurysm* (p. 68),
  — *Hemorrhoids* (phlebosclerosis),
  — *Esophageal varices* (phlebosclerosis).

— Vascular *necrosis* can occur
  — *Cystic medial necrosis* of the aorta (p. 58),
  — *Myocardial infraction* and lead to a ventricular perforation (► C), in which case bleeding into the pericardium creates a cardiac tamponade (► D) that causes cardiac arrest.

— Vascular *erosion*
  Can occur as the result of one of the following three processes in perivascular tissue.
  — Perivascular *inflammation* can occur in a pulmonary cavity in tuberculosis, in acute pancreatitis with liquefactive necrosis (p. 132), and in erosive gastritis.
  — *Encephalomalacia* in a cerebral infarction,
  — *Gastroduodenal ulcer* with peptic necrosis.

— Perivascular *neoplasms*
  — *Bronchogenic carcinoma,*
  — *Glioblastoma* with a tendency to produce spontaneous necrosis can cause tumorous vascular erosion (p. 358).

■ Over-Stretching of Vascular Structures

Can occur as a result of
— Trauma, such as a laceration and contusion, and of
— *hypertension.*

✚ **Clinical presentation:** *Cerebral stroke* (apoplexia) occurs as the result of the following pathogenetic chain reaction: Hypertension leads to reactive sclerosis of the vessel wall, especially in the cerebral vessels. The lenticulostriate branches of the middle cerebral artery are predisposed to such lesions in hypertensive vasculopathy disease (p. 388). This leads to rupture of the vessel wall with massive cerebral hemorrhage occurring primarily in the basal ganglia of the brain and in the cerebrum (► B). The hemorrhage creates a cavity in the brain tissue and occasionally penetrates into the cerebral ventricle, causing a stroke initially characterized by unilateral flaccid paralysis and later by unilateral spastic paralysis.

☺ **Prominent patients** who died of cerebral stroke include German composer Felix Mendelssohn (1809–1847) and Russian revolutionary Vladimir Ilich Lenin (1870–1924).

— Over-stretching of surrounding tissue can lead to the same result.

✚ **Clinical presentation:** *Mallory-Weiss syndrome* is caused by paroxysmal vomiting with simultaneous antiperistalsis and cardial spasm in a stomach affected by prior gastric disease (alcohol, cortisone, radiation therapy, shock, or carcinoma). This results in longitudinal mucosal tears in the cardial and fundic region that lead to gastric bleeding.

Diapedesis Bleeding

Definition: Passage of blood through the intact walls of histologically normal capillaries in the form of diffuse punctate bleeding (purpura) or patches of extravasated blood (ecchymosis).

Pathogenetic principle: The various forms of diapedesis are attributable to ultrastructural microvascular damage. Four processes can cause such lesions:
— *Hypoxia:*
  — Asphyxiation with elevated venous pressure leads to Tardieu ecchymoses on serous membranes.
  — *Fat embolisms* can cause ischemia and lead to cerebral microhemorrhages (cerebral purpura).

— *Toxic and infectious* processes:
  — *Influenza viruses* cause endothelial toxicity with hemorrhagic tracheitis and pneumonia.
  — *Meningococci* produce endotoxins that lead to purpura fulminans (► E; testicular purpura).
  — *Streptococcal toxins* cause scarlet fever, leading to petechiae.

— *Toxic allergic* processes
  — can cause purpura.

— *Chemical toxins*
  — such as in chemotherapy for neoplastic disease can cause symptoms such as gastric diapedesis (► F).

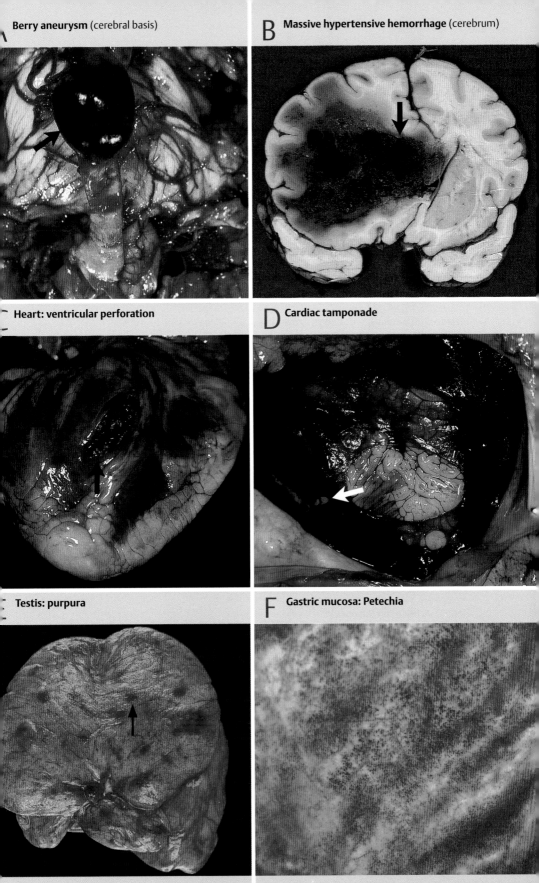

A Berry aneurysm (cerebral basis)

B Massive hypertensive hemorrhage (cerebrum)

Heart: ventricular perforation

D Cardiac tamponade

Testis: purpura

F Gastric mucosa: Petechia

Hemorrhagic Diathesis

Definition: Abnormally increased or extended bleeding due to an otherwise adequate cause or a generalized propensity to bleed in the absence of an adequate cause.

> **Note:** Hemorrhagic diathesis leads to diapedesis. In the absence of any histologic changes to the vessel wall, the etiology and pathogenesis of hemorrhagic diathesis and diapedesis overlap.

Causal pathogenesis: the following three vascular forms of hemorrhagic diathesis are differentiated:
— Congenital or acquired weakness in the vessel wall;
— Toxic-infectious vascular injury;
— Toxic-allergic vascular injury.

■ Osler-Weber-Rendu Disease

Synonym: hereditary hemorrhagic telangiectasia.

Definition: Hemorrhagic diathesis resulting from hereditary occurrence of multiple angiomatous telangiectasias.

Pathogenetic basis of this disease is a mutation of TGF-β-binding proteins including the endothelial endogelin, which disturbs the signal pathway involved in capillary development.

Morphology: Visible tangles of blood vessels measuring 1–2 mm are present in the skin and mucosa of the head; trunk; and respiratory, intestinal, and urogenital tracts (► A, B). Minor injuries cause bleeding.

➕ **Clinical presentation:** This very rare disorder exhibits an autosomal dominant inheritance pattern with irregular penetrance. Initial manifestations in puberty include nosebleeds that are difficult to control as well as bleeding in the skin, mucosa, oral cavity, nasopharyngeal space, and digits. Intestinal bleeding and hematuria also occur and lead to mild hypochromic anemia.

▦ Henoch-Schoenlein Purpura

Definition: Generalized purpura or ecchymoses as a result of a type III hypersensitivity (p. 170).

Pathogenesis: Several different antigens may act as pathogens depending on the patient's age:
— In *infants,* parvovirus B19 infection causes infectious erythema (p. 250).
— In *children* and especially boys, bacterial antigens (often streptococcus) are the pathogens.
— In *older persons,* allergens (p. 166) are the pathogens.

In each case, an antigen-antibody reaction leads to leukocytoclastic vasculitis (see p. 170, ► D).

➕ **Clinical presentation and morphology:** This disorder is less common. Symptoms include:
– skin and mucosal bleeding;
– *purpura,* generalized punctate bleeding (► C, skin bleeding);
– *ecchymoses,* small patches of bleeding (► D, conjunctiva).

Other symptoms include:
– alveolar hemorrhage;
– bleeding into the abdominal cavity;
– *bleeding from the wall of the intestine* leading to abdominal colic and melena;
– *renal bleeding* due to glomerulonephritis, leading to hematuria (often accompanied by serous polyarthritis).

> **Note:** The vascular forms of hemorrhagic diathesis are characterized by spontaneous purpura and a positive Rumpel-Leede test with a normal thrombocyte count and normal bleeding and coagulation times.

■ Thrombocytopenic Forms

General definition: Hemorrhagic diathesis resulting from thrombocyte deficiency.

General pathogenesis: The disorder is due to an abnormally low thrombocyte count or deficient thrombocyte function. In terms of causal pathogenesis, two forms are differentiated:

Aplastic forms occur as a result of genetically determined delayed thrombocytopoiesis in the bone marrow or toxic, radiation-induced, or tumor-induced bone marrow lesions.

Cytoclastic forms may occur as a result of *idiopathic increased destruction of thrombocytes* (as in idiopathic thrombocytopenic purpura Werlhof's disease). Here, viral infection or pharmaceutical incompatibility results in autoreactive antibodies against thrombocytes. Histocytes in the splenic pulp phagocytize the thrombocytes, leading to follicular enlargement (a sign of B-cell activation) and splenomegaly.

Cytoclastic forms may also occur as a result of *secondary increased destruction of thrombocytes* due to increased depletion or toxic injury.

➕ **Clinical presentation and morphology:**
Bleeding tests include a positive Rumpel-Leede test with increased bleeding time and normal coagulation time.
Skin and organ bleeding in the form of focal accentuated punctate bleeding (petechiae) occurs following minor trauma or spontaneously. Examples include petechial hemorrhage of the gastric mucosa (► E) and petechial pericardial hemorrhage (► F).

■ Thrombasthenic Forms

General definition: Rare hemorrhagic diathesis due to a congenital or acquired derangement of thrombocyte function with a normal thrombocyte count.

➕ **Clinical presentation and morphology:** This lesion is very rare.
– *Blood tests* show increased bleeding time.
– *Skin and organ bleeding* includes petechiae or ecchymosis.

> **Note:** Hemarthrosis is almost never observed in thrombocytopenia.

> **Note:** Critical threshold in number of thrombocytes: number in blood with adequate hemostasis: ca. 30,000 thrombocytes per mm³.

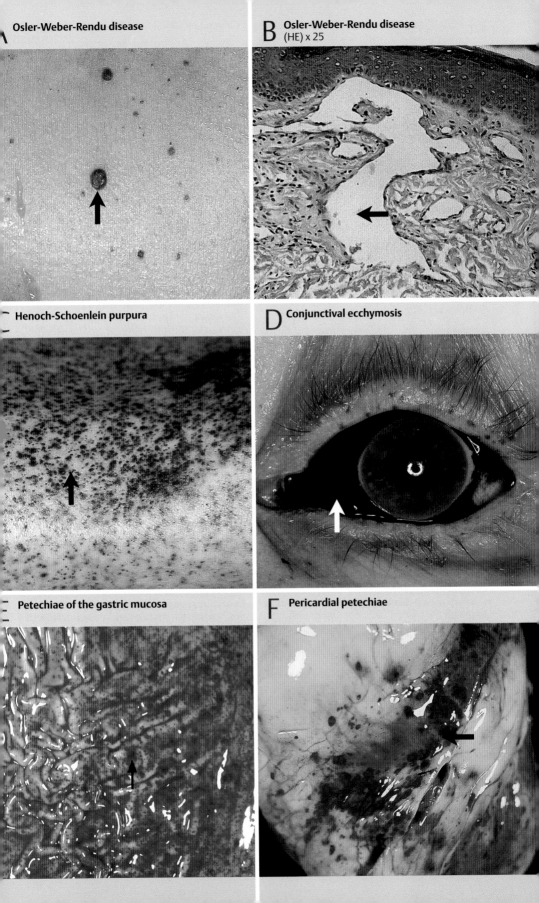

Osler-Weber-Rendu disease

B Osler-Weber-Rendu disease
(HE) x 25

Henoch-Schoenlein purpura

D Conjunctival ecchymosis

Petechiae of the gastric mucosa

F Pericardial petechiae

23

Generalized Cardiovascular Disorders

■ Coagulopathic Forms

General definition: Hemorrhagic diathesis due to a congenital or acquired defect of the coagulation system.

✚ **General clinical presentation:** All forms of coagulation disorders are characterized by widespread bleeding such as ecchymoses (► A; petechiae are characteristically absent). Hematomas in soft tissue (such as bleeding into the psoas) are occasionally present.

▦ Hemophilia A (rare)

Textbook example of an X-linked recessive defect.

Definition: Hereditary coagulation disorder involving a factor VIII deficiency.

Factor VIII is composed of the following components:
— Factor VIII – C is the active coagulant component.
— Factor VIII – R is the regulator carrier protein.
— Factor VIII – VWF is the platelet adhesion factor.

Pathogenesis: The disorder involves factor VIII – C dysplasia (type A+) or deficient synthesis of factor VIII – C (type A−).

✚ **Clinical presentation and morphology:** The disease is passed from female carriers to their sons. Several types of bleeding typically occur.
Hemarthrosis occurs in 95 % of all cases. Everyday activities such as climbing stairs lead to microtrauma with recurrent bleeding into the joint space. The blood diffuses into the synovial membrane (► B) and into the articular cartilage. There it is absorbed, leading to deposits of hemosiderin in the synovial membrane and joint capsule with brown discoloration (► C). This results in irreversible damage to the articular cartilage with progressive degenerative joint disease and deformity leading to stiffening of the joint (► B).
Muscular hematomas occur in 60 % of all cases. This usually takes the form of bleeding into the psoas after blunt microtrauma from everyday activities.
Bleeding in the gums occurs in 50 % of all cases.
Urogenital bleeding occurs in 40 % of all cases. This manifests itself as hematuria, menorrhagia, and metrorrhagia (► D, uterine bleeding).
Intestinal bleeding occurs in 40 % of all cases. This manifests itself as melena (bloody stools).
Epistaxis (nosebleed) occurs in 30 % of all cases.

☺ **Prominent patients:** Queen Victoria of Britain (1819–1901) was a carrier of the disease. Intermarriage among European royalty brought forth manifestations of hemophilia A among the czars of Russia and the house of Bourbon in Spain.

❗ **Note:** *Spontaneous hemarthrosis in children* may be a sign of hemophilia. Verification of the child's coagulation status is indicated in such cases.

▦ Disseminated Intravascular Coagulation

Definition: Hemorrhagic diathesis due to depletion of clotting factors (abbreviation: DIC).

Etiologic factors include hereditary intravascular coagulation (common) and idiopathic plasma inactivation with simultaneous proteolysis of clotting factors (rare).

Pathogenetic chain reaction: Excessive activation of clotting factors in nearly the entire circulatory system, leading to endothelial injury, occurs as a result of the following processes:

— *Procoagulant activity* resulting from generation of procoagulant substances such as histamine, adrenaline, serotonin, and endotoxin;
— *Action of thromboplastin* released from tissue with a high thromboplastin content, such as in premature separation of the placenta;
— *Platelet activation* due to contact of blood with a "foreign surface," such as in dialysis;
— *Thrombin activation* due to the release of proteolytic substances that act like thrombin, such as snake venom.

The result of these processes is intravascular coagulation (see Shwartzman-Sanarelli reaction, p. 394) with formation of microthrombi. Cells of the RES continue to intercept the thrombi until their receptors are saturated, resulting in an RES blockade (p. 26, 350). The microthrombi remain in the bloodstream and obstruct the capillary structures, injuring the erythrocytes mechanically and leading to microangiopathic hemolytic anemia (► E). This leads to hypoxic endothelial and tissue damage. A plasma activator in the tissue activates the fibrinolysis system.

✚ **Result:** Activation of the clotting and fibrinolysis system leads to hemorrhagic diathesis and multiple thrombi in the microvasculature. This results in a shock syndrome with multiple microinfarcts and/or larger infarcts, primarily in the brain and renal cortex.

Experimental examples of disseminated intravascular coagulation (DIC) include the Shwartzman-Sanarelli reaction (p. 394) and experiments *in vitro*. In the latter, a frozen section of lung tissue from a DIC patient is covered with a layer of fibrin and incubated. Because the fibrinolysis system is activated, the fibrin film over the blood vessels will be lysed (► F).

❗ **Note:** *Complications of bleeding* include anemia. *Iron deficiency anemia* results from chronic blood loss. The erythrocytes contain insufficient iron to synthesize hemoglobin. This has several consequences.
– In the *peripheral blood,* the erythrocytes are reduced in number and size (microcytes), and their hemoglobin content is diminished (hypochromasia).
– *Bone marrow* exhibits compensatory hyperplasia with an increased number of immature erythropoiesis precursor cells.

Sequelae of anemia include chronic hypoxemic hypoxia with corresponding organ changes (p. 68).

❗ **Note:** *Anemia is defined* as a hemoglobin concentration of less than 130 g/l in men and less than 120 g/l in women.

Aside from these generalized cardiovascular disorders in the form of deranged blood pressure or coagulation, localized disorders can also occur in individual vascular regions. These disorders will be discussed in the next chapter.

A Ecchymosis

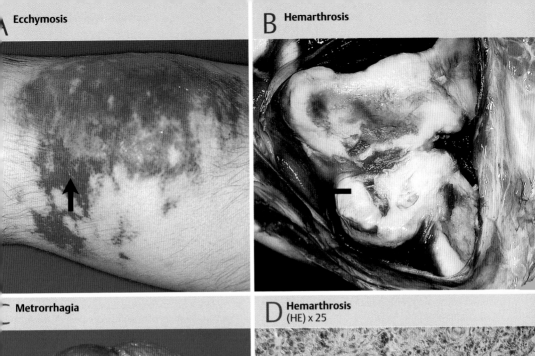

B Hemarthrosis

C Metrorrhagia

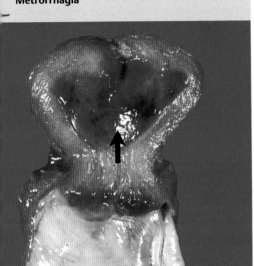

D Hemarthrosis
(HE) x 25

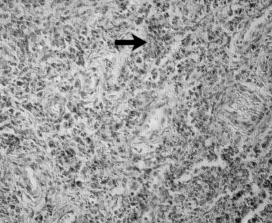

E DIC: Microthrombosis in lung vessels
(PAS) x 150

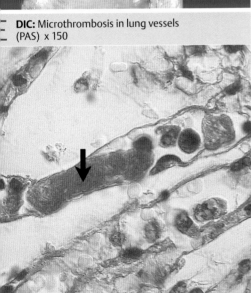

F DIC: Fibrinolysis in lung vessels
(lung tissue coated with fibrin) x 15

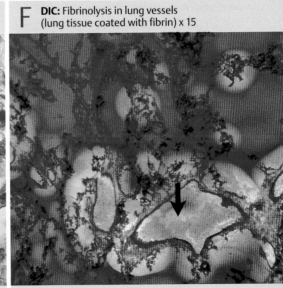

Traffic Jams on Major and Secondary Routes
Localized Circulatory Disorders

Summary

The efficiency of the circulatory system is based on normal fluid dynamics of blood. Deviations from the normal state have several consequences.

▶ **Thrombosis:** Formation of intravascular thrombi *in vivo* may be aptly described as hemostasis at the wrong site. This occurs as a result of defects in the vessel wall, abnormal blood flow, and blood hypercoagulability. Different types of thrombosis will form depending on which of these three components (known as Virchow's triad) initiates the process. Types of thrombi include red, mixed, and hyaline thrombi.

▶ **Embolism:** This refers to substances such as of thrombi, fat, and air carried by the blood to sites distant from their point of origin. The venous forms most often lead to pulmonary embolism, the arterial forms to organ infarction.

▶ **Arterial hemodynamic disorders** involve hypoperfusion with resulting hypoxia and reduced clear-

ance of waste products. This is referred to as ischemia. Three distinct subtypes may be identified according to their duration and severity:

— *Absolute persistent ischemia* is complete occlusion of the terminal artery over an extended period of time, resulting in necrosis in the region supplied by the artery.
— *Absolute temporary ischemia* is complete occlusion of the terminal artery for a limited period of time, resulting in minor hypoxic injury.
— *Relative ischemia* or functional ischemia is a mismatch between the amount of blood the vessels can supply and the oxygen demands of the tissue supplied.

▶ **Venous hemodynamic disorders** are caused by impaired drainage of venous blood, which leads to venous stasis or a hemorrhagic infarction.

Thrombosis

Definition: Occlusion of the vascular or cardiac lumen by a thrombus, a fibrinous aggregate of thrombocytes and/or clot occurring *in vivo*. This disorder is very common.

Causal Pathogenesis

Thrombosis is hemostasis at the wrong site and is attributable to what is known as Virchow's triad:
— Endothelial lesion of the vessel wall;
— Hemodynamic abnormality;
— Hypercoagulability.

■ Endothelial Lesion ("wall factor")

This occurs as a result of a *pathogenetic chain reaction.* Damage to the vascular endothelium (such as can occur in inflammation, ▶ A) leads to deficiency of the endothelial factors that inhibit coagulation. It also exposes the microfibrillar subendothelial tissue. This allows the thrombocyte adhesion and coagulation activation factors in that tissue to take effect (p. 407, ▶ A).

■ Hemodynamic Abnormality ("flow factor")

Both high and low rates of flow promote thrombosis.
Decelerated blood flow (▶ B) causes venous thrombosis. *Etiologic factors* include:
— Widening of the vessels (varicose veins; ▶ C, D);
— Increased hematocrit levels (as in desiccation);
— Increased viscosity (as in paraproteinemia);
— Vascular impingement (as in bedridden patients).

This leads to agglutination of erythrocytes and aggregation of thrombocytes (▶ B). Stagnating blood flow also causes an oxygen deficit leading to endothelial injury.

Accelerated blood flow in combination with turbulence causes arterial thrombosis.

Etiologic factors include local vascular stenosis.

This presses thrombocytes against the surface of the endothelium, creating a platelet thrombus (p. 407 B).

Maelstrom in the blood flow. Etiologic factors include:
— Local widening of the vessel (such as an aneurysm);
— Impaired passage (such as calcified venous valves);
— Vascular bifurcations.

The resulting turbulence in the blood flow develops shear forces that can cause the endothelium to separate from underlying tissue.

■ Hypercoagulability ("blood factor")

Hereditary etiologic factors include:
— Mutated factor V (Leiden's factor);
— Mutated prothrombin;
— Hereditary deficiency in anticoagulants.

Acquired etiologic factors include:
— Tissue injury with release of clotting factors, hyperlipidemia, pregnancy, oral contraceptives, thrombocytosis;
— *Heparin-induced thrombocytopenic syndrome* with antibodies against heparin-platelet-factor IV-complex after treatment with unfractionated heparin;
— *Antiphospholipid-antibody syndrome:* antibodies against phospholipids are generated as a sequela of autoimmune diseases (SLE, p. 180), drug or bacterial exposition.

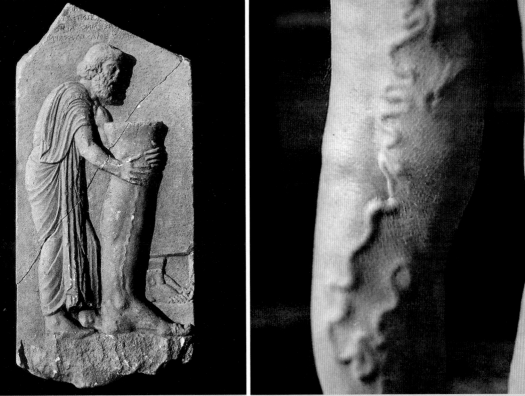

A **Wall factor:** Thrombus on an endothelial defect: polyarteritis nodosa (PAS) x 75

B **Flow factor:** Slowed blood flow (intravital microscopy) x 40

C **Varicose veins in the leg** in ancient votive sculpture

D **Varicose veins in the leg**

Forms of Thrombi

The structure of thrombi varies according to the causative mechanism.

■ Laminated Thrombus (depository Thrombus)

Etiologic factors include endothelial injury in:
- Atherosclerotic plaque rupture;
- Vasculitis and endocarditis;
- Arterial and cardiac aneurysm.

Pathogenesis: Endothelial injury exposes the subendothelial microfibrils (► A1). These microfibrils come into contact with the flowing blood and cause thrombocytes to precipitate on to them (► A2). This creates a "white platelet thrombus" (or primary platelet thrombus) (► B) and activates the coagulation cascade. Fibrin is then precipitated over the platelet thrombus, and large numbers of erythrocytes and a few leukocytes become caught in the fibrinous mesh. The thrombus grows as these deposits increase, and projects into the bloodstream. This creates turbulence in the blood flow that causes additional thrombocytes, fibrin, and bloods cells to precipitate. The net result is progressive growth of the thrombus with characteristic periodic layering (► D) of white structures (aggregations of thrombocytes; ► D1) and red structures (fibrin erythrocytes; ► D2).

The cut surface of mural thrombi (thrombi on a vessel wall) exhibits a pattern resembling tree rings as a result of this process.

Morphology:

- **Platelet thrombi** are brittle gray thrombi that adhere to the vessel wall. They consist of a uniformly alternating pattern of aggregated thrombocytes and erythrocytes interspersed with fibrin.
  Result: These thrombi are *brittle,* with little fibrin.
- **Intermediate thrombi** are produced by uniform deposition of aggregates of thrombocytes and erythrocytes perpendicular to the direction of blood flow. This creates a pattern of surface laminations referred to as lines of Zahn (► C, atrial appendage). The thrombus exhibits a coral-like arrangement of thrombocyte aggregates admixed with granulocytes, resulting in a white and red pattern of laminations perpendicular to the direction of blood flow (► D).
  Result: These thrombi are *elastic* and exhibit a certain degree of mechanical resistance.

■ Red Thrombus (stagnation thrombus)

Etiologic factors include reduced blood flow in:
- Ligated blood vessels;
- Vascular occlusion due to a laminated thrombus in a previously compromised blood vessel or blood-filled cavity;
- Slowed blood flow as a result of abnormal irreversibly widened venous walls (varices).

Pathogenesis: Various etiologic factors lead to stagnating blood flow. Within the stagnant blood, hypoxia (p. 22, 68) leads to thrombocyte injury. The injured thrombocytes release substances that activate coagulation, resulting in precipitation of fibrin.

Morphologic findings include a thrombus with the same homogeneous red color as the blood from which it formed (► E). A red thrombus usually becomes deposited on an intermediate thrombus or the head of a laminated thrombus. This thrombus is loosely held together by a sparse random mesh of fibrin. *Later,* the fibrin retracts, producing a thin, flattened thrombus that is again able to float in the vascular lumen. The result is that all or part of the thrombus can be torn loose by simple actions such as pressing on the abdomen or defecation. The thrombus then travels through the bloodstream where it can form an embolus.

Result: These thrombi are low in fibrin and therefore *brittle and inelastic* with low mechanical resistance.

■ Mixed Thrombus

Primary etiologic factor: persistent stasis of the blood.

Morphologic findings include a thrombus composed of one or more laminated thrombi with interspersed or apposed red thrombi. These thrombi appear as long occlusive casts of the vascular lumen.

■ Hyaline Thrombus

Primary etiologic factor: disseminated intravascular coagulation (p. 400).

Morphologic findings include a homogeneous eosinophilic red thrombus in minor vessels such as capillaries, arterioles, and venules (► F). The thrombus is composed of disintegrated thrombocytes and fibrin. These thrombi are hyaline micro-thrombi.

> **Note:** The *clinical rule of thumb* for a red thrombus is that it arises unnoticed in the lee; a gust of wind will carry it away.

> **Note:** The *clinical rule of thumb* for thrombus adhesion is that a *red thrombus* "floats" (hardly adheres at all), a *white thrombus* "sticks" (adheres slightly), and an *intermediate thrombus* "adheres".

> **Note:** The *commonest site* for thrombi is in the veins of the lower legs of bedridden patients.

> **Note:** *Signs of thrombosis* include:
> - tenderness of veins to palpation;
> - foot pain upon dorsiflexion;
> - edema in the leg (demonstrated by comparative measurements).

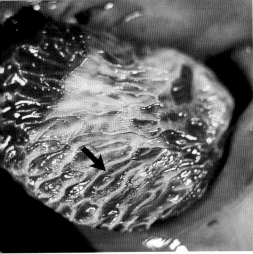

A Thrombocyte on an endothelial defect
(TEM) x 20000

2 →
1 →

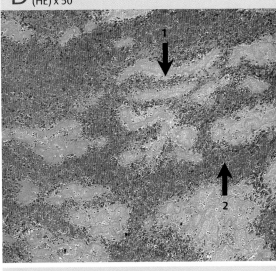

B Platelet thrombus
(intravital microscopy) x 25

C Intermediate thrombus: cardiac auricle
lines of Zahn

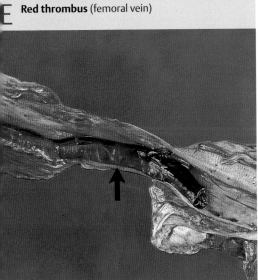

D Intermediate thrombus
(HE) x 50

1

2

E Red thrombus (femoral vein)

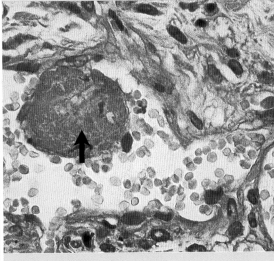

F Hyaline thrombus (lung)
(PAS) x 100

24

Localized Circulatory Disorders

Forms of Thrombosis

■ Venous Thrombosis

Occurrence: Most common form of thrombosis.
Etiologic factors:
— **Right heart failure**, especially in bedridden patients, leads to slowed blood flow with deep venous thrombosis in the thigh and the pelvic veins (▶ A). This can produce a pulmonary embolism.
— **Varices** (widened veins) lead to slowed blood flow with superficial venous thrombosis that can lead to thrombophlebitis.
— **Cerebral sinus thrombosis** due to post-traumatic or septic thrombus can lead to hemorrhagic cerebral infarction (p. 422).

■ Arterial Thrombosis

Etiologic factors:
— **Aneurysm** (▶ C1): causes turbulence, resulting in formation of a mural thrombus on the interior surface of the vessel wall (▶ C2). This can lead to arterial embolism.
— **Compromised arterial wall** in atherosclerosis (p. 90) can lead to a mural thrombus.

■ Cardiac Thrombosis

Etiologic factors:
— **Endocardial lesions** in endocarditis lead to formation of thrombi on the margins of the valves known as vegetations. These can lead to arterial embolism.
— **A myocardial aneurysm** in myocardial infarction (p. 418) leads to localized ventricular immobility and lesion of the heart wall. This in turn causes mural thrombus.
— **Dilation of the cardiac auricle** slows the blood flow (p. 404), producing a ball thrombus.
— **Atrial dilation** in mitral stenosis and atrial fibrillation leads to mural thrombus.

Sequelae of Thrombosis

Thrombus organization occurs according to the following timetable:

Day 1: The thrombus arises.
Day 2: The thrombus (▶ E1) becomes endothelialized (▶ E2).
Day 3: The leukocytes in the thrombus disintegrate, leaving only vestiges of the cells.
Day 4: The thrombus has become completely homogenized, with hyalinization of the fibrin-erythrocyte aggregates.
Day 7: Organization of the thrombus begins. Capillary-rich granulation tissue (▶ F1) branches outward from the vascular wall (▶ B1) into the thrombotic fibrin (▶ F3). This leads to proteolytic lysis and phagocytosis of the thrombus. The capillaries establish connections to the vascular system, and the thrombus becomes recanalized.
Day 28: Subintimal myofibroblasts trigger the sclerosis process.

Several conditions may occur secondary to impaired thrombus organization:

■ Recurrent Thrombus

Pathogenesis: Scarring sclerosis of the vascular intima can cause a residual mesh of strands of connective tissue to remain after the thrombus is lysed. These strands can act as a "seed crystal" for a recurrent thrombus.

■ Obliteration of the Vessel

Pathogenesis: The thrombus becomes transformed into scarring that occludes the vascular lumen.

■ Post-thrombotic Syndrome

Pathogenesis: Organization of the thrombus with scarring of the venous valves leads to venous stasis. This has several consequences. The resulting varices lead to recurrent thrombi, which in turn exacerbate the venous stasis. This leads to edema with sclerosis and skin atrophy, which in turn causes necrosis of the skin and venous ulcer (often an ulcer of the leg).

■ Puriform Thrombolysis

Pathogenesis: Reactive post-thrombotic inflammation of the vessel wall leads to granulocytic and proteolytic lysis of the thrombus.

This manifests itself clinically as thrombophlebitis.

■ Thrombus Calcification

Pathogenesis: Delayed organization of the thrombus leads to thrombus calcification. The calcified area later ossifies to form a phlebolith (p. 134).

■ Thromboembolism (p. 410)

A thrombus that becomes detached from the wall of the vessel is carried away by the blood. This body then lodges in a vascular bifurcation or in a branch of the vessel, where it produces tissue necrosis (p. 128).

✚ **Complications** of thromboembolism vary according to the specific vascular system involved:
Arterial thromboembolism: The arterial system narrows from the aorta to the arterioles. This means that a dislodged thrombus will occlude a small artery.
Venous thromboembolism: The venous system widens in the direction of flow from the venules to the vena cava. This means that a dislodged thrombus will occlude a large vein (often a pulmonary vein). The *result* is a systemic cardiovascular disorder (see below).

! **Note:** In *therapeutic thrombolysis,* hyaline thrombotic foci can remain for years but will still respond to fibrinolysis.

! **Note:** *Differential diagnosis* of clotting *post mortem.*
Cruor: *Pathogenesis:* rapid postmortem clotting.
Morphology: This is a smooth elastic homogeneous red clot of all blood components, primarily erythrocytes admixed with fibrin. The clot does not adhere to the vessel walls, and cruor can be drawn out of all vessels as a cast of the vascular lumen at autopsy (▶ B).
Bacong clot: *Pathogenesis:* Erythrocytes precipitate due to a coagulation disorder or high blood sedimentation rate, and clots form over them.
Morphology: This is a smooth elastic postmortem clot not adhering to the vessel walls, having a glassy yellowish appearance and lacking erythrocytes.

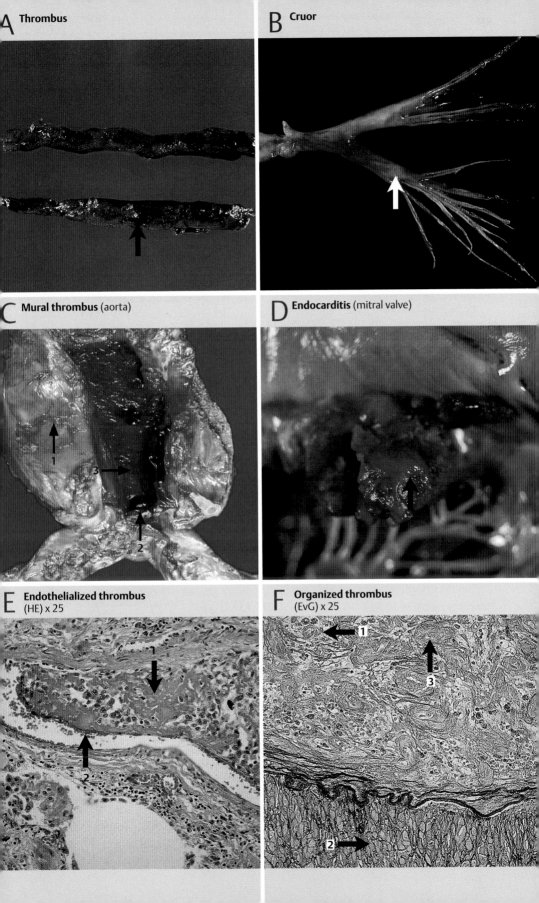

A Thrombus

B Cruor

C Mural thrombus (aorta)

D Endocarditis (mitral valve)

E Endothelialized thrombus
(HE) x 25

F Organized thrombus
(EvG) x 25

Embolism

Definition: Process in which certain substances enter the bloodstream in larger vessels as coherent bodies (emboli) and lodge in and occlude smaller vessels.

Several types of embolisms may be differentiated according to the *material* forming the embolus. In descending order of incidence, these include:
— *Thrombotic embolus*;
— *Fat embolus* of plugs of fat or bone marrow;
— *Air embolus* of air bubbles or foam;
— *Parasitic embolus* of parasitic larvae;
— *Bacterial embolus* of fibrin-coated bacteria;
— *Tumor embolus* of fibrin-coated tumor cells (▶ p. 348 E);
— *Amniotic fluid embolus*;
— *Foreign body embolus,* such as the tip of a venous catheter;
— *Organ embolus*, such as liver cells in ERCP.[1]

Embolisms are also differentiated according to the underlying *hemodynamic mechanism:*
— *Orthograde embolism* (direct embolisms) is an embolism occurring in the direction of blood flow. This is common. As the veins become wider in the direction of blood (except for the branches of the portal vein), this type of embolism usually occurs in the arteries (▶ A).
— *Retrograde embolism* is very rare. One example of such an embolism is an embolus of tumor cells carried opposite to the direction of blood flow from the prevertebral venous plexus toward the spinal column due to increased abdominal pressure.
— *Crossed embolism* (paradoxical embolism) is rare. Such embolism may occur in the presence of an open foramen ovale (▶ B1) or defect in the septum of the left atrium. Where the pressure in the right atrium also greatly exceeds that of the left atrium (as in right heart insufficiency), an embolus (▶ B2) from the pulmonary vessels can pass into the extrapulmonary vessels.

Thromboembolism

Definition: Passage of thrombus material into the arterial or venous system.

■ Venous Thromboembolism (very common)

This type of embolism usually occurs as a pulmonary embolism, less often as a portal vein embolism.

▦ Pulmonary Embolism

Occurrence: In 20% of all hospital patients.

Definition: Passage of thrombus material into the pulmonary veins, resulting in vascular occlusion and life-threatening venous thrombosis.

Thrombogenetic factors:
— Weight: Obese patients are more often affected than slender patients.
— Gender: Men are twice as like to develop pulmonary embolisms as women.

— Age: Older patients are more often affected than younger patients.
— Meteorology: Passage of atmospheric fronts affects thromboembolism.

Location of source thrombus:
The thrombus originates in veins of the thigh or pelvis in 90% of all cases; in 10%, it originates in the deep veins of the calf or in the periprostatic or periuterine venous plexus.

Dislodging factors of the source thrombus:
— Abrupt alternating dorsiflexion and plantar flexion of the foot acts as a pump and accelerates blood flow in the calf.
— The inguinal ligament can cut off a red thrombus as the patient sits up in bed.
— Venous pressure is increased when the patient defecates and coughs.
— Fibrinolysis leads to thrombus loosening and fragmentation.

Morphology of pulmonary embolism:
— *Peripheral pulmonary embolism* is painless in the case of right heart insufficiency but produce pain and expectoration of blood in the case of left heart insufficiency.
  Result: A small (peripheral) embolism.

— *"Shrapnel" embolism* is brittles red thrombi that fragment upon breaking free of the vessel wall or as they hits a vascular bifurcation. These fragments then occlude central and peripheral pulmonary arteries.
  Result: A central and peripheral embolism.

— *Straddling embolism* is pliable laminated thrombi that straddle a vascular bifurcation (▶ C), occluding the trunk of the pulmonary artery of the entire outflow tract.
  Result: A central embolism (▶ A).

+ Complications of pulmonary embolism:
Acute cor pulmonale results where an embolism occludes more than 85% of the cross-section of the pulmonary flow tract. Death occurs due to right heart failure.
Chronic cor pulmonale may occur secondary to massive pulmonary embolism with subtotal occlusion of the central branches of the pulmonary artery or as a result of recurrent peripheral embolisms.
Pulmonary infarction (▶ D): The lungs have a double vascular supply via the right heart and pulmonary arteries and via the left heart and bronchial arteries. As a result, pulmonary infarction occurs only where embolic occlusion of a branch of the pulmonary artery occurs in the presence of left heart insufficiency such as mitral stenosis. The slight residual flow through the bronchopulmonary anastomoses causes extravasation of capillary blood in the walls of the dying alveoli. As a result, a pulmonary infarction is always hemorrhagic (with few exceptions) and exhibits a characteristic wedge shape.
Recurrent embolism: Pulmonary embolisms become organized into stranded structures (p. 408). These strands can trap smaller emboli (▶ E, F), causing occlusion of a branch of the pulmonary artery. In this manner, a peripheral embolism may become a central embolism.

! Note: Venous thromboembolism is far more common than arterial thromboembolism.

---

[1] ERCP = endoscopic retrograde cholangiopancreatography.

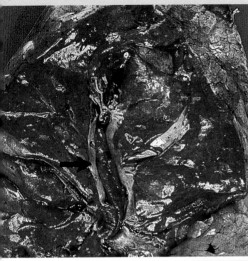

A Pulmonary embolism

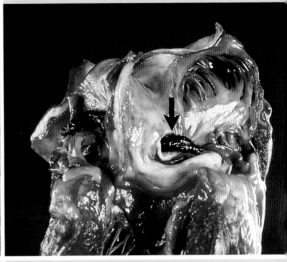

B Crossed embolism

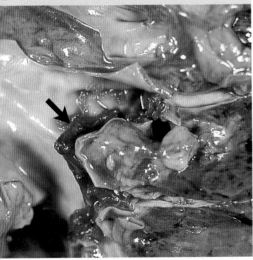

C Straddling embolism

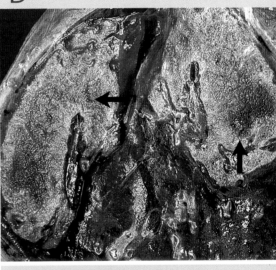

D Pulmonary infarction

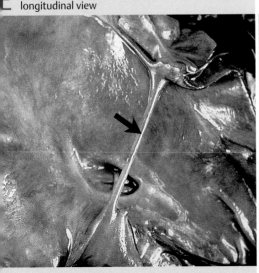

E Strand of organized embolism:
longitudinal view

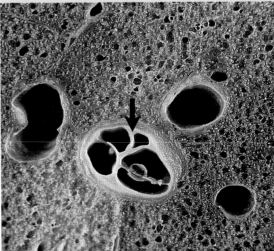

F Strand of organized embolism:
cross-sectional view

■ Arterial Thromboembolism

Pathogenesis and sequelae vary according to the source of the thrombus.

Source thrombi in the left heart can occur:
— In the left atrium with atrial fibrillation;
— In the left ventricle due to myocardial infarction;
— In the left ventricle due to parietal endocarditis;
— In the heart valves in bacterial endocarditis.

Source thrombi in the aorta can occur in atherosclerosis
— With plaque rupture, creating microembolisms (often in the form of cholesterol embolisms; see below). This results in the release of thrombotic material into the arterial bloodstream, and the embolism lodges in a peripheral arterial bifurcation.

✚**Complications** vary according to the vessel affected.
Encephalomalacia (p. 420) results from cerebral arterial embolism.
Infarction of the small bowel results from mesenteric arterial embolism.
Renal infarction (hematuria) results from renal arterial embolism.
Gangrene of the leg results from femoral arterial embolism.

Fat Embolism

Definition: These are lipid aggregations carried by the bloodstream to the lungs, from which they enter systemic arterial circulation.

■ Traumatic Fat Embolism (common)

Etiologic factors for the occurrence of fat embolisms:
— **Multiple fractures** or cortical bones lead to the release of fatty bone marrow and occasionally medulla as well (► A).
— **Impingement of subcutaneous fat** by crush injuries or cramps leads to the release of fat droplets into the bloodstream.
— **Burns** involving the skin and subcutaneous fatty tissue can result in liquefaction of fat with release of fat droplets into the bloodstream.

Pathogenesis: The fat droplets are initially released into the lymph system from which they are transported via the venous bloodstream into the lung. There, enzymes act on the fat.

Result of this enzymatic action depends on the quantity of fat.
— *Small quantities* are broken down by endothelial lipase.
— *Large quantities* cannot be sufficiently broken down by enzymatic action. They occlude the pulmonary flow tract (► B) and cause acute cor pulmonale.

■ Fat Emboli Syndrome (rare)

Pathogenesis: This disorder occurs in traumatic shock following a clinically asymptomatic interval of several days. The origin of the fat embolism is not yet understood.

Possible mechanism: A compensatory sympathetic adrenergic response in the hyperdynamic phase of shock causes catecholamines to be released. This leads to lipo-

lysis with release of fatty acids from the fatty tissue, which in turn leads to re-esterification of the fatty acids to triglycerides in the liver. These triglycerides are released into the venous bloodstream, which transports them to the lung. There, epithelial damage and lack of endothelial lipase prevents lipid breakdown.

Result: Formation of fatty microthrombi that cause fat embolisms in the brain and cerebral purpura (punctate bleeding areas of necrosis; ► C).

Air Embolism (rare)

Definition: Occlusion of the pulmonary microvasculature by air bubbles.

Etiologic factors for entry of air into the venous system include:
— Induction of air into a gaping vein during a goiter operation or as a result of separation of the placenta In an atonic uterus;
— Air drawn into a vein as a result of improper intravenous infusion technique;
— Air pressed into a vein in an explosion injury.

Pathogenesis: A quantity of air exceeding 5 ml rapidly enters the venous bloodstream and triggers the following chain reaction. Foam forms in the blood and collects in the right ventricle of the heart. From there, the foam is carried via the branches of the pulmonary artery to the pulmonary microvasculature. There, air bubbles interrupt the continuity of blood flow, producing hypoxic injury to the capillary endothelium. This in turn triggers platelet adhesion and degranulation, and these processes generate inflammation mediators (p. 202).

Result: Exudative alveolitis (p. 40) that leads to interstitial pulmonary edema and increases the load on the right heart (ARDS).

Cholesterol Embolism (rare)

Pathogenesis: Rupture of a plaque in atherosclerosis (p. 90) or placement of a stent in the presence of an atherosclerotic aortic aneurysm releases cholesterol-containing detritus into the bloodstream, causing embolism, which:

Results in arterial microembolisms (primarily occurring in the abdominal organs) that exhibit characteristic cholesterol crystal gaps (► D).

Amniotic Fluid Embolism (rare)

Pathogenesis: A tear in the myometrium occurring during amniorrhexis results in induction of amniotic fluid into the mother's bloodstream. Thrombokinase in the fluid causes hypercoagulability. Fibrinolytic substances lead to fibrinolysis, and vasoactive substances cause shock.

Result: Disseminated intravascular coagulation (p. 402).

Parasite Embolism (rare)

Pathogenesis: The release into the venous bloodstream of substances of parasitic origin such as *Echinococcus* cysts (p. 282) in cardiac echinococcosis (► E), which can lead to embolism.

Result: Occlusion of the pulmonary artery (► F).

A Bone marrow embolism (lung)
(silver stain) x 25

B Fat embolism (lung)
(toluidine blue) x 200

Cerebral purpura (brain)
(HE) x 50

D Cholesterol embolism
(EvG) x 50

E Cardiac echinococcosis

F Echinococcal hydatid embolism (lung)

Arterial Circulatory Disorders

Recapitulation: See ischemia and tissue necrosis (p. 22, 68, and 128).

Several types of ischemia are differentiated according to their duration and severity. These include:

— *absolute persistent ischemia;*
— *absolute temporary ischemia;*
— *temporary acute ischemia;*
— *chronic relative ischemia.*

Absolute Persistent Ischemia

General definition: Ischemic hypoxidotic tissue necrosis in the area supplied by a terminal artery due to complete, persistent occlusion of this artery in the absence of sufficient collateral circulation.

Etiologic factors of absolute persistent ischemia involves.

Structural occlusion of an artery with impaired supply may occur due to:

— Thromboembolic disease;
— Arteriosclerosis;
— Vasculitis with thrombosis;
— Vascular compression (as in vessels surrounded by tumors);
— Ligature.

Result: Occlusive vascular disease in the form of obturation infarction.

Functional occlusion of an artery with hypoperfusion of the area it supplies (► A, B) may occur for several reasons.

— *Hemodynamic factors* include sudden hypotension secondary to subtotal arterial stenosis.
— *Hematogenous factors* include sudden increased oxygen consumption (exertion such as climbing stairs), sudden reduced oxygen saturation of the blood, and sudden thickening of the blood (for example due to cryoglobulins).
— *Vasogenic factors* causing persistent vascular spasms of anatomically patent vessels (► A1) include toxic factors such as cardiac glycosides (► A), ergot alkaloids, and lead or nicotine poisoning; hypotensive crises; and hypothalamic dysregulation with increased sympathetic vascular tone (as in Raynaud's syndrome).

Results: Include non-occlusive vascular disorders such as a non-obturation infarct in the heart or small bowel (► A2, B) and gangrene in the extremities.

Pathogenetic chain reaction: Absolute persistent ischemia produces an area of tissue necrosis known as an infarct. The size of the infarct depends on several factors, including:

— The diameter of the occluded artery;
— The quality of existing collateral vessels;
— The elasticity of the collateral vessels.

Acute occlusion of a major artery in an organ with sufficient collateral circulation overburdens these collateral vessels. The collateral circulation becomes insufficient to nourish the area normally supplied by the occluded artery, and the flow of blood comes to a standstill in the periphery.

The *result* is ischemic tissue necrosis (usually in the form of coagulative necrosis that preserves the tissue structure, except in the brain where liquefactive necrosis occurs) and infarction.

■ Anemic Infarct

General definition: Tissue necrosis due to persistent loss of blood supply from an anatomic terminal artery (without collateral circulation) or a functional terminal artery (with insufficient collateral circulation).

General morphology: The earliest macroscopic sign of infarction occurs after 6 hours in the form of a yellowish area of tissue. The infarct has several distinct sections:

— The *center* exhibits complete tissue necrosis (example: ► C1, D; bone infarct).
— The *periphery* exhibits a hemorrhagic margin with incomplete tissue necrosis with masses of erythrocytes in the capillaries resulting from the slight, insufficient residual blood supply (► C2).
— An *edematous area surrounding the necrosis* is the result of exudative inflammation with sublethal cell injury.

The organ tissue surrounding the necrosis responds to an infarct as it would to an injury. The lesion triggers the wound healing process, and the necrotic area is organized by granulation tissue and heals with scarring. The further development of the infarct depends on the load the affected tissue has to bear. Infarcted areas subject to compressive loads dilate; infarcted areas that do not bear such loads shrink.

■ Hemorrhagic Infarct

General definition: Tissue necrosis due to persistent occlusion of a terminal artery with slight, insufficient residual blood supply.

General pathogenesis: There are several sources of the residual blood supply to the infarct.

Arterial occlusion:

— Collateral circulation supplies blood (for example in a mesenteric infarct).
— Retrograde venous blood flow may occur due to increased venous pressure (for example in a mesenteric infarct).
— In anatomic regions with a double vascular supply, secondary vessels provide some supply to the area where primary vessels are occluded (for example in a hemorrhagic pulmonary infarct; ► E, F).

Venous occlusion (p. 422):

— Venous thrombosis prevents drainage of blood. This produces tissue ischemia with necrosis and locally increased blood pressure that leads to bleeding into tissue.

General morphology: Findings include a dark red cyanotic area of necrosis projecting above the normal anatomic plane due to engorgement with blood (► E, F). The infarct heals with granulation tissue and scarring, with characteristic brown discoloration due to hemosiderin.

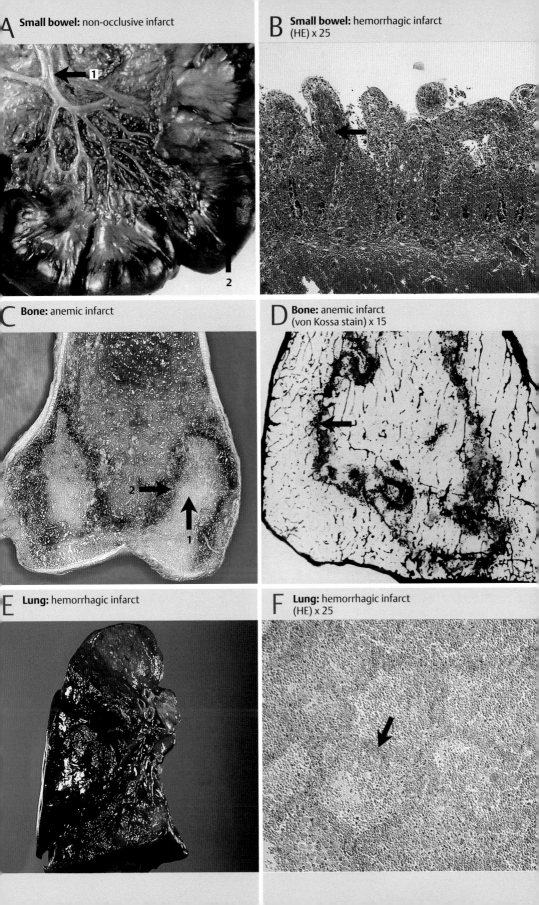

A **Small bowel:** non-occlusive infarct

B **Small bowel:** hemorrhagic infarct (HE) x 25

C **Bone:** anemic infarct

D **Bone:** anemic infarct (von Kossa stain) x 15

E **Lung:** hemorrhagic infarct

F **Lung:** hemorrhagic infarct (HE) x 25

Absolute Temporary Ischemia

General definition: Minor tissue injury in the form of disseminated necrosis or hypoxic cell changes due to brief loss of blood supply.

General pathogenesis: The extent of tissue injury is usually only minimal (▶ A), and it depends on the specific organ's or tissue's tolerance of ischemia, which also determines its recovery time. Tissue injury can normally be repaired by normal regeneration if the blood supply is restored to the affected area within its recovery time by:

— Thromboembolectomy;
— Spasmolysis;
— Releasing the hemostat in a transplanted organ.

Relative Ischemia

Synonym: oligemia.

General definition: Disproportion between the currently available blood supply and the current demand for oxygen of an organ or tissue.

This may be illustrated by the analogy of the "farthest field":

A certain supply of water is sufficient to irrigate an area of farmland. A reduction in the flow of water means that there will barely be enough to irrigate the farthest field. When the volume of water required increases in hot weather, the farthest field is the one that dries out.

General pathogenesis: Here, the oxygen deficit is the result of two limiting factors: (a) the volume of blood flow and/or the oxygen content of the blood and (b) the tissue's demand for oxygen.

These factors determine the severity of the relative ischemia and therefore of the oxygen deficit as well.

Two forms of relative ischemia are differentiated according to the duration of the oxygen deficit.

■ Acute Temporary Relative Ischemia

General definition: Barely sufficient blood supply to a tissue at rest and during moderate exercise due to stenosis of a functional terminal artery (▶ B).

Pathogenesis: This involves a latent relative insufficiency of the blood supply in the presence of increased physical activity. Such a situation triggers the following pathogenetic chain reaction: An increase in the demand for oxygen in the area supplied by a functional terminal artery leads to a relative oxygen deficit. The cells adapt by shifting from aerobic to anaerobic glycolysis.

This results in accumulation of acidic metabolites such as lactic acid and CO_2 and a lack of high-energy substances such as ATP.

In muscles, this situation stimulates the nociceptive nerve endings, producing stabbing pain, and impairs relaxation of the musculature.

Morphologic findings include ischemic cell injury.
— Minor injury produces mitochondrial swelling (p. 18).
— Severe injury leads to coagulative necrosis of individual cells or small groups of cells (p. 130). In parenchymatous organs, the necrosis heals as disseminated calluses; in the brain, it heals as focal areas of softening, primarily in the basal ganglia and internal capsule.

✚ **Clinical presentation** depends on the organ involved.
Coronary arteriosclerosis causes angina pectoris (radiating chest pain) with exercise and/or nicotine use.
Femoral arteriosclerosis leads to intermittent claudication (pain spasms) with exertion of the leg muscles such as while climbing stairs.
Mesenteric arteriosclerosis leads to abdominal angina (colicky abdominal pain) in patients who have consumed large meals and experience increased intestinal demand for blood.
Cerebral arteriosclerosis leads to hypotension during sleep with transitory ischemic attacks. These are painless, as the brain does not possess sensory nerves.

■ Chronic Relative Ischemia

General definition: Ischemic disorder due to stenosis of a terminal artery or arteriole (arteriosclerosis) that is so severe that the blood supply is insufficient even at rest (▶ C).

General pathogenesis: Chronic relative ischemia causes generation of oxygen and nitrogen metabolites that lead to apoptosis (p. 128, 132) of parenchymal cells vulnerable to ischemia. The stromal cells tolerate ischemia better and survive.

Morphologic sequelae include numeric atrophy of the organ or tissue (p. 124) and reparative interstitial fibrosis (p. 40, 69).

Result: Development of smaller infarcts or nodular to diffuse fibrosis.

A Absolute temporary ischemia

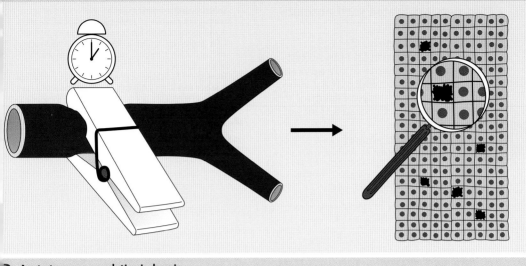

B Acute temporary relative ischemia

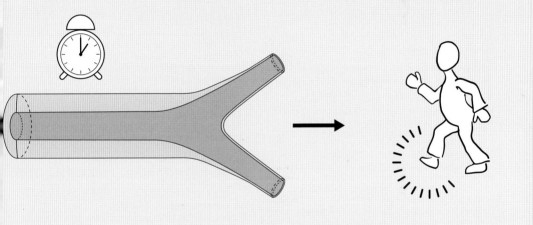

C Chronic relative temporary ischemia

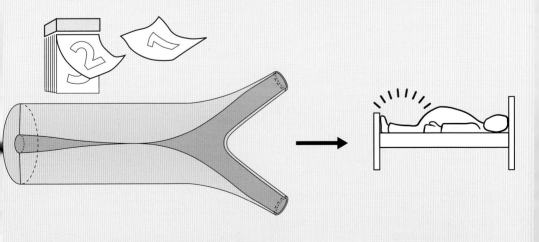

Disorders Associated with Absolute Persistent Ischemia

■ Myocardial Infarction

Textbook example of an arterial ischemic disorder.

Definition: Commonly known as a heart attack, this is an anemic infarct with coagulative necrosis of a large area of the myocardium due to occlusion of one of the three main trunks of the coronary arteries.

Factors in causal pathogenesis:

— **Insufficiency of collateral coronary arteries** usually occurs due to atherosclerotic stenosis (▶ A, B1). This is the underlying disorder that precedes coronary artery insufficiency and gives rise to the following lesions:

— **Endothelial erosion at an atheromatous plaque** may occur in the setting of an accompanying inflammatory reaction mediated by lipid-phagocytizing macrophages (and occasionally cytotoxic T-lymphocytes as well).

— **Rupture of an atheromatous plaque** may occur as a result of hemodynamic stress that exceeds the strength of the plaque. Plaques with high lipid content and few myocytes in their walls are particularly at risk.

— **Coronary artery spasm** is rare but may occur as an isolated event or in combination with a complication of an atheromatous plaque.

Result: Occlusive thrombosis (▶ B2) leading to absolute persistent ischemia.

Formal pathogenesis: See acute hypoxia.

Morphologic findings of a heart attack develop according to the following timetable:

6 hours (acute infarction): The cytoplasm in the area of infarction is eosinophilic and fuchsinophilic with wave-like arrangement of myocytes ("myocyte weaving"; ▶ D). Cytoplasmic enzymes (GOT, LDH, and CPK) are released, providing diagnostic evidence of the lesion.
Reperfusion after ischemia overloads the tissue surrounding the necrotic area with calcium. This produces a continuous spasm leading to necrosis with contraction bands.
Macroscopic findings include a yellow-tan infarct (▶ C).

24 hours: Necrosis triggers an exudative inflammatory reaction in the tissue surrounding the necrotic area. This leads to hyperemia and leukocyte migration, creating a hemorrhagic border around the infarct.

4 days (subacute infarction): Necrosis triggers the wound healing process. This leads to proteolytic breakdown of the necrosis and organization by granulation tissue from the tissue surrounding the necrotic area.
Macroscopic findings include a yellow-tan infarct with a hemorrhagic halo.

6 weeks (old infarction): The area of infarction has been replaced with scar tissue.
Macroscopic findings include a whitish-gray callus (▶ E) and compensatory hypertrophy of the rest of the myocardium.

Infarcts are classified according to topographic location of the stenosis (variations according to left or right type of blood supply):

— **Anterior wall infarcts** result from occlusion of the anterior interventricular artery.

— **Posterior wall infarcts** occur near the base of the heart and result from occlusion of the right coronary artery.

— **Lateral wall infarcts** result from occlusion of the left circumflex coronary artery.

Infarcts are also classified according to the type of ischemia involved:

— **Subendocardial infarcts** involve worsening of acute temporary relative ischemia as a result of stenosis of one or more main trunks of the coronary arteries. This produces multiple focal infarcts measuring about 1 mm (a mosaic infarct) in the inner third of the myocardium.

— **Transmural infarcts** involve absolute persistent ischemia as a result of stenosis of one main trunk of a coronary artery. This produces an infarct measuring about 1 cm in all three layers of the wall of the heart.

✚ **Clinical presentation:** Men are affected significantly more often than women, and the disorder is often fatal.
Symptoms include sudden angina, severe apprehension with a sense of impending doom, and cardiogenic shock. *Later,* leukocytosis with a left shift, increased temperature and transaminase levels, and ECG changes.

✚ **Complications** of myocardial infarction:
Sudden cardiac death is caused by ventricular fibrillation resulting from impaired conduction induced by necrosis.
Pericarditis epistenocardica is a fibrinous inflammatory reaction of the epicardium overlying an area of necrosis; auscultatory findings include a pericardial friction rub. *Later,* adhesions develop between the layers of the pericardium.
Myocardial aneurysm (p. 408) develops where ischemic myocardial damage leads to ventricular akinesis. This in turn results in systolic expansion.
Parietal endocardial thrombosis is mural thrombus overlying an area of endocardial necrosis. It also occurs in myocardial aneurysm (p. 408) and involves increased risk of embolism.
Cardiac rupture occurs as a result of necrotic and granulocytic softening of the myocardial wall (myomalacia). A tear in the ventricular wall causes bleeding into the pericardium, successively leading to cardiac tamponade and cardiac arrest.
Mitral valve insufficiency can result from necrosis of the papillary muscle.

■ Anemic Splenic Infarct

Definition: Coagulative necrosis in the spleen resulting from loss of blood supply (absolute persistent ischemia) in a branch of the splenic artery.

Morphologic findings include a well-circumscribed infarct, initially dark red and later yellow with a hemorrhagic halo (▶ F).

Infarcts are classified according to etiologic factors:

Wedge-shaped infarcts with their base on the capsule of the spleen:

Usually due to thromboembolic occlusion of the splenic artery and occasionally to stenosis of the splenic artery from leukemic infiltrate.

Spotted spleen with multiple small infarcts may result from several disorders including:

— Polyarteritis nodosa in the splenic artery (p. 58);
— Arteritis of the splenic artery in the setting of Wegener granulomatosis (p. 184);
— Hypertensive arteriolar necrosis;
— Disseminated intravascular coagulation with intravascular microthrombi (p. 400);
— Sickle-cell anemia with intravascular agglutination of cells.

✚ **Clinical presentation:** Patients report "sudden pain" beneath the left costal arch.

A Coronary artery: stenosis

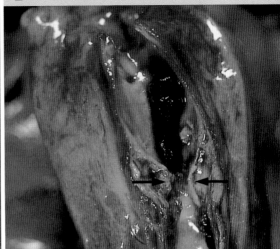

B Coronary artery: thrombus

C Heart: acute infarct

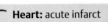

D Myocardium: acute infarct
(Luxol fast blue) x 50

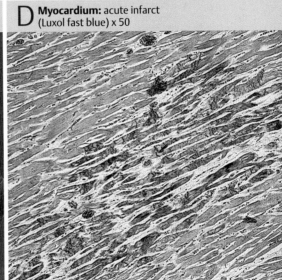

E Heart: infarct scar

F Spleen: infarcts

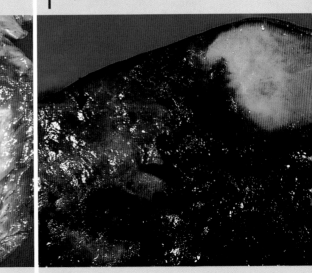

24

Localized Circulatory Disorders

■ Anemic Cerebral Infarction

Definition: Liquefactive necrosis of a region of the brain due to loss of blood supply in the main trunk of one of the three cerebral arteries.

Etiologic factors of such a loss of blood supply include insufficiency of cerebral collateral circulation in the presence of rupture of an atheromatous plaque (common) or cerebral thromboembolism in cardiac thrombosis.

Formal pathogenesis: See acute hypoxia (p. 22, 68).

Morphologic findings of a cerebral infarction develop according to the following timetable:

Up to 3 days (demarcation stage): Liquefactive necrosis produces slight swelling of the necrotic area. The infarct exhibits a softened doughy consistency (encephalomalacia), stains only slightly, and is demarcated by perifocal edema (► A, C).

2–14 days (absorption stage): Macrophages migrate from the surrounding tissue into the necrotic area. There they phagocytize myelin detritus and break it down in phagocytic vacuoles (lipid vacuoles). These vacuole accumulate in the macrophage cytoplasm, turning these cells into lipophages (► D).

Result: Liquefaction of the necrotic area into a whitish substance, leading to encephalomalacia.

1–8 weeks (cystic stage): Elimination of the necrosis by macrophages leaves behind a tissue defect.

Result: Formation of a cavity lined with glial and connective tissue (► B).

Infarcts are classified according to topographic location of the stenosis as follows:

▦ Total Infarct

Synonym: massive malacia.

Pathogenesis: Loss of blood supply from the basal arteries of the brain and/or the three major arteries of the brain (middle cerebral, anterior, and posterior arteries) produces absolute persistent ischemia in the areas supplied by these vessels.

Morphologic findings include a sharply demarcated wedge-shaped focus of liquefactive necrosis in the affected cortical and medullary region that becomes transformed into a cystic lesion.

✚ **Clinical presentation:** Patients present with a cerebral stroke involving hemiparalysis and/or extrapyramidal symptoms and aphasia (loss of speech). Symptoms become less severe as the perifocal edema regresses.

✚ **Special form of total infarct:**
Wallenberg syndrome (posterior inferior cerebellar artery syndrome) results from thrombotic occlusion of the origin of the vertebral artery from the subclavian artery. This thrombus spreads to the posterior inferior cerebellar artery, producing myelomalacia (medullary softening) of the posterolateral medulla oblongata. Symptoms failure of cranial nerves: trigeminal nerve paresthesia, facial nerve palsy, paralysis of the soft palate, hoarseness, and ataxia.

☺ **Prominent patients** who died of cerebral infarctions include the German painter Caspar David Friedrich (1774–1840) and Czech composer Antonín Dvořák (1841–1904).

▦ Border Zone Infarct

Definition: Compromised blood supply with acute temporary relative ischemia in the most distal fields of the area supplied by the three major cerebral arteries.

Morphologic findings include multiple focal areas of cortical softening measuring several millimeters occurring primarily in the troughs of the gyri. Later, these lead to necrosis and scarring with a fine granular change in the cortex (granular atrophy).

▦ Microinfarcts

Definition: Compromised blood supply with acute temporary relative ischemia in the areas supplied by the minor cerebral arteries and arterioles.

Morphologic findings include multiple tiny focal areas of cortical softening up to 1 mm in size occurring primarily in the cerebral medulla and basal ganglia.

■ Anemic Renal Infarct

Definition: Liquefactive necrosis due to loss of blood supply with absolute persistent ischemia in the area supplied by the renal artery or one of its branches.

The morphologic correlate of a renal infarction develops according to the following timetable:

1 day after occlusion of the artery, only traces of the cells remain in a grayish yellow infarct (► E1, F).

3 days later, the necrosis appears organized, with a hemorrhagic halo of capillary-rich granulation tissue (► E2).

4 weeks later, the necrotic area appears as a sunken grayish-white scar.

Infarcts are classified according to topographic location of the stenosis:
— **Trapezoidal cortical infarcts** occur due to peripheral occlusion of the arcuate artery.
— **Triangular cortical infarcts** occur due to occlusion of one of the radiating arteries (► E1).
— **Cortical and medullary infarcts** occur due to central occlusion of the arcuate artery.
— **Subtotal and total renal infarcts** occur due to occlusion of the trunk of the renal artery (► F).

❗ **Note:** *Clinical symptoms of renal infarction* include sudden lumbar pain with hematuria.

❗ **Note:** Absolute persistent ischemia leads to renal infarction; chronic relative ischemia leads to ischemic injury characterized by severe parenchymal atrophy without necrosis.

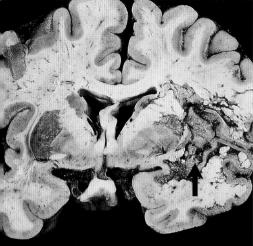

A Central nervous system: acute infarct

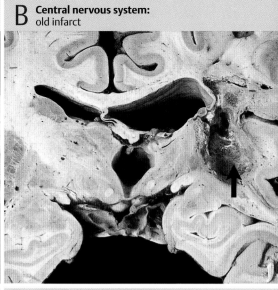

B Central nervous system: old infarct

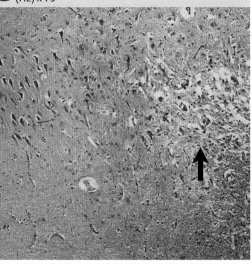

C Cerebellum: acute infarct (HE) x 75

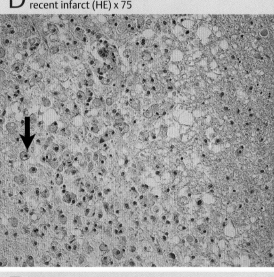

D Central nervous system: recent infarct (HE) x 75

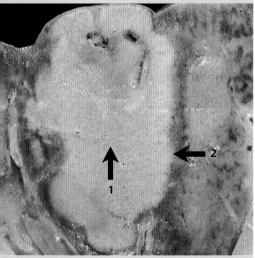

E Kidney: infarct

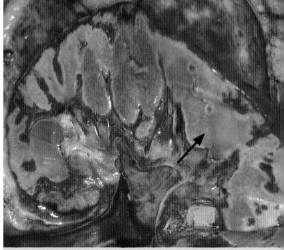

F Kidney: subtotal infarct

Venous Hemodynamic Disorders

Venous Stasis

Definition: Engorgement of capillaries and veins due to impaired drainage.

Etiologic factors include:
— *Right heart insufficiency* leading to hyperemia;
— *Stenosing venous disease* (obliteration of a vein);
— *Dilatative venous disease* (varices).

Morphologic findings vary according to the duration of stasis.

Acute venous stasis involves hypoxic injury only. This includes cyanotic organ enlargement with sublethal cell injury.

Chronic venous stasis involves hypoxic injury and increased hydrostatic pressure. This includes proliferation of collagen fibers in the organ stroma (congestion fibrosis; p. 40, 69). *Later,* this leads to widespread cell death in the organ in the form of cyanosis and numeric atrophy (p. 124).

Associated Disorders

■ Hepatic Congestion

Etiologic factors include right heart insufficiency and constrictive pericarditis.

Morphologic findings vary according to the duration of stasis.
— **Acute hepatic congestion** lasts for a period of hours. Findings include cyanotic hepatomegaly with focal depressions on the cut surface and congested sinusoids in the central regions of the lobules.
— **Subacute hepatic congestion** lasts for a period of days. Findings include a network of cyanotic lines of congestion between the central veins.
— **Chronic hepatic congestion** lasts for several weeks. Findings include cyanotic lines of congestion bordered by hepatocellular cords exhibiting hypoxia, fatty degeneration, and compressive atrophy. Liver cells die and release transaminases into the serum. The lines of congestion run between the central regions of the lobules, forming a "nutmeg liver" pattern (► A, B).

Long-term chronic congestion leads to fibrosis of the necrotic parenchyma that produces nodular parenchymal pathology (congestive cirrhosis; p. 42).

Hemorrhagic Infarct

Definition: Tissue destruction resulting from the complete interruption of venous drainage as a result of total occlusion of a major organ vein.

Etiologic factors include venous thrombosis and strangulation of a vein, such as can occur in torsion of a cord of vascularized fibrous tissue (for example testicular torsion; ► C, D).

Pathogenesis: Congestion resulting from complete venous stasis causes necrosis and extravasation of capillary blood.

Morphologic findings include blood-saturated distended dark red tissue from cyanosis (► C, F).

Associated Disorders

■ Hemorrhagic Cerebral Infarction

Definition: Cerebral infarction resulting from thrombosis of cerebral venous or dural sinus thrombosis.

Etiologic factors include non-septic thrombosis (without thrombophlebitis) and septic thrombosis (with thrombophlebitis).

Morphologic findings (► E) include an initially red, swollen, and softened infarcted area (red malacia). *Later,* histiocytes clear the necrosis and clot material, and hemosiderin accumulates within the histiocytes (siderophages). This imparts a brown color to the infarcted area (brown malacia).

> ✚ **Clinical presentation:** Patients present with blood in the cerebrospinal fluid, convulsions, and symptoms of cerebral stroke.

■ Mesenteric Infarction

Definition: Hemorrhagic infarction of a segment of the bowel due failure of arterial supply or venous drainage.

Etiologic factors:
— *Occlusion of one of the mesenteric veins* may result from thrombosis or torsion of the vascular pedicle.
— *Embolism of one of the mesenteric arteries* may occur. Collateral circulation exists between the celiac trunk, superior mesenteric artery, and inferior mesenteric artery. At least two of these vessels must be occluded before infarction will occur. This means that the mesenteric arteries are not terminal arteries; occlusion will cause blood to flow through the collateral vessels into the infarcted area, resulting in a hemorrhagic infarction.

Morphology (► F): The infarcted bowel appears distended and dark red (cyanotic). The walls are fragile, and the lumen is filled with fluid (*radiographic findings* include fluid shadows; *auscultatory findings* include a metallic lapping sound). This necrosis of the wall of the bowel is accompanied by reactive fibrinous peritonitis.

Histologic findings include a blood-saturated mucosa, which is barely discernible as a result of the concurrent necrosis.

> ✚ **Clinical presentation:** Patients present with a *triad of symptoms* including acute abdomen, shock, and bloody diarrhea.

> ✚ **Complications** include purulent migrating bacterial peritonitis and rupture of the bowel wall.

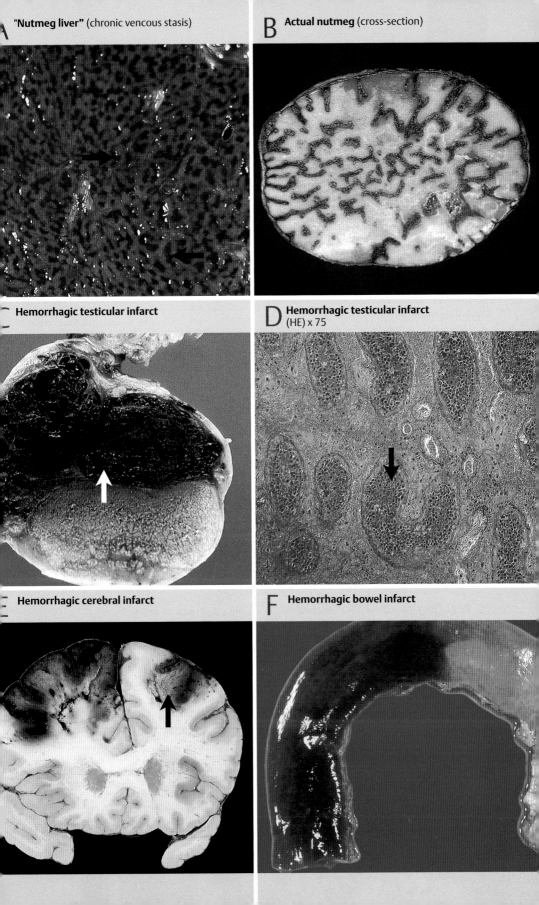

A **"Nutmeg liver"** (chronic vencous stasis)

B **Actual nutmeg** (cross-section)

Hemorrhagic testicular infarct

D **Hemorrhagic testicular infarct** (HE) x 75

E **Hemorrhagic cerebral infarct**

F **Hemorrhagic bowel infarct**

25 Edema

Flooding Through Breached Dikes

Summary

Half of the body consists of water. Two-thirds of this water is contained within the cells, and one third is outside the cells. The extracellular space thus forms the watery environment in which the cells live. It follows that the intake and discharge of body water as well as its distribution and passage back and forth between the cells and the extracellular space must be finely coordinated. Accordingly, normal blood vessels release only the quantity of fluid that is required to nourish tissue. Edema occurs where more fluid than normal is released into tissue. Edemas occur in accordance with Starling's hypothesis (1909). This states that the normal exchange of fluid between the intravascular and extravascular spaces is such that water from the blood passes into the interstitium at the level of the arteriolar capillary branches and from there re-enters the bloodstream either directly at the level of the venular capillary branches or indirectly via the lymph system.

General definition: Edema is the abnormal accumulation of fluid in the extravascular portion of the extracellular space.

General pathogenetic factors as described by Starling's hypothesis may occur individually or in combination. These include:
- Increased hydrostatic pressure in the capillaries (► A1);
- Increased oncotic pressure in the blood (► A2);
- Increased permeability of the capillaries (► A3);
- Impaired lymph drainage (► A4).

In pathologic terms, an edema is the result of an "exudation process".

> **Note:**
> An *inflammatory edema* or effusion is an exudate with a specific gravity exceeding 1.018, as it contains large quantities of protein.
> A *noninflammatory edema* is a transudate with a specific gravity less than 1.018, as it contains only small quantities of protein.

> **Note:** Inflammatory edema contains large quantities of protein.

Hydrostatic Edema

■ Cardiac Edema

Definition: This edema occurs as a result of congestion in the systemic or pulmonary vessels due to insufficient output of the right and/or left ventricles.

Etiologic factors:
- **Left heart failure** increases the pressure upstream of the left heart, causing congestion in the pulmonary capillaries. This presses blood serum through the alveolar capillary membrane (► B1) into the lumina of the alveoli (► B2).
  Result: An alveolar pulmonary edema and often edematous congestion in the form of a pleural effusion.

- **Right heart failure** impairs drainage in the pulmonary vessels, which manifests itself as pulmonary hypertension. This causes congestion in the vena cava and thoracic duct, increasing the pressure in the venular capillary branches and impairing pleural lymph drainage. This is often complicated by secondary hyperaldosteronism with sodium retention. *Result:* A peripheral edema in one or more of the following organs and tissues.
  - In the *skin,* anasarca occurs in dependent parts of the body (primarily in the lower extremities) in the form of mobile edemas (► C) in the subcutaneous fatty tissue that empty into incisions made in the skin (► D).
  - In the *pleura,* such an edema occurs in the form of a pleural effusion.

■ Portal Edema

Definition: Edema in the region drained by the portal vein (primarily the intestinal region) occurring in the setting of portal hypertension.

Ascites only occurs where the postsinusoidal vessels are constricted, as can occur in cirrhosis of the liver.

■ Venous Edema

Definition: Edema occurring in regions with impaired venous drainage.

Etiologic factors:
- **Venous occlusion** may occur due to thrombosis or compression.
- **Venous insufficiency** may occur due to widening or defective venous valves in varicose veins.

■ Osmotic Edema

Definition: Edema resulting from an imbalance of sodium chloride and water in the blood.

Etiologic factors:
- **Hypotonic hydration** may occur due to excessive intake of water or secretion of antidiuretic hormone (occurring in Schwartz-Bartter's syndrome). This leads to hyponatremia.
- **Hypertonic hydration** may occur due to excessive intake of hypotonic saline solution or hyperactivity of the adrenal cortex with increased reabsorption of sodium (occurring in Conn's syndrome and Cushing's syndrome, p. 122). This leads to hypernatremia.

Pathogenesis of edema

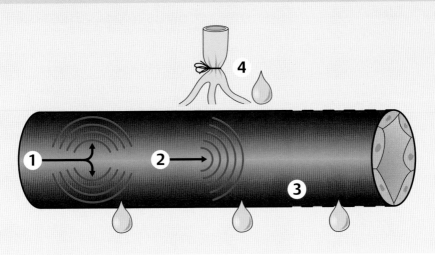

B Alveolar pulmonary edema
(EvG) x 25

C Cutaneous edema

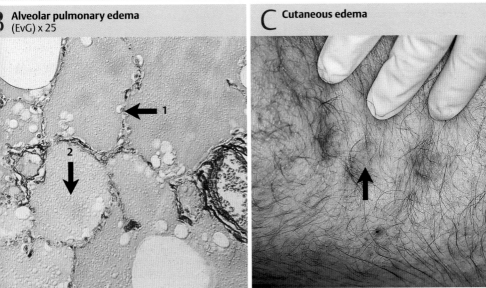

D Cutaneous edema (skin incision)

E Peripheral edema (subcutaneous tissue)
(HE) x 50

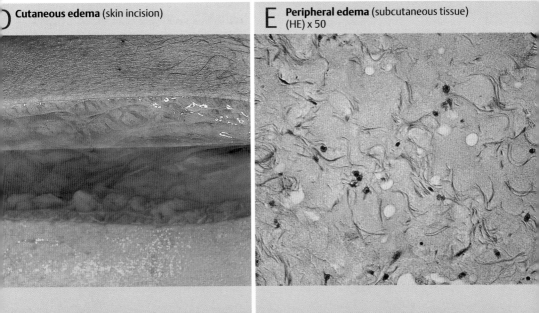

Oncotic Edema

Definition: Edema resulting from excessively low colloidal osmotic pressure due to protein deficiency. In rare cases, this edema may occur due to improper plasma replacement.

Etiologic factors include:
— *Proteinuria* with renal protein loss;
— *Enteropathy* with protein loss;
— *Starvation* (p. 124) with insufficient protein intake;
— *Cirrhosis of the liver* (p. 42) with deficient albumin synthesis.

Vascular Edema

Definition: Edema resulting from the generation of inflammation mediators that increase vascular permeability and/or damage capillaries (see p. 196).

Etiologic factors include:
— *Pathogen toxins* (as in toxic shock) leading to an exudative inflammatory reaction;
— *Immune complex vasculitis* (as in an anaphylactic reaction);
— *Physical and chemical noxious agents* (such as the mustard gas used in World War I);
— *Toxic metabolites* (such as uremic toxins produced in uremia);
— *Release of mediators* in inflammations (such as insect stings);
— *Persistence of complement factors* in antagonist deficiency (such as in Quincke edema, ▶ A).

Lymphedema

Physiology of lymph drainage: Approximately half of the circulating plasma proteins leave the blood capillaries and after passing through the interstitium, are reabsorbed into the lymph capillaries. From there they are carried into the lymph vessels and venous blood.

The "lymph load" is the quantity of protein that must be removed from the interstitium per unit of time.

Definition: Edema that occurs as a result of functional and/or obstructive impairment of lymph drainage from tissue.

— *Primary lymphedema* is caused by congenital defects or sclerosis of lymph vessels.
— *Secondary lymphedema* is caused by blockage or inefficiency of otherwise functional lymph vessels.

Pathogenesis: Failure of lymph drainage leads to milky-yellowish widening of the lymph vessels (lymphangiectasia, ▶ B). Proteins from capillary blood accumulate in lymph channels and vessels in the interstitium (▶ C). This mobilizes histiocytes, which phagocytize the protein. Protein accumulations occur where it is present in quantities that exceed the histiocytes' capacity to phagocytize it. This increases oncotic pressure and causes water to accumulate in the tissue, creating a lymphedema.

✚ **Clinical presentation and morphology:**
Primary lymphedema occurs in these disorders:
— *Milroy's disease* is hypoplasia of the lymph vessels of the leg with an autosomal dominant inheritance pattern;
— *obliterative lymphatic disease* involves congenital stenosing sclerosis of the lymph vessels of the calves.
Secondary lymphedema occurs in these disorders:
— *lymphangiosis carcinomatosa* and/or metastatic obliteration of the lymph nodes with lymph congestion;
— *recurring lymphangitis* (as in erysipelas) with inflammatory obliteration of the lymph vessels;
— *lymph vessel scarring* following skin burns;
— *elephantiasis* with massive swelling of the legs due to parasitic obstruction of the lymph vessels in the setting of filariasis (p. 284);
— *post-thrombotic syndrome* and/or sclerotherapy with reactive fibrotic obliteration of lymph vessels;
— *Meigs' syndrome,* ascites occurring due to unknown causes in the setting of a benign ovarian tumor (usually a fibroma) accompanied by unilateral pleural effusion.

❗ **Note:** *Special forms of lymphedema* include the following disorders:
— **Cellular edema** (Greek *oidema,* swelling) occurs due to abnormal inflow of water into the cell.
— **Anasarca** involves extensive accumulation of fluid in the subcutaneous tissue.
— **Hydrops** is excessive accumulation of watery fluid in existing organ cavities (such as the gall bladder). Special forms of hydrops include *hydrocephalus* (fluid accumulation in the cranium) and *ascites* (fluid accumulation in the peritoneal cavity).

Sequelae of Edema

■ **Sclerosis:** Persistence of lymphedema stimulates proliferation of stromal fibroblasts, which form collagen fibers. This leads to fibrotic hardening of tissue that was formerly soft and edematous.

■ **Dermatopathy:** Atrophy of the skin, and occasionally hyperkeratosis in the vicinity of the edema, predisposes patients to erysipelas.

■ **Recurrent Erysipelas** (p. 212).

■ **Nodal Vascular Sinus Transformation:** Lymph congestion transforms the lymph node sinuses into an anastomotic network of capillary-like vessels (▶ D) with stromal sclerosis (p. 40).

■ **Stewart-Treves Syndrome:** This rare syndrome involves a lymphangiosarcoma that usually arises in the upper arm affected by chronic postmastectomy lymphedema and spreads centripetally.

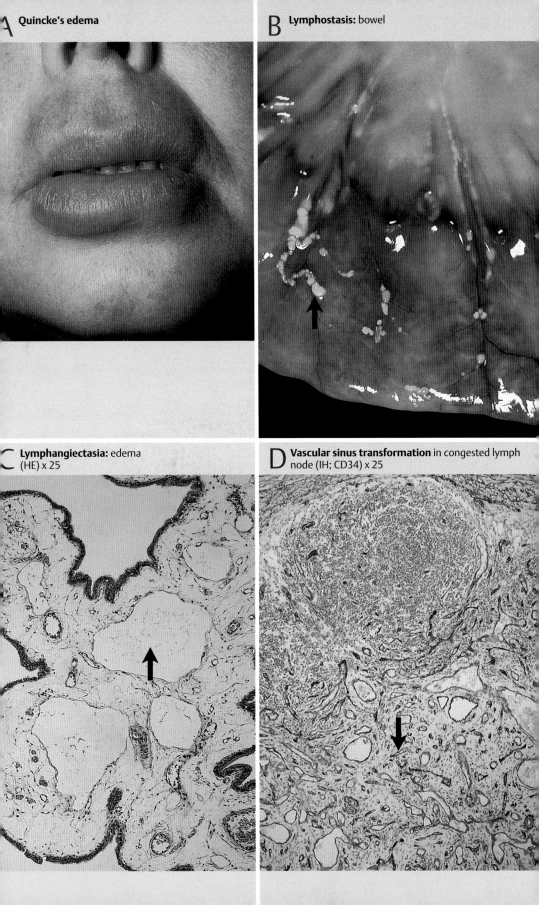

A Quincke's edema

B Lymphostasis: bowel

C Lymphangiectasia: edema (HE) x 25

D Vascular sinus transformation in congested lymph node (IH; CD34) x 25

Cerebral Edema

Physiology of the blood-brain barrier: The cerebral vascular endothelium with its adhesive structures forms the blood-brain barrier. This endothelium controls the exchange of fluid and other substances between the intravascular and extravascular spaces in the central nervous system. A breach in the endothelial barrier results in extravasation of blood plasma into the extracellular space.

General definition: Diffuse or local accumulation of fluid in the brain with a resulting increase in the volume of the brain tissue.

Cerebral edema is differentiated according to magnitude as either:
— *Generalized cerebral edema* diffusely disseminated over the entire brain, or
— *Perifocal cerebral edema* around a focal process.

Cerebral edema is also differentiated according to cause. These include:
— Vasogenic cerebral edema;
— Cytotoxic cerebral edema;
— Interstitial cerebral edema;
— Hyposmotic cerebral edema.

■ Vasogenic Cerebral Edema

Definition: Cerebral edema resulting from functional disruption of the blood-brain barrier, usually in the vicinity of a focal process.

Etiologic factors include:
— Brain tumors (p. 368);
— Cerebral infarcts (p. 420);
— Focal cerebral injuries (p. 316);
— Massive cerebral hemorrhages (p. 398);
— Cerebral abscesses (p. 214).

Pathogenesis: A focal process leads to continuous spread of the edema via the extracellular space along the white matter (cerebral medulla). *Later*, the edema spreads along the gray matter.

Regression of the edema depends on its duration.
— Cerebral edemas of *short duration* regress completely.
— *Persistent cerebral edemas* produce myelin injury, successively leading to demyelination and necrosis.

■ Cytotoxic Cerebral Edema

Definition: Cerebral edema resulting from functional disruption of the blood-brain barrier due to collapse of cerebral energy metabolism.

Etiologic factors include:
— Acute ischemia in cerebral infarction;
— Hepatogenic encephalopathy;
— Cerebral intoxication (cyanide poisoning).

Pathogenesis: Collapse of cerebral energy metabolism leads to the loss of the ATP-dependent ion pump. This in turn results in passive inflow of water into the ganglion cells, glial cells (especially astrocytes), and endothelial cells. This increases the volume of the cells while decreasing the volume of the extracellular space.

■ Interstitial Cerebral Edema

Synonym: hydrocephalic edema.

Definition: Cerebral edema resulting from impaired drainage of cerebrospinal fluid characterized by formation of hydrocephalus with accompanying increased intraventricular pressure.

Etiologic factors:
— Impaired drainage of cerebrospinal fluid,
— Obstructive hydrocephalus.

Pathogenesis: Impaired drainage of cerebrospinal fluid leads to passive passage of CSF through the ependyma into brain tissue and reduced drainage of extracellular fluid into the ventricular system.

■ Hyposmotic Cerebral Edema

Definition: Cerebral edema resulting from hypervolemia with secondary hyponatremia.

Pathogenesis: Passive inflow of fluid into the brain tissue along an osmotic gradient.

✚ Complications of cerebral edemas and intracranial masses:

Filling of reserve space: A diffuse, subacute increase in volume effectively means that there is too much brain tissue for the cranium to accommodate. This displaces the brain into "reserve cavities," specifically the subarachnoid space and ventricles.
Morphologic findings include flattened gyri and closed sulci (► A, B). A slowly expanding mass will produce cerebral atrophy.

Subfalcine herniation: A focal mass and/or cerebral edema can displace the midline of the brain to the contralateral side (► C1, D). This causes the cingulate gyrus to herniate under the falx cerebri.
Clinical symptoms include headache, nausea, and impaired vision.

Transtentorial herniation: Axial displacement of brain tissue from the middle cranial fossa into the posterior cranial fossa through the tentorial notch (► C2). The herniated tissue primarily includes uncus of the parahippocampal gyrus (uncal herniation).
Clinical symptoms include anisocoria (pupils of unequal size), impaired vision, and hemiparesis and hemiplegia progressing to a decerebrate state.

Tonsillar herniation results from the most severe cerebral edema. Portions of the cerebellum are forced through the foramen magnum into the vertebral canal (► C3, E).
Clinical symptoms include cardiac arrest and respiratory paralysis.

A **Normal brain**
(unfixed specimen)

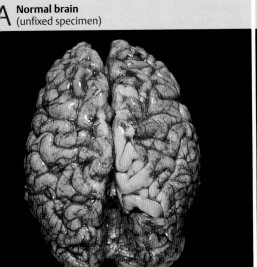

B **Cerebral edema**
(fixed specimen)

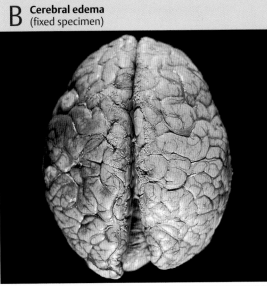

C **Types of cerebral herniation**

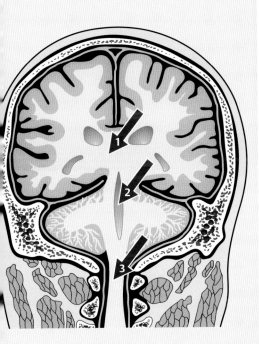

D **Subfalcine herniation**

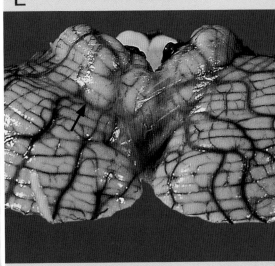

E **Tonsillar herniation** (cerebellum)

Subject Index

Note:

Page numbers in **bold** indicate major discussions.
Page numbers in *italics* refer to figures, or tables.